DRIPPS / ECKENHOFF / VANDAM

INTRODUCTION TO ANESTHESIA

EIGHTH EDITION

DRIPPS / ECKENHOFF / VANDAM

INTRODUCTION TO ANESTHESIA

DAVID E. LONGNECKER, MD

Chairman
Department of Anesthesia
University of Pennsylvania
School of Medicine
Philadelphia, Pennsylvania

FRANK L. MURPHY, MD

Associate Professor of Anesthesia
Hospital of the University of Pennsylvania
Department of Anesthesia
Philadelphia, Pennsylvania

W.B. SAUNDERS
Harcourt Brace Jovanovich, Inc.
Philadelphia, London, Toronto, Montreal, Sydney, Tokyo

W. B. SAUNDERS COMPANY
Harcourt Brace Jovanovich, Inc.

The Curtis Center
Independence Square West
Philadelphia, PA 19106

Editor: Richard Zorab

Dripps, Eckenhoff, Vandam
INTRODUCTION TO ANESTHESIA ISBN 0-7216-3525-3

Printed in the United States of America.

Last digit is the print number: 9 8 7 6 5 4 3 2 1

Contributors

CHRISTIAN M. ALEXANDER, M.D.
Assistant Professor of Anesthesia, Veterans Affairs Medical Center, Philadelphia, Pennsylvania
Positioning the Surgical Patient

STANLEY J. AUKBURG, M.D.
Associate Professor of Anesthesia, Hospital of the University of Pennsylvania, Philadelphia, Pennsylvania
The Anesthesia Machine

JAMES E. BAUMGARDNER, M.D., Ph.D.
Assistant Professor of Anesthesia and Bioengineering, University of Pennsylvania, Philadelphia, Pennsylvania
Interpretation of Arterial Blood Gas and Acid Base-Data

EUGENE K. BETTS, M.D.
Associate Professor of Anesthesia, The Children's Hospital of Philadelphia, Philadelphia, Pennsylvania
Pediatric Anesthesia

FREDERICK W. CAMPBELL, M.D.
Associate Professor of Anesthesia, Hospital of the University of Pennsylvania, The Children's Hospital of Philadelphia, Philadelphia, Pennsylvania
Cardiopulmonary Resuscitation

ANGELINA D. CASTRO, M.D.
Associate Professor of Anesthesia, Hospital of the University of Pennsylvania, Philadelphia, Pennsylvania
Management of Anesthesia for Specialty Procedures

THEODORE G. CHEEK, M.D.
Associate Professor of Anesthesia, Hospital of the University of Pennsylvania, Philadelphia, Pennsylvania
Obstetric Anesthesia and Perinatology

THOMAS J. CONAHAN, M.D.
Associate Professor of Anesthesia, Hospital of the University of Pennsylvania, Philadelphia, Pennsylvania
Outpatient Anesthesia

BENJAMIN G. COVINO, M.D., Ph.D.*
Chairman, Department of Anesthesia, Brigham and Women's Hospital; Professor of Anaesthesia, Harvard Medical School, Boston, Massachusetts
Pharmacology of Local Anesthetics

JOHN J. DOWNES, M.D.
Professor of Anesthesia and Pediatrics, University of Pennsylvania, Philadelphia, Pennsylvania
Pediatric Anesthesia

RODERIC G. ECKENHOFF, M.D.
Assistant Professor of Anesthesia and Physiology, University of Pennsylvania, Philadelphia, Pennsylvania
The Medical Gases

McIVER W. EDWARDS, Jr., M.D.
Associate Professor of Anesthesia, Veterans Affairs Medical Center, Philadelphia, Pennsylvania
Premedication

NORIG ELLISON, M.D.
Professor of Anesthesia, Hospital of the University of Pennsylvania, Philadelphia, Pennsylvania
Managing Fluids, Electrolytes, and Blood Loss

DENNIS M. FISHER, M.D.
Professor of Anesthesia and Pediatrics, University of California Medical Center, San Francisco, California
Muscle Relaxants

SARAH M. FISHER, M.D.
Assistant Professor of Anesthesiology, Temple University, Philadelphia, Pennsylvania
Neuroanesthesia and Neurologic Diseases

RALPH T. GEER, M.D., F.C.C.M.
Associate Professor of Anesthesia and Internal Medicine, Hospital of the University of Pennsylvania, Philadelphia, Pennsylvania
Critical Care of the Surgical Patient

---

* Deceased.

D. ERIC GREENHOW, M.D., Ph.D.
Associate Professor of Anesthesia, Hospital of the University of Pennsylvania, Philadelphia, Pennsylvania
Recovery from Anesthesia: The Postoperative Visit

DAVID M. GUARNIERI, M.D.
Instructor in Anesthesiology, Jefferson Medical College, Philadelphia, Pennsylvania
Preoperative Evaluation

BRETT B. GUTSCHE, M.D.
Professor of Anesthesia, Professor of Obstetrics and Gynecology, Hospital of the University of Pennsylvania, Philadelphia, Pennsylvania
Obstetric Anesthesia and Perinatology

C. WILLIAM HANSON, III, M.D.
Assistant Professor of Anesthesia and Internal Medicine, University of Pennsylvania, Philadelphia, Pennsylvania
Managing the Desperately Ill Patient: Trauma and Shock

SEAN K. KENNEDY, M.D.
Associate Professor of Anesthesia, Hospital of the University of Pennsylvania, Philadelphia, Pennsylvania
Pharmacologic Principles of Anesthetics; Nonopioid Intravenous Anesthetics

WILHELMINA C. KOREVAAR, M.D.
Assistant Professor of Anesthesia, Hospital of the University of Pennsylvania, Philadelphia, Pennsylvania
Diagnosis and Therapy of Chronic Pain

DONALD H. LAMBERT, Ph.D., M.D.
Anesthesiologist, Brigham and Women's Hospital, Associate Professor of Anaesthesia, Harvard Medical School, Boston, Massachusetts
Pharmacology of Local Anesthetics

DAVID E. LONGNECKER, M.D.
Robert Dunning Dripps Professor of Anesthesia, University of Pennsylvania, Philadelphia, Pennsylvania
Anesthesiology as a Medical Specialty

BRYAN E. MARSHALL, M.D., F.F.A.R.C.S., M.R.C.P.
Horatio C. Wood Professor of Anesthesia, University of Pennsylvania, Philadelphia, Pennsylvania
The Inhaled Anesthetics

RONALD M. MEYER, M.D.
Assistant Professor of Clinical Anesthesia, Northwestern University Medical School; Attending Anesthesiologist, Columbus Hospital, Chicago, Illinois
Airway Management

THOMAS A. MICKLER, M.D.
Assistant Professor of Anesthesia, University of Pennsylvania, Philadelphia, Pennsylvania
Patients with Metabolic and Endocrine Disorders

FRANCIS L. MILLER, M.D., Ph.D.
Assistant Professor of Anesthesia, Hospital of the University of Pennsylvania, Philadelphia, Pennsylvania
The Inhaled Anesthetics

FRANK L. MURPHY, M.D.
Associate Professor of Anesthesia, Hospital of the University of Pennsylvania, Philadelphia, Pennsylvania
Conduct of General Anesthesia; Hazards of Anesthesia; The Further Study of Anesthesiology

STANLEY MURAVCHICK, M.D., Ph.D.
Associate Professor of Anesthesia, Hospital of the University of Pennsylvania, Philadelphia, Pennsylvania
Geriatric Patients

CONSTANCE F. NEELY, M.D.
Assistant Professor of Anesthesia, University of Pennsylvania, Philadelphia, Pennsylvania
Cardiovascular Disease

GORDON R. NEUFELD, M.D.
Associate Professor of Anesthesia, University of Pennsylvania, Philadelphia, Pennsylvania
Anesthesia and Respiratory Disease

DORENE A. O'HARA, M.D., M.S.E. (Engineering)
Assistant Professor of Anesthesiology, Robert Wood Johnson Medical School, New Brunswick, New Jersey
Opioids in Anesthesia Practice

ALAN J. OMINSKY, M.D., J.D.
Bernstein, Bernstein & Harrison, Philadelphia, Pennsylvania
The Law and Anesthesia Practice

ANDRANIK OVASSAPIAN, M.D.
Professor of Clinical Anesthesiology, Northwestern University Medical School, Chicago, Illinois
Airway Management

STEPHEN J. PREVOZNIK, M.D.
Professor of Anesthesia, Hospital of the University of Pennsylvania, Philadelphia, Pennsylvania
Preoperative Evaluation

FRANCIS X. RIEGLER, M.D.
Assistant Professor of Anesthesia, University of Pennsylvania, Philadelphia, Pennsylvania
Spinal and Epidural Anesthesia; Nerve Blocks

JOSEPH S. SAVINO, M.D.
Assistant Professor of Anesthesia, Hospital of the University of Pennsylvania, Philadelphia, Pennsylvania
Monitoring the Anesthetized Patient

DAVID S. SMITH, M.D., Ph.D.
Associate Professor of Anesthesia, University of Pennsylvania, Philadelphia, Pennsylvania
Neuroanesthesia and Neurologic Diseases

MITCHELL D. TOBIAS, M.D.
Assistant Professor of Anesthesia, University of Pennsylvania, Philadelphia, Pennsylvania
Hepatic and Renal Disease

TIMOTHY R. VADEBONCOUER, M.D.
Instructor in Anesthesia, Brigham and Women's Hospital, Harvard Medical School, Boston, Massachusetts
Management of Postoperative Pain

MARIE L. YOUNG, M.D.
Assistant Professor of Anesthesia, Hospital of the University of Pennsylvania, Philadelphia, Pennsylvania
Outpatient Anesthesia

PREFACE

Introduction to Anesthesia began in 1949 as a manual for the anesthesia housestaff at the Hospital of the University of Pennsylvania. Robert D. Dripps, who died in 1972, James E. Eckenhoff and Leroy D. Vandam edited seven editions of this popular and influential introductory textbook. With the eighth edition, Drs. Eckenhoff and Vandam have transferred the editorial responsibility for the book to us. The second generation of editors are both at the University of Pennsylvania and are firmly grounded in the traditions that guided the previous editions. In particular, we believe that the student of anesthesia must acquire routines and habits of safe practice, yet must understand the scientific principles that form the basis for that practice and be aware of areas of uncertainty and debate as well. Our goal remains unchanged: to provide in a concise and affordable volume the fundamentals of anesthesiology. Although the book is oriented to the beginning student of anesthesia, it also provides a succinct but comprehensive source for those with more experience who seek a concise review of an area.

The style of the present edition differs somewhat from that of its predecessors. Double-column text and the liberal use of tables, boxes and shaded type are all designed to speed access to important ideas and to improve comprehension. As before, references are meant to identify material for further study and not to document the authors' every assertion. Rather than separate sections on basic science and clinical applications, we have presented important basic concepts together with the corresponding clinical material, to improve comprehension and to emphasize the close correlation of basic science and clinical practice.

As in the previous revisions, the eighth edition reflects current anesthesia practice. Some clinical material has been omitted because it is unlikely to be encountered in the the first year of anesthesia study: anesthesia for patients undergoing cardiac surgery, or for neonates, for example. Some topics that formerly warranted separate chapters have been incorporated with other material: deliberate hypotension, the management of arterial hypotension and the anesthesia record. Other subjects have been added or emphasized: acute and chronic pain treatment outside the operating room now receive individual chapters; the management of patients suffering from shock or massive trauma and the management of patients with severe disorders of liver and renal function receive special treatment because of the increasing prevalence of these problems, especially in teaching hospitals. Two new chapters are directed to the beginning student of anesthesia. One, "The Conduct of General Anesthesia," presents in text some of the oral traditions concerning the art and craft of anesthesia. The other, "The Further Study of Anesthesia," describes patterns of study that apply during training and forever after.

Experts in special areas of anesthesia have provided many of the chapters. Their hard work forms the foundation of this book, but we altered significantly all of their contributions, for the sake of a uniform editorial style. The errors that remain are those of the editors and not of the contributing authors.

We are grateful to Drs. Dripps, Eckenhoff and Vandam, not only for bringing this book through its first forty years, but for providing so much of the leadership that has brought the specialty of anesthesia to its present stature in caring for patients. It is our hope that this edition will contribute as much to the training of new generations of anesthesiologists as its predecessors did to ours.

DAVID E. LONGNECKER
FRANK L. MURPHY

Contents

SECTION 3
Drugs Used in General Anesthesia

SECTION 4
Administering General Anesthesia

SECTION 5
Conduction Anesthesia

SECTION 6
Patients with Special Requirements

SECTION 1

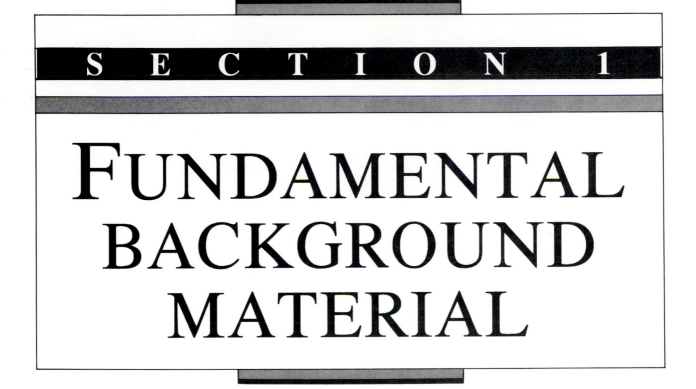

FUNDAMENTAL BACKGROUND MATERIAL

CHAPTER ONE

Anesthesiology as a Medical Specialty

Anesthesiology has advanced as a medical specialty during the past decade. Anesthesiologists now participate actively in both inpatient and outpatient care, working in operating rooms, recovery rooms, outpatient clinics, outpatient surgery centers, and intensive care units (ICUs). Anesthesiologists are also active in medical research, in the administration of their hospitals, and in national organized medicine. However, this was not always the case. Earlier, the specialty experienced significant difficulties in establishing its position in medical practice, in medical schools, and in organized medicine. The limited number of medical personnel in the specialty contributed greatly to these problems. A limited view of the scope of anesthesia practice held by some anesthesiologists (and others in the medical community) also presented barriers to growth of the specialty. The key to the continued success and development of the specialty lies not in the development of new drugs or a new area of practice, but in the continued development of a philosophy of anesthesia practice.

Anesthesiology will continue to thrive as long as its practitioners fulfill a commitment to care for all patients that may benefit from the medical expertise of anesthesiologists. The application of this expertise is most evident in the classical practice of anesthesia; that is, the care of surgical patients in the operating rooms. However, this expertise extends into numerous other areas as well including the preoperative and postoperative care of surgical patients, and the care of other medical conditions that anesthesiologists are uniquely prepared to address. Examples include the care of those with chronic pain, and the treatment of acute drug overdose. The most important element of this approach is the philosophy that anesthesiologists are partners in the care of medical and surgical patients, and not simply technical consultants who participate in specific procedures only. Wherever the partnership philosophy prevails, anesthesiologists are valued and respected as physicians by their medical and surgical colleagues; wherever it has been ignored or not practiced for whatever reasons, then, anesthesiologists have been viewed as specialists with a limited role in overall health care. The philosophy demands dedication and enthusiastic commitment, but the rewards of personal satisfaction, patient satisfaction, and professional recognition more than justify the effort. Indeed, the recent development of anesthesiology as a specialty, the promise of its immediate future, and the satisfaction of its practitioners, reflect the application of this philosophy.

A Concise View of the Development of Anesthesiology in the United States

Although surgical anesthesia was discovered in the 1840s, the real emergence of the specialty began in the early 1900s, and achieved recognition during and after World War II; the results of these efforts have been most evident since the early 1980s. It is clear that anesthesiology reached "maturity" as a medical specialty earlier than the 1980s in several institutions, and it is also apparent that it has not yet reached this position in some centers; yet the impression appears reasonable if the profession is viewed overall.

The first organization of anesthesia practitioners in the United States was the nine-member Long Island Society of Anesthetists, formed in 1905. The name was changed to the New York Society of Anesthetists in 1911 to reflect the interest of the Society that extended well beyond Long Island. Efforts to form a section of anesthesiology within the American Medical Association were begun by the New York Society in 1912 but, despite repeated efforts, the Section was not approved until 1940. Although numerous factors contributed, this long delay reflected attitudes about the value of the specialty in the first part of the twentieth century. The fact that large numbers of both medical and nonmedical personnel were allowed to administer anesthesia with little formal training did nothing to enhance the reputation of the specialty.

The years immediately before, during, and after World War II were associated with great changes in the discipline, and with the introduction of organizations that today represent the specialty. The New York Society of Anesthetists became the American Society of Anesthetists in 1936, and the American Society of Anesthesiologists in 1945. The growth of this organization has been dramatic, from 568 members in 1940 to 28,507 in 1990 (Fig. 1–1). The American Board of Anesthesiology (ABA) was formed in 1938 as an affiliate board of the American Board of Surgery (nine diplomates were certified after the first examination); the ABA became an independent board in 1941. The number of ABA diplomates increased from 105 to 19,061 between 1940 and 1990 (see Fig. 1–2).

While the academic growth of the specialty has paralleled the growth in numbers of practitioners, the academic development of the specialty has lagged behind that of many other disciplines in universities and medical schools. The first certificate for formal graduate medical training in anesthesiology was awarded at the University of Iowa in 1923. Dr. Ralph Waters, of the University of Wisconsin, became the first university professor of anesthesiology in 1927. However, most institutions did not establish departments of anesthesiology until the 1940s to the 1960s, and many university departments have had no more than two chairpersons. (The Veterans Administration has only accepted the concept of independent depart-

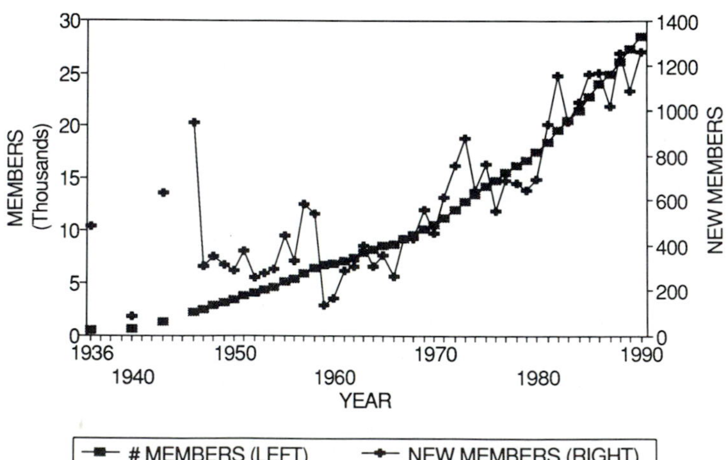

FIGURE 1–1. Annual and cumulative growth in membership of the American Society of Anesthesiologists. Values for initial years are discontinuous because data by year are not available.

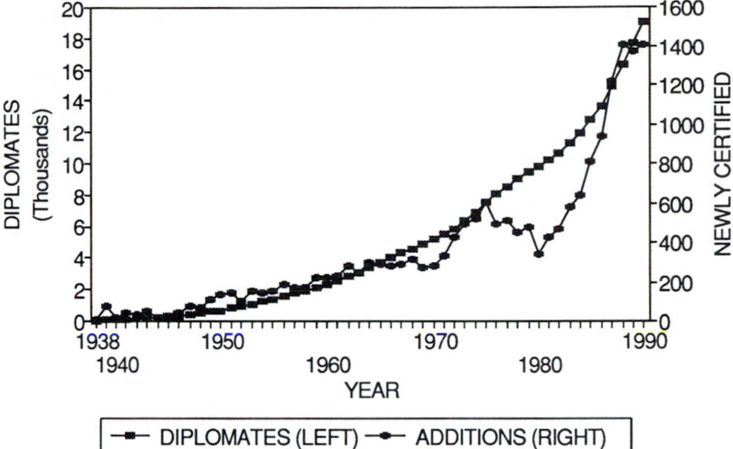

FIGURE 1–2. Annual and cumulative growth in numbers of diplomates certified by the American Board of Anesthesiology.

ments of anesthesiology very recently, and anesthesiology remains a section of surgery in most Veterans Administration hospitals).

The value and prowess of physician anesthesiologists was recognized most dramatically during World War II, when the importance of anesthesia became evident in the care of wounded soldiers. Many physicians returned from World War II to enter training programs in anesthesiology, and these individuals became the leaders of the emergence of the specialty in the 1950s and 1960s. A small number of individuals developed elite university departments that supplied large numbers of leaders and practitioners to the specialty during this interval; prominent among these were Robert D. Dripps of the University of Pennsylvania (one of the editors of the earlier editions of this textbook), Emanuel M. Papper of Columbia University, and Stuart F. Cullen of the University of Iowa and later the University of California at San Francisco. These, and a small group of others, formed the nucleus for the development of the scientific foundations of the specialty in the three decades immediately after World War II. Several of these leaders in anesthesiology were appointed to leadership positions (dean or vice president for health affairs) in university medical centers, attesting to the fact that anesthesiology had become a respected medical discipline in the view of the larger medical community.

BREADTH OF THE SPECIALTY

Initially, nearly all anesthesiologists practiced in all areas of the discipline, an understandable necessity in a new specialty with few practitioners. This emphasis remains the basis of practice for the vast majority of anesthesiologists, but there is a growing trend for subspecialization in major universities and medical centers. The principal subdisciplines include obstetric anesthesia, pediatric anesthesia, cardiothoracic anesthesia, neuroanesthesia, anesthesia for outpatient surgery, and acute and chronic pain management.

Obstetric Anesthesia

Obstetric anesthesia has emerged as a subdiscipline that is highly regarded by patients and obstetricians alike. Anesthesia-related factors such as anesthetic mishaps, or associated factors such as pulmonary aspiration of gastric contents, have been prominent causes of maternal morbidity and mortality for many years, emphasizing the need for subspecialty practice in obstetric anesthesia. The role of anesthesiologists in preventing neonatal morbidity and resuscitating the newborn also has become apparent in recent years. Further, the dramatic pain relief and safety provided by epidural analgesia for labor and delivery is well recognized by large numbers of patients. Indeed, hospital administrators even use the presence of obstetric anesthesia subspecialty practice as evidence of the quality of their hospitals, and as enticements for patients in their marketing programs. Anesthesiologists have played a prominent role in neonatal care also; one of the most prominent among these was Virginia Apgar, the creator of the Apgar score that is used internationally to evaluate the condition of the newborn. Obstetric anesthesiologists have formed a society for their subdiscipline, and fellowship training in obstetric anesthesia is offered by many training programs.

Pediatric Anesthesia

Pediatric anesthesia has emerged as a highly developed subspecialty, and pediatric anesthesiologists have achieved positions of prominence in the training of anesthesiologists and pediatricians who practice pediatric critical care medicine. Many prominent pediatric anesthesiologists have training and board certification in both pediatrics and anesthesiology, and fellowships in pediatric anesthesia are available to those who have completed anesthesiology training programs. Pediatric anesthesia is a recognized section within the American Academy of Pediatrics, and pediatric anesthesiologists have formed their own subspecialty society as well.

Cardiothoracic Anesthesia

Cardiothoracic anesthesia is one of the largest subdisciplines within the specialty of anesthesiology. Anesthesiologists have contributed prominently to the development of the safety of cardiac surgery, including coronary bypass operations and open heart procedures. The development of narcotic anesthesia, a technique that permitted cardiac operations even in those with poor myocardial function, is an example of the role of anesthesia care in the development of cardiac surgery; others include recent studies that defined the influences of anesthetic techniques or underlying myocardial ischemia on the morbidity and mortality associated with cardiac operations. Cardiothoracic anesthesiologists have continued to lead in the transfer of technology into the operating room; a recent example is the intraoperative use of transesophageal echocardiography (TEE). There are two major organizations for cardiothoracic anesthesiologists, and fellowships in cardiothoracic anesthesia are offered in numerous major universities and medical centers.

Neuroanesthesia

Neuroanesthesia is a smaller subdiscipline of anesthesia practice. Although neuroanesthetists participate in all the operations performed by neurosurgeons, their special expertise usually involves intracranial procedures. Anesthetics have significant influences on cerebral blood flow, cerebral metabolism, intracranial pressure, and the extent of tissue hypoxia that is tolerated by the central nervous system, and anesthesiologists have been leaders in developing scientific information regarding the influences of these factors on outcome following cerebral ischemia or hypoxemia. Neuroanesthesiologists often are involved in the care of neurosurgical patients postoperatively, because both ventilation and systemic hemodynamics (and thus cerebral perfusion) have important influences on outcome, and because many of the principles of neuroanesthesia are extended into the postoperative period. Neuroanesthetists have their society, and enjoy joint membership with their colleagues in neurosurgery. Fellowships in neuroanesthesia are offered at major universities and centers, and may well become even more common with the further development of vascular neurosurgery, an area that tests the skills of both neurosurgeons and neuroanesthetists.

Anesthesia for Outpatient Surgery

Anesthesia for outpatient surgical procedures has developed rapidly in recent years, as outpatient surgical centers have become increasingly common. These centers were developed in response to efforts to lower costs by reducing the length of hospital stays for surgical patients. Procedures that were once restricted to hospital inpatients are now performed on outpatients routinely. The development of new drugs and approaches to anesthesia care has done much to further the trend for outpatient operations. Many anesthesiologists now offer outpatient clinics that provide preanesthetic evaluation for surgical outpatients, an approach that enhances both the quality and the efficiency of anesthesia care in busy outpatient surgical facilities. The development of new anesthetic drugs and techniques that are associated with rapid induction and emergence from general anesthesia has done much to expand the range of possible candidates for outpatient procedures. Anesthesiologists interested in outpatient surgery have also formed a society devoted to their subdiscipline, and some training programs offer extended subspecialty training in outpatient anesthesia.

Regional Anesthesia

Regional anesthesia has developed into an area of special interest for many anesthesiologists, several of whom have been prominent in the development of new drugs and techniques for this subspecialty. Some of the more interesting new developments have included the use of prolonged regional anesthesia for initial postoperative pain, especially in children or outpatients. For example, it is common for anesthesiologists to perform field blocks or regional anesthesia (such as caudal anesthesia after lower extremity operations) in pediatric surgical patients, and regional anesthesia is used with increasing frequency to provide initial postoperative pain relief after upper extremity operations. Obstetric anesthesiologists and those who provide anesthesia for orthopedic patients are prominent contributors to the subdiscipline of regional anesthesia.

Anesthesia for Pain Management

Anesthesia for pain management has become increasingly prominent in recent years. Chronic pain management developed in the 1970s, whereas acute pain management has gained popularity in the 1980s. The importance of the subdiscipline of pain management was recognized by the American Board of Anesthesiology, which received approval from the American Board of Medical Specialties in 1991 to offer subspecialty board certification in pain management.

CHRONIC PAIN MANAGEMENT

Chronic pain management is directed to the care of those with a history of chronic pain, or with acute pain that is known to lead to chronic pain and disability (such as that associated with reflex sympathetic dystrophy). The subdiscipline requires the knowledge and skills associated with expertise in regional anesthesia, combined with expertise in behavioral medicine; in exercise physiology (many treatment plans include an important exercise component); in the pharmacology of sedatives, antidepressants, narcotics, and analgesics; and an understanding of neurological disease and neurological diagnosis. This has led to the development of multidisciplinary clinics, and multidisciplinary training is an important component of the fellowship training in pain management.

ACUTE PAIN MANAGEMENT

Acute pain management is a rapidly expanding aspect of perioperative care, and now forms a major component of the pain management activities of many anesthesiology departments. The most prominent aspect of this activity involves the management of acute postoperative pain. The techniques for acute pain management are many and varied. They include patient-controlled intravenous narcotic analgesia, epidural analgesia with combinations of narcotics and local anesthetics, and less common regional anesthesia approaches such as interpleural analgesia. Both patients and surgeons have noted the remarkable decrease in postoperative pain associated with these techniques, and some have observed decreased stays in ICUs as well as an overall decrease in the duration of hospital stays.

Critical Care Medicine

Critical care medicine is a logical subspecialty of anesthesiology, especially because it is a natural extension of the intensive care that is provided in the operating rooms. The American Board of Anesthesiology was authorized to issue subspecialty certification in critical care medicine in 1985, and by the end of 1989, 421 ABA diplomates had achieved subspecialty certification. Anesthesiologists participate in patient care and administration in surgical, pediatric, and medical ICUs. Anesthesiologists participate in the training of those from other disciplines that offer subspecialty certification such as surgery, internal medicine, obstetrics, pediatrics, and neurosurgery.

Preanesthetic Evaluation

Modern anesthesiology departments are involved in several other areas of activity as well. Prominent among these is the preanesthetic evaluation clinic. These clinics are designed to provide preanesthetic evaluation for patients scheduled to come to the hospital on the day of operation, who otherwise would not be seen by an anesthesiologist in advance of the proposed procedure. This assures that the patient is evaluated medically for the demands of anesthesia, and that the patient understands the plans for anesthesia care. It may be a cost-saving mechanism as well, for it eliminates delays and cancellations in the operative schedule and the anesthesiologist may be able to curtail preoperative tests and consultations to only those that are essential for quality care.

Anesthesiologists are also active in clinical hyperbaric medicine, blood banking, and trauma care.

Research

Anesthesiologists have become increasingly involved in clinical and laboratory research. The breadth of clinical research ranges from health care policy and allocation of health care resources, to drug and device testing for perioperative or intensive care. Laboratory research spans similarly broad areas, ranging from cardiopulmonary physiology to molecular genetics. Although pursued by only a fraction of practitioners, the future of anesthesiology depends to a great extent on the advances made by those in clinical or laboratory research.

THE FUTURE

Anesthesiologists' ambitions for their specialty were once limited by the attitudes of patients and other medical specialists, and by a shortage of medical personnel in the discipline. Now, anesthesiologists' participation in the full range of patient care, administration, education, and research is limited only by their training, ambition, and willingness to be full-fledged partners in medical care.

REFERENCES

American Board of Anesthesiology. Quality anesthesia care: A model of future practice of anesthesiology. Anesthesiology 1977; 47:488–489.

American Board of Anesthesiology: A modification in the training requirements in anesthesiology: Requirements for the third clinical anesthesia year. Anesthesiology 1985; 62:175–177.

Eckenhoff JE. A wide-angle view of anesthesiology: Emory A. Rovenstine memorial lecture. Anesthesiology 1978; 48:272–279.

Little DM Jr. The founding of the specialty boards. Anesthesiology 1981; 55:317–321.

Little DM Jr, Betcher AM. The Diamond Jubilee 1905–1980. Park Ridge, Ill: American Society of Anesthesiologists, Inc, 1980.

Vandam LD. American Society of Anesthesiologists Rovenstine Lecture-1979: Anesthesiologists as clinicians. Anesthesiology 1980; 53:40–48.

Volpitto PP, Vandam LD. The genesis of contemporary American Anesthesiology. Springfield, Ill: Charles C Thomas, 1982.

CHAPTER TWO

Interpretation of Arterial Blood Gas and Acid-Base Data

Routine and frequent arterial blood gas measurements have placed the clinical management of respiratory and acid-base disorders in anesthetized and critically ill patients on a firm scientific foundation. Astrup and Severinghaus (1987) provide an account of the development of blood gas measurements and their interpretation. This chapter provides a pragmatic introduction to interpreting data obtained from the blood gas laboratory. Related material is covered in later chapters on medical gases (see Chapter 12), pulmonary disease (see Chapter 22), and on critical care (see Chapter 37).

Arterial Oxygen Tension

Arterial oxygen tension, Pa_{O_2}, is defined as the partial pressure of oxygen present in a hypothetical gas phase in equilibrium with a sample of arterial blood. Normal values of 90 to 100 mm Hg decrease with age (see Chapter 27). Although intra-arterial measurement is possible, most often a sample of arterial blood is drawn into a syringe and taken to the blood gas laboratory, where it is placed in a chamber separated by an oxygen-permeable membrane from an electrolyte solution bathing a platinum cathode and a silver anode. The electric current flowing through this polarographic oxygen electrode at a fixed potential is a function of the oxygen tension. Errors in obtaining and handling the blood sample may invalidate the data. First, blood may be drawn from a vein by mistake. Second, large air bubbles left in the syringe containing the blood sample may exchange oxygen and carbon dioxide with the sample. Third, if the syringe is not placed in ice, cell metabolism may consume enough oxygen to decrease the P_{O_2}; because white cells are especially metabolically active, this problem is accentuated in patients with leukocytosis.

Although there are hazards to increased arterial oxygen tension, especially in neonates, usually the patient's Pa_{O_2} is less than expected. Thus, the interpretation of arterial P_{O_2} more commonly requires explaining a decreased P_{O_2}. The difference between inspired oxygen tension and the Pa_{O_2}

mainly reflects factors involving regional pulmonary blood flow, regional ventilation and gas diffusion (see Chapters 12, 22, and 37).

Hypoventilation usually is described in pulmonary physiology texts as an unlikely cause of arterial hypoxemia, which is quite true in a normal subject whose minute ventilation changes slowly. In the practice of anesthesia, the patient's minute ventilation often changes rapidly and profoundly, as after the intravenous administration of muscle relaxants, narcotics, sedatives, or anesthetics. Because the body stores for oxygen are very small and primarily limited to the oxygen stores in the functional residual capacity in the lung, sudden depression of ventilation commonly leads to hypoxia; hypoventilation must be considered in the differential diagnosis of decreased Pa_{O_2}.

ARTERIAL CARBON DIOXIDE TENSION

The partial pressure of carbon dioxide in an arterial blood sample, Pa_{CO_2}, like the Pa_{O_2}, represents the partial pressure in a hypothetical gas phase in equilibrium with the blood. In the Severinghaus CO_2 electrode, carbon dioxide in the blood sample diffuses through a membrane to an electrolyte solution, the pH of which is measured by a pH electrode and corresponds to the Pa_{CO_2}.

Pa_{CO_2} is closely regulated around a normal value between 37 and 43 mm Hg. Deviations may reflect changes in minute ventilation, rate of CO_2 production, and the efficiency of gas exchange in the lungs (see Chapter 22). Interpretation of Pa_{CO_2} depends on whether the CO_2 tension is greater than normal or less than normal; the discussion here is divided accordingly.

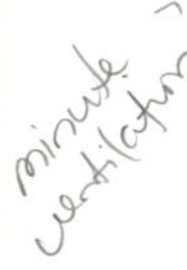

Causes of hypercarbia include increased CO_2 production, decreased minute ventilation, and decreased efficiency of ventilation (i.e., how well the lung uses the minute ventilation to exchange gases). Conversely, low Pa_{CO_2} can be the result of decreased CO_2 production or increased minute ventilation, but supra-normal lung efficiency does not occur. Decreased CO_2 production most commonly results from hypothermia, whether induced or unintentional. Patients receiving mechanical ventilation who are in shock, with extremely low cardiac outputs and peripheral vasoconstriction, may become hypocarbic and give the appearance of decreased CO_2 production because of failure to deliver carbon dioxide from the unperfused tissue to the lungs. Physiologic compensation for metabolic acidosis or alkalosis includes increased or decreased minute ventilation, and hypocarbia or hypercarbia, respectively (Table 2–1).

Isolated abnormalities of P_{CO_2} are relatively well tolerated so long as associated hypoxemia or extreme abnormalities of pH are avoided. When time permits, successful treatment of the underlying abnormality corrects the P_{CO_2} as well. In more urgent circumstances, the patient is likely to be receiving

TABLE 2–1. Changes in Arterial CO_2 Tension

Causes of Increased Pa_{CO_2}	Causes of Decreased Pa_{CO_2}
Increased CO_2 production	Decreased CO_2 production
Hyperthermia (malignant hyperthermia, fever, sepsis)	Hypothermia
Reperfusion of hypercarbic tissue, (after vascular procedure or removing pneumatic tourniquet)	Extreme circulatory collapse
Bicarbonate administration	
CO_2 insufflation (laparoscopy)	
Decreased minute ventilation	Increased minute ventilation
Mechanical ventilator adjusted incorrectly	Mechanical ventilator adjusted incorrectly
Inadequate manual ventilation	Excess manual ventilation
Ventilator or breathing circuit malfunction	Early shock
Airway obstruction	Early pneumonia
Respiratory depression (anesthetics, narcotics, sedatives)	Stroke or head trauma
Muscle weakness (residual neuromuscular blockade, neuromuscular disease)	
Chest wall abnormalities (kyphoscoliosis)	
Splinting from pain after abdominal or chest operations	
Compensation for metabolic alkalosis	Compensation for metabolic acidosis
Decreased efficiency of ventilation	
Extremes of ventilatory failure (severe COPD, asthma)	
Increased dead space (pulmonary embolism)	

controlled ventilation; altering minute ventilation promptly change Pa_{CO_2} (see Chapter 12). Therapy for abnormalities of Pa_{CO_2} is directed toward changes in minute ventilation. Thus, even when an increased CO_2 is the result of increased production, increases in arterial CO_2 are by definition hypoventilation, and are treated by increasing the minute ventilation, usually mechanically.

ARTERIAL pH

The human body employs a complex array of mechanisms, including the lungs, blood, and kidneys, which are integrated with other physiologic systems, to maintain acid-base status. This presentation emphasizes a pragmatic approach to the interpretation of arterial data. To describe the patient's acid-base status, one first defines the pathophysiology (respiratory or metabolic; acidosis or alkalosis), then assesses the severity of the disorder, and then deduces from the overall clinical picture the pathologic process that led to the acid-base derangement.

The variables we measure to define acid-base status are arterial CO_2 tension and hydrogen ion concentration, or more commonly pH, the negative logarithm to the base 10 of the hydrogen ion concentration. Serum bicarbonate concentration ($[HCO_3^-]$) is not measured, but is calculated from the arterial pH and CO_2 measurements; the values are accurate as long as the plasma bicarbonate buffer system is near equilibrium, which is usually the case.

RESPIRATORY ACIDOSIS AND ALKALOSIS

Interpretation of respiratory acid-base status is straightforward, and depends solely on the measured Pa_{CO_2}. An increased Pa_{CO_2} is by definition respiratory acidemia, and reduced CO_2 tension is by definition respiratory alkalemia. So long as minute ventilation, CO_2 production, and pulmonary function do not change for several minutes before the arterial blood sample is obtained, it is reasonable to assume that arterial CO_2 tension reflects P_{CO_2} throughout the body.

Assessing the degree of derangement is also straightforward. Alveolar CO_2 ($F_{A_{CO_2}}$), CO_2 production ($\dot{Q}_{CO_2}$), and alveolar ventilation ($\dot{V}_A$) are related by:

$$\dot{Q}_{CO_2} = F_{A_{CO_2}} \times \dot{V}_A. \tag{1}$$

Over the short term, alveolar CO_2 and arterial CO_2 are directly related, as are the alveolar and expired minute volumes. Because CO_2 production also changes little over the short term in anesthetized patients or those in the Intensive care unit (ICU), this equation may also be written as:

$$\text{(expired minute ventilation)} \times (\text{arterial } CO_2) = \text{constant}$$

or

$$\dot{V}_E \times Pa_{CO_2} = k. \tag{2}$$

Thus, for a constant CO_2 production, Pa_{CO_2} and alveolar ventilation are hyperbolically related (Fig. 2–1). This allows us to quantify directly derangements of the respiratory acid-base status and to adjust mechanical ventilators accordingly. For example, if arterial CO_2 is two times normal, then ventilation is half the needed value.

METABOLIC ACIDOSIS AND ALKALOSIS

It would be convenient if metabolic acid-base status could be quantified by comparing the serum bicarbonate concentration to its normal value, 26 mM. The $[HCO_3^-]$ alone does give a partial ap-

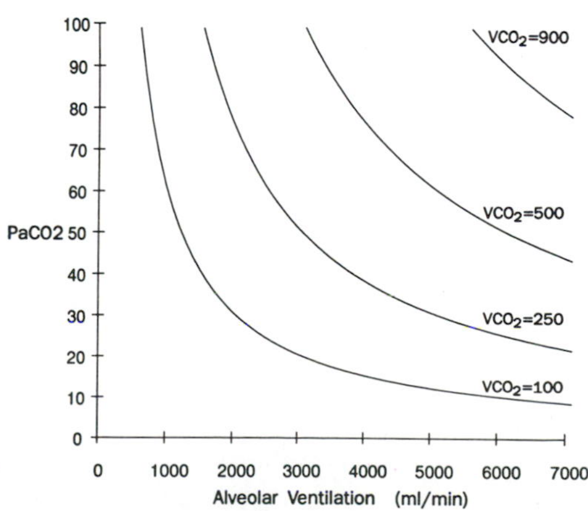

FIGURE 2–1. The relationship between arterial CO_2 tension and alveolar ventilation is a hyperbola for each value of minute CO_2 production (V_{CO_2}).

proximation of the metabolic acid-base status, but interpretation is complicated by buffering of metabolic acids and bases by a variety of noncarbonate buffers, especially hemoglobin. Because of these noncarbonate buffers, we must make a correction (usually fairly small) to the deviation of bicarbonate concentration from normal, as outlined below. The most common such correction is the *base excess,* used frequently, yet often misunderstood.

The bicarbonate buffer system is central to any discussion of metabolic acid-base status, not only because it is an important physiologic buffer, but also because two of the components of the system, arterial pH and $Paco_2$, are readily measured. Recall that carbonic acid (H_2CO_3) is in equilibrium with its conjugate base, bicarbonate or HCO_3^-:

$$CO_2 + H_2O \rightleftarrows H_2CO_3 \rightleftarrows HCO_3^- + H^+. \quad (3)$$

Therefore

$$\frac{[H^+] \times [HCO_3^-]}{[CO_2]} = K \quad (4)$$

which gives the familiar Henderson-Hasselbach relationship

$$pH = pK + \log \frac{[HCO_3^-]}{\alpha Pco_2} \quad (5)$$

where alpha (α) is a solubility coefficient for CO_2 in plasma.

For plasma, in which CO_2, hydrogen ion, and HCO_3^- are in equilibrium, any of the three variables is uniquely determined by the other two. For example, if this equation is plotted as in Figure 2–2, with separate curves for each value of $Paco_2$, for any given pH and $Paco_2$, the $[HCO_3^-]$ is uniquely determined. Therefore, by knowing Pco_2 and pH, one can calculate $[HCO_3^-]$, regardless of any other buffers of the system. The curves of Figure 2–2 always hold, so long as the system includes H^+, HCO_3^- and CO_2 in equilibrium.

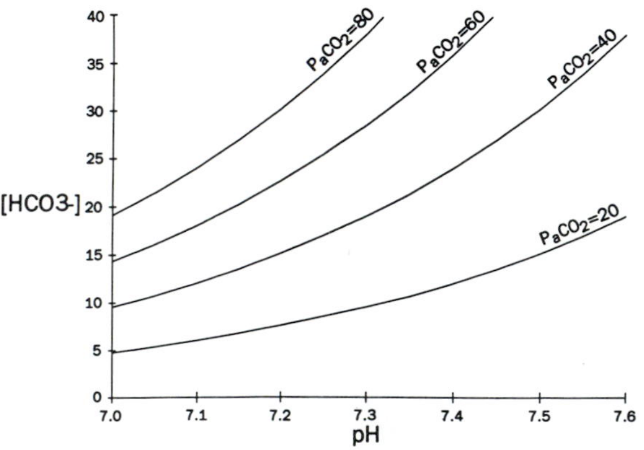

FIGURE 2–2. Plots of the Henderson-Hasselbach relationship. $[HCO_3^-]$ can be uniquely determined for any $Paco_2$ and pH.

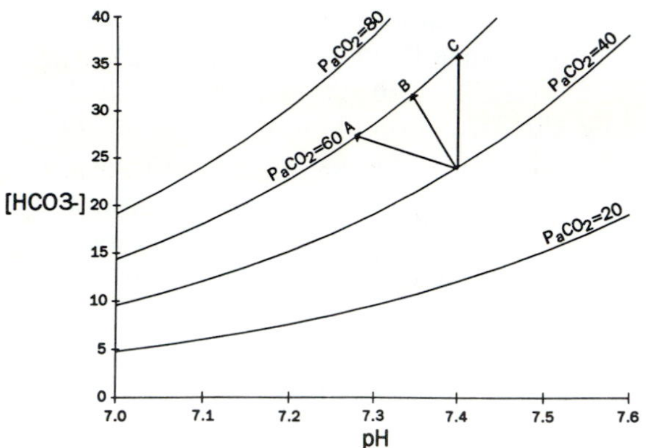

FIGURE 2–3. As $Paco_2$ is increased from 40 to 60, equation (4) predicts an increase in $[HCO_3^-]$ and in $[H^+]$. However, the Henderson-Hasselbach relationship does not predict whether the result is point A, B, or C.

However, the Henderson-Hasselbach relationship does not reveal how $[Hco_3^-]$ and pH change when $Paco_2$ increases or decreases from normal, corresponding to hypo- or hyperventilation. For example, without any additional information, we cannot tell in Figure 2–3 if increasing CO_2 will take us to point A, B, or C. We see from equation (3) that adding CO_2 to the buffer system will increase both HCO_3^- and H^+ (i.e., decrease pH).

Adding CO_2 in the physiologic range of pH, however, has practically no effect on $[HCO_3^-]$ if there are no other buffers in the system. At a pH of 7.4, the absolute concentration of H^+ is about 4×10^{-8} mol per L, whereas the concentration of HCO_3^- is about 2.6×10^{-2} mol per L, a ratio of 6.5×10^5, or nearly 1 million. If there were no other buffers, the equal amounts of H^+ and HCO_3^- formed from the added H_2CO_3 would change the pH much more than the $[HCO_3^-]$; in fact, the change in $[HCO_3^-]$ could be neglected completely. Therefore, if the system included only the HCO_3^- buffer, the buffer line for CO_2 would be flat, as in Figure 2–4.

If changes in $Paco_2$ do not change the $[HCO_3^-]$ for a pure bicarbonate buffer system, the corollary is that at any $Paco_2$ the $[HCO_3^-]$ reflects only the

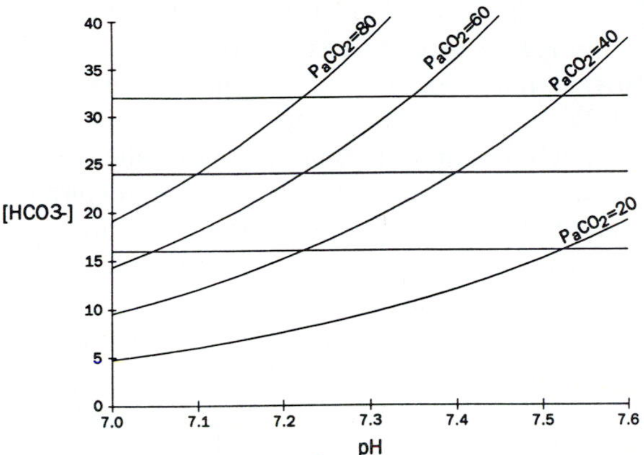

FIGURE 2–4. The "buffer curve" for a CO_2 titration determines the results of $Paco_2$ changes. The buffer curves are the nearly horizontal lines, each corresponding to a given $[HCO_3^-]$. For a pure bicarbonate buffer system at physiologic pH, the slopes of the buffer curves are nearly zero; For example, a bicarbonate buffer system with $[HCO_3^-]$ of 24 (middle line) will have a pH of 7.4 at a $Paco_2$ of 40, as shown at the intersection of the lines. If CO_2 is added to bring the $Paco_2$ to 60, the pH decreases to 7.2. Bicarbonate concentration is changed only by adding or removing metabolic acid.

amount of metabolic acid added to or subtracted from the system. For a pure bicarbonate system at a pH around 7.4, the $[HCO_3^-]$ alone would be a simple indicator of metabolic acid-base status. The buffer lines for CO_2 titration would be a family of flat curves with the vertical distance between the curves reflecting metabolic acid-base status.

In reality, however, there are other buffers for H^+ in the body, each obeying a relationship similar to equation (6)

$$H^+ + B^- \rightleftarrows HB \qquad (6)$$

where B^- represents other buffers. As metabolic acid is added to the system, some of the H^+ also ends up as hemoglobin (Hb), which is not reflected by changes in $[HCO_3^-]$. Since concentrations of HB are not measured in assessing metabolic acid-base status, how can one determine how much H^+ has been added or taken away from the system? Even though the amount of Hb or of B^- are unknown, if the system were somehow adjusted to a normal $[H^+]$, then the ratio B^-/Hb would also be normal. And, if this titration of H^+ were performed with an acid that produces a change of one HCO_3^- (for every H^+ ion), then the change in $[HCO_3^-]$ during this titration would directly reflect how much H^+ had been in the system as HB. The acid to use for this imaginary titration is CO_2.

This is one way of viewing the concept of base excess. Base excess is the difference between a normal $[HCO_3^-]$ and the $[HCO_3^-]$ that results from titrating the blood sample to a normal pH by adjusting the $Paco_2$. The deviation of this corrected $[HCO_3^-]$ from normal can be viewed as having two components: the amount that $[HCO_3^-]$ has changed from normal due to buffering of metabolic acid by the bicarbonate system (recall that this component will not change during the CO_2 titration, because the $[HCO_3^-]$ for a pure bicarbonate system is independent of $Paco_2$), and the amount $[HCO_3^-]$ has changed from normal due to buffering by other buffers. This latter component can be considered a correction factor to the measured bicarbonate concentration, and although much has been written on the best way to correct the $[HCO_3^-]$, in reality, this correction is usually small.

Of course, one cannot carry out this titration in the patient, so the correction factor is calculated. Given the actual slope of the CO_2 buffer line, illustrated in Figure 2–5, one can then imagine correcting any measured arterial blood gas to a normal pH by adding CO_2. For a pure HCO_3^- system (Fig. 2–4), the slope of this line is essentially zero; the buffer line is steeper when there are more noncarbonate buffers in the system, as found in patients (Fig. 2–5).

Unfortunately, in any given patient, the slope of the buffer line is unknown. Typical slopes for typical patients, the slope for normal whole blood, and how the slope for whole blood changes with variations in hemoglobin concentration are all known,

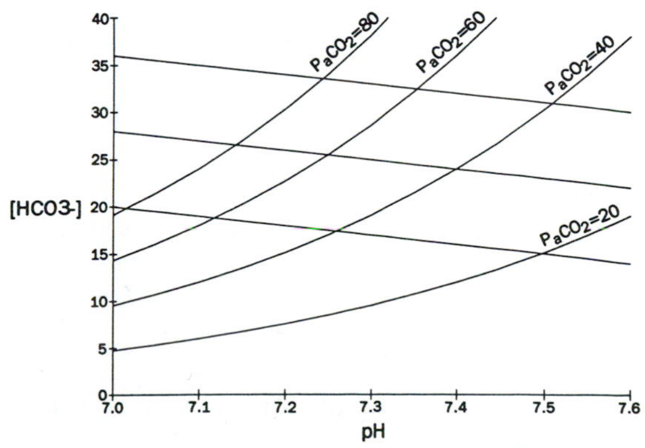

FIGURE 2–5. In a real patient, the slope of the CO_2 buffer curve is small but not negligible, because of the effects of non-bicarbonate buffers.

but there is no assurance that in a particular patient the buffers will be typical or present in normal concentrations. In fact, the slope varies depending on the duration of the acid-base disturbance, and the buffer curve is not really linear even in normals. The end result is that despite the importance frequently attached to the base excess, the number is always calculated, not measured, and the calculation is always approximate. It is inappropriate to prescribe bicarbonate therapy based only on a quantitative interpretation of the base excess.

In summary, if the $Paco_2$ has increased, the patient has a respiratory acidosis; if it has decreased, the patient has a respiratory alkalosis. The degree of ventilatory abnormality is proportional to the deviation of $Paco_2$ from normal. If the base excess is positive, the patient has a metabolic alkalosis; if negative, a metabolic acidosis. The magnitude of the base excess reflects the severity of the abnormality, but only approximately.

Defining the direction and severity of the acid-base abnormality, however, is only the first part of interpreting the data. Each of these disturbances may be primary or compensatory, and in mixed disturbances several processes occur simultaneously, with combinations of primary and secondary changes. The underlying pathology is not defined by the blood gas and pH data alone, but by an understanding of the patient's overall condition. An example may help to clarify the importance of assessing other clinical data in determining the causes of acid-base disturbances.

Case History

A 72-year-old man with a history of chronic obstructive pulmonary disease (COPD) and peripheral vascular disease presents to the emergency room with the sudden onset of abdominal pain, breathing at a respiratory rate of 28. As an anesthesiologist, you go to the emergency room to evaluate the patient before a planned exploratory laparotomy. Among the data is the analysis of an arterial blood sample taken while the patient was breathing room air: Pao_2, 57; $Paco_2$, 40; pH, 7.12; and $[HCO_3^-]$, 12.

One can estimate the alveolar Po_2 from an approximate form of the alveolar gas equation (see Chapter 22):

$$P_{A_{O_2}} = F_{IO_2} \cdot 713 - (Pa_{CO_2}/R)$$

$$P_{A_{O_2}} = 0.21 \cdot 713 - (40/0.8) = 100.$$

The alveolar-arterial O_2 difference is 100 − 57 = 43 mm Hg, clearly increased (normal is <10). The Pao_2 is much decreased; given the history of COPD, this is likely due to ventilation/perfusion mismatch and an unknown degree of shunt.

The $Paco_2$ is normal, but much more respiratory compensation (hyperventilation, diminished $Paco_2$) might be expected for this degree of metabolic acidosis (see below).

To assess the metabolic acid-base status, one estimates the base excess. One convenient estimate predicts that for every increase in pH of 0.1 as the CO_2 is decreased, the $[HCO_3^-]$ will decrease by 1. In this patient, one would like to increase the pH from 7.12 to 7.42 by removing CO_2, a change of 0.3 pH units, predicting that $[HCO_3^-]$ will decrease by 3 mEq during this titration. The corrected $[HCO_3^-]$ is then 12 − 3 = 9. The base excess is given by (base excess) = (corrected $[HCO_3^-]$) − (normal $[HCO_3^-]$), or base excess = 9 − 25 = (−16). This patient has a severe metabolic acidosis.

This defines the patient's acid-base and oxygen disorders and the severity of each, but determining the causes of these disorders requires considering other data. The severe metabolic acidosis suggests organ ischemia, especially if the anion gap is large or the measured lactate is elevated. The nature of the pain and the patient's history suggest a dissecting aortic aneurysm or mesenteric artery disease. Other surgical causes of an acute abdomen and metabolic acidosis include bowel obstruction and pancreatitis. The patient clearly needs further evaluation, but very likely has a surgical problem and may come to the operating room soon.

The tachypnea and inability to compensate for severe metabolic acidosis suggests significant COPD, abdominal splinting, fatigue, and impending respiratory failure. He may benefit from immediate mechanical ventilatory support despite the normal $Paco_2$. Also, bicarbonate therapy would be hazardous before ventilation is controlled, as he may not be able to excrete the additional CO_2 load, owing to his lung disease.

Although there is no way to be sure without baseline data, the suggestion of severe COPD raises the possibility that this patient chronically retains CO_2. Also, the Pao_2 would be depressed even more if the CO_2 were elevated, raising the possibility that this patient chronically depends on hypoxic drive to ventilation. Both of these points will be important in planning weaning from mechanical ventilation after the operation.

REFERENCES

Astrup P, Severinghaus JW. The history of blood gases, acids, and bases. Copenhagen: Munksgaard International Publishers, 1987.

Davenport HW. The ABC of acid-base chemistry. 6th ed. Chicago: University of Chicago Press, 1974.

Hindman BJ. Sodium bicarbonate in the treatment of subtypes of acute lactic acidosis: Physiologic considerations. Anesthesiology 1990; 72:1064–1076.

Shapiro BA, Harrison RA, Walton JR. Clinical application of blood gases. 3rd ed. Chicago: Year Book Medical Publishers, 1982.

SECTION 2

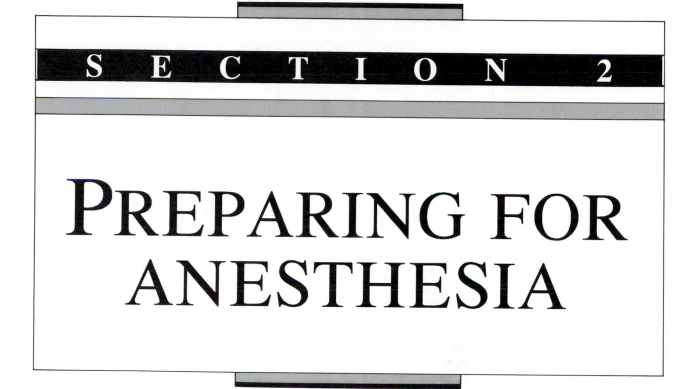

PREPARING FOR ANESTHESIA

CHAPTER THREE

PREOPERATIVE EVALUATION

Every anesthetic begins with the preoperative evaluation. This meeting of patient and anesthesiologist allows for an exchange of information, an assessment of physical status, and the formulation of an anesthetic plan. The aim is to have the patient in the best possible condition, both mental and physical, prior to surgery. The preoperative visit is as important as any aspect of intraoperative management in providing a safe, effective anesthetic.

To become familiar with the patient requires a careful history of the surgical illness and any concomitant medical problems, a review of the patient's chart, and a physical examination directed at the concerns of anesthetic intervention. Laboratory tests are then obtained to augment the findings of the history and physical examination; they rarely uncover new abnormalities. These data, along with the patient's American Society of Anesthesiologists physical status class, constitute a summary of the anesthesiologists's assessment of the patient's state of well-being, and provide a basis for preparations aimed at improving the patient's preoperative condition.

Beyond gathering information, the anesthesiologist establishes a doctor-patient relationship that reduces patient anxiety by building a foundation of trust and respect. Educating the patient about anesthesia, outlining a schedule of upcoming events, and discussing risks and options in an objective manner leads naturally to informed consent for the anesthetic management plan. A comforting and informative preoperative visit completes the psychological preparations of the patient.

Cost containment has engendered several striking changes in preoperative evaluation. To shorten hospital stays, anesthesiologists have begun to evaluate patients before admission in preanesthetic clinics. In this outpatient setting, the anesthesiologist acts as a consultant and formulates a plan for a smooth perioperative course. In addition, there is now general agreement that the history and physical examination are the best means of detecting significant disease before surgery, and that routine screening laboratory tests, in the absence of a significant positive history, do little to affect patient outcome. The ordering and interpreting of laboratory data are undergoing review with an eye toward reducing costs.

As the modern preoperative evaluation is streamlined to save money, it is vital to the cause of good care that the anesthesiologist not abandon the goal of establishing a degree of rapport with each patient, no matter how brief the contact with the patient may be.

The remainder of this chapter describes a method of preoperative evaluation that incorporates the preferred methods of the past into the more streamlined anesthetic practice of the future.

The Patient Interview

The anesthesiologist who is to administer the anesthetic should perform the preoperative evaluation, although this may not be possible for patients scheduled in ambulatory clinics or for admission on the day of operation. Under these circumstances, preanesthetic evaluation may occur days before admission; the patient arrives at the hospital just before the operation, and then is either discharged from the hospital or admitted as an inpatient depending upon the nature of the operation and the patient's response. The anesthesiologist performing the evaluation informs the patient that he will meet other members of the anesthesia staff in the operating room, minimizing surprises on the day of operation. To build the patient's confidence, anesthesia team members introduce themselves to the patient and acknowledge that they have reviewed the chart. Important items must be relayed to the anesthesiologists caring for the patient in the operating room; the written summary must be unusually thorough and intact.

In order to establish the appropriate bond between patient and anesthesiologist, the interview is carried out in private with the utmost consideration for the impression created in the patient's mind. An unhurried, well-organized, and reassuring interview fosters a sense of cooperation in the patient that may be needed on the day of operation. The setting for the preanesthetic interview must project the confidential nature of what is to be discussed, and provide privacy for an adequate physical examination. Although this interview traditionally was performed in the patient's hospital room late in the afternoon on the day prior to operation, this was more a matter of necessity than design. Commonly, asking for additional tests or therapy meant postponing the operation, and this setting involved a host of distractions, and others competing for the patient's time. Often, anesthesiologists now see patients in a preoperative clinic a week or two prior to operation, allowing consultant anesthesiologists to make timely recommendations for the patient's management. The office setting precludes unwanted interruptions, and allows an effective interchange between patient and anesthesiologist.

Frequently, the need for an emergency operation requires that the anesthesiologist meet the patient for the first time in the hallway outside the operating room. Even under such circumstances, preoperative evaluation must cover all pertinent issues. This versatility is fundamental to anesthesia practice.

ELEMENTS OF THE PREANESTHETIC HISTORY

- **Age**
- **Sex**
- **Vital signs, height, weight as recorded in chart**
- **Planned operation (compare patient's expectations with schedule)**
- **Patient's sense of overall health and list of illnesses**
- **Medications**
- **Drug allergies, adverse reactions**
- **Previous surgery and anesthesia**
  - **Patient satisfaction with anesthetic**
  - **Any complications of anesthesia: sore throat, spinal headache, etc.**
  - **History of fever, severe myalgia, or other signs of malignant hyperthermia**
  - **Prolonged emergence or intraoperative awareness**
  - **Awakening paralyzed; pseudocholinesterase deficiency**
- **Family history of difficulties with anesthesia**
- **Review of systems, with questions designed to test function**
  - **Cardiovascular**
    - **Cardiac or coronary artery disease**
    - **High blood pressure**
    - **Exercise tolerance**
  - **Pulmonary, including smoking history, asthma, exercise tolrance**
  - **Renal**
  - **Hepatic, including hepatitis or jaundice after anesthesia**
  - **Endocrine, especially diabetes**
  - **Neurologic: stroke, numbness, weakness, sciatica**
- **Dental**
  - **Dental damage, loose teeth**
  - **Dental prostheses**
- **Airway**
  - **Snoring**
  - **History of difficulty breathing**
  - **History of neck stiffness**
- **Pregnancy: is the patient pregnant?**

Patient's special fears, wishes about anesthesia

General versus regional

Premedication

Nausea

Intraoperative awareness

"Not waking up"

Note: Rarely would an anesthesiologist raise all of these questions with a single patient. For example, a thin young athlete with no medical history might be asked only a handful of questions.

THE MEDICAL HISTORY

The importance of a medical history lies in its ability to uncover and assess the severity of any pathology that would influence the selection and management of an anesthetic. The present surgical illness, any current medical problems, and a review of systems are explored for their contribution to any physiologic, metabolic, or anatomic derangements. The inpatient hospital course, if applicable, is studied for the most recent developments of the disease processes. Specific positive findings are sought, and followed up by in-depth questioning. Pertinent negatives, especially for common diseases such as hypertension, diabetes, atherosclerotic vascular disease, and congestive heart failure, are important. Generalities of physical condition, such as exercise tolerance or significant weight loss, provide clues to the degree of dysfunction.

The medical history may be elicited by questioning the patient directly, by following a checklist, or by asking the patient to complete a questionnaire, written or automated. Questionnaires cover all of the essential items and provide a brief summary of the patient's health history. A typical questionnaire appears in Figure 3–1. With a completed health survey in hand, the anesthesiologist can focus on preanesthetic problem areas instead of spending large amounts of time confirming the absence of disease. More attention can be devoted to counseling the patient on the anesthetic options that are available and providing instruction that will lead to a safer anesthetic. Patient acceptance of this approach is still unproven. One preliminary report has found the written responses to be accurate.

The practice employed at the University of Pennsylvania Admissions Evaluation Center is a tripartite approach involving a health survey questionnaire (Fig. 3–1), a nurse practitioner, and an anesthesiologist. The patient initially completes the health survey, and then discusses the results with a nurse practitioner, who questions the patient to elicit details concerning each abnormal response. Medical problems are characterized by date of onset, severity, functional significance, and response to therapy. A problem list is then compiled, and a physical examination is performed to confirm the presence of disease. The anesthesiologist who completes the evaluation concentrates on anesthesia-related matters and reviews the patient's general health.

Certain aspects of the medical history always require additional questioning by the anesthesiologist because of their crucial role in planning an anesthetic. Current medications must be defined with respect to dose, schedule, patient compliance, and results achieved. Patients' medications are usually continued unchanged, but it may be appropriate to alter the dose, change to a shorter acting preparation, or even discontinue the drug temporarily depending on the potential for drug interactions, the effects of drug withdrawal, and the drug's pharmacokinetic properties. Individual assessment is warranted in each case.

Allergy history also requires a systematic approach in order to outline the magnitude of the problem. Allergic reactions are frequently misunderstood, and appropriate documentation often is lacking. Severity ranges from asymptomatic rashes to generalized urticaria to life-threatening anaphylaxis, but too commonly the reported allergy actually represents drug intolerance, usually to an opioid. As a general rule, all drug reactions are recorded because many nonanesthetic drugs with potential for serious allergic responses are administered in the operating room. If an allergic response seems likely, the offending drug is not repeated without formal immunological testing or pretreatment with antihistamines and corticosteroids is indicated (as in the case of contrast dye allergies).

The patient's previous anesthetic experiences are invaluable in choosing the next anesthetic, but close questioning is usually required to elicit useful

☐ **DAY SURGERY UNIT (Yellow)**

☐ **AM ADMIT UNIT (Pink)**

☐ **SHORT STAY UNIT (Blue)**

HISTORY NO.

NAME

RACE

AGE

SEX

Imprint with Name Plate or Print Patient's Name, Hosp. No. & Physician

TO BE COMPLETED BY SURGEON

MINIMUM STUDIES FOR PHYSICAL STATUS I & II PATIENTS.

(When in doubt about need for a study, contact one of the designated anesthesia consultants)

	Under Age 40	Over Age 40	Over Age 60	Diuretic or Antihypertensive Use
☐ CBC	YES	YES	YES	YES
☐ EKG	NO	YES	YES	YES
☐ Chest X-Ray	NO	NO	YES	YES
☐ SMA-6	NO	NO	YES	YES
☐ OTHER				

OPERATIVE PROCEDURE: ______________________ ______________________

Requesting Physician's Signature
(Must be present to obtain studies)

SURGEON TO COMPLETE FOR AM ADMIT AND SHORT STAY PATIENTS ONLY

PATIENT'S OLD RECORDS REQUESTED ☐ YES ☐ NO INITIALS/DATE ____________

OLD RECORD FORWARDED TO AM ADMIT-SHORT STAY UNIT ☐ YES ☐ NO INITIALS/DATE ____________

HISTORY AND PHYSICAL EXAM:

SENT TO ADMISSIONS WITH PATIENT ☐ YES ☐ NO INITIALS/DATE ____________

TO BE FORWARDED BY SURGEON'S OFFICE ☐ YES ☐ NO INITIALS/DATE ____________

HEALTH SURVEY QUESTIONNAIRE – TO BE COMPLETED BY ALL PATIENTS

Dear Patient:

We welcome the opportunity to participate in your medical care. To save you an extra trip to the hospital, we depend on your surgeon to evaluate your health and to order appropriate studies. We depend on you to provide accurate health screening information on this form.

To help us, please complete the following survey.

Thank you for your help and we look forward to caring for you.

Hospital of the University of Pennsylvania

NAME				DATE SURVEY FILLED OUT
STREET ADDRESS		CITY	STATE	ZIP CODE
AGE	HEIGHT	WEIGHT	HOME TELEPHONE	OTHER TELEPHONE

HOSPITAL OF THE UNIVERSITY OF PENNSYLVANIA

FIGURE 3–1. The health evaluation questionnaire used in the Preadmission Evaluation Clinic at the Hospital of the University of Pennsylvania. After the patient completes the health survey, a nurse practitioner reviews it with the patient, after which an anesthesiologist reviews the form and the nurses notes, performs a physical examination and the preanesthesia visit. Illustration continued on following page.

List All Allergies (Including medication allergies)

____

____

____

____

List All Medications You Have Taken In The Past Five Years.

____

____

____

____

List All Medicines You Now Take

____

____

____

____

List All Medical Illnesses You Have Had

____

____

____

____

List All Operations You Have Had

OPERATION	DATE

	NO	YES	
1. Have you ever had a problem with anesthesia other than nausea or vomiting?	☐	☐	______________
2. Has anyone related to you ever had a problem with anesthesia other than nausea or vomiting?	☐	☐	______________
3. Could you be pregnant?	☐	☐	______________
4. Do you smoke? If so, how many packs per day?	☐	☐	______________
5. Do you have a cough?	☐	☐	______________
6. Do you bring anything up when you cough?	☐	☐	______________
7. Have you had asthma?	☐	☐	______________
8. Do you have a cold?	☐	☐	______________
9. Can you walk up two flights of stairs without getting short of breath?	☐	☐	______________
10. Have you had any difficulties with breathing?	☐	☐	______________
11. Do you have any bleeding tendencies?	☐	☐	______________
12. Have you ever been anemic?	☐	☐	______________

FIGURE 3–1. Continued.

	NO	YES	
13. Do you have a heart murmur?	☐	☐	________
14. Have you ever had a heart attack?	☐	☐	________
15. Have you ever had angina or pain in the chest related to your heart?	☐	☐	________
16. Have you ever had high blood pressure?	☐	☐	________
17. Do you ever wake up short of breath at night?	☐	☐	________
18. Do you have diabetes?	☐	☐	________
19. Have you had significant weight loss in the past 4 months without trying to diet?	☐	☐	________
20. Have you ever had thyroid problems?	☐	☐	________
21. Have you ever had an abnormal chest x-ray?	☐	☐	________
22. Have you ever had a stroke?	☐	☐	________
23. Have you ever had epilepsy, seizures or falling out?	☐	☐	________
24. Do you have frequent headaches?	☐	☐	________
25. Have you ever had eye problems?	☐	☐	________
26. Have you ever had kidney disease?	☐	☐	________
27. Have you ever been jaundiced?	☐	☐	________
28. Have you ever had hepatitis?	☐	☐	________
29. Have you ever had an arm or leg become numb or weak ?	☐	☐	________
30. Do you have any physical disabilities?	☐	☐	________
31. Do you have any chipped or loose teeth, dentures, caps, bridgework or braces?	☐	☐	________
32. Would you describe yourself as being extremely anxious about your pending procedure?	☐	☐	________
33. Have you ever been under the care of a psychiatrist?	☐	☐	________

FIGURE 3–1. Continued.

information. Less dangerous problems, such as awakening with the endotracheal tube in place, or postoperative nausea and vomiting are prevalent and often easily recalled by patients. Understandably, patients usually cannot recall life-saving interventions. Clues to an adverse reaction to previous anesthetics may be ambiguous, and may consist only of a stay in an intensive care unit or a lengthy postoperative course with several new physicians participating in the patient's care. The family's history of anesthetic complications may disclose inheritable diseases, such as malignant hyperthermia or pseudocholinesterase deficiency. Vital information can be found in the records of prior anesthetics: the effect of the premedication, the response to anesthetic agents and techniques, details of laryngoscopy, and any untoward outcomes. A close review of a recent anesthetic provides the most reliable guide to planning the next.

THE PHYSICAL EXAMINATION

The emphasis of the preanesthetic physical examination is on those elements necessary in a given patient. Without exception, evaluation of the airway is in order. Beyond that, anticipation of forthcoming events in the operating room, and the patient's history dictate the examination to be performed and the expected yield in diagnosing inconspicuous disease. A prudent approach to care includes a primary anesthetic plan and one or more contingency plans for each case. The physical exam must be directed according to the patient's history and the plans for operation and anesthesia.

The anesthesiologist might measure the blood pressure in both arms (or possibly the legs) when asymmetry is likely, as in congenital, atherosclerotic, or postsurgical changes of the aorta or its major branches. Orthostatic changes in heart rate and blood pressure are of importance when volume status is in question, as in diuretic use, prolonged fasting, or blood loss. The cardiopulmonary exam may be expanded to include a walk down the hallway to assess fatigue and dyspnea. A deliberate inspection of the fingertips for cyanosis, clubbing, or nicotine stains, and an inspection of the lower extremities for signs of vascular insufficiency or edema is helpful. Respiratory drive and coordination of thoracoabdominal musculature may be affected by altered body habitus, such as obesity, cachexia, or kyphoscoliosis. These simple observations are examples of the supplementary measures that are added to the general physical examination to clarify the patient's preoperative status and functional reserve.

EXAMINING THE AIRWAY

(1) Overall appearance
- **Neck: stout or thin, long or short?**
- **Sunken cheeks suggesting poor mask fit**

(2) In mouth
- **Mouth opening**
- **Anterior displacement of mandible**
- **Tongue size**
- **Uvula visible**
- **Protruding upper incisors**
- **Loose, damaged teeth**
- **Prostheses**

(3) Movement
- **Flexion/extension of neck**
- **Sniffing position**

(4) Palpation
- **Trachea in midline**
- **Distance from mentum to hyoid (5 cm)**

(5) Nose
- **Both nares patent**
- **Protubrant nose suggesting poor mask fit**

(6) Recognizable syndromes with airway abnormalities (see Chapter 13)

Examining the area of the proposed operation may provide an estimate of the extent of surgery. Inspection of both venous and arterial access sites assists in planning intravenous fluid administration and invasive monitoring, and may avert difficulties in the operating room. When regional anesthetics are planned, examining the site of needle insertion confirms landmarks and rules out local skin infection. A brief neurological examination may uncover preexisting nerve dysfunction, essential to planning regional anesthetics. The position that the patient will assume during the operation may not be tolerated because of circulatory, respiratory, or musculoskeletal problems. This may justify a brief trial during the preoperative evaluation to find a suitable position.

Airway evaluation merits a unique place in the preanesthetic assessment. The systematic evaluation described in the sidebar and in Chapter 13 is essential not only to predict the degree of difficulty of tracheal intubation, but to gauge the level of effort that will be required to manage and support the airway in the absence of an endotracheal tube. Any potential for damage to the teeth must be documented in the patient's chart and discussed with the patient beforehand, as the most common litigation after anesthetic care involves dental damage. Clear documentation of existing problems and of the likelihood of further damage not only promotes good care, but limits awards if injury to the teeth should occur.

The ingredients for a complete physical examination vary from patient to patient; it is likely that no two patients receive exactly the same examination.

LABORATORY TESTING

Few quibble over laboratory testing for an appropriate clinical indication. However, there is serious doubt about the usefulness of preoperative testing in the asymptomatic patient prior to elective surgery. The high cost and low yield of such screening investigations have led to a reappraisal of the practice of ordering a fixed battery of preoperative laboratory tests for all surgical patients. Physicians order laboratory tests for many reasons, some of which have little to do with improving the patient's health (Table 3–1). These biases have impeded the development of a nationwide policy regarding preoperative screening tests. An understanding of some of the mathematical principles of screening, in conjunction with a brief review of the major advances in this area of research, will guide proper selection of laboratory testing for the preoperative patient.

TABLE 3–1. Reasons Why Physicians Order Laboratory Tests*

Screening
Peer pressure
Personal reassurance
Ease of performance with ready availability
Hospital policy
Medicolegal need
Documentation
Hospital profit
Curiosity
Insecurity
Habit
Establish a baseline

* Reproduced with permission from Lundberg GD. Is there a need for routine preoperative laboratory tests? (editorial) JAMA 1985;253:3589.

TABLE 3–2. Characteristics of an Ideal Screening Test*

The patient is asymptomatic, with no evidence on history or physical examination of the condition for which they are being screened.
The condition will potentially alter the outcome of surgery.
The preoperative diagnosis will aid perioperative management.
The prevalence and severity of the condition are great enough to warrant the expense of screening.
The tests are sufficiently sensitive to allow detection and specific enough to avoid over-diagnosis.

*Reproduced with permission from Carson JL, Eisenberg JM. The preoperative screening examination. *In* Goldmann DR, Brown FH, Levy WK, Slap GB, Sussman EJ, eds. Medical care of the surgical patient. 1st ed. Philadelphia: JB Lippincott Company, 1982:16–30.

Not only must screening tests be limited to those which will detect abnormalities that might affect patient management, but the prevalence of the disease and the sensitivity, specificity, and positive predictive value of the proposed test must also be known, so that the test results can be interpreted (Table 3–2).

Table 3–3 describes a hypothetical test with a sensitivity of 95 per cent and a specificity of 95 per cent. The positive predictive value of the test decreases dramatically as the hypothetical prevalence of the disease declines from 50 per cent to 10 per cent to 1 per cent, because the number of false-positive test results overwhelms the number of true-positive results, even though the test enjoys good sensitivity and specificity. A practical example of this occurs in the use of a barium enema as a test for detecting gastrointestinal (GI) pathology. Among patients older than 60 years of age and having a history of anemia and bright red blood per rectum, the prevalence of significant GI disease is about 50 per cent. Under these circumstances, barium enema performs reliably as a test for diagnosing such findings as GI malignancy or diverticular disease. On the other hand, among pa-

Table 3–3. How the Positive Predictive Value of a Test Varies Depending Upon the Prevalence of Disease*

Distribution of Patients (%) for a Test with a Sensitivity of 95% and Specificity of 95%				
Prevalence	*TP†*	*FP†*	*TN†*	*FN†*
50%	47.5	2.5	47.5	2.5
10%	9.5	4.5	85.5	0.5
1%	0.95	4.95	94.05	0.05

Prevalence	*Positive Predictive Value*
50%	47.5/(47.5 + 2.5) = 0.95
10%	9.5/(9.5 + 4.5) = 0.68
1%	0.95/(0.95 + 4.95) = 0.16

* Modified from Goldman L. Quantitative aspects of clinical reasoning. *In* Braunwald E, Isselbacher KJ, Petersdorf RG, Wilson JD, Martin JB, Fauci AS, eds. Harrison's principles of internal medicine. 11th ed. New York: McGraw-Hill Book Company, 1987:5–11.

† *Abbreviations*: TP, true-positive; FP, false-positive; TN, true-negative; FN, false-negative.

Definitions: sensitivity = TP/(TP + FN); specificity = TN/(TN + FP); positive predictive value = TP/(TP + FP); prevalence = (TP + FN)/(TP + FP + TN + FN).

tients of all ages without any GI complaints, the prevalence of GI disease is approximately 1 per cent. Using the barium enema as a screening test in this group yields a large number of false-positive results that cannot be distinguished easily from the true-positive results, and leads to further evaluation, with concomitant risk and additional expense.

In the realm of preoperative screening, these calculations often yield startling results when a test such as the partial thromboplastin time (PTT) is examined closely. The PTT has a sensitivity of 99 per cent and a specificity of 72 per cent for detecting clotting disorders. Since the prevalence of asymptomatic clotting disorders is 1:100,000, only one individual with real disease will be found out of 100,000 patients, but 28,000 patients will be falsely labeled as having a coagulation defect. The burden imposed by delaying or canceling operation, and retesting to determine if any bleeding disorder does exist, argues against the use of this test in the asymptomatic patient.

Most studies in this area consist of retrospective review of hospital charts and concern to a single

Table 3–4. Simplified Strategy for Preoperative Investigations

	T/S	Hb	PT/PTT	PLT/BT	Elect	Creat/BUN	Gluc	X-ray	ECG
Surgical Procedure									
Minor									
Major	X	X							
Age (yr)									
<40									
40–70									X
>70					X	X			X
Associated Conditions									
Cardiovascular								X	X
Pulmonary								X	X
Malignant			X						
Hepatobiliary			X						
Renal					X	X			
Bleeding disorder			X	X					
Diabetes					X	X	X		
Medications									
Diuretics					X	X			
Digitalis					X				
Corticosteroids					X		X		
Anticoagulants			X						

* Reproduced with permission from Blery C, Szatan M, Fourgeaux B, Charpak Y, Darne B, Chastang C, Gaudy JH. Evaluation of a protocol for selective ordering of preoperative tests. Lancet 1986;1:139–141.

Abbreviations: T/S, type and screen; Hb, hemoglobin determination; PT, prothrombin time; PTT, partial thromboplastin time; PLT, platelet count; Elect, Na^+, K^+, Cl^-, CO_2, proteins; Creat, creatinine; BUN, blood urea nitrogen; Gluc, glucose; x-ray, chest film; ECG, electrocardiogram.

test. A few have evaluated both prospectively and jointly the major preoperative tests. One such study (Blery et al., 1986) stands out because of its use of a previously established protocol to order selectively preoperative tests (Table 3–4). The protocol took into account the clinical status of the patient (age plus associated medical conditions), the scheduled operation, and the likely yield of information of the tests involved. In 3866 consecutive surgical patients, only 0.2 to 0.4 per cent of the tests not ordered would have influenced patient management. Use of the protocol did not put any patient's life at risk.

This study demonstrates not only that routine testing performed without indication yields few significant abnormalities, but that omission of such tests seldom leads to regrets. Routine preoperative investigations, when ordered without clinical indication, rarely produce new diagnoses that will affect patient management or outcome. The abnormalities that are uncovered tend to be unexpected, often lack clinical relevance, and seldom lead physicians to alter their decision-making strategies. The current consensus is that the medical history and physical examination provide the greatest yield in terms of discovering new disease. Laboratory testing is appropriate for confirming and quantifying suspected disease, for assessing the effects of treatment, and as a screening measure only when the potential benefit has been proven.

The development of a protocol for the selective ordering of laboratory tests is still in evolution, but the chart given here provides a reasonable starting point for the exercise of clinical judgment.

Informed Consent

Before undertaking an anesthetic, the anesthesiologist is obliged to obtain the patient's informed consent. A prudent approach is to inform the patient of the reasonable anesthetic options, to cite the risks and benefits as plainly as possible, and to agree on a course of action that covers most common contingencies. The patient's response to this discourse may range from a request for more specifics, to an expression of trust with no further doubts concerning the procedure. The anesthesiologist must be prepared to answer all questions posed by the patient in a manner that provides the appropriate information for a reasonable and educated decision. Written documentation of the informed consent is included in the patient's chart. It may consist either of a statement detailing the patient's acceptance of the proposed anesthetic plan or a standardized consent form that summarizes the appropriate issues and is signed by the patient or their representative.

Physical Status Classification

Every patient is assigned an American Society of Anesthesiologists physical status classification prior to the administration of anesthesia (Table 3–5). This serves as a general measure of the state of well-being of the patient, taking into account all of the problems the patient brings to the operating room, including systemic disturbances that may have been caused by the surgical illness.

Although studies of anesthetic mortality show a correlation with the physical status classification,

Table 3–5. Patient Physical Status Modified Slightly from ASA Definitions

Physical Status

1. The patient has no systemic disease, including the pathologic process for which surgery is needed, which is only localized. Example: A healthy young man requires inguinal herniorrhaphy.
2. The patient suffers mild or moderate systemic disease, due either to the surgical condition or to a concomitant disease. Example: The patient described above takes oral medication for diabetes, but has no end-organ damage and has never suffered severe ketoacidosis.
3. Severe systemic disease limits the patient's activity. Example: The patient above had an myocardial infarction last year and now has angina usually controlled by medical treatment.
4. Severe life-threatening disease markedly limits the patient. Example: The patient above has congestive heart failure and can walk less than half a block.
5. The moribund patient has a 50 percent 24-hour mortality, regardless of the planned surgery. Example: Our patient has infarcted bowel and is anuric, comatose, and has a blood pressure of 70/40 on a dopamine infusion.
6. The patient has been declared dead and will undergo surgery for organ donation. Example: 72 hours after a motorcycle accident, a PS I patient comes to the OR liver and kidney donation.
7. When the patient requires emergency surgery, an E is appended to the PS number. Example: The diabetic patient described suffered a strangulated hernia during the years before he developed coronary occlusion and sought attention promptly; he was rated PS 2E.

this categorization does not describe risk directly. The risks of any operation are determined not only by those factors that are patient-related, but those related to the specific operative procedure (a craniotomy is associated with a higher mortality than a hysterectomy), the experience of the surgical team and of the medical institution with a given procedure, and to a degree, the choice of anesthetic agents and techniques.

THE PREANESTHETIC NOTE

The summation of the evaluation process is the preoperative note in the patient's chart. Like any consultant's note, it omits needless repetition of data and presents instead a logical explanation of the anesthesiologists's findings, diagnoses, and plans, with a brief explanation. It is a legal document through which anesthesiologists communicate their assessment and plans to others; it must be ordered, concise, and logical.

ANESTHESIOLOGIST'S PREOPERATIVE NOTE

(1) Heading, labeling it as "Anesthesia Preoperative Note"

(2) Patient identification

- **Name**
- **Age, sex, occupation, race if relevant**
- **Planned surgery**
- **Statement that anesthesiologist has seen patient and reviewed the chart.**

(3) Problem-oriented list of major disease processes, giving for each:

- **Disease**
- **Severity, in functional terms**
- **Present treatment**
- **Likely effect on perioperative course**
- **Management plan**

(4) Special issues for anesthesia management

- **Drug allergies, reactions**
- **Review of previous anesthetics**
- **Airway, dentition**

(5) Outline of anesthetic plan

- **Regional versus general versus local; reasons**
- **Special management, such as awake intubation, and reasons**
- **Monitoring; why chosen**
- **Special preoperative recommendations:**
  - **Add or delete medications**
  - **Consultations**
  - **Studies**
- **Postoperative care anticipated, if out of the ordinary**

(6) Physical status

(7) Statement of informed consent

(8) Legible signature

EXAMPLES OF TWO PREOPERATIVE NOTES

The preoperative note varies in length and complexity depending on the case. Abbreviations and sentence fragments save space and time, but important findings, plans, and reasoning must all be covered. For example, a healthy patient coming for a brief ambulatory procedure who has passed through a preadmission clinic such as the one described in this chapter might have a preoperative note like this one:

9/15/91 ANES PREOP NOTE

James Roe, a healthy 22-year-old college track athlete, requires removal of screws from ankle fracture. I have interviewed Mr. Roe and examined him, his old chart, and his health survey. No diseases, allergies, medications, dental, or airway problems. Previous GA with isoflurane was uneventful. PS I; after discussion including spinal or local, he prefers and consents to GA.

Joan Q. Doe, M.D.

For a more complex case, the note would be longer:

9/15/91, 11:00 AM
ANESTHESIA PREOPERATIVE NOTE

Mrs. Roe is a 68-year-old woman, for ORIF today of hip Fx sustained yesterday at 0900. No allergies, no previous anesthetics.

Meds:	**Valium 5 mg po hs for sleep** **morphine 5 mg IM q 4 hour prn pain**
Allergies:	**None**
Airway:	**Good mobility, opens mouth, all of uvula visible**
Teeth:	**Edentulous**
Food:	**NPO since accident**

Problems include:

(1) ***Mild dehydration, blood loss, hypovolemia:*** **urine output 20 cc per hour since admission, Hb 14.6, Na 144, K 3.3, tongue dry. Volume to be restored before anesthesia begins. Intravenous fluids ordered by surgeon. Plan tilt test before induction, bladder catheter to follow urine output.**

(2) ***Obesity:*** **5′1″ tall, 244 pounds, central obesity. No Hx of snoring or sleep apnea. ABG shows P_{O_2} 88 on room air, P_{CO_2} 41, pH 7.44. Chest film clear. Will need oxygen postoperatively, but respiratory failure or ICU care not likely. May need A-line to obtain bp; pt accepts.**

(3) ***Diabetes:*** **DM × 6 years, takes 28 NPH q AM, glucose 295 at 7:00 AM today, no ketones, no Hx ketoacidosis or hypoglycemia. No signs end-organ damage: BUN 18, Cr 1.2, EKG normal. Plan: monitor glucose and treat PRN in OR and RR.**

(4) ***Full stomach:*** **Full stomach possible, as she reports nausea and pain since the fall and is getting narcotics. Plan H_2 blocker and rapid sequence induction.**

The patient prefers GA, after discussion, as she fears being awake in OR. With no special cardiac risk factors and easy airway for rapid sequence induction, this is acceptable and will produce unconsciousness. ASA PS II.

John Doe, M.D.

ANESTHESIA ORDERS:

(1) For OR at 2:00 PM

(2) NPO

(3) Hold insulin

(4) Morphine 10 mg IM now

(5) IV: NS at 250 cc per hour

(6) Cimetidine 300 mg po now

J. Doe, M.D.

The note begins by stating the proposed surgical procedure. Next, the pertinent findings of the medical history, physical examination, and previously obtained laboratory values are listed with an assessment of the anesthetic implications for each issue identified. Next is a discussion of the anesthetic plan with recommendations for further testing, invasive monitoring, or needed therapy. At times, a consultant may be needed to answer a specific question or recommend treatment. Statements regarding informed consent and physical status classification follow. Recommendations to delay the scheduled procedure must always be made with ample reasoning and pursued through personal contact with the surgical staff.

CONCLUSION

The classic preoperative visit, conducted at the patient's bedside on the evening before operation, is passing from the scene under the pressures of day surgery, same-day admissions, and the needs of cost containment. This change may bring improvement in patient care if practitioners and institutions substitute a system of preadmission consultation that allows adequate time for patient and anesthesiologist to talk and which incorporates well-chosen preoperative studies. For the foreseeable future, the goal of optimum preparation of the patient for operation and anesthesia will be met only by a thorough history and physical examination, by good rapport between patient and physician, and by selecting tests indicated by the medical history and clinical judgment.

REFERENCES

Blery C, et al. Evaluation of a protocol for selective ordering of preoperative tests. Lancet 1986; 1:139–141.

Goldberger AL, O'Konski M. Utility of the routine electrocardiogram before surgery and on general hospital admission. Ann Intern Med 1986; 105:552–557.

Kaplan EB, et al. The usefulness of preoperative laboratory screening. JAMA 1985; 253:3576–3581.

Sox HC, Garber AM, Littenberg B. The resting electrocardiogram as a screening test. Ann Intern Med 1989; 111:488–502.

Suchman AL, Mushlin AI. How well does the activated partial thromboplastin time predict postoperative hemorrhage? JAMA 1986; 256:750–753.

Tape TG, Mushlin AI. The utility of routine chest radiographs. Ann Intern Med 1986; 104:663–670.

Turnbull JM, Buck C. The value of preoperative screening investigations in otherwise healthy individuals. Arch Intern Med 1987; 147:1101–1105.

CHAPTER FOUR

PREMEDICATION

In the early years of anesthesia practice there was little or no use of preanesthetic medicines, but by 1920 it was common for anesthesiologists to prescribe some medication before anesthesia, and the term "premedication" began to be used. Induction of anesthesia with ether was often slow, punctuated by coughing and struggling with excessive salivation and bronchial secretions; it was unpleasant for both patient and anesthetist. Routine premedication with morphine, a barbiturate, and atropine or scopolamine made the patient sleepy, cooperative, dry-mouthed, and amnestic for most perioperative events.

Thiopental and other rapid-acting intravenous anesthetics have made these precautions unnecessary: patients pass almost instantly through the stage of excitement and struggling. Instead of relying on a fixed regimen of premedication, anesthesiologists now combine the psychological effects of a reassuring preoperative visit with medication chosen for specific purposes to meet each patient's needs before anesthesia and operation.

When writing orders for premedication, the anesthesiologist seeks to improve the patient's comfort, blunt harmful reflexes, reduce the chance of aspiration of gastric contents, and ensure that patients receive the medications needed to treat chronic illnesses, allergies, or perioperative infections. This chapter discusses these goals and the means available to meet each (Table 4–1). The special needs of infants and children are discussed in Chapter 25.

Patient Safety and Preoperative Medication

All of the drugs used for preoperative medication produce unwanted side effects. Opioids and sedatives, and especially combinations of them, can cause hypotension, respiratory depression, loss of consciousness, upper airway obstruction, hypercarbia, and hypoxemia. Although these harmful effects can be limited by assessing patients for such risk factors as obesity, a history of sleep apnea, old age, or intercurrent cardiopulmonary disease, unanticipated relative overdose can still occur. When these drugs are given intravenously in small doses with appropriate monitoring and in the presence of a trained observer, these complications can be avoided or treated. When the medications are given orally or intramuscularly and the patient is left for some time unobserved, the risks increase.

To reduce the hazards of preoperative sedatives and opioids, they are avoided completely or used in greatly reduced doses in the elderly, those at risk from airway compromise or respiratory depression, and in patients liable to hypotension. Patients are not told that they will be "knocked out" before coming to the operating room, as the

TABLE 4–1. Goals of Premedication

Patient comfort
- Relief of anxiety
- Sedation
- Amnesia
- Analgesia

Begin managing anesthesia problems
- Salvation
- Bronchial secretion
- Vagal reflexes
- Analgesia and sedation for general or regional anesthesia
- Control of hypertension and tachycardia
- Anticonvulsant effect

Prevent nausea and vomiting
Prevent aspiration of gastric contents
Prevent infection
Continue treatment of intercurrent disease

small doses of premedicants are chosen deliberately, thereby keeping to a minimum the risk of overdose at the cost of undertreating some patients. Those who arrive anxious in the operating suite may receive additional sedatives intravenously before going to the operating room.

PATIENT COMFORT

Anxiety

The principal goal of premedication is to calm the patient, who is naturally anxious about the coming operation. Originally, this was done for pragmatic reasons: it was easier to induce anesthesia by mask or open drop techniques in a calm patient, and during chloroform inductions, "excited" patients, with their greater catecholamine levels were thought to be more susceptible to possibly fatal ventricular arrhythmias. There are few clear data at present to support the idea that freedom from preoperative anxiety improves postoperative outcome, but to make operation and anesthesia less frightful remains an important humanitarian aim.

Relieving Anxiety Without Drugs

It is not always necessary to give medication to make a patient more calm. In Egbert's classic 1963 study, patients who received a preoperative visit felt less nervous than those who received no visit or those who received pentobarbital alone (Table 4–2). Many other studies since then have confirmed that patients' anxieties are greatly relieved by a reassuring visit during which they are advised of what is to come (see Chapter 3). More sophisticated techniques such as self-hypnosis, meditation, or learned relaxation responses are of great value, but are too time consuming for routine use.

Not all patients are calmed by sedatives; those who are both anxious and by nature most comfortable when in control of themselves and their surroundings may respond paradoxically to the effects of sedatives and become more openly anxious. All patients benefit from a preoperative visit by the anesthesiologist. After such a visit, medication can be prescribed if the patient requests it or if the anesthesiologist anticipates some specific benefit, or can be withheld if that seems best.

Drugs to Relieve Anxiety

As shown in the Egbert study and many others, moderate doses of hypnotic drugs are likely only to make patients sleepy, but not to relieve anxiety. This important distinction is made simply by asking the somnolent patient about his feelings. At present, benzodiazepines are the drugs that have been shown to produce specific antianxiety effects with the least severe side effects such as respiratory depression. They are not without hazards, as evidenced by the deaths attributed to midazolam

TABLE 4–2. Value of Preoperative Interview Compared with Pentobarbital*

	Percentage of Patients Reporting the Effect			
	Preoperative Treatment			
Effect	*Interview*	*Pentobarbital*	*Both*	*Neither*
Feel nervous	40	61	38	58
Feel drowsy	26	30	38	18
Adequately sedated	65	48	71	35

* Reproduced with permission from Egbert LD, Battit GE, Turndorf H, Beecher HK. The value of the preoperative visit by an anesthetist. JAMA 1963;185:553–555.

Note: This study compared the effects observed in patients receiving pentobarbital or a sympathetic preoperative interview or both or neither.

given to older patients when the drug was first released (and likely used in excessive doses).

Medication to relieve preoperative anxiety can be given both the night before operation and again several hours before the patient goes to the operating room: appropriate times are on awakening, for morning operations; and a few hours later in the morning, for afternoon operations. Benzodiazepines are well absorbed from the stomach, eliminating the need for intramuscular injections if enough time (one hour) is allowed for the drug to reach the bloodstream. Sedative premedications given just before the patient comes to the operating room are likely to have no beneficial effects, and are best replaced by intravenous sedation administered in the operating suite.

DIAZEPAM

Diazepam can be given orally. The usual dose is 0.15 mg per kg body weight, given several hours before operation, but in patients habituated to benzodiazepines or who are unusually anxious, up to 0.25 mg per kg can be used. Smaller doses are appropriate for older, frailer patients. Diazepam can no longer be considered appropriate for parenteral use, because of inconsistent absorption from intramuscular sites, and pain and phlebitis on intravenous injection.

MIDAZOLAM

Midazolam can be given intramuscularly without discomfort and with reliable effect an hour or two before operation in doses of 0.07 to 0.1 mg per kg. For intravenous premedication before taking a patient into the operating room, repeated doses of 0.5 to 1.0 mg are given to effect.

LORAZEPAM

Lorazepam, four times as potent as diazepam, is well absorbed orally and is so long acting in its effects that it may produce unwanted sedation and amnesia after surgical procedures of ordinary duration. It is most useful for patients undergoing major or lengthy procedures following which prompt emergence is not essential. Lorazepam produces remarkable amnesia for many patients, an effect that can be an advantage for some and a source of concern for others.

PHENOTHIAZINES

The phenothiazine promethazine is often used for its sedative, drying, and antiemetic effects. It is commonly combined with meperidine as a premedicant for invasive diagnostic procedures, including radiologic studies and cardiac catheterization. Hydroxyzine has similar properties and an additional bronchodilator effect. Other phenothiazines, particularly chlorpromazine, have been used extensively to produce sedation. Chlorpromazine potentiates opioids without causing further respiratory depression; its alpha-adrenergic blocking action is a troublesome side effect that produces unwanted hypotension during general or regional anesthesia, however.

Amnesia

Amnesia for perioperative events can add to the patient's comfort, but it also has undesired effects. Some patients may find it distressing to be unable to recall events, and worry about having done something embarrassing. As a rule, it is better to put patients at ease and make them comfortable rather than give a drug to make them forget later their fears and discomfort. For distasteful and uncomfortable procedures such as awake intubation, insertion of central venous catheters, positioning on a fracture table, or long operations under regional anesthesia, or when a patient asks not to remember events, amnesia is most reliably produced by drugs given intravenously although they may be given intramuscularly before the patient comes to the operating room. Midazolam, lorazepam, or scopolamine (0.4 to 0.6 mg intravenously) each produce effective anterograde amnesia; there is no reliable way to produce safely retrograde amnesia for events preceding drug administration.

Amnesia after midazolam is dose related: at 0.05 mg per kg intravenously, 60 per cent of patients are amnesic for endoscope insertion, while after 0.15 mg per kg, 96 per cent are amnesic. The lesser of these doses is just greater than the doses usually used for routine sedation during surgery under local anesthesia. The amnesia from midazolam is greatest two to five minutes after intravenous injection and lasts 20 to 30 minutes, while that from intravenous lorazepam is delayed 15 to 20 minutes, but lasts six to eight hours.

Analgesia

Patients in pain can receive opioids as part of their premedication. There is no need for the patient with a painful abdomen, an ischemic foot, or a fracture to suffer during the trip to the operating room. Morphine is a good choice, provided its side effects are taken into account and it is not given without close supervision to patients at special risk for airway obstruction or respiratory depression (see Chapter 10). Other opioids offer no advantages over morphine in this application.

Patients who have received morphine are likely to be nauseated by movement. Typically, premedication will be followed by transportation, so that when morphine is given it is usually accompanied by an antiemetic.

PREMEDICATION AS THE BEGINNING OF ANESTHESIA.

Blockage of Salivation and Bronchial Secretions

The routine use of drugs to produce a dry mouth has become less common because of the wide use of intravenous induction followed by rapid tracheal intubation, and because of the nonirritating qualities of modern inhalational agents. It is not necessary to give an anticholinergic drug before every anesthetic. Nevertheless, induction of anesthesia is sometimes associated with the accumulation of excessive saliva and bronchial secretions, especially in smokers, provoking coughing and laryngospasm. It is good practice to give a drying agent before applying a topical anesthetic to the airway for laryngoscopy or bronchoscopy, so that the anesthetic is not washed away by saliva.

When drying of secretions is necessary, glycopyrrolate 0.2 mg intramuscularly as a premedicant is the drug of choice. It is less apt to cross the blood-brain barrier than are scopolamine or atropine; thus it avoids the confusion associated with the central anticholinergic syndrome that occurs in some elderly patients. Atropine also produces more tachycardia than does glycopyrrolate. To delay giving the anticholinergic until the patient comes to the operating room does not allow time for the mouth to dry.

Blockage of Vagal Reflexes

Children, and some well-conditioned young athletes, may respond to airway manipulation, visceral stimuli, and halothane anesthesia with bradycardia, sometimes abrupt and profound (see Chapter 25). This can be prevented by premedication with an anticholinergic, but treatment can be delayed until the patient reaches the operating room.

Beginning Anesthesia Before Reaching the Operating Room

Other reasons sometimes given for prescribing opioids or sedatives as premedicants include relieving the discomfort of needles used for intravenous access or regional anesthesia, initiation of a planned balanced anesthetic, or their antitussive actions. These are all desirable effects, but they can be achieved more reliably and safely by administering the drug intravenously to the patient in the operating room, where their effects can be monitored, rather than by intramuscular injection. The dangers and undesirable effects of opioids and sedatives make it best to give premedicants in modest doses only for problems that will arise before the patient arrives in the operating room, thus erring towards producing modest effects that can be supplemented by additional intravenous drug, as opposed to excessive premedication in patients who are not monitored.

Control of Hypertension

As compared to normotensive patients, those with hypertension respond to the stimuli of laryngoscopy, intubation, and operation with exaggerated increases in blood pressure. Clonidine, sympathetic antagonists, and narcotics all obtund these responses and have been used as premedicants for this purpose. However, these drugs can produce unwanted hypotension, bradycardia, or respiratory depression. As argued previously, these purposes are best achieved by administering the drugs intravenously to patients in the operating room. Clonidine is not available in an intravenous formulation in the United States. It has the advantage of blunting catecholamine responses perioperatively, presumably as a result of its central alpha-2 adrenergic action. It has numerous other actions that are important to anesthesiologists: it reduces narcotic or inhalation requirements by approximately 40 per cent; it can produce significant bradycardia or hypotension when combined with beta blocking drugs or calcium channel blockers; it may result in prolonged sedation and drowsiness postoperatively.

Providing Anticonvulsant Effect

Some authors recommend premedication with benzodiazepines to reduce the chance of central nervous system toxicity from local anesthetics. In mice, moderate doses of benzodiazepines that did not cause sedation or loss of the righting reflex reduced the incidence of deaths and convulsions from the local anesthetics lidocaine, bupivacaine, or etidocaine given intraperitoneally. Benzodiazepines are used to treat local anesthetic toxicity, but the benefits of prophylaxis for this purpose have not been proven in humans; optimum effects can be expected from intravenous administration just before the block is performed, not from intramuscular or oral administration before coming to the operating room.

Nausea and Vomiting

Nausea, retching, and vomiting are common before and after operation; the incidence reported in various studies ranges from 10 to 55 per cent. Aside from the distress it causes patients, retching and vomiting can endanger the results of eye, ear, facial, or neurological surgery by increasing the chance of venous bleeding, and by raising intraocular and intracranial pressures. Antiemetic premedicants have been advocated to reduce the incidence of this distressing complication.

Droperidol

The most effective antiemetic now used in anesthesia practice is droperidol, which has been shown in numerous studies to have major antiemetic effects. Children undergoing strabismus surgery had an incidence of nausea or vomiting of 47 per cent, but preoperative droperidol reduced this to 10 per cent. Patients undergoing termination of pregnancy exhibited nausea and vomiting related to the use of a prostaglandin pessary; a small dose of droperidol (0.25 mg intravenously) decreased the incidence of postoperative nausea from 41 per cent to 21 per cent. As a premedicant it sometimes causes dysphoria or agitation that is extremely unpleasant for some patients, even leading to refusal of the operation on rare occasions. Extrapyramidal reactions are not as likely to occur as with prochlorperazine.

To avoid preoperative dysphoria, yet reduce the incidence of postoperative nausea and vomiting, droperidol is best given in small doses (0.125 to 0.25 mg) intravenously during the anesthetic, and not as a premedicant. It may be appropriate to reserve this drug for patients in whom vomiting poses special hazards (those who have undergone the operations listed above and patients with mouths wired closed after oral surgery) or who give histories of severe vomiting after anesthesia.

Aspiration of Gastric Contents

Given that precautions are taken for patients at special risk of regurgitation and aspiration (Rapid Sequence Induction and Intubation or Awake Intubation, Chapter 13), skilled management of general anesthesia results in few cases of severe aspiration. Nevertheless, preanesthetic treatment that reduces gastric acidity or the volume of gastric contents is expected to reduce the incidence and the severity of the consequences of aspiration of gastric contents, especially in high-risk patients.

Fasting

Common practice dictates that adult patients take nothing by mouth for at least eight hours before induction of anesthesia. Recent studies have questioned this tradition, showing that 150 ml water given an hour before anesthesia may actually promote gastric emptying and decrease activity. On the other hand, gastric emptying times for solid food are much longer than for fluids, and aspiration of solid food particles is particularly devastating. Pain, anxiety, and opioids, all found in patients coming for operation, delay gastric emptying. Further studies may validate the idea of giving liquids until very near the time of operation to healthy patients who are without extra risk factors for aspiration.

Although prolonged fasting is not needed, the discomfort of a few hours of fasting is so slight, and the damage done by pulmonary aspiration is so great, that a conservative approach to the matter is justified. Before elective operation, it is recommended that healthy adult patients abstain from solid food for eight hours. Clear liquids may be taken until three hours before operation unless there is some reason to expect delayed gastric emptying. Oral medication with up to 30 ml of water is permitted until the anesthesia begins.

H_2 Blockers

As many as 80 per cent of patients undergoing elective operation have gastric contents of pH less than 2.5, so that acid aspiration syndrome is possible. Aspiration of a volume greater than 25 ml is probably necessary for serious pneumonitis to develop. Gastric pH can be maintained greater than 2.5 by giving cimetidine 300 mg hs and 300 mg orally or intramuscularly an hour or two before operation (Fig. 4–1).

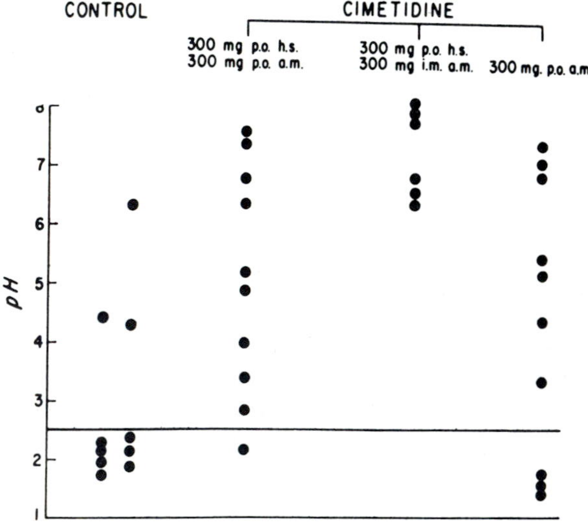

FIGURE 4–1. Distribution of Gastric Fluid pH in Control and Cimetidine-Treated Adults. (Reprinted with permission from Weber L, Hirshman CA. Cimetidine for prophylaxis of aspiration pneumonitis: Comparison of intramuscular and oral dosage schedules. Anesth Analg 1979; 58:426–427.)

Disadvantages of cimetidine include decreased hepatic metabolism of diazepam, lidocaine, and propranolol; sedation; bronchoconstriction; and arrhythmias. Ranitidine 150 mg orally lasts longer than cimetidine and may have fewer adverse side effects. Famotidine, 40 mg orally given one to two hours before anesthesia, has an effect like that of ranitidine; both produce gastric volumes of less than 25 ml and acidity of pH greater than 2.5.

Antacids

Orally administered antacids may also be used as premedicants to reduce the acidity of the stomach contents, especially before emergency operations. A few milliliters of sodium bicarbonate 8.4 per cent given orally neutralizes gastric acidity, though complete mixing with the stomach contents may take 20 minutes. Particulate antacids, which contain magnesium and aluminum hydroxides, cause serious pneumonitis themselves. Magnesium citrate, 0.3 M, or sodium citrate, 0.3 M, 10 to 20 ml given 15 to 60 minutes before induction, or the commercial product Bicitra (magnesium citrate and citric acid) reliably neutralize gastric contents.

Antacid therapy can only ameliorate the sequelae of aspiration, should it occur, since it does nothing to reduce the volume of stomach contents or to eliminate the effects of aspiration of solid food particles. It is most useful in emergency situations when histamine blockers do not have time to act.

Metoclopramide

Metoclopramide (10 mg orally or intravenously) increases gastric motility and relaxes the gastroduodenal sphincter, promoting gastric emptying. It acts within one to three minutes after intravenous administration and 30 to 60 minutes after oral administration. Large doses of the drug are tolerable; side effects are usually mild and include abdominal cramps and the central nervous system effects of dopaminergic blockade. Its effect may be diminished by atropine. It is an effective adjunct to H_2 blockers or antacids; the combination of cimetidine 300 mg the night before operation with oral cimetidine 300 mg and metoclopramide 10 mg on the morning of operation reduces gastric vol-

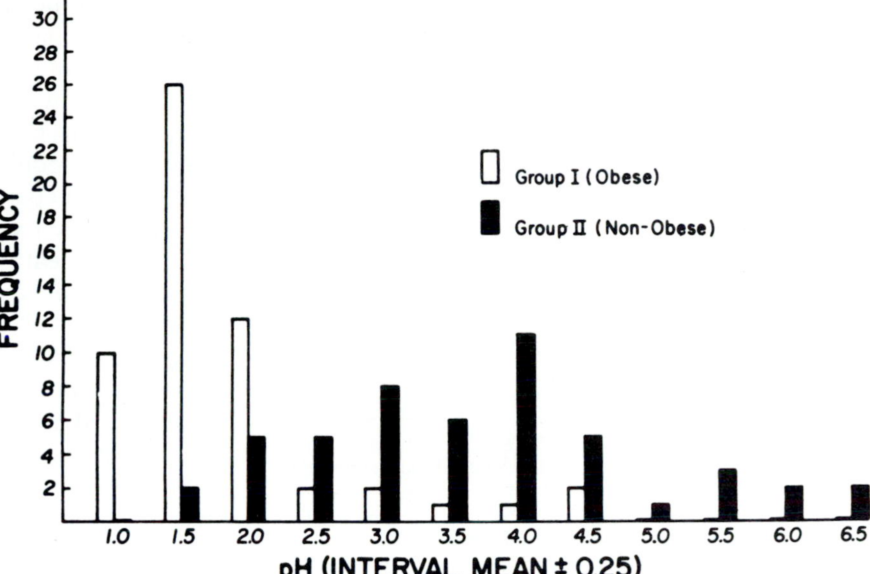

FIGURE 4–2. Frequency Distribution of Gastric Fluid pH in Obese and Non-Obese Patients. (Reprinted with permission from Vaughan RW, Bauer S, Wise L. Volume and pH of gastric juice in obese patients. Anesthesiology 1975; 43:686–689.)

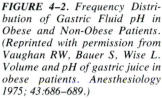

ume to less than 25 ml and the acidity to a pH of greater than 2.5.

The short-term use of all of these drugs, including H_2 blockers, antacids, and metoclopramide, is virtually without risk of serious side effects. Because the risk of aspiration pneumonitis is also small in healthy patients without risk factors, it is difficult to determine whether their routine use is justified. However, many patients can be predicted to be at special risk for aspiration because of increased volume or acidity of gastric contents, or because of increased likelihood of regurgitation. These include obese patients (Fig. 4–2), pregnant patients, diabetics with gastroparesis, emergency patients, and probably those with gastroesophageal reflux.

In these cases, rational combinations of these three therapies are justified. For elective surgery, a regimen consisting of an H_2 blocker taken by mouth on the night before operation and with metoclopramide on the morning of operation is effective. For emergency surgery, a soluble antacid 15 to 30 minutes before induction at least reduces acidity. Metoclopramide is also appropriate, but not if enhanced gastric emptying might harm the patient, as in abdominal trauma. H_2 blockers cannot be expected to be effective before induction, but may increase the intragastric pH by the end of operation.

Premedication to Prevent Infection

Many patients undergoing surgery now receive prophylactic antibiotics, which have been shown to reduce the rate of wound infections if given just before incision. At times, antibiotics are ordered to be given intramuscularly in the patient's room before coming to the operating suite. Because of uncertain absorption and irregular timing, this is not as effective as intravenous administration of antibiotics with the induction of anesthesia. It is best for the anesthesiologist to consult the surgeon about the dose and timing of prophylactic antibiotics used in this fashion.

Patients with cardiac valvular disease or prosthetic devices have an increased susceptibility to bacterial endocarditis during procedures that produce bacteremia of 15 minutes or more duration. The current recommendations of the American Heart Association outline the patients considered to be at risk (Table 4–3). The antibiotic regimen is recommended by an appropriate consultant.

Before administering any antibiotic, the prudent anesthesiologist takes a careful history of drug allergy. Rapid intravenous administration of vancomycin (giving a typical dose intravenously in less than 60 minutes) may cause histamine release with flushing, edema, rash, and hypotension.

TABLE 4–3. Procedures and Conditions that Require Endocarditis Prophylaxis*

Procedures
Dental procedures
Procedures with subgingival manipualtion
Procedures involving muscosal incisions or bleeding
General procedures
Rigid endoscopy
Endoscopy with biopsy
Urological procedures with infected urine or prostate
Incision and drainage of infected sites
Renal lithotripsy with infected urine
Gallstone lithotripsy
Conditions
Lesions of native valves
Mitral valve prolapse with insufficiency (holosystolic murmur and/or left atrial enlargement)
Heavily calcified valves
Valves previously damaged by endocarditis
Patients with transvalvular pacing wires or catheters
Other cardiac conditions
Conditions with a jet-lesion effect, such as coarctation of the aorta, arteriovenous fistulae, and ventricular septal defects.
Idiopathic hypertrophic subaortic stenosis
Prostheses
Prosthetic cardiac valves
Synthetic vascular grafts

* See Bayer AS. New concepts in the pathogenesis and modalities of the chemoprophylaxis of native valve endocarditis. Chest 1989;96:893–899; and Bayer AS, Nelson RJ, Slama TG. Current concepts in prevention of prosthetic valve endocarditis. Chest 1990;97:1203–1207.

Large blood concentrations of some antibiotics may cause ototoxicity or nephrotoxicity. Interactions with neuromuscular blockers can occur also (see Chapter 11).

CONTINUATION OF PREOPERATIVE THERAPY

Almost any medication a patient takes routinely is best continued up until operation, assuming it was effective and necessary in the first place. Exceptions may be drugs with narrow therapeutic indices such as digoxin and aminophylline, which can produce toxicity, and which can be given intraoperatively if needed. Monoamine oxidase (MAO) inhibitors present a troublesome dilemma: their presence makes the patient's response to adrenergic agents unpredictable and exaggerated; but eliminating these hazards requires weeks of abstinence, and exposes the patient to considerable risk from untreated depression. Several studies have shown that patients receiving MAO inhibitors can be given anesthesia safely; great caution is required in using sympathomimetic drugs, and meperidine must not be used, because it is associated with hypertension, hyperthermia, coma, and death in patients taking MAO inhibitors. Tricyclic antidepressants (imipramine) also block uptake of norepinephrine, but their effects largely dissipate within three days of being discontinued. Precautions for their use are similar to those for MAO inhibitors. Other antidepressants, antihypertensives, and antiparkinsonian drugs are continued up to an hour or two before surgery, given parenterally or with 30 ml of water.

It is especially important to continue drugs whose omission could cause a serious withdrawal syndrome: clonidine, beta-adrenergic blockers,

TABLE 4–4. General Approach to Premedication

Assess the patient's levels of insomnia, anxiety, pain, risk factors for aspiration, endocarditis, allergies, and medications already prescribed

Insomnia
- A benzodiazepine PO the night before operation

Anxiety
- Reassurance first of all
- If medication is needed
  - Diazepam 10 to 15 mg PO the night before operation
  - Diazepam 5 to 15 mg PO early in the morning of operation and again if the operation is delayed until afternoon
  - Substitute midazolam 5 mg IM for diazepam above

Pain
- If the patient suffers from pain preoperatively, add IM morphine, choosing dose according to patient size, severity of pain, and opioid habituation; starting dose: 10 to 15 mg

If a dry mouth is needed
- Glycopyrrolate 0.2 mg IM an hour before OR

If risk factors for full stomach are present
- Cimetidine 300 mg po hs before operation
- Cimetidine 300 mg po morning of operation
- Metoclopramide 10 mg po morning of operation

If prophylaxis for postoperative emesis is needed
- Droperidol 0.25 mg IV intraoperative
- Reduce amounts of other sedatives and narcotics

If risk factors for endocarditis are present
- Seek consultation regarding antibiotic prophylaxis

If the patient takes other medications
- Continue the medication on the normal schedule, with the exceptions of insulin, steroids, and at times, digoxin or aminophylline (depending on measured levels or signs of toxicity)

barbiturates, and opioids are examples. The patient on methadone maintenance can be given methadone as a premedicant. Alcoholics are treated with a benzodiazepine to prevent delirium tremens and convulsions.

OVERALL RECOMMENDATIONS

Simple guidelines for premedication are summarized in Table 4–4. The habits of relying on reassurance in place of sedatives, of giving important medications intravenously in the operating room instead of as premedicants, and of considering each patient's needs individually instead of following fixed policies are the keystones of safe, effective prescription of medications before anesthesia and operation.

REFERENCES

Egbert LD, Battit GE, Turndorf H, Beecher HK. The value of the preoperative visit by an anesthetist. JAMA 1963; 185:553–555.

Goresky GV, Maltby JR. Editorial. Fasting guidelines for elective surgical patients. Can J Anaesth 1990; 37:493–495.

McCammon RL. Prophylaxis for aspiration pneumonitis. Can Anaesth Soc J 1986; 33:S47–53..

Mirakhur RK. Anticholinergic drugs. Br J Anaesth 1979; 51:671–679.

Palazzo MGA, Strunin L. Anaesthesia and emesis I: Etiology. Can Anaesth Soc J 1984; 31:178–187.

Palazzo MGA, Strunin L. Anaesthesia and emesis II: Prevention and management. Can Anaesth Soc J 1984; 31:407–15.

CHAPTER FIVE

The Anesthesia Machine

The anesthesia machine is divided into two major components. The first is the gas delivery system, which provides mixtures of oxygen, other gases, and anesthetics via the fresh gas outlet to the second component, the patient breathing circuit, and ventilator. This chapter describes the gas delivery system, the breathing system, the anesthesia ventilator, and the devices that monitor their function. In addition to serving as a desk and storage cabinet, the modern anesthesia machine often includes physiologic monitors such as capnographs, described in Chapter 6.

The Gas Delivery System

The anesthesia machine meters out gases stored under pressure or vaporizes volatile liquids to provide gas mixtures of known concentrations. Hospitals provide a central supply system for oxygen, nitrous oxide, and often air and nitrogen, which are distributed to operating rooms via pipes and flexible hoses. Small gas cylinders mounted on the anesthesia machine provide emergency gas supplies or less commonly used gases, such as helium.

Anesthesia Gas Cylinders

The cylinders mounted on anesthesia machines are usually "E" size, containing 650 to 700 L of gas at a pressure of 2200 pounds per square inch (psi). Cylinders filled with nitrous oxide contain liquid and gas at room temperature and a pressure of 750 psi; they deliver about 1550 L of gas.

Cylinders are attached to the anesthesia machine with yokes equipped with pin indexing systems that permit attaching only cylinders containing the appropriate gas to each yoke. The position of the pins (yoke) and matching holes (cylinder outlet) is specific for each gas. The indexing system must not be compromised by altering the fittings or using adapters to attach inappropriate gas cylinders.

Yokes include check valves to prevent the reverse flow of gases from the machine, as might occur when replacing an empty cylinder. Check valves also prevent escape of gas when a hose is disconnected from the machine.

Pressure-Reducing Valves

The pressure within gas cylinders varies with temperature and decreases as the gas is used. Pressure regulators convert the high cylinder pressure to a constant working pressure (usually 45 psi), which remains constant as the tank empties. The pressure regulator contains an outlet chamber and a smaller inlet chamber separated by a valve. The valve is held open by pressure from a spring, which is adjusted to set the desired pressure in the outlet chamber. Gas pressure in the outlet chamber acts through a diaphragm to close the valve. Thus, when downstream pressure decreases, the valve opens to supply more gas and maintain the pressure constant. Pressure gauges display the pressures found in gas cylinders and supply lines.

Control of Gas Flow

Gas at the regulated pressure passes next to flow controllers, each of which contains a needle valve and a flowmeter.

The needle valve employs a screw with a fine thread to drive a gently tapered stem that fits into a seat with a matching taper, providing precise control of the resistance to gas flow. The flow control knobs are color coded, and the oxygen knob is fluted as well, to make it easier to identify.

Anesthesia machines are designed at present to deliver 150 to 500 ml per minute of oxygen when the oxygen flow control knob is in the full "off" position, in order to guarantee a minimal supply of oxygen to the breathing circuit. This is usually accomplished by placing a fixed flow bypass in parallel with the needle valve (Fig. 5–1).

The usual flowmeters are calibrated glass tubes with a barely perceptible internal conical taper, with the narrowest end at the bottom; a float rides freely in the bore of the tube. Gas flowing from the bottom upwards in the tube buoys the float. The resistance to the flow of gas through the gap between the float and the wall of the tube creates a pressure drop across the float. Opening the needle valve allows more gas to flow into the tube,

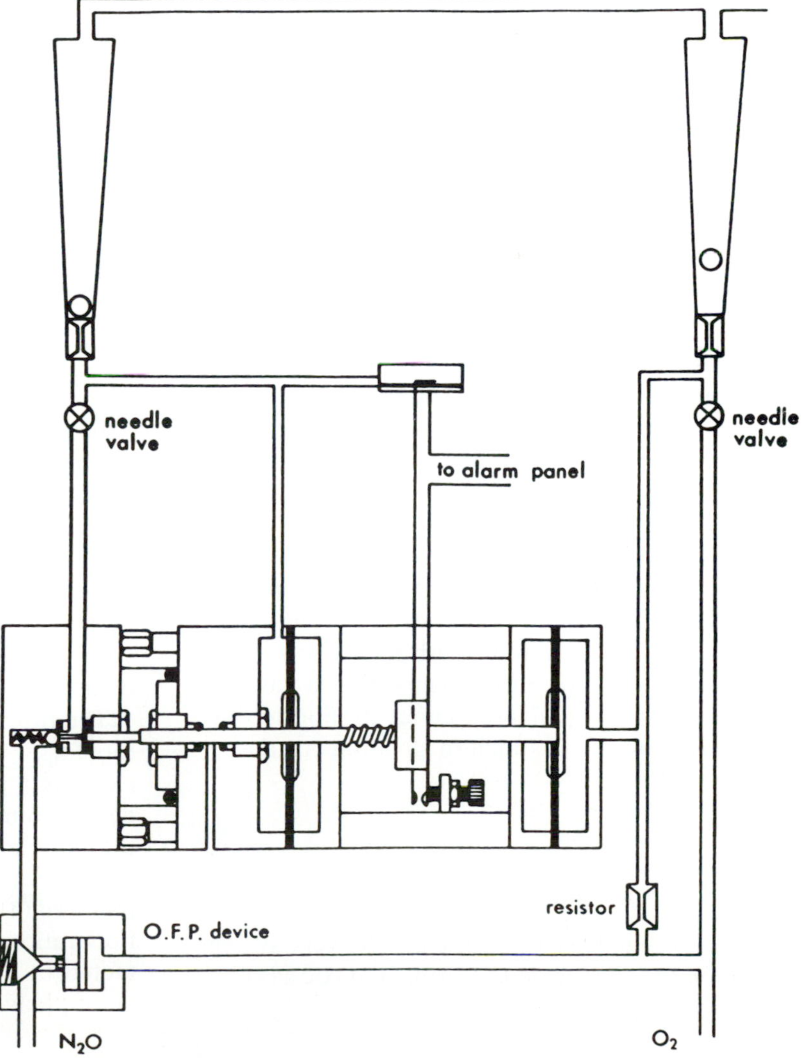

FIGURE 5–1. Gas flow control and safety systems. This diagram shows the high-pressure gas system, including the needle valves, flow tubes, bypass resistors for oxygen, the oxygen nitrous oxide ratio controller and the oxygen pressure fail-safe device. Oxygen enters at the lower right corner from a pressure regulator. The fail-safe system (OFP) stops the flow of N_2O if the O_2 supply pressure fails. The bypass resistor allows a small flow of oxygen, even when the oxygen needle valve is closed. (Reproduced with permission from Technical Service Manual. North American Drager, Telford, PA, 1985.)

which causes the float to rise, so that the cross-sectional area between the float and the inner tapered wall of the glass tube increases. At an equilibrium position, the force created by the pressure difference across the float equals the weight of the float, and the gas flow can be read from the adjacent calibrated scale. A spherical float is read at its center; all other shapes are read at the top of the float.

The minimum flow that can be accurately determined from a flow tube with a linear taper is approximately one tenth of its full scale, which may not provide adequate resolution or accuracy for both high and low flow rates. This can be solved by using a single tube with a dual taper or a pair of flow tubes for a single gas. In some obsolete machines, the two tubes lie parallel, a separate needle valve supplies each tube, and the total flow is the sum of the two indicated flows. In modern machines, the tubes lie in series, a single needle valve supplies both tubes, and gas flow is read from the tube giving the best estimate (Fig. 5–1).

Flow tubes are calibrated for 20° C and sea level atmospheric pressure, and are accurate to 10 per cent of the reading under these conditions. Flowmeters read falsely high at high altitude and falsely low when pressures exceed 760 mm Hg, owing to back pressure from vaporizers or accessories or use of the machine in a hyperbaric chamber. The changes in outlet pressure during positive-pressure breathing cause the float to bob up and down; accurate flows are indicated at end expiration. Each flowmeter must be used only with the specific gas for which it is calibrated, and with the calibrated scale supplied with the tube.

The outflow of the various flowmeters is mixed in a manifold and then delivered to the vaporizer assembly. By convention, gases flow from left to right within the manifold, with O_2 always at the right. This minimizes the chance that a gas leak will decrease the delivered concentration of oxygen and provides a standard position for the O_2 flowmeter.

Additional Safety Features

Other design features of the gas delivery system decrease the chance of delivering hypoxic gas mixtures as well.

OXYGEN FLUSH

The oxygen flush valve delivers about 50 L per minute of oxygen directly to the common gas outlet, bypassing flowmeters and vaporizers. Intermittent flushes of oxygen may be used to compensate for large leaks in the breathing system while the cause of the leak is corrected, in order to rapidly increase the inhaled oxygen concentration and decrease the inhaled anesthetic concentration, and to speed the emergence from anesthesia by allowing rapid refilling of the breathing system reservoir bag after venting the exhaled gas into a scavenger system. Because of the very high flow rates, pressing the O_2 flush button during the inspiratory phase of mechanical ventilation can result in dangerous peak airway pressures.

OXYGEN FAIL-SAFE SYSTEM

To prevent administration of hypoxic gas mixtures, fail-safe systems halt or proportionately decrease the flow of other gases when the O_2 supply pressure fails. During the machine check, this feature is tested by setting flows of oxygen and nitrous oxide and then shutting off the supply of oxygen to the machine. A properly functioning fail-safe system will shut off nitrous oxide flow as the oxygen pressure falls.

O_2–N_2O FLOW RATIO CONTROLLER

Fail-safe systems respond to loss of oxygen supply pressure, but do not guard against setting the flow meters to deliver a hypoxic mixture, as might happen when the oxygen flow control valve is turned off by mistake. Standards now require that anesthesia machines not deliver gas mixtures of O_2 and N_2O containing less than 25 per cent oxygen. This is accomplished by a nitrous oxide:oxygen flow ratio monitor or controller.

The flow ratio monitor incorporates flow detectors for N_2O and O_2. When the N_2O:O_2 flow ratio exceeds a predetermined value (usually 7:3), the device sounds an alarm signal. On some machines, the audible alarm can be switched off to allow high concentrations of nitrous oxide, as is sometimes required in closed system anesthesia. Although the flow ratio monitor protects against errors not detected by the fail-safe system, it only sounds an alarm, leaving the operator to correct the flows.

Nitrous oxide: oxygen flow ratio controllers limit oxygen concentrations in the delivered gas mixture to 25 per cent or greater (Fig. 5–1). When oxygen flow is decreased or N_2O flow is increased so as to reduce the concentration of oxygen below 25 per cent, the flow ratio controller automatically adjusts the flow of the other gas to maintain the oxygen concentration at 25 per cent.

OXYGEN ANALYZERS

Although effective, any of these fail-safe design features may malfunction, allowing the delivery of hypoxic gas mixtures. To protect against this, the anesthesia machine has an oxygen analyzer in the patient breathing circuit, usually a self-polarizing polarographic electrode. This consists of a lead anode, an alkaline electrolyte solution, and a gold cathode, separated from the gas phase by a Teflon membrane. The reduction of oxygen produces hydroxyl ions, which react with the lead cathode to induce a voltage proportional to the oxygen concentration. So that oxygen analyzers ensure reliably against hypoxic gas mixtures, they have reserve power supplies, they are calibrated against room air daily, and the low-oxygen alarm cannot be switched off. Because condensation of liquid on the barrier membrane significantly slows the response time of these cells, they are mounted above the gas path in the inspired (dry) limb of the breathing circuit.

Vaporizers

Modern precision vaporizers convert liquid anesthetics such as halothane, enflurane, and isoflurane into measured amounts of vapor that are added to the fresh gas mixture to produce known concentrations of anesthetic.

The first such vaporizers were the "copper kettles." Through a needle valve and flowmeter, a known flow of oxygen was passed through a kettle that produced a saturated vapor mixture of oxygen and anesthetic. Knowing the oxygen flow and the saturated vapor pressure of the anesthetic at the temperature of the kettle allowed calculation of the amount of vapor produced. These devices required complicated calculations to determine output anesthetic concentrations, and they could deliver excessive concentrations of anesthetic if misadjusted. Because of these problems, kettle-type vaporizers are no longer offered for sale, although some are still in use.

Kettles have been replaced by agent-specific vaporizers, which add to the fresh gas mixture the concentration of volatile anesthetic indicated on the dial of the vaporizer. Gas delivered to the vaporizer is proportioned into two streams—a vaporizer stream and a bypass stream—according to the setting on the dial. Gas flowing through the vaporizer is saturated with the anesthetic, and is then diluted to the set concentration by the bypass stream (Fig. 5–2).

Inaccuracies can be introduced by a number of factors. Changes in room temperature and cooling owing to vaporization alter the vapor pressure of the anesthetic and thereby the amount of anesthetic vapor added to the vaporizer stream. Modern vaporizers provide nearly constant output over a wide range of temperatures by employing materials with appropriate temperature expansion coefficients in the bypass valve assembly.

The composition of the gas mixture influences the output of vaporizers by at least two mechanisms. First, the solubility of nitrous oxide in halogenated agents (approximately 4 ml of N_2O gas per ml of volatile liquid) causes the volatile liquid to act as a reservoir when the N_2O concentration is changed. After an increase in delivered N_2O, N_2O is taken up by the volatile liquid, transiently decreasing the volume of gas flowing through the vaporization chamber and thus decreasing the output concentration of volatile anesthetic. Conversely, decreases in the concentration of N_2O cause a temporary increase in the vaporizer's output. Second, changes in the viscosity of the carrier gas alter the performance of the flow-dividing valve and also cause output to decrease when N_2O concentration is increased. These effects of nitrous oxide are most significant with low flow or closed breathing systems. Changes in carrier gas rate and back pressure have negligible effects on the output of modern, well-designed vaporizers.

Even the best-designed vaporizers can be unsafe if used improperly. Filling an agent-specific vaporizer with the wrong agent causes it to deliver not only the wrong agent, but the wrong concentration as well. This is most dangerous when a vaporizer designed for an anesthetic of low vapor pressure is filled inadvertently with one having a greater vapor pressure. A system of vaporizer filling ports that are keyed to matching rings on bot-

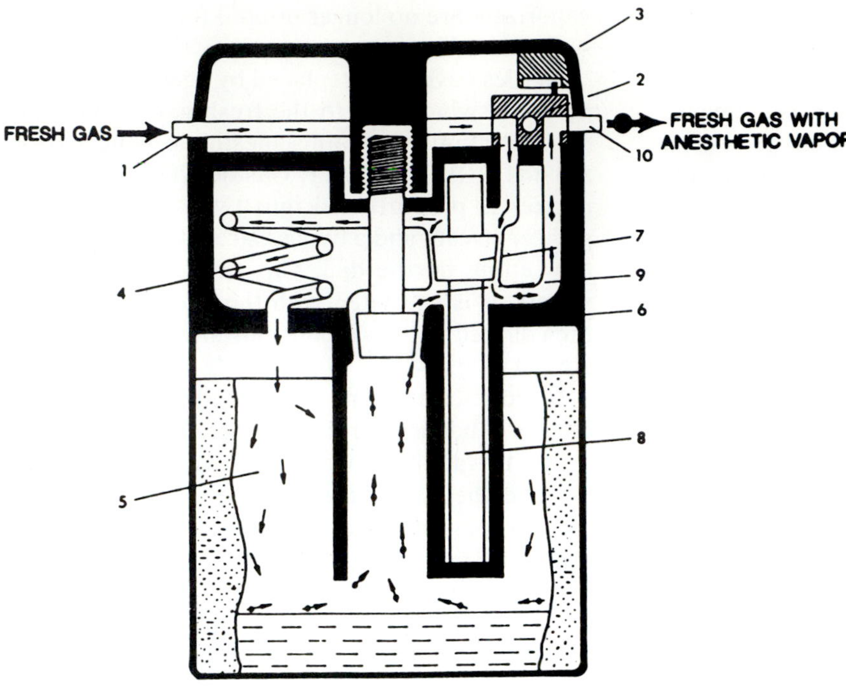

FIGURE 5–2. Precision vaporizer. The precision vaporizer allows output concentration to be set with a single concentration knob. Gas delivered to the fresh gas inlet is proportioned into two streams which flow through two parallel passages. Each passage contains a control cone that creates resistance to flow. The bypass cone resistance is fixed. The vaporization chamber cone resistance is controlled by rotating the concentration knob. Gas flowing through the vaporizing chamber becomes saturated with the anesthetic agent and is diluted by the bypass stream. Standards dictate that anesthetic concentration increase with counterclockwise rotation of the concentration knob. (Reproduced with permission from Technical Service Manual. North American Drager, Telford, PA, 1984.)

tles of liquid anesthetic can prevent using the wrong agent, but it has proven impractical and unpopular. Agent-specific gas analyzers (see Chapter 6) can identify both the type and the concentration of anesthetic emanating from a vaporizer, protecting against filling the vaporizer with the wrong anesthetic or against vaporizer malfunction. Vaporizers have low-mounted filling ports to prevent overfilling, and they are mounted rigidly to the machine to prevent overturning. Both of these accidents can introduce liquid anesthetic into the output of the machine. When a machine has several vaporizers, they are linked by a system that prevents switching on more than one at a time, to avoid contamination of the downstream vaporizer by vapor from the one upstream. Vaporizers are calibrated and serviced at regular intervals.

The most prevalent misuse of agent-specific vaporizers consists simply of administering a higher concentration of anesthetic than the patient requires. Although agent-specific vaporizers are limited to delivering concentrations no more than a few times the minimum alveolar concentration (MAC), a safety feature which has made these vaporizers more popular than the older kettles, even these concentrations are too great for some patients.

After passing through the vaporizer assembly, the gas mixture is piped to the common gas outlet of the anesthesia machine, and thence to the breathing circuit.

BREATHING CIRCUITS

Breathing circuits supply the lungs with a tidal flow of gas of appropriate composition, volume, and pressure, allowing either spontaneous, assisted, or controlled ventilation; they may also conserve heat, water vapor, and anesthetics by allowing rebreathing of exhaled gas from which CO_2 is removed. Two breathing circuit designs dominate modern anesthesia practice: circle systems and various modifications of the Mapleson D system. Both systems employ reservoir bags, breathing tubes, a fresh gas inlet, and a pop-off device (adjustable positive pressure relief valve) for release of excess gas; the circle system also incorporates a CO_2 absorption canister and permits rebreathing of some or all of the exhaled gas. These constituent parts are discussed below, followed by an analysis of the function of both circuit types.

Reservoir Bags

Although a normal adult patient rarely requires a total minute ventilation greater than 12 L per minute, the instantaneous inspiratory flow often exceeds 30 L per minute. Because the anesthesia machine delivers fresh gas at lesser flow rates, these transitory peak demands are met by a compliant reservoir bag (3 to 5 L). The bag also serves as a safety device because its distensibility limits circuit pressures to less than 60 cm H_2O, even when the pop-off valve is closed.

Breathing Tubing

The reservoir bag and the patient's airway (mask or endotracheal tube) are connected by breathing tubing, made of rubber or plastic and about 1 meter in length, with a volume of 400 to 500 ml per meter. Corrugations provide flexibility, resist kinking, and promote turbulent instead of laminar flow. During positive pressure ventilation, some of the delivered gas distends the tubing and some is compressed within the breathing circuit; thus, the resulting tidal volume is less than the delivered gas volume. Because of its wide bore, a breathing tube offers essentially no resistance to breathing (less than 1 cm H_2O per L per minute).

Breathing tubing is connected to the patient by a curved elbow with a connector having an outside diameter of 22 mm to fit standard face masks and an inside diameter of 15 mm to fit endotracheal tube connectors.

The possibility that breathing circuits might transmit bacterial infections from one patient to the next has led to the use of disposable tubing and rebreathing bags or bacterial filters. Postoperative respiratory infections seem to occur no less frequently with disposable equipment than with reusable circuits that have been cared for properly. Proper care includes washing with soap and water or germicides, followed by thorough drying.

Respiratory Valves

Valves in the breathing circuit limit gas to flowing in one direction, preventing unintended rebreathing of exhaled gas, and permit positive pressure breathing. The large orifices of the valves are closed by light disks of mica, ceramic, or plastic so that resistance to breathing is negligible even when water condensate causes the disk to stick to its seat, increasing the opening pressure slightly. The valves are enclosed in a clear dome housing so that the operator can monitor their function.

Adjustable Pressure-Limiting Valve

The adjustable pressure-limiting valve (APL valve) allows venting of excess gas from the breathing system. It consists of a disk held against an orifice by a spring that can be adjusted to vary the positive circuit pressure required to open the valve.

CO_2 Absorption Canisters

In a circle system, gas that is to be reused is cleared of carbon dioxide by passing through a canister containing a chemical CO_2 absorbent. Hydroxides of potassium, sodium, lithium, barium, and calcium all have clinical use. The reaction between CO_2 and the alkaline metal hydroxides, Na and K^+, involves the intermediate formation of a hydrate, and thus requires water.

$$2NaOH + 2H_2O \rightarrow 2NaOH \cdot H_2O \quad (1)$$

$$2NaOH \cdot H_2O + CO_2 \rightarrow Na_2CO_3 + 3H_2O \quad (2)$$

The reaction produces both heat and water. Solid granules of calcium hydroxide combine with CO_2 through a different reaction, too slow to be of practical use. However, a combination of 70 to 80 per cent $Ca(OH)_2$, 3 to 5 per cent NaOH (or KOH), and 10 to 20 per cent water with small amounts of sodium silicate produces a granule with acceptable reaction speed, capacity, and durability. A pH-sensitive dye is added to indicate when the chemical absorbent has been consumed. Although other agents have been used, such as barium hydroxide or lithium hydroxide, this mixture, sold as soda lime, is the most popular.

The 2-liter canister in modern absorbers has a gas volume of nearly 1 L when filled with granules of CO_2 absorbent. It contains about 1000 gm of absorbent and is capable of eliminating over 100 L of CO_2, giving a fresh canister more than eight hours of useful life in a low-flow system employed for a normal adult. Respiratory resistance is typically less than 1 cm H_2O for a 60 L per minute flow rate. Flow direction through the canister is from top to bottom, with a dust and moisture trap at the bottom to avoid introduction of dust or wet alkali into the inspiratory limb of the breathing circuit. The dye changes color in the top canister first; when the color change reaches the bottom canister, it is moved to the top, and the top canister is refilled with fresh absorbent and moved to the bottom.

The Circle System

The circle breathing system contains a CO_2 absorption canister to remove CO_2 from the expired gas, all or part of which is reused as inspired gas, allowing very low fresh gas flows with virtually total rebreathing (closed system). As fresh gas flows are increased, rebreathing is reduced; when fresh gas flow exceeds the minute ventilation, rebreathing of expired gas approaches nil, and the canister is unnecessary.

A circle breathing system contains an inspiratory and an expiratory limb, each with a one-way valve, and a reservoir bag (Fig. 5–3). The valves may be mounted anywhere between the patient and the bag with little difference in their function; in practice, they reside on the absorber. Three more components make up a functional system: a carbon dioxide absorber, a fresh gas inflow site, and a pop-off valve. These may be placed anywhere within the circle, but only a few locations are practical.

The absorber offers some resistance to breathing; so that the operator can assist inspiration, it is placed in the inspiratory limb on the bag side of the inspiratory valve. Fresh gas is introduced to the inspiratory limb, upstream of the inspiratory valve. This provides fresh gas for most or all of the inspired gas in high-flow techniques and most efficiently restores oxygen and anesthetic gas to the inspired gas mixture in low-flow techniques.

The pop-off valve usually resides on the bag side of the expiratory valve opposite the bag mount. During spontaneous ventilation, it is usually left wide open to minimize the effort the patient must make to exhale; gas leaves the circuit by the pop-off valve during the latter phases of exhalation. During manually controlled or assisted ventilation, the valve is partially closed so that some gas enters the patient's lungs and some leaves the system via

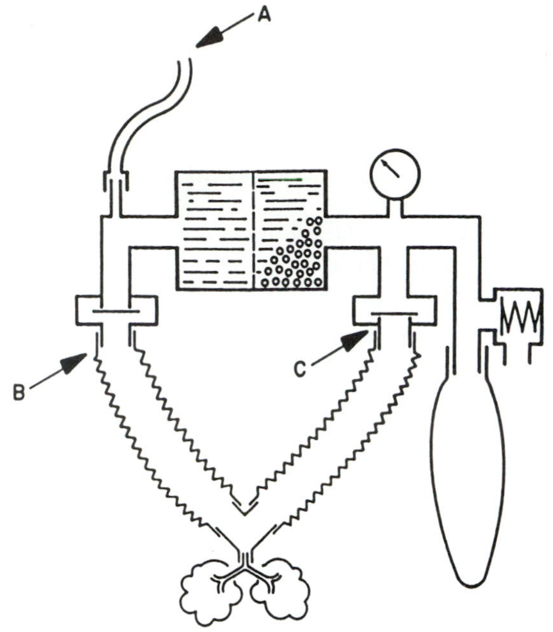

FIGURE 5–3. *Circle breathing system. The circle breathing system derives its name from the two limbs of breathing tubing linking the patient's airway to a compliant reservoir (rebreathing bag or ventilator bellows) in which exhaled gas is collected. One-way valves in the breathing tubing divide the circle into patient and reservoir sides and limit each limb of tubing to ether inhalation or exhalation. A CO_2 absorption canister allows for safe rebreathing of the exhaled gas. The composition of inhaled gas is altered by the introduction of fresh gas (A) to the circle. A pop-off valve exhausts excess gas to the atmosphere via a scavenging system. To provide efficient replenishment of oxygen and anesthetic gas, fresh gas is introduced close to the inspiratory valve (B) on its bag side. Since the absorber offers some resistance to breathing, and the anesthetist can assist inspiration, the canister is placed between the breathing reservoir and the inspiratory valve. The inspiratory and expiratory valves are mechanically attached to the absorber for durability and convenience. For efficient CO_2 elimination the pop-off valve is positioned on the bag side of the expiratory valve (C). (Schreiber, P. Anesthesia systems, p. 27. Telford, PA: North American Drager, 1985.)*

the pop-off valve during positive-pressure inspiration.

Mapleson D Circuits

The Mapleson D breathing system consists of a reservoir bag connected to the patient's airway by a single breathing tube with a fresh gas inlet at the patient end of the tube and a pop-off valve at the bag end (Fig. 5–4). This configuration places the pop-off valve where the greatest CO_2 concentration is present during the phase of breathing when

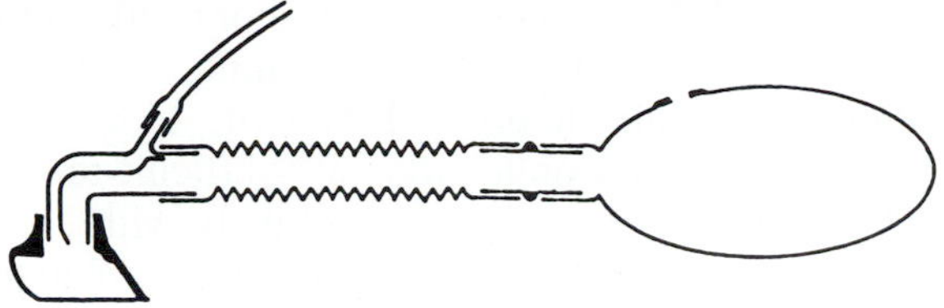

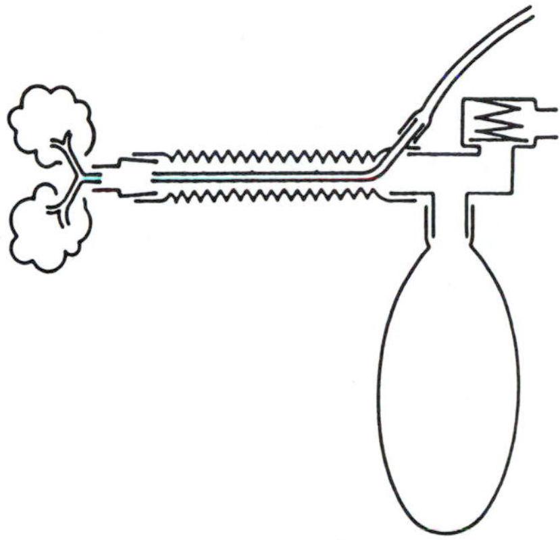

FIGURE 5–4. Mapleson D breathing systems. Two variations of Mapleson D systems are depicted, the Jackson-Rees system above, and the Baine modification below. The Jackson-Rees version vents excess gas through an aperture in the rebreathing bag; in the Baine version, a spring-loaded pop-off valve serves this function. (Schreiber, P. Anesthesia systems, p. 27. Telford, PA: North American Drager, 1985.)

excess gas escapes. Due to their light weight, minimal volume, and mechanical simplicity, Mapleson D-based systems are popular for pediatric use.

Humidity and Heat Exchange in Breathing Circuits

Tracheal intubation by-passes the natural heat and water exchange that occurs in the nose and pharynx, placing the burden of humidification on the tracheobronchial tree. Breathing only the cool, dry, fresh gas from the anesthesia machine results in water losses of about 10 ml per hour, with a concomitant heat loss due to evaporation of about 5 Kcal per hour. With circle systems and minimal fresh gas flows, heat loss can be reduced to as little as 1 Kcal per hour and water loss to 3 ml per hour by allowing the patient to reuse relatively warm, humid exhaled gas. Because systems based on the Mapleson D circuit require high flows to eliminate CO_2, arrangements for heating and humidifying inspired gas are common, especially in pediatric anesthesia.

PRESSURE AND FLOW MONITORS IN THE BREATHING CIRCUIT

In additional to monitoring the oxygen content of the gas in the breathing circuit, modern anesthesia machines also display pressure and often expiratory flow. As a minimum requirement, a mechanical pressure gauge measures peak, plateau, and end expiratory pressures; adding a flowmeter gives information about the tidal volume. When these gauges are attached to a microprocessor, it can provide automatic display and monitoring of these values, along with monitoring for apnea, breathing-circuit disconnections or sustained high pressures. Sustained high pressures occur most frequently when a spontaneously breathing patient is mistakenly connected to a circuit with a fully closed pop-off valve. The workings of these devices have not been standardized and must be learned for each anesthesia machine.

SCAVENGING OF EXCESS GAS

Gases escaping from the pop-off valve and around a loose-fitting face mask contaminate the operating room atmosphere with measurable concentrations of anesthetics. To reduce exposure of operating room workers, modern pop-off valves and ventilator relief valves discharge exhaust gas to a waste gas scavenger. Excess gas is usually aspirated from the scavenger by the operating room suction system at flows of 15 to 20 L per minute. Because pop-off flow rates may reach brief peaks of 50 L per minute, the scavenger includes a reservoir, the volume of which is greater than a single tidal volume. To protect the breathing circuit from the negative pressure of the suction system or from obstruction of the pop-off valve, scavengers provide for both positive and negative pressure relief.

THE ANESTHESIA VENTILATOR

Patient breathing circuits permit manual ventilation by compression of the reservoir bag; this not only allows control of the ventilatory pattern, but

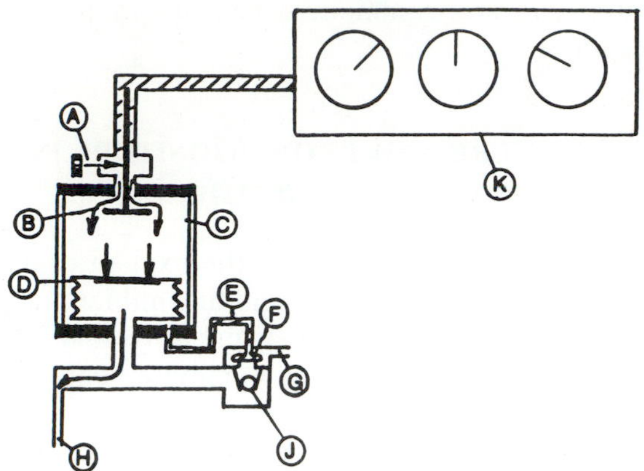

FIGURE 5–5. A typical anesthesia ventilator. The bellows (17) in its sealed chamber (16) empties into a T, one arm of which (22) is connected to the anesthesia breathing circuit. The other arm is connected to the mushroom valve (21), which is closed during inspiration by pressure (20) from the sealed chamber and which permits venting to the atmosphere (23) at end expiration, while a check valve prevents entrainment of room air during spontaneous breathing (ball valve below [21]). The bellows is driven by oxygen (2) metered into the chamber by the electronic and pneumatic circuitry shown. A stop (19) limits bellows filling and thus regulates tidal volume. (Adapted from Technical Service Manual. North American Drager, Telford, PA, 1985.) (17=D, 16=C, 22=H, 21=F, 20=E, 23=G, ball valve below [F]=J, 2=B and 19=A.)

the sensation of air passing to and from the lungs to the bag provides imprecise but useful clues to changes in compliance and resistance. However, during long procedures, a mechanical ventilator frees the operator for other tasks. Anesthesia ventilators are simpler than their ICU counterparts. They consist of three parts: a bellows assembly, a pop-off valve, and the pneumatic drive (Fig. 5–5). The bellows is the functional equivalent of the rebreathing bag, sealed in a box. The pneumatic drive applies pressure to the inside of the box, substituting for manual compression of the bag. The box is usually a clear plastic cylinder, so that the bellows is visible. An adjustable stop limits the excursion of the bellows, thereby determining the volume to be delivered. The mouth of the bellows is attached to a T-connector, one limb having an automatic pop-off valve and the other connected to the bag mount of the breathing circuit or to a selector valve. The valve allows connection to the breathing circuit of either the ventilator bellows with its integral pop-off valve or the usual rebreathing bag and manual pop-off valve.

If the bellows is mounted with its opening pointed upward, refilling during exhalation is aided by gravity. When small partial disconnections or leaks occur, this design helps maintain bellows volume, a small theoretical benefit. However, major leaks or disconnections are difficult to detect because the bellows fills passively with each breathing cycle. For this reason it is preferable to mount the bellows with its opening facing downward. In this case, positive pressure is required to fill the bellows during exhalation, creating an obligatory positive end-expiratory pressure (PEEP) of 1 to 3 cm H_2O. Any leak in excess of fresh gas flow, such as a disconnected endotracheal tube, leads to emptying of the bellows, providing a visible signal.

The automatic APL valves found in ventilators resemble one-way dome valves, with a flexible membrane replacing the rigid disk (''mushroom valves''). When one side of the membrane is pressurized, the annulus of the valve is occluded, and gas cannot escape from the circuit. The chamber above the membrane is connected by tubing to the chamber enclosing the bellows. During inhalation, the same pressure that compresses the bellows also acts on the membrane to close the mushroom valve, directing the gas exiting from the bellows into the breathing circuit.

Anesthesia ventilators use oxygen from the regulated supply forced through an air-entraining venturi to compress the bellows. If small leaks appear in the bellows, the breathing circuit will be contaminated with oxygen-enriched air, thus offering a margin of safety. The driving gas is metered into the bellows housing through valves and solenoids controlled by logic and timing circuitry. Venting the chamber to the atmosphere begins exhalation, a passive process. The respiratory rate is controlled by a timer.

The switch from inhalation to exhalation may be triggered either by a timer or by the appearance of a large pressure difference between the inside and outside of the bellows. While the bellows is being compressed, this difference is only a few centimeters of H_2O, but it rises to nearly the pressure of the drive source when the bellows is empty. If the change from inhalation to exhalation occurs after a fixed time interval, the inspiratory flow rate must be adequate to fully compress the bellows in the time available. With pressure triggering, adequate exhalation time must remain between inhalations for passive exhalation of the entire tidal volume without trapping air in the lungs, which involves adjusting the inspiratory:expiratory (I:E) ratio.

Although tidal volume is adjusted by setting the volume displaced from the bellows, the bellows displacement is not the same as the tidal volume. Volume is lost to compression of gas in the breathing system and to expansion of the breathing tubing. Fresh gas inflow during the inspiratory phase also contributes to delivered tidal volume. Direct measurement with a flowmeter placed as close to the Y-connector as possible is required for accurate measurement of tidal volume.

Disconnect Alarms

Use of a mechanical ventilator removes the tactile feedback provided during manual ventilation, eliminating one warning of inadvertent breathing circuit disconnection. Listening continuously to breath sounds and observing chest wall movement are part of good practice, but lapses occur. Monitoring of exhaled volume in the breathing circuit and of airway CO_2 concentration helps overcome this problem, but a separate disconnection alarm is provided with anesthesia ventilators. When the ventilator is functioning and connected, these alarms sense the periodic positive pressure excursions above a threshold value, manually selected to be slightly below the peak inspiratory pressure. If no pressure peak is detected during a given interval, then an alarm is sounded. These alarms may fail to detect a complete disconnection if partial occlusion of the disconnected fitting (by pinching or other obstruction) allows pressure peaks to continue.

THE ANESTHESIA MACHINE CHECK

Before beginning an anesthetic, one must complete a checklist procedure to ensure that the anesthesia machine is in working order and that all necessary equipment and supplies are available. Failure to inspect the anesthesia machine is a critical factor in many anesthesia accidents, and a written checklist reduces the chance of overlooking an important item (see Appendix). An abbreviated check may be sufficient between cases when the same anesthesia machine is to be reused immediately, but it is never proper to induce anesthesia without first examining the breathing circuit, oxygen supply, suction, and airway equipment. Although the similarities among modern anesthesia machines outweigh the differences, a thorough testing of an unfamiliar machine will reveal its important idiosyncracies and make safe operation possible.

Regular preventive maintenance of anesthesia machines is required by state and national hospital certifying agencies. Hospital biomedical engineering departments, manufacturers, or independent service agencies all may offer service contracts that include regular inspection. Detailed checks of the anesthesia machine provide opportunities to identify deficiencies between preventive maintenance visits. Each malfunction must be recorded in writing, and defective machines must be removed from service immediately until repaired. Malfunctions must be reported as required by the Safe Medical Device Act of 1990 (Public Law 101–629).

CONCLUSION

In recent years, anesthesia machines have become increasingly complex as manufacturers have incorporated not only safety devices but ventilators and physiologic monitors that are controlled by microprocessors that present data on video displays. The confusing welter of data can overwhelm an operator unfamiliar with the machine. Integrated computer-based monitoring systems help interpret data and relieve the operator of some vigilance tasks, but it remains the operator's responsibility to understand the system and to interpret the data correctly. To use these machines safely, anesthesiologists, whether beginners or experienced consultants, can take several steps.

First, study each machine thoroughly. Employ the manual supplied by the manufacturer and follow the machine check-out procedure given in this chapter. This will make the machine's behavior predictable rather than mysterious.

Second, perform the complete check-out procedure daily and an abbreviated version between cases. This will prevent the use of an anesthesia machine with an undetected malfunction.

Third, when a machine malfunctions or an alarm occurs during the case, the anesthesiologist can most quickly and safely resolve the situation by focusing attention on the patient's condition. This means taking steps to ensure that the patient is well ventilated with oxygen and has a normal blood pressure, ECG, and peripheral oxygen saturation before undertaking to diagnose a possible machine malfunction.

Fourth, have available at each anesthetizing location an alternate source of oxygen and a means of ventilating the patient. This can save the patient if the breathing system or the anesthesia machine should fail.

Fifth, a regular program of maintenance and repair will forestall machine failures.

Without the operator's vigilance, careful study, and regular maintenance, a modern anesthesia machine is a dangerous instrument; with these precautions, it is a safe, reliable device with which to trust patients' lives.

REFERENCES

American Society of Anesthesiologists. Check-out, a guide for preoperative inspection of an anesthesia machine, Park Ridge, IL: ASA Patient Safety Videotape Program, 1986.

Dorsch JA, Dorsch SA, eds. Understanding anesthesia equipment. 2nd ed. Baltimore: Williams & Wilkins, 1984.

Eger EI, Ethans CT. The effects of inflow, overflow and valve placement on economy of the circle system. Anesthesiology 1968; 29:93.

Petty C, ed. The anesthesia machine, New York: Churchill Livingstone, 1987.

Schreiber P. Anaesthesia equipment: Performance, classification, and safety. New York: Springer-Verlag, 1972.

APPENDIX

Anesthesia Machine Check-out and Immediate Pre-anesthesia Preparation

Room:

1.* ____ Table: tilts head-down, locked
2.* ____ Suction hose: within arm's reach, in working condition
3.* ____ Suction catheter or wand
4. ____ Scavenger system: connected, adequate air flow

Machine:

5. ____ Battery test; power on
6. ____ GASES: verify correct tank/correct yoke.
7. ____ GASES: correct hoses securely connected to correct wall outlets.
8. ____ Close flow valves before opening cylinders, connecting hoses.
9.* ____ Test O_2, N_2O flows for full range.
10. ____ Tank wrench
11. ____ O_2 reserves in cylinders if piped O_2 to be used: 500 psi in one; if cylinder O_2 to be used: 500 psi in one; 1500 psi in second
12. ____ N_2O reserves in cylinder(s): 740 psi
13. ____ Turn *off* all cylinders; leave tank wrench on closed O_2 cylinder.
14. ____ FAIL-SAFE/O_2 RATIO SYSTEMS:
    a) Set O_2 1.5 L/min; increase $N_2O > 5$ L/min. If ratio controller present, O_2 flow will increase; if alarm is present, it will sound.
    b) If (a) fails, check fail-safe: run N_2O, disconnect O_2 supply, and bring O_2 pressure to zero. O_2 low-pressure alarm should sound, N_2O should shut off.
15. ____ Vaporizers properly filled: not above over-fill line, some liquid present
16. ____ Vaporizers labeled
17. ____ Vaporizer filler caps and drain cocks closed tightly
18. ____ Vaporizers completely shut off at the end of check-out procedure
19. ____ Low pressure system leak check according to manufacturer's instructions

Breathing Circuit:

20. ____ Oxygen analyzer: calibrate, verify electrode in circuit.
21.* ____ Soda lime present and not exhausted.
22. ____ CO_2 absorber bypass valve closed, if present
23. ____ Reservoir bag, corrugated tubing and Y piece, elbow connector
24. ____ Warmer/humidifier, if used
25. ____ Unidirectional valves competent and patent: disconnect each corrugated tube from the Y piece, inhale and exhale into each limb, ensure that the inspiratory valve allows only inspiration and that the expiratory valve allows only expiration; reassemble circle and breathe through it with Y piece and angle connector in place.
26.* ____ Check for leaks: close APL valve, occlude Y piece, inflate system to 30 to 40 cm H_2O, *using O_2 flush valve*. If pressure remains steady with no inflow of gas, system is free of leaks. The flow required to maintain pressure is the leak rate.
27.* ____ Release pressure via APL valve, not the Y piece.
28.* ____ Proper sequence in checking circle: no connections broken in circle after it is checked for leaks

Airway:

29.* ____ Masks of appropriate sizes
30.* ____ LARYNGOSCOPE: light is bright and does not flicher when laryngoscope is shaken
31.* ____ Spare laryngoscope blade & handle
32.* ____ Oral and nasal airways: appropriate sizes
33.* ____ Endotracheal tube, proper size, check cuff
34.* ____ Spare endotracheal tube, next size smaller
35.* ____ Lubricant
36.* ____ Stylet
37.* ____ Pillow or pad to position patient's head

Monitoring:

Locate, turn on, warm up, calibrate as needed:

38. ____ Precordial, esophageal stethoscope
39. ____ EKG
40. ____ Blood pressure cuff or automated equivalent
41. ____ Temperature monitoring device
42. ____ Pulse oximeter
43. ____ Capnograph, CO_2 analyzer, or mass spectrometer, if used.

Drugs, IVs:
44.* ____ Thiopental or other IV hypnotic
45.* ____ Atropine
46.* ____ Succinylcholine
47.* ____ Extra syringes and needles
48.* ____ IV set, IV supplies
49.* ____ Drugs or supplies for the specific patient
50.* ____ Standard stock of drugs, if used

51. ____ Know location of resuscitation equipment and drugs, including emergency oxygen, bag/mask assembly

This method of preparing to give anesthesia is appropriate for the first case of the day. When using the same equipment for successive cases, it may be appropriate to repeat only the items marked (*). Item (43) is standard in many practices, but not all.

CHAPTER SIX

MONITORING THE ANESTHETIZED PATIENT

Monitoring during anesthesia includes monitoring of the anesthesia machine and ventilator, discussed in the preceding chapter, and monitoring of the patient, the subject of this chapter. Careful observation of the anesthetized patient serves several purposes. First, the patient responds to anesthesia and operation with predictable changes in breathing, heart rate, blood pressure, or other variables. By monitoring the patient's responses, and at times such information as the inspired and end-tidal concentrations of anesthetic gases, the depth of anesthesia can be adjusted appropriately. Second, patients undergoing anesthesia and operation suffer physiologic derangements, such as blood loss, hypothermia, hypertension, arrhythmias, organ ischemia, metabolic changes, or pulmonary dysfunction. Systematic assessment of these changes permits accurate treatment. Third, unexpected catastrophes such as myocardial infarctions or airway obstruction threaten patients' lives. Vigilant observation supplemented by mechanical alarms can minimize or prevent damage from these accidents. Fourth, to give a successful anesthetic, as well as to defend against charges of malpractice, requires an accurate and complete record over time of the events of the operation and anesthesia, the drugs given, and the patient's responses.

The selection of monitors must take into account the utility of the generated data, the expense, and patient risk. Routine or essential monitors include pulse oximetry, noninvasive blood pressure, capnography, temperature, electrocardiography, precordial or esophageal stethoscope, oxygen analyzers, and inspection of the patient. The use of these essential monitors is required by present standards of care in all surgical patients, if circumstances permit, because of the minimal risk and potential for life-saving information. Present standards are summarized in Table 6–1. Other noninvasive and invasive monitoring is used only with clear indication.

Modern monitoring devices are expensive; the complex balance among costs, added risks of monitoring, and possible benefits to patient safety govern not only the use of a technique in a given patient, but the decision to invest in equipment and training. Whereas a monitor that does not influence medical or surgical management cannot be justified, even some quite expensive techniques can save money in the long run for patients, physicians, hospitals, and insurance companies. Improved safety implies lessened morbidity and mortality for patients, reduced costs for third-party payers, diminished legal costs, and less costly insurance premiums and malpractice settlements.

Monitors are categorized as invasive or noninvasive. The former penetrate the body through the

TABLE 6–1. Essential Monitors for All Patients Undergoing Anesthesia

Observation
- A trained individual present at all times
- Observe movement, skin color, pattern of breathing, tearing, position, events in the surgical field, blood loss
- Patient's report of comfort/discomfort
- Monitor, interpret, and act on continually all of the data listed below

Stethoscope
- Breath sounds
- Heart sounds: amplitude, rhythm

Pulse oximeter
- Pulse
- Peripheral oxygen saturation

Oximeter
- Inspired oxygen concentration (not used if patient not breathing from breathing circuit)

Capnograph
- End-tidal CO_2
- Shape of capnogram
- Respiratory rate
- Delivery of CO_2 to lungs by cardiac output

EKG
- Cardiac rate
- Rhythm
- Ischemic changes

Blood pressure
- Continuous or intermittent, according to need

Airway pressure (if applicable)
- Cyclic changes indicate breathing
- Disconnection of endotracheal tube
- Breathing circuit malfunction

Temperature (if applicable)
- Hypothermia
- Hyperthermia

Neuromuscular
- Peripheral nerve stimulator, if muscle relaxants are in use

Fluid balance
- Blood, urine, and other fluids lost
- Blood and other fluids given

Other
- The automatic alarms provided with the anesthesia machine and ventilator

Anesthesia record
- A contemporaneous record, complete and accurate for all of the above data, the drugs given and the events of surgery

Note: These recommendations are more stringent than those of the American Society of Anesthesiologists' House of Delegates (1989), but reflect a careful standard of practice. When patients are breathing room air, or receiving oxygen by nasal cannulae, it may not be practical to measure inspired oxygen tension or airway pressure. For short procedures, temperature monitoring may not be needed.

skin or via an orifice. The degree of invasiveness is variable, and the separation of monitors into these categories is not rigid. A peripheral nerve stimulator is considered noninvasive, but it is rarely used while the patient is awake. Likewise, although the standard echocardiogram is noninvasive, transesophageal echocardiography is invasive and associated with morbidity and mortality.

Monitors do not interpret data and do not substitute for sound clinical judgment. In this sense, the most important monitor of the patient's condition is an observant and thoughtful anesthesiologist. To make the most of the data available, one must constantly question their interpretation.

PRECORDIAL OR ESOPHAGEAL STETHOSCOPE

Those administering anesthesia often wear a custom-molded earpiece that is connected either to a stethoscope placed on the chest (precordial) or to a sealed tube inserted into the midesophagus (esophageal). This provides continuous monitoring without sophisticated electronics; it is noninvasive, inexpensive, reusable, and easy to use. Listening continuously to heart tones warns of changes in volume status and contractility (loudness and pitch), the occurrence of venous air embolism (mill-wheel murmur), and the onset of dysrhythmias. As a monitor of ventilation, the stethoscope detects wheezing, rhonchi, and stridor. During anesthetic induction the precordial stethoscope provides information about airway patency, secretions, respiratory rate and indirectly, about depth of anesthesia.

A conventional binaural stethoscope provides higher quality sound transmission, useful when listening closely to breath sounds or heart sounds, or when verifying positioning of an endotracheal tube, but it is cumbersome and impractical for continuous use.

BLOOD PRESSURE

The repeated measurement of arterial blood pressure is standard practice during anesthesia because operations and anesthetics are associated with changes in blood pressure great enough to do harm unless anticipated and treated.

Blood pressure is not uniform throughout the arterial circulation. Gravity influences blood pressure because the weight of a column of blood increases or decreases the hydrostatic pressure within a vessel. Assuming the density of blood is equal to that of water, a 1 cm column of blood is equal to 0.74 mm Hg. In the upright or sitting position, arterial blood pressure in the head may be 20 or 30 mm Hg less than central aortic pressure. Likewise, blood pressure in the lower extremities is increased depending on the height of the fluid column from the heart to the site of measurement. Differences in blood pressure are less in the recumbent position.

Blood is a fluid in motion, and the pressure at a given point is a function of flow, viscosity, and vessel diameter. Blood viscosity does not change appreciably from the aorta to smaller peripheral arteries. In contrast, vessel diameter decreases abruptly over short distances and accounts for the differences in blood pressure in the aorta and radial artery. With each cardiac cycle a stroke volume is ejected into the aorta creating an incident pressure wave that propagates downstream and is reflected at the artery-arteriolar junction. The contour of the arterial pressure wave at a specific site represents the summation of the incident and reflected pressure waves. The pressure wave in the ascending aorta is less affected by reflected waves than the pressure wave in more distal arteries. Peripheral sites of blood pressure measurement are closer to the artery-arteriole interface and are more affected by reflected waves (Fig. 6–1).

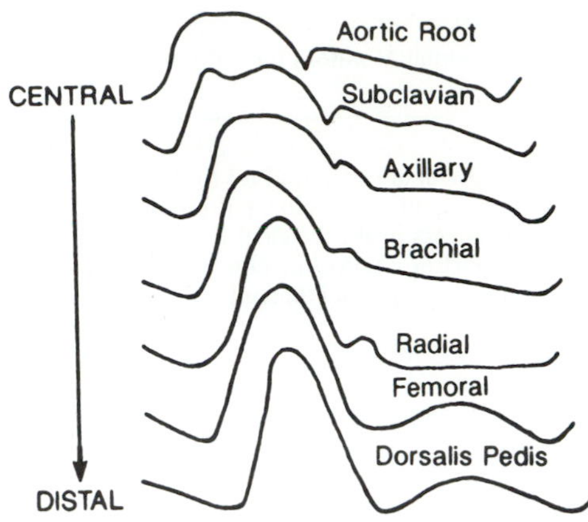

FIGURE 6–1. As compared to the aortic trace, the pressure waveform from the radial artery is changed by a delay in transmission, steeper upstroke, loss of high frequency components, increases in systolic and pulse pressures, and a decrease in mean arterial pressure. (Reproduced with permission from Bedford R. Invasive blood pressure monitoring. In *Blitt CD, ed. Monitoring in anesthesia and critical care medicine. New York: Churchill Livingstone, 1990.)*

Noninvasive blood pressure monitoring suffices for most patients during routine operations. A cuff wrapped around the patient's arm or leg is connected to a manometer and is inflated to a pressure greater than systolic blood pressure; during gradual deflation the observer detects signs of blood flow distal to the cuff. The simplest method of detection is palpation of a distal artery with the return of a pulse corresponding to the systolic blood pressure. Listening for Korotkoff sounds provides systolic and diastolic blood pressures. Unfortunately, the auscultatory method requires a quiet work place and is less sensitive at lower pressures, when the Korotkoff sounds are faint.

Oscillometry bypasses the need for auscultation. The oscillometric method senses blood flow by changes in cuff pressure as the cuff is deflated. When the pressure in the cuff is just below systolic blood pressure, the cuff pressure begins to oscillate at the same frequency as the pulse rate. Further deflation of the cuff permits more blood flow through the now partially occluded artery and results in oscillating changes in the volume of tissue within the cuff. The cyclic volume changes produce corresponding amplitude changes in the cuff pressure. The oscillations dissipate with further deflation because the volume changes are not transmitted to the more loosely fitting cuff. The point of maximum oscillation corresponds to the mean arterial blood pressure.

Automated devices that measure blood pressure noninvasively automatically inflate and deflate the cuff and detect distal flow. Automatically measuring blood pressure at frequent intervals decreases the incidence of undetected hypotension. Oscillometric devices are most common. Their major disadvantage is sensitivity to motion artifact. Other automated techniques include Doppler ultrasonography to detect motion in the walls of the artery, a microphone and amplifier to detect Korotkoff sounds, and finger plethysmography to detect changes in the volume of digital arteries with each pulse.

The size of a blood pressure cuff influences the pressure reading. The ideal cuff width is approximately 40 per cent of the circumference of the extremity. Too narrow a cuff does not transmit the cuff pressure to the underlying artery and results in a falsely high blood pressure reading. Too large a cuff does not distort the pressure measurement, but may compress neural structures at the axilla or elbow.

Cuff measurements of systolic and mean arterial pressure are accurate when compared to invasive methods. However, fluctuations in blood pressure related to respiration are common. Because the slowly deflated cuff measures the systolic and diastolic pressure during different portions of the respiratory cycle, the pulse pressure may be inaccurate. The pulse pressure will be artificially decreased if the minimum systolic and maximum diastolic pressures are measured. This is true whether a manual or automated device is used.

Continuous intra-arterial monitoring of blood pressure is useful when small changes in blood pressure may produce organ ischemia (as in unstable angina pectoris) and when major operations produce large, rapid changes in blood pressure. The measuring system includes an intra-arterial catheter, low-compliance pressure tubing, a pressurized low-flow continuous flush system, a transducer with a pressure-sensing diaphragm, and the display unit that converts an electrical signal into a numerical value. After it is assembled and filled with heparin-saline solution, all air bubbles must be cleared from the system to prevent damping of the signal or air embolism.

Although smaller arterial cannulae are more likely to kink or limit the rate of blood sampling, small 20-gauge Teflon catheters are preferred for the radial artery because they are also less likely to cause thrombosis and vascular injury.

If cannulation results in thrombosis of the radial artery, it is feared that inadequate ulnar blood flow or an incomplete palmar arch may lead to ischemia of the hand. Often, Allen's test is performed before placing a radial artery catheter to assess ulnar and palmar arch blood flow. However, the predictive value of Allen's test has been challenged by reports in which the ulnar artery was cannulated after multiple punctures of the ipsilateral radial artery, with no evidence of subsequent hand ischemia.

"Ringing" results in these measuring systems when their natural resonant frequencies (20 to 25

Allen's Test

The operator compresses the patient's radial and ulnar arteries at the wrist while the patient makes a tight fist for 20 seconds. After the patient relaxes the hand, it remains blanched until the ulnar artery is released. If the entire hand, including the thumb and thenar eminence, does not appear well perfused within five seconds, the ulnar supply is inadequate. A pulse oximeter on the thumb can be used instead of skin color to judge adequate perfusion.

Placing a Catheter in the Radial Artery

A large number of acceptable techniques have been described for placing a catheter in the radial artery; none is foolproof and all depend on skill and experience. These paragraphs describes one workable method.

Gently fix the patient's hand and forearm to a board, with the wrist held in moderate dorsiflexion by a bolster under the wrist (Fig. 6–2). To reduce the risk of local infection and to minimize contact with the patient's blood, prepare the skin aseptically and use appropriate sterile precautions, including gloves. Infiltrate the skin over the radial artery at the middle or proximal skin crease, where it is prominent. If the artery is small, or puncture is difficult, make a small aperture in the skin with an 18- or 19-gauge needle, to reduce drag on the arterial catheter. Using a 20-gauge catheter-over-needle assembly, advance the needle directly at the artery, with the hub raised at an angle of 30 degrees from the horizontal, until the pulsatile flow of blood into the hub of the needle signals that the tip of the needle has entered the artery.

At this point, two techniques are possible. If it seems easy to do so, depress the hub of the needle, advance the needle in the artery for a few millimeters, and slide the catheter into the artery, just as when placing an intravenous catheter. If this is not feasible, pass the needle through the artery, transfixing it, and then remove the needle from the catheter. Withdraw the catheter slowly until arterial blood appears; the catheter can sometimes be threaded into the artery or a flexible wire (.025-inch for the usual 20-gauge catheter) advanced into the lumen to serve as a guide. If the first attempt fails, apply pressure to the artery for a few minutes before trying again, to prevent the formation of a large hematoma. The connection between the hub of the catheter must be very secure; accidental disconnection can cause disastrous bleeding. Apply a transparent sterile dressing and remove the bolster under the wrist or replace it with a smaller one, to prevent compression of the median nerve.

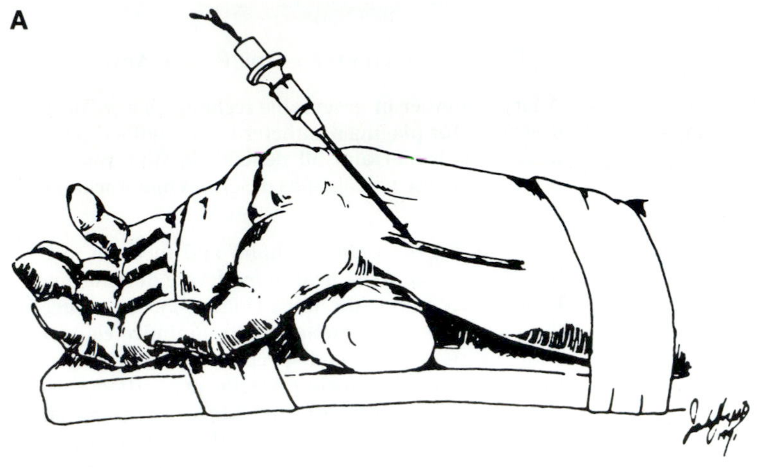

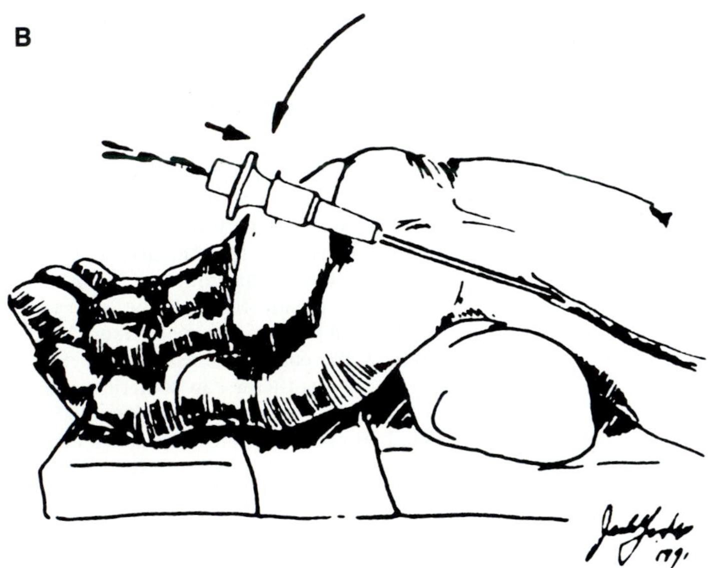

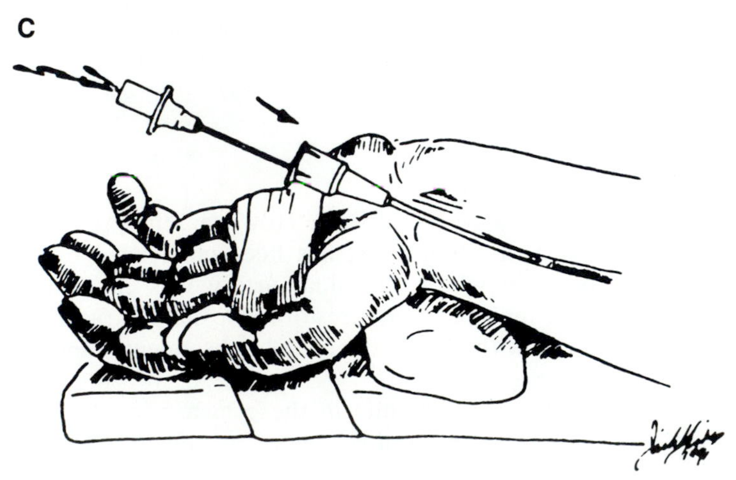

FIGURE 6–2. *Radial artery cannulation.* A, *A small pad under the wrist maintains extension. The catheter and needle assembly approach the artery at about a 45-degree angle from the horizontal.* B, *After the needle enters the artery, the hub of the needle is depressed and the catheter and needle are advanced together a few millimeters into the lumen.* C, *With the needle fixed, the catheter is advanced fully into the artery.*

Hz) are near those found in the arterial tree at the site of cannulation. This accentuation of peak pressures exaggerates the pulse pressure but produces little inaccuracy in the mean arterial pressure. Higher resonant frequencies give less trouble with ringing and are produced by using tubing that is larger in diameter, less compliant, or shorter. If peaks are blunted instead of accentuated, the signal is said to be damped, usually due to constriction in the tubing produced by stopcocks or kinks, or to air bubbles in the tubing or transducer. Overdamped systems underestimate systolic blood pressure and overestimate diastolic blood pressure, but mean pressure is unaffected. An underdamped system does not distort pressure waveforms if the natural frequency of the system is high enough to prevent ringing. These problems are usually not present in the systems as manufactured, but when using long lengths of tubing or when ringing is evident, deliberate damping may improve the accuracy of the arterial waveform.

The pressure-sensing transducer consists of a stiff diaphragm that is displaced by intravascular pressure. This displacement is sensed by a strain gauge that is connected to electronic circuitry, which converts the signal to a pressure trace, and a digital display of systolic, mean, and diastolic pressures. Transducers require a zero reference. The level of the right atrium is appropriate in most circumstances, but if the measurement of perfusion pressure to a specific organ (such as brain) is indicated, then the zero reference is adjusted accordingly (such as to the base of the skull). Mounting the transducer at the zero reference level can be cumbersome; an alternate method uses a pressure offset. The transducer is mounted; during "zeroing," fluid-filled tubing is connected between the (distant) transducer and the desired zero point. This creates an offset zero pressure level which is valid until the patient is moved.

The risk of infection with reusable transducers has led to the use of disposable systems. Miniature transducers placed at the tips of intra-arterial catheters produce high fidelity signals that are independent of the catheter, extension tubing, and stopcocks. They are not used routinely for arterial pressure monitoring because of expense.

CENTRAL VENOUS PRESSURE

Cannulating the central venous circulation provides a large-bore cannula for the rapid administration of fluids, or a port for blood sampling or passage of catheters into the heart, and permits the measurement of central venous pressure (CVP). Every pathway anatomically possible has been used for access to the central circulation. In anesthesia practice, cannulation of the right internal jugular vein is popular because of the ease of access to the neck and the straight path from the internal jugular vein to the right heart (Fig. 6-4). The subclavian route or an antecubital vein are sometimes used. As with arterial cannulae, the intravascular pressure is transduced into an electrical signal and displayed on a physiological monitor in both analog and digital forms. Risks have been reduced to acceptable rates, but include pneumothorax, hemothorax, and inadvertent puncture of the subclavian or carotid arteries.

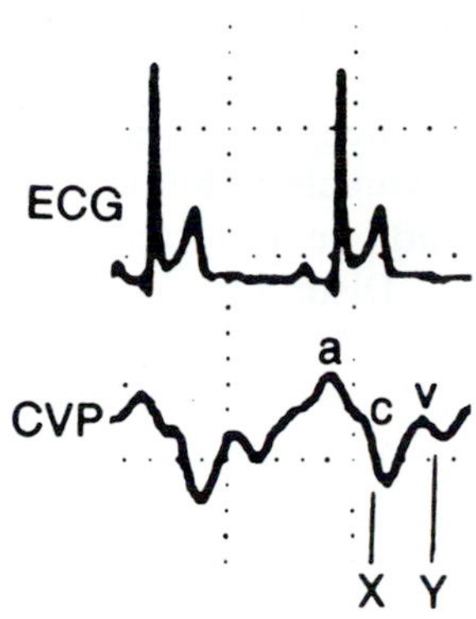

FIGURE 6–3. The ECG and a simultaneous central venous waveform, which consists of the components labeled a, c, V, X, and Y. a wave, right atrial contraction; X descent, right atrial relaxation; c wave, bulging of tricuspid into right atrium during right ventricular contraction; V wave, passive filling of the right atrium; Y descent, rapid emptying of the right atrium into the right ventricle.

Central venous pressure is an index of the circulating blood volume and preload to the right ventricle. The pulsatile characteristics of the CVP are a function of the uninterrupted return of venous blood to the right atrium, right atrial size and compliance, intrathoracic pressure, and the mechanical properties of the tricuspid valve and right ventricle (Fig. 6–3).

A decreased CVP suggests hypovolemia or an increase in venous capacitance, as with vasodilatation following sympathetic blockade. An increased CVP with normal cardiac function suggests hypervolemia, vasoconstriction, or increased intrathoracic pressure. Central venous pressure is increased by positive pressure ventilation and positive end-expiratory pressure, and is measured only at end-expiration. An increased CVP in the presence of arterial hypotension suggests cardiac dysfunction, but left ventricular dysfunction may not be reflected promptly by increased CVP. Disorders that increase right ventricular afterload (pulmonary emboli) or impair diastolic filling (cardiac tamponade) also increase CVP, as does incompetence of the tricuspid valve, which also results in large V waves.

PULMONARY ARTERY PRESSURE

Pulmonary artery (PA) catheters measure pulmonary artery pressure (PAP), pulmonary artery occlusion pressure (PAOP), cardiac output, mixed venous oxygen saturation, and the derived values of systemic and pulmonary vascular resistance (Fig. 6–4).

In addition to the risks of jugular puncture, the

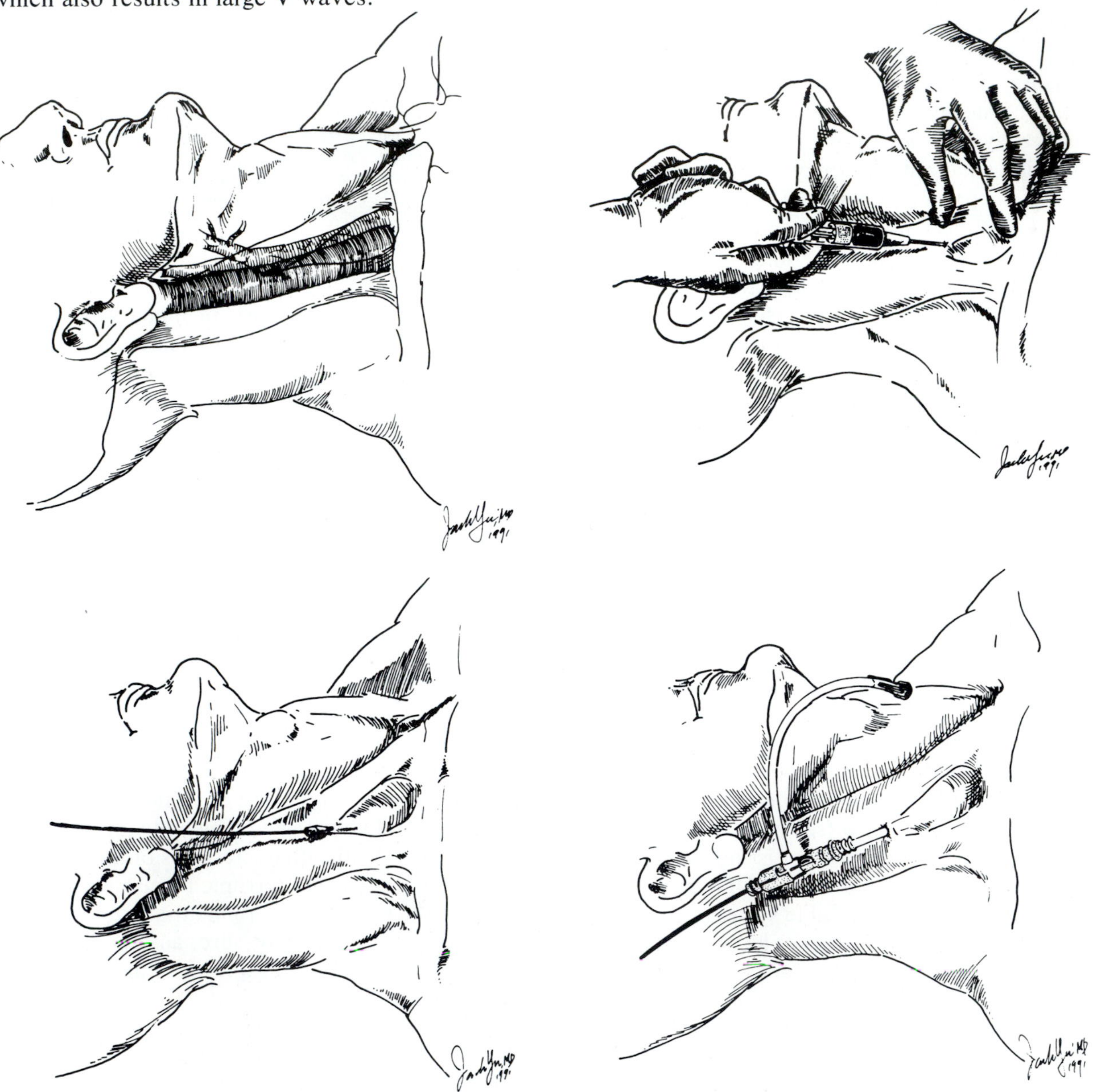

FIGURE 6–4. Anatomical relationship between internal jugular vein, carotid artery, and sternocleidomastoid muscle and the Seldinger technique demonstrating cannulation of the internal jugular vein and passage of a guide wire.

Technique of Placing Pulmonary Artery Catheter: Right Internal Jugular Route

Most PA catheters used for intraoperative monitoring are inserted via the right internal or external jugular vein. The internal jugular vein is located immediately lateral to the carotid artery and beneath the medial border of the clavicular head of the sternocleidomastoid muscle (Fig. 6–4). Place the patient head-down to distend the jugular vein, with the head turned to the left. Using sterile technique and local anesthesia, insert a 20-gauge catheter-over-needle assembly, with a syringe attached, near the apex of the triangle formed by the lateral border of the medial head and the medial border of the lateral head of the sternocleidomastoid muscle. Direct the needle dorsad, in the direction of the ipsilateral nipple, advancing while aspirating until venous blood flows freely into the syringe; then advance the cannula into the vein. When this or any other catheter is open from the air to the central circulation, precautions to prevent air embolism include the head-down position, Valsalva maneuver, or occluding the hub of the catheter with the gloved finger. Connect the catheter via a fluid-filled tube to the transducer and verify that the pressure trace is not that of the carotid artery. Then pass a wire to serve as a guide for an 8.5 French introducer that will accommodate a 7 French PA catheter.

Flush the PA catheter with heparinized saline, cover it with a catheter contamination shield, test the distal balloon for asymmetry or leaks, and connect the lumen from the distal opening to a transducer. Insert the catheter to a depth of 20 cm (the junction of the right atrium and superior vena cava), inflate the balloon and watch the pressure trace while advancing the catheter into the right ventricle and pulmonary artery until a PAOP tracing is obtained (Fig. 6–5). Advance the catheter only while the balloon is inflated, do not pass the catheter deeper than 60 cm, and after attaining the PAOP tracing, withdraw the deflated balloon a few centimeters to remove redundancy or loops in the right atrium or right ventricle.

To avoid dangerous pulmonary hemorrhages, do not leave the balloon inflated for longer than is needed to obtain a PAOP reading, or exceed the manufacturer's recommended volume of inflation (1.0 to 1.5 ml). Because PA catheters tend to migrate distally, monitor pressure at the tip of the catheter; if a PAOP trace appears with the balloon deflated, withdraw the catheter and do not inflate the balloon until a PA trace again is obtained.

pulmonary artery catheter itself may cause right ventricular perforation, pulmonary embolus, pulmonary artery rupture, dysrhythmia, infection, and pulmonary infarction.

The pulmonary artery occlusion pressure is an indirect measurement of left atrial pressure and an index of left ventricular preload. Usually, changes in PAOP precede changes in CVP, but the two change in the same direction (hypovolemia, heart failure). Isolated right heart failure is an exception, and produces an increase in the CVP and a decrease in the left atrial pressure.

Pulmonary artery catheters detect myocardial ischemia but lack sensitivity and specificity. Myocardial ischemia results in a decrease in ventricular compliance and an increase in left ventricular end-diastolic pressure (LVEDP). In the absence of mitral stenosis, the increased LVEDP results in an increase in PAOP and PAP. In addition, mitral regurgitation due to ischemia of the papillary muscles may be detected by the appearance of a V wave on the PAOP tracing. Although commonly used for ischemia monitoring, the PA catheter is a less sensitive monitor for myocardial ischemia than the ECG or transesophageal echocardiography. Increases in PAP and PAOP are not specific for myocardial ischemia and are affected by changes in intravascular volume, sympathetic nervous system activity, and the mode of ventilation.

Cardiac Output

The standard estimate of cardiac output in the operating room is obtained by measuring pulmonary blood flow by thermodilution. Other methods, not dependent on an indwelling PA catheter, include dye dilution, aortic pressure pulse methods, transthoracic bioimpedance and echocardiography, but all have proven cumbersome, impractical, or unreliable for routine intraoperative use. The thermodilution pulmonary artery catheter is equipped with multiple ports and a tip thermistor to permit measurement of the change in blood temperature in the PA after injection of cold solution into the central venous circulation. Cardiac output is related to the volume of blood in which the indicator (cold solution) is diluted, and is measured by integrating the change in pulmonary blood temperature over time. The measurements are not continuous and are influenced by the speed of in-

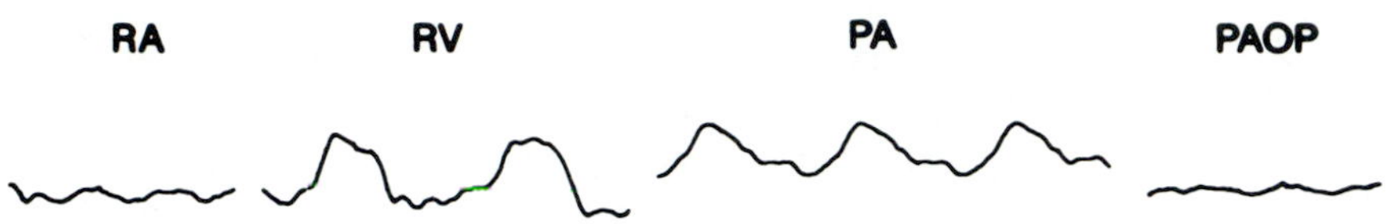

FIGURE 6–5. The typical waveform recorded from the distal port of a PA catheter as it is advanced from the right atrium (RA), to the right ventricle (RV), to the pulmonary artery (PA), and to the pulmonary occlusion position (PAOP). Notice the increase in diastolic pressure after passing from RV to PA.

jection, the relationship of injection to the phase of the respiratory cycle, the volume of injectate, the concomitant administration of cold intravenous fluids, and technical errors. Further, the pulmonary artery catheter measures right ventricular cardiac output, which is not an accurate estimate of left ventricular cardiac output in patients with intracardiac shunts.

CALCULATING PERIPHERAL RESISTANCE

Where:

CO = cardiac output, (2.5 to 4.0 L per min per m^2)*

MAP = mean arterial pressure, (80 to 120 mm Hg)*

CVP = mean central venous pressure, (0 to 8 mm Hg)*

SVR = systemic vascular resistance, (1200 to 1500 dyne-cm per sec^5)*

$$SVR = 80\ (MAP - CVP)/CO$$

*** (Normal values)**

The most important application of intraoperative cardiac output monitoring is in the management of hypotension. Hypotension is caused either by low cardiac output (heart failure, hypovolemia) or low systemic vascular resistance (sepsis). Cardiac output monitoring differentiates the causes of hypotension by permitting the calculation of SVR. Diminished cardiac output is treated with volume expansion, inotropes, or chronotropes. Decreased SVR may be treated with a vasoconstrictor (phenylephrine).

Pulmonary artery catheters permit the measurement of mixed venous saturation ($M\bar{v}O_2$), either by sampling or by continuous measurements using oximetric pulmonary artery catheters. Measurements of $M\bar{v}O_2$ are useful in evaluating shock states and determining optimum PEEP settings.

ANESTHETIC GAS MONITORING

The most commonly used instrument to measure the concentration of anesthetic gases is the mass spectrometer. A gas sample is retrieved from the breathing circuit and analyzed in a central off-line spectrometer. The sample is ionized by electrons, which are accelerated through a magnetic field, dispersing onto a collecting plate. The degree of deflection by the magnet is a function of the mass and charge of the ions. The site of impact is specific for a gas species, and the number of impacts at each site represents the relative concentration in the sample. Mass spectrometers are used to measure concentrations of oxygen, nitrogen, carbon dioxide, and anesthetic gases. The anesthetic concentration in the airway during the plateau (end-tidal) phase of the carbon dioxide expirogram reflects the alveolar concentration of anesthetic.

A mass spectrometer can be placed in each anesthetizing location, providing continuous measurements. Shared systems sample gas from the separate operating rooms sequentially, introducing intervals of several minutes between sequential measurements for each patient.

Other methods used to measure anesthetic and respiratory gases include infrared spectroscopy, Raman spectroscopy, electrochemical and polarographic sensors, and piezoelectric absorption. Most anesthetic gases and carbon dioxide absorb light in the infrared spectrum. The concentration of a known gas can be derived from the light energy absorbed, the path length of the emitted signal, and the absorption coefficient of the gas. Conventional infrared spectroscopy cannot identify the specific anesthetic vapor in a breathing circuit because there is considerable overlap in the absorption spectra of halothane, enflurane, and isoflurane in the near infrared (310 nm). More sophisticated (and expensive) light sources are available that emit light in the far infrared and permit identification of the specific halogenated agents by their characteristic absorption pattern.

Molecules of a gas can absorb light to excite specific unstable vibrational and rotational energy states, which collapse to emit light (Raman scattering) in spectra specific to the species of molecules and of intensity proportional to their concentrations. Measuring this scattered light, the Raman spectrometer can distinguish and measure the concentration of the potent anesthetic vapors, nitrous oxide, oxygen, nitrogen, and carbon dioxide. Although not widely used, optical systems are relatively inexpensive compared to the machinery needed in a mass spectrometer.

At first blush, monitoring the inspired, expired and end-tidal concentrations of anesthetic gases seems to add precision to the administration of general anesthesia. However, using moderately high fresh gas flows (3 L per minute or more) to reduce the time constant for circle breathing systems and familiarity with the principles of uptake and distribution of anesthetics, assures accuracy adequate for clinical purposes, especially in view of the need to adjust concentrations to account for interpatient variability. In practice, the most valuable contribution of anesthetic gas monitoring is to guard against inadvertent overdose.

Oxygen

Monitoring of inspired oxygen tension is described in Chapter 5. Although anesthesia machines are reliable, separate monitoring of the concentration of oxygen in the inspired gas is necessary and dictated by present standards of care.

Carbon Dioxide

Carbon dioxide in respiratory gases can be measured by infrared light absorption or mass spectrometry. Nitrous oxide strongly absorbs infrared light near the same wavelength as carbon dioxide and its presence in the gas mixture must be taken into account. The sample chamber may lie within the breathing circuit (mainstream) or be connected to the breathing circuit by a sampling tube through which a pump aspirates a small flow of gas (sidestream).

End-tidal P_{CO_2} approximates arterial P_{CO_2} in normal people. However, end-tidal P_{CO_2} underestimates arterial P_{CO_2} when physiologic deadspace is increased. The difference changes significantly with induction of anesthesia, changes in position, or pathologic factors that affect matching of pulmonary ventilation and perfusion, such as pulmonary embolism.

The capnogram is the graphic display of airway P_{CO_2} as a function of time. Changes in its contour reflect disorders of ventilation. Many factors influence the shape of the capnogram, including the expiratory flow rate, the distribution of pulmonary blood flow, the distribution (both spatial and temporal) of ventilation, and the gas sampling rate when using a sidestream analyzer. The interplay of all these factors render capnography a relatively nonspecific monitor of disease. Nonetheless, abrupt change in the shape of the capnogram always signifies an acute change in the patient's physiologic state (Fig. 6–6).

Capnography effectively detects breathing circuit problems. Breathing circuit disconnections during mechanical ventilation, accidental extubation, and airway obstruction produce acute changes in the CO_2 expirogram. Tracheal intubation can be distinguished from esophageal intubation by the consistently high CO_2 concentration in the exhaled gas from the trachea. A slow rise in the exhaled CO_2 concentration suggests partial airway obstruction, either mechanical (tube kinking) or physiologic (bronchospasm). A progressive decrease in the end-tidal CO_2 occurs with hyperventilation, low cardiac output, increase in physiologic deadspace ventilation (pulmonary emboli consisting of air or thromboemboli) or low CO_2

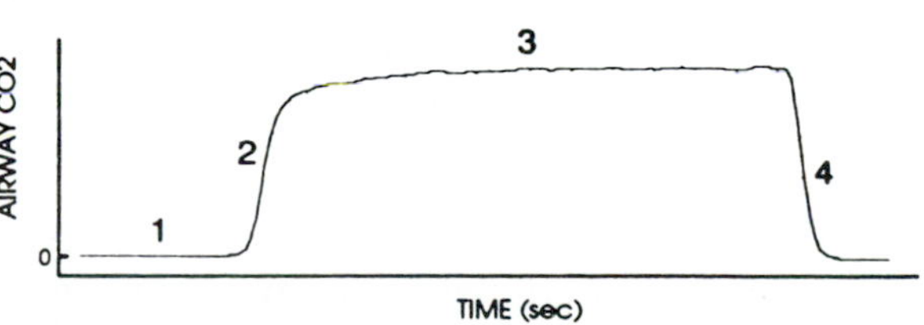

FIGURE 6–6. A typical capnogram. 1, Inspired CO_2 is zero. 2, washout of anatomic deadspace and appearance of alveolar CO_2. 3, Plateau representing alveolar gas CO_2 content. 4, Beginning of inhalation.

production (hypothermia). A progressive increase in end-tidal P_{CO_2} occurs with hypoventilation or an increase in CO_2 production (malignant hyperthermia).

PULSE OXIMETRY

Hypoxemia results in irreversible organ injury if not detected and treated within minutes. Pulse oximeters continuously measure arterial hemoglobin saturation, warning of deteriorating Sa_{O_2} before changes in the color of the patients' skin or blood are evident. Pulse oximeters are noninvasive, cost-effective, and reusable. These devices were adopted almost immediately and universally in the United States, without the benefit of studies show that they improve outcome, because they are cheap when compared to the human and financial costs of hypoxic episodes. Further, a number of studies using them have demonstrated unexpected hypoxemia in patients undergoing sedation for local anesthesia, and following general anesthesia.

Pulse oximetry is likely to decrease the incidence and duration of perioperative hypoxemia, and is useful in the titration of oxygen therapy, weaning patients from ventilators, reducing the risk of retrolental fibroplasia in neonates, and in the monitoring of pulse rate. Other controversial uses include measuring systolic blood pressure in combination with a sphygmomanometer, detecting perfusion in Allen's test, and detecting brachial or subclavian artery compression during shoulder or chest procedures. These are questionable applications because these devices were designed to detect oxygen saturation in low flow states, not to detect inadequate perfusion.

The pulse oximeter is not an early warning monitor for esophageal intubation, breathing circuit malfunctions, or the administration of hypoxic gas mixtures. Capnography, pressure-volume alarms, and inspired oxygen concentration monitors permit earlier recognition of these common critical incidents.

Pulse oximetry measures the oxygen saturation of hemoglobin in arterial blood by transillumination and detection of differences in the optical absorption properties of hemoglobin. The patterns of light absorption at the two wavelengths used by pulse oximeters are significantly different for the two forms of hemoglobin. The ratio of light absorbance at 660 nm to absorbance at 940 nm is a function of the relative proportions of oxyhemoglobin and deoxyhemoglobin. The contribution of arterial hemoglobin to this absorption is isolated by examining only the pulsatile component of the transmitted signal, which is due to incoming arterial blood and is independent of the light absorbance from venous blood and tissue. Arterial hemoglobin saturation is calculated from data obtained in healthy volunteers; accuracy fails at lower saturations because these experimentally derived curves do not extend below Sa_{O_2} values of 70 per cent.

Pulse oximeter signal processing is affected by electrical interference and motion. Oximeter probes need not be shielded from ambient light because the oximeter detects and corrects for background light by interspersing short intervals when no signal is emitted. Motion artifact is common and difficult to filter if it occurs at a frequency similar to that of the arterial pulse.

ELECTROCARDIOGRAPHY

The intraoperative monitoring of the electrocardiogram (ECG) was described in 1918 and remains the most sensitive and practical monitor for the detection of disorders of cardiac rhythm and conduction. Multilead monitoring and the ability to select a frequency response range have improved its diagnostic value, as have computerized signal processing and automated ST segment analysis. A permanent recording permits more leisurely analysis, comparison with the preoperative ECG, and documentation of findings. The inability to monitor 12 leads continuously, the lack of specificity of ST and T wave changes, and interference associated with shivering and electrocautery are the major limitations of intraoperative ECG monitoring.

Standardization of the ECG tracing is required before evaluating ST segment changes; a 1-mV signal must produce a 10-mm deflection. The configuration of the ECG waveform frequently is distorted by extraneous electrical activity. A baseline trace width of greater than 2 mm suggests electrical interference, most commonly caused by 60 Hz power lines. In the diagnostic mode, filters eliminate signals with a frequency of less than 0.05 Hz;

in the monitor mode, filters pass only frequencies greater than 0.5 and less than 40 Hz. The monitor mode minimizes baseline drift and the effects of respiration and muscle movement on the ECG but may result in distortion of the ST segment and T wave. Because the restricted bandwidth of the monitor mode may produce artifactual ST segment elevation or depression, the diagnostic mode is used in patients at risk for myocardial ischemia. Other filters with even narrower bandwidths (0.5 to 20 Hz) are useful when electrical interference produces an unrecognizable ECG, but leave little information of value in the ST segments.

Operating room ECG equipment counts heart rate by averaging several RR intervals. This is unreliable in patients with irregular rhythms such as atrial fibrillation. The device may not sense R waves if the electrical vector of the heart is isoelectric in the monitored lead. Because the R and T wave have the same electrical axis in normal patients, it is not unusual for the beat detector to be triggered by both waves, resulting in a calculated heart rate of twice the actual. Adjusting sensitivity or monitoring a different lead resolves both these problems.

Disturbances of rhythm in patients under anesthesia may be supraventricular or ventricular. The differentiation is important because rhythm disturbances differ in their etiology, effect on the cardiovascular system, treatment, and prognosis. Tachycardia caused by atrial or AV node reentry is common during anesthesia and usually not associated with significant hemodynamic instability. Ventricular tachycardia is a medical emergency, associated with hypotension and low cardiac output and requiring immediate intervention. Supraventricular arrhythmias originate in the atria or A-V junction and, unless associated with aberrant conduction, are characterized by QRS complexes of normal axis and duration. Ventricular arrhythmias originate in the lower conduction system or ventricular myocardium and appear as wide QRS complexes. Ventricular arrhythmias most commonly have a left bundle branch block (BBB) pattern. The association of P waves and QRS complexes does not exclude the possibility of ventricular arrhythmias if the ectopic locus is high in this bundle or there is retrograde conduction to the atria. QRS complexes with constantly related upright P waves suggest a supraventricular origin. All available leads are inspected when diagnosing a rhythm disorder. Lead II and V_1 are the most useful because P waves have the largest amplitude in these leads and lead II is parallel to the electrical vector of the heart.

Analysis of intervals and QRS configuration permit the detection and diagnosis of conduction disorders. Conduction blocks, like ectopic electrical activity, can be acute or chronic in onset, be a variant of normal (right BBB), or associated with severe disease (see Chapter 21).

ST segments are examined for their shape and position relative to the preceding TP interval. Normal ST segments are slightly curved with a smooth transition to the T wave. Flat or horizontal ST segments that form an acute angle with the T wave, and down-sloping ST segments are suspicious for myocardial ischemia (Fig. 6–7). ST segment depression of greater than 1 to 2 mm is associated with subendocardial injury and is never normal. ST segment elevation results from transmural ischemia, but may also occur after DC cardioversion and in normal adults; marked ST segment elevation in the precordial leads has been described in otherwise young healthy black men. Factors other than myocardial ischemia that produce abnormal ST segments include drug therapy, electrolyte disturbance, cardiomyopathy, pericarditis, myocarditis, mitral valve prolapse, and cerebrovascular accidents. The most sensitive lead for the detection of perioperative myocardial ischemia is V_5. The simultaneous display of leads II and V_5 permits monitoring of a large portion of the left ventricle. The presence of left or right BBB places significant limitations on the diagnostic value of ST segment analysis. Finally, a normal ECG does not exclude the presence of coronary artery disease or myocardial ischemia.

The T wave represents ventricular repolarization and is inspected for axis, shape, and height. The T wave axis is in the same general direction (50 degrees) as the QRS axis. Inverted T waves with an upright QRS complex are almost always

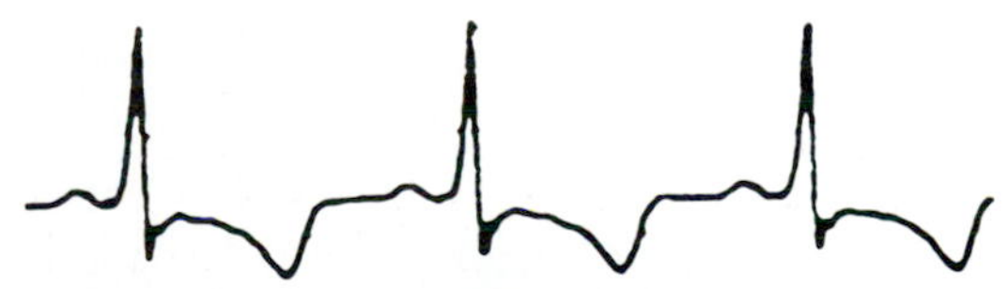

FIGURE 6–7. ST segment depression and inverted T wave in a patient with myocardial ischemia.

associated with a myocardial abnormality. The normal T wave has a smooth rounded contour. Notched and pointed T waves occur with pericarditis and myocardial infarction, respectively. The height of normal T waves is less than 5 mm in the standard limb leads and less than 10 mm in the precordial leads. Tall T waves may occur with myocardial ischemia, infarction, hyperkalemia, or stroke. Small or flat T waves occur with hypokalemia.

QT interval measurement is practical only if a printed tracing of the ECG is available. A normal QT interval is less than half of the RR interval. However the QT interval must be corrected for heart rates greater than 90 or less than 65 beats per minute. Prolongation of the QT interval may be idiopathic or associated with hypokalemia, stroke, hypothermia, mitral valve prolapse, and drug effect (quinidine, procainamide, and phenothiazine). Prolonged QT intervals are associated with increased risk of reentrant ventricular tachydysrhythmias because of the delay in ventricular repolarization.

The ECG is most valuable if monitored beginning before induction of anesthesia. Any abnormal or marginal ECG finding is less worrisome if it is present in the preoperative ECG and remains unchanged throughout the perioperative period, and is more troubling if it first appears, or worsens, intraoperatively.

Temperature

Intrinsic temperature regulation by the hypothalamus fails during general anesthesia. Hypothermia is common during major operations in modern, cold operating rooms, and may produce cardiac dysrhythmia, potentiation of anesthetic drugs and neuromuscular blockade, coagulopathy, increased vascular resistance, decreased availability of oxygen, and postoperative shivering. Small children and infants are especially prone to hypothermia because of their increased ratio of body surface area to weight; the elderly are susceptible because of their limited compensatory mechanisms. The use of low fresh gas flows, warm inspired gas, warmed intravenous fluids, blankets, warm rooms, and minimizing skin exposure reduce heat loss. Intraoperative hyperthermia is less common and may result from malignant hyperthermia, fever, and inappropriate efforts to warm the patient.

Temperature monitoring is appropriate in all patients unless the procedure is very brief (less than 15 minutes). However, increases in body temperature do not provide the earliest warnings of malignant hyperthermia, whose first sign is increased CO_2 production.

Temperature is measured with electronic thermometers. The site of temperature measurement is important because body temperature is not uniform. Core temperature reflects the temperature of vital organs and is measured in the nasopharnyx, external auditory canal, midesophagus, or central blood. Rectal temperature is not a reliable measure of core temperature. Temperature measurements at peripheral sites reflect perfusion and heat loss at the site being monitored.

Even temperature monitoring is not without risk. Temperature probes meant to lie in the external auditory canal may perforate the tympanic membrane if placed too deep. Nasopharyngeal probes may cause epistaxis. Esophageal temperature may be falsely low if the probe is left high in the esophagus, exposed to the cooling effect of gases in the adjacent trachea.

References

Barker SJ, Tremper KK. Pulse oximetry: Application and limitations. Int Anesthesiol Clin 1987; 25(3):155–175.

Blitt CD. Monitoring in anesthesia and critical care medicine. New York: Churchill Livingstone, 1990.

Gravenstein JS, Paulus DA. Clinical monitoring practice. 2nd ed. Philadelphia: JB Lippincott, 1987.

Kelleher JF, Pulse oximetry. J Clin Monit 1989; 5(1):37–62.

Norton HN. Biomedical sensors, fundamentals and application. Park Ridge: Noyes Publication, 1982.

Weinfurt PT. Electrocardiographic monitoring: An overview. J Clin Monit 1990; 6(2):132–128.

Wiedermann HP, McCarthy K. Noninvasive monitoring of oxygen and carbon dioxide. Clin Chest Med 1989; 10(2):239–254.

SECTION 3

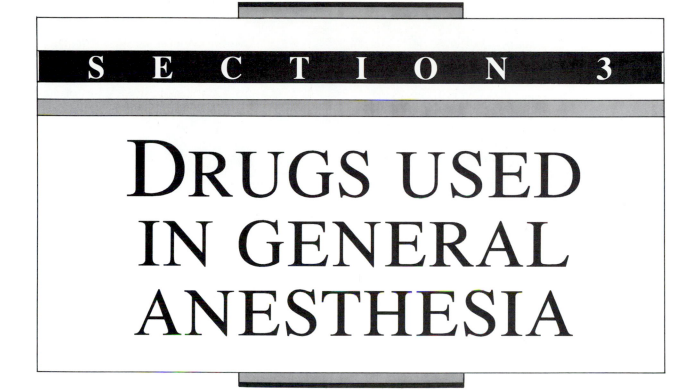

DRUGS USED IN GENERAL ANESTHESIA

CHAPTER SEVEN

PHARMACOLOGIC PRINCIPLES OF ANESTHETICS

Anesthetic drugs may be administered in a single dose, or titrated in a series of smaller increments to achieve a desired effect. In either case, the anesthesiologist must be aware of the factors that determine how the administered dose will achieve a resulting blood concentration of drug (pharmacokinetics), and how that concentration of drug will affect the patient (pharmacodynamics). The relationship between a dose of drug and the resulting physiologic effect, the dose-response curve, represents the summation of both pharmacokinetics and pharmacodynamics.

The factors governing responses to a single drug are complex. The practice of anesthesia requires the simultaneous administration of multiple drugs, demanding considerable understanding of pharmacologic principles.

PHARMACOKINETICS

The pharmacokinetics of a drug may be separated into three major categories: absorption, distribution, and elimination. All these processes involve the movement of a drug across cell membranes, controlled by a variety of physical-chemical properties of molecules and cell membranes. The movement of a drug depends on its molecular size; its solubility at the site of administration; its lipid solubility and ability to cross the cell membrane; and the fraction of drug in the ionized to un-ionized forms and the lipid solubility of each form.

The cell membrane may be thought of as a dynamic, fluid mosaic of globular proteins penetrating either partially or completely through a phospholipid bilayer. The lipid molecules are quite mobile, making the bilayer a flexible structure. Although the phospholipid bilayer is impermeable to polar molecules, specific hydrophobic or hydrophilic channels may be formed by lipid or protein complexes in the membrane. Water diffuses easily through most physiologic membranes, and may take with it small ($<$100 to 200 molecular weight) water-soluble compounds such as urea.

Larger, nonpolar molecules may diffuse passively across the cell membrane driven by the concentration gradient across the membrane and depending on the lipid solubility of the drug, expressed as the lipid : water partition coefficient of the drug. The greater the lipid : water coefficient, the greater is the concentration of drug in the membrane and the faster equilibrium is achieved. At equilibrium, the concentrations of polar compounds will not be equal on either side of the membrane. Differences in pH across the membrane will influence the ionization state on either side, producing an electrochemical gradient that affects the final equilibrium concentrations on each side of the membrane (Fig. 7–1).

Drugs also may be carried across the cell membrane by carrier-mediated active transport. In contrast to passive diffusion, this process is specific for certain molecules, requires energy, may move compounds against an electrochemical gradient, and may be inhibited competitively. Facilitated diffusion is a similar process that requires no energy input, but cannot move compounds against an electrochemical gradient.

Absorption

In its broadest sense, bioavailability refers to the fraction of administered drug that reaches either its site of action or a biologic fluid with access to the site of action. For example, after oral administration, a large fraction of drug absorbed from the gastrointestinal tract and then through the portal circulation may be inactivated by the liver. This phenomenon, called the first pass effect, results in decreased bioavailability of the drug.

Molecular properties of a drug may influence absorption. Most drugs are weak acids or bases in a solution containing both ionized and un-ionized forms. The pK of the drug and the pH of the environment determine how much of the drug is in the un-ionized, lipid-soluble form available to cross cell membranes. In the stomach, for instance, weak acids exist predominantly in their un-ionized, readily absorbable forms. In the intestine, at pH 7 to 8, the same drug is ionized and does not readily cross the membrane.

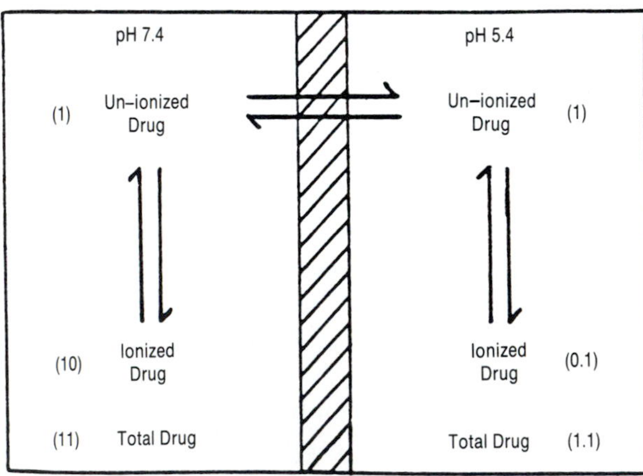

FIGURE 7–1. A concentration difference of total drug can develop on two sides of a membrane that separates fluids with different pHs. At steady state, the nonionized (un-ionized) drug concentration on both sides of the membrane is similar, but the concentration of ionized drug differs. (From Hug CC. Pharmacokinetics of drugs administered intravenously. Anesth Analg 1978; 57:704–723. Reproduced by permission of the author and the International Anesthesia Research Society.)

The route of administration determines bioavailability. The oral route is often the simplest for the patient, but offers several impediments to absorption, including the first pass effect discussed earlier. Variations in gastric pH, gastrointestinal motility, and the presence of food and enzymes all modify the extent of absorption. Some drugs may be dissolved and absorbed in the mouth, minimizing the first pass effect and destruction by gastric enzymes. Similarly, rectal administration reduces the impact of the first pass effect.

Subcutaneous injection usually produces a gradual absorption of drug. Epinephrine may be added to further delay uptake, a technique often used to prolong the effects of local anesthetics. Injections of aqueous solutions are more rapidly absorbed from intramuscular sites than after subcutaneous injections. The intravenous route eliminates impediments to absorption, providing drug to the circulation immediately upon injection. This is the fastest way to provide drug effect, and is usually the route chosen for drugs given during anesthesia (except for inhalation anesthetic agents). The inhalation route is nearly as fast as the intravenous, because of the large alveolar surface area and its ready access to the pulmonary blood flow. In an emergency, epinephrine instilled through an endotracheal tube reaches the circulation nearly as fast via mucosal absorption as via the intravenous route.

Other factors influence the rate of absorption. Drugs in aqueous solution are more rapidly absorbed than solids, suspensions, or oily solutions. Drugs given in greater concentration are absorbed more rapidly, as are those exposed to a large surface area for absorption. Blood flow at the site of drug administration influences the rate of absorption as well. For example, local anesthetics are taken up especially rapidly from well-perfused areas such as the face or scalp, but the addition of vasoconstrictors such as epinephrine slows absorption.

Distribution

Once a drug has reached the systemic circulation, either through absorption or intravenous injection, it distributes itself throughout the body, ultimately coming to equilibrium within all accessible tissues. Immediately following administration, distribution is determined principally by lipid solubility and regional blood flow. Thus, lipid-soluble drugs are rapidly distributed to brain, heart, and kidney, all organs with substantial blood flow. With more time, muscle tissue will receive its share, and much later, the poorly perfused fat and bone tissue. While it is possible for peripheral tissue to have a greater drug concentration than blood (from ion trapping, tissue binding, or tissue solubility, for instance), the blood concentration usually exceeds tissue concentration during this early phase of distribution.

For a drug that equilibrates freely between blood and its site of action (effect compartment), the effects of small intravenous doses dissipate because the circulation redistributes the drug to other more slowly equilibrating compartments, not because of metabolism or elimination. This is often the case for drugs given in anesthesia practice; a good example is thiopental, which has a pKa of 7.6 and is quite lipid soluble. Following initial intravenous administration, effective brain concentrations are achieved almost immediately, because cerebral blood flow is great and the drug remains mostly un-ionized and lipid soluble. As the drug distributes into other, less well-perfused organs, the blood concentration declines and thiopental diffuses out of brain tissue, back into the central circulation. As the brain concentration decreases, the patient regains consciousness. The brevity of the effect of thiopental is the result of redistribution, not metabolism or elimination.

Protein binding, usually reversible, also influences distribution of drugs. Plasma albumin is the most important binding agent, especially for acidic drugs (alpha 1-acid glycoprotein tends to bind basic drugs). Because the bound fraction of the drug is unavailable for pharmacologic activity or metabolism, only the free fraction determines drug effect. The bound portion, in effect, functions as a drug reservoir, releasing drug as the plasma concentration declines through redistribution or metabolism. This may prolong the effect as well as the half-life of the drug. Plasma proteins have only a limited number of binding sites, and protein bound drugs tend to compete for those sites. Administration of a new drug with affinity for the same binding sites displaces a previously administered protein-bound drug, effectively raising the blood concentration of free drug. Such effects are seen after thiopental (70 to 85 per cent bound to plasma albumin) is administered to a patient taking other protein-bound drugs, such as phenylbutazone or aspirin (see Chapter 9).

Fat tissue may also act as a reservoir of fat-soluble compounds. Following prolonged administration of such a drug, the fat stores may accumulate a large amount of drug, which will be released to the central circulation as the blood level decreases from drug metabolism. The blood supply to fat is relatively poor, so that accumulation of the drug takes a long time, and the subsequent release of the drug is slow. This effect accounts for the small but measurable concentrations of anesthetics found in blood for days after anesthesia, which in turn may produce prolonged impairment of cognitive function or significant degrees of hepatic metabolism of the drug.

Elimination

The elimination of drugs from the body is usually a two-step process of metabolism and excretion. In some cases, such as inhalation anesthetics, metabolism is a minor element, and elimination depends almost exclusively on excretion via the lungs.

Most metabolism of drugs takes place in the liver. Phase I reactions convert the drug to a more polar metabolite by oxidation, reduction, or hydrolysis. Usually, the metabolite is inactive, but it may be even more active than the parent compound. Hydrolysis is an important mechanism for inactivating such drugs as succinylcholine and procaine. Phase II synthetic reactions join the drug or its metabolite to an endogenous molecule (e.g., glucuronate, sulfate) creating a water-soluble substance that is more readily excreted.

Most drugs are eliminated via renal or hepatobiliary excretion. Renal excretion is the net result of filtration, reabsorption, and excretion of substances in the kidney. Driven by mean arterial pressure, the ultrafiltrate of plasma in Bowman's capsule contains water and low molecular weight substances filtered from the blood. Hydrophilic substances remain in the tubule and are excreted. Lipophilic substances are reabsorbed across the tubule and reenter the systemic circulation along with any substances that are actively reabsorbed. Passive reabsorption of lipophilic substances occurs in the presence of a concentration gradient, enhanced by tubular reabsorption of water in the tubules. Un-ionized small molecules tend to be easily reabsorbed. In the usually acidic environment of the renal tubule, weak acids are un-ionized and more readily reabsorbed.

Clinical Pharmacokinetics

Simple physiologic and mathematical models that may fail to represent all of the complexities of pharmacokinetics nevertheless make it possible to understand and predict the behavior of drugs in the body.

Physiologic models group together organ systems that behave similarly from a pharmacokinetic perspective when dealing with the specific drug being modeled. For instance, to simplify predicting the behavior of inhaled anesthetics, organs are grouped together depending on their relative blood supply, rather than grouped by category of organ function. Thus, organs of the vessel-rich group, including heart and brain, tend to show similar patterns of drug accumulation and distribution. Similarities of drug solubility and blood perfusion are the common denominators that define organ groups in physiologic models, but these are usually complex models, which require extensive analysis and may be difficult to apply to individual patients.

Mathematical models, on the other hand, do not follow anatomic definitions when assigning compartments. Rather, the models describe observed drug levels over time in hypothetical pharmacokinetic compartments that do not have any direct anatomic correlates. The apparent volume of distribution, for instance, may be less than or greater than the blood volume or extracellular fluid compartment.

One-Compartment Model

In the simplest one-compartment model, the concentration of a drug decreases a fixed fraction from the equilibrium level during each equal time period. In Figure 7–2, a hypothetical curve demonstrates this relationship of drug blood level to

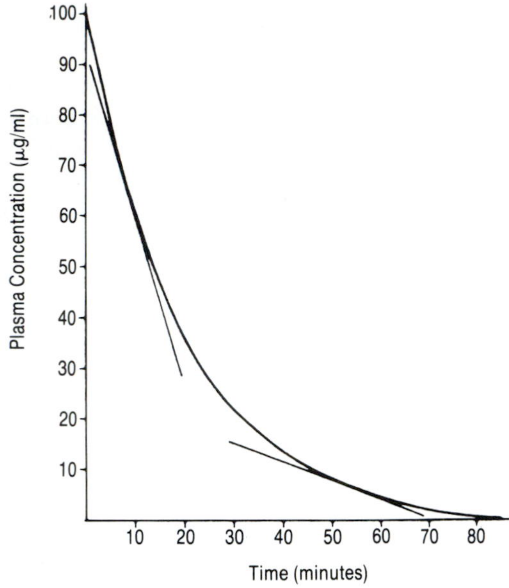

FIGURE 7–2. The exponential decay of drug concentrations at a fixed rate from a single compartment generates the curve shown. The tangents represent the slopes, or rates of decay, of drug concentration at 10 and 50 minutes after injection. (Reprinted with permission from Stanski DR, Watkins WD. Drug disposition in anesthesia. New York: Grune & Stratton: 1982:7.)

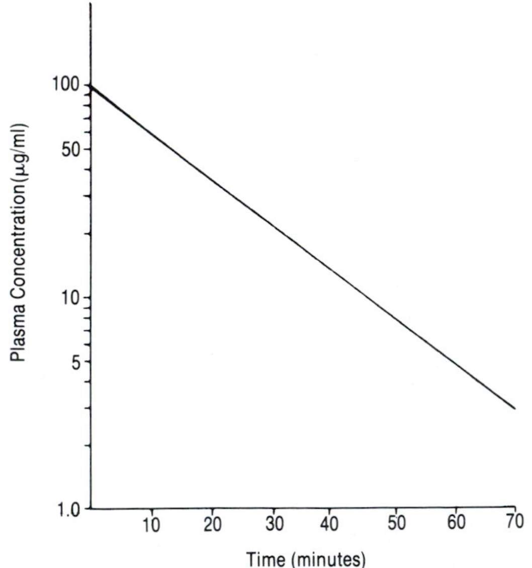

FIGURE 7–3. Plotting the logarithm of the drug concentration on the ordinate yields a straight line for monoexponential decay of drug concentrations in a single-compartment model with first-order kinetics. (Reprinted with permission from Stanski DR, Watkins WD. Drug disposition in anesthesia. New York: Grune & Stratton, 1982:7.)

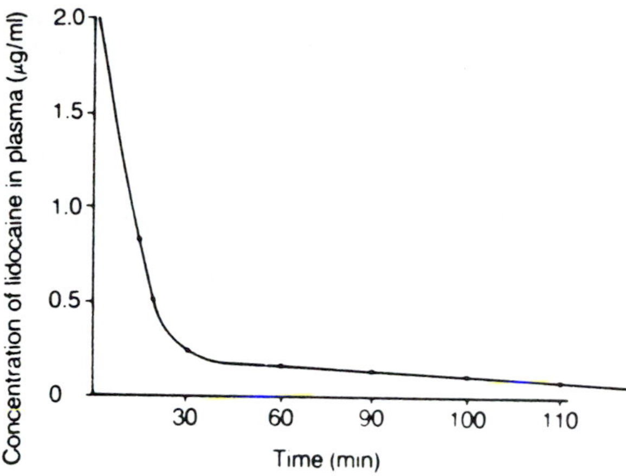

FIGURE 7–4. Expected concentrations over time for an intravenously administered drug with kinetics that fit a two-compartment model.

time. Figure 7–3 shows the same data with drug level displayed on a logarithmic scale; decay of drug levels at constant rates (single exponential decline) is portrayed as a straight line on such a plot. The elimination half-life is the time required for the concentration to decrease by one half. After five half-lives, the drug level has decreased to about 3 per cent of its original value.

Two-Compartment Model

The pharmacokinetics of most anesthetic drugs given intravenously can be described with a two-compartment model. Figure 7–4 illustrates the simulated behavior of a drug in two compartments, the concentration of which decays exponentially. Two distinct phases are apparent: the first is a sharp decline from the peak following administration, representing rapid distribution of the drug into tissue spaces; the second is a much slower decay representing elimination.

The distribution phase behaves as if a drug were introduced into a central compartment of relatively small volume (analogous to, but not anatomically equivalent to, the blood and richly perfused organs such as heart, lung, and brain). The slower phase of elimination corresponds to the behavior of a drug in a peripheral compartment of much larger volume. In Figure 7–5, the same data are presented with drug concentrations on a logarithmic scale. Two distinct phases are apparent and can be defined mathematically by the equation:

$$C_p = Ae^{-\alpha t} + Be^{-\beta t}$$

where CP = plasma concentration at time t
α = rate constant of the distribution phase
β = rate constant of the elimination phase
A = intercept at time 0 of the distribution phase line
B = intercept at time 0 of the elimination phase line
t = time

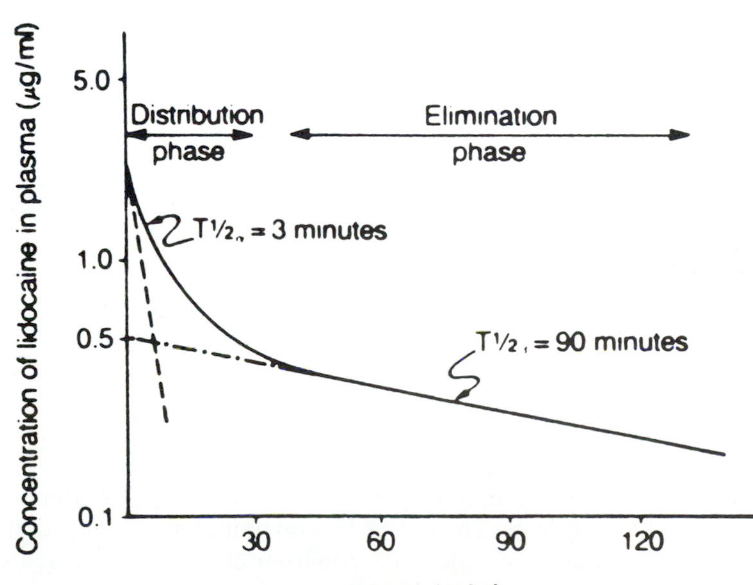

FIGURE 7–5. The same data as in Fig. 7–4, plotted on logarithmic scale.

In this biexponential expression, the first exponential term describes distribution, and the second term describes elimination. The rate constants α and β are determined from the slopes, and are used to calculate the distribution half-life ($t\frac{1}{2}_{\alpha}$) and the elimination half-life ($t\frac{1}{2}_{\beta}$).

Elimination

Although distribution of anesthetic drugs often requires a two-compartment model to describe behavior, elimination usually follows first order kinetics; that is, a constant percentage of the drug is eliminated in a given time period. As long as the mechanisms for metabolism and excretion are not saturated, this is generally the case. Should those mechanisms become saturated, then elimination would follow zero-order kinetics: a constant amount of drug would be eliminated during each time period. This situation might occur during constant infusion of a drug such as vecuronium, a nondepolarizing neuromuscular blocking agent.

Because elimination follows first-order kinetics, the elimination rate constant is equal to the fraction of drug eliminated in that time period. If 15 per cent of a barbiturate is eliminated each hour, then k = 0.15 hour.

For many anesthetic drugs, such as the inhalation agents, elimination is often described in terms of the elimination time constant ($T_{1/e}$). In one time constant, the drug concentration will change by a factor of 1/e, or 63 per cent. The elimination time constant (measured in units of time) is equal to the reciprocal of the elimination rate constant.

$$T_{1/e} = 1/k$$

The half-life of the drug is related to the time constant by

$$t = 0.693\ T_{1/e}$$

Clearance

In pharmacokinetic terms, clearance of a drug is analogous to the concept of creatinine clearance in renal physiology. Creatinine clearance does not refer to the amount of creatinine cleared in a given time period, rather it defines the volume of blood that would have to be cleared of its creatinine in a given time period in order to account for all the creatinine excreted in that period. Drug clearance, expressed as volume per unit time (flow), similarly equals that volume of a biologic fluid (plasma) that would have to be totally cleared of the drug in order to account for all the drug eliminated in that time period. Total drug clearance is the sum of all the component clearance rates, such as renal, hepatic, etc., and represents that part of the volume of distribution cleared of drug per unit time.

$$Cl = V_d \times k$$

where: Cl = clearance
V_d = the volume of distribution
k = the elimination rate constant

Hepatic elimination clearance may be expressed as

$$Cl_H = Q \times E$$

where: Cl_H = the hepatic elimination clearance
Q = hepatic blood flow
E = the hepatic extraction ratio

Drugs with larger hepatic extraction ratios (>0.7) are cleared at a rate that depends on hepatic blood flow and not changes in enzyme activity, a phenomenon referred to as perfusion-dependent elimination. Hepatic disease tends not to influence the extraction ratio. Drugs with a small extraction ratio (<0.3) are not greatly influenced by changes in hepatic blood flow. With small hepatic extraction, a large amount of drug remains available for metabolism by hepatic enzyme systems. A decrease in hepatic blood flow will not have much of an influence on clearance, because the altered flow will result in very slight change in the amount extracted (low extraction ratio), and the amount available for metabolism is already excessive. Thus, total clearance changes very little. An increase in enzyme activity, however, will produce a corresponding increase in hepatic clearance. Hepatic elimination of drugs with small extraction ratios is referred to as capacity-dependent elimination. Figure 7–6 demonstrates the effect of liver blood flow on hepatic clearance at various values of the hepatic extraction ratio.

Pharmacokinetics and Disease

Renal disease with resulting loss of glomerular filtration reduces renal clearance of drugs, the decreased drug clearance usually paralleling the decrease in creatinine clearance. Many nondepolar-

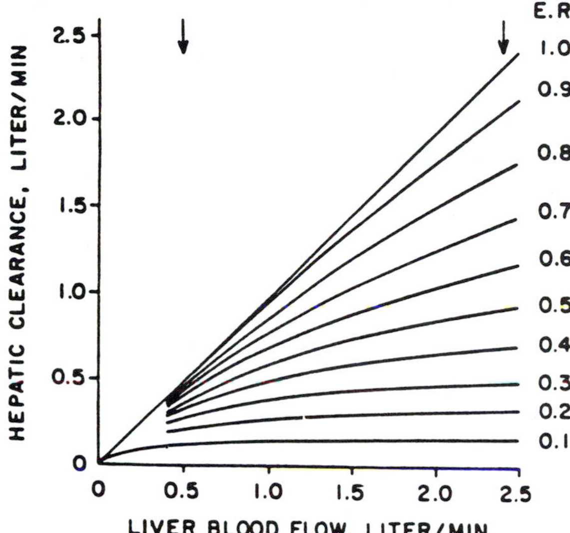

FIGURE 7–6. Hepatic blood flow varies between 0.5 and 2.5 L per minute, denoted by the arrows. Within this range, hepatic clearance of drugs poorly extracted by the liver (low extraction ratio [E.R.]) are not much affected by changes in blood flow; the clearances of those with larger values for E.R. do change with hepatic blood flow. (Reproduced with permission from Wilkinson GR, Shjand DG. A physiologic approach to hepatic drug clearance. Clin Pharm Ther 1975; 18:377.)

izing neuromuscular blockers are excreted unchanged in the urine, and decrease of creatinine clearance predicts the decreased excretion seen with these drugs in patients with renal disease (Fig. 7–7). If the only effect of renal disease is on elimination, then the initial dose of the drug need not be reduced, but subsequent maintenance doses are reduced to take into account the decreased elimination of drug. In fact, renal disease may affect pharmacokinetics by mechanisms other than diminished renal clearance of drugs. Urea competes with other drugs for protein binding sites, especially on albumin. In some forms of renal disease there is protein wasting. Both of these features of renal disease reduce the number of protein binding sites available for drugs, making more free drug available in the plasma. Uremic patients have a reduced dose requirement for thiopental because of decreased protein binding of the drug.

Hepatic disease may also influence drug action. Decreased production of albumin may decrease plasma protein levels and make more free drug available, as described earlier. These patients would be more sensitive to a "standard" dose of a protein-bound drug. On the other hand, patients with cirrhosis or ascites are more resistant to an initial dose of pancuronium, due to an increased apparent volume of distribution. This increased volume of distribution leads to a prolonged elimination half-life as well.

Hepatic enzyme and synthetic function tests are unreliable predictors of decreased capacity to metabolize and excrete drugs. The functions of the liver are numerous and complex, making any one synthetic test an unlikely predictor of some other hepatic function.

Hepatic clearance may be unaffected by hepatic disease, probably owing to the large margin of reserve in hepatic function. Decreased clearance of diazepam and midazolam (metabolized by Phase I oxidation) is seen in viral hepatitis and cirrhosis; while clearance of oxazepam and lorazepam (metabolized by Phase II glucuronide conjugation) is unchanged.

In cases of decreased cardiac output, hepatic blood flow is likely to decrease, so clearance of drugs with larger hepatic extraction ratios decreases. For instance, infusion rates of lidocaine (E = 0.7 to 0.9) must be reduced in patients with congestive heart failure. Similar reductions in subsequent doses are made with fentanyl (E = 0.6), etomidate (E = 0.9), propofol (E = 1.0), ketamine (E = 1.0), and methohexital (E = 0.5).

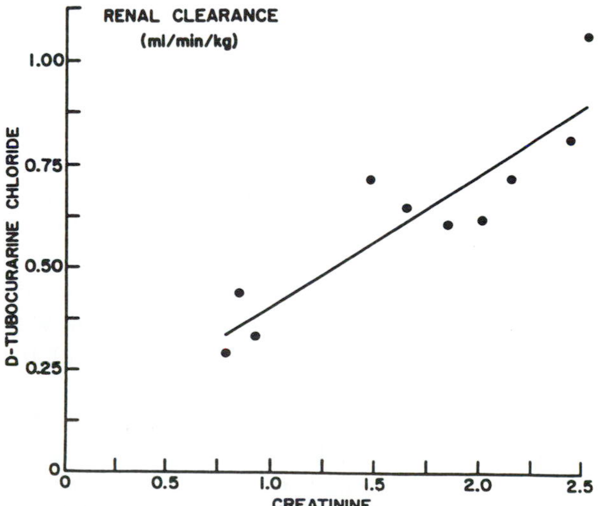

FIGURE 7–7. Renal curare clearance parallels creatinine clearance. (Reproduced with permission from Shanks CA, Avram MJ, Ronai AK, Bowsher DJ. The pharmacokinetics of d-Tubocurarine with surgery involving salvaged autologous blood. Anesthesiology 1985; 62:161.

PHARMACODYNAMICS

Once a drug has been delivered to the target organ, it can exert its pharmacologic effect. The pharmacodynamics of a drug describe the interaction of that drug with the target cell, usually in the form of a specific interaction with a protein macromolecule, a receptor. Receptors are classified on the basis of observed responses to specific agonists and antagonists. Multiple subtypes of receptors are often identified, such as alpha-1 and alpha-2 adrenergic receptors.

Some receptors, such as the steroid hormone receptors, are located in the cytoplasm, but most are within the cell membrane. Their receptor sites face outward from the cell membrane; substances with poor lipid solubility do not need to cross the cell membrane in order to exert their effect. (Many endogenous catecholamines and polypeptide hormones have poor lipid solubilities.)

Because the density of receptors in the cell membrane may change, the response to a given concentration of drug may vary widely, depending on the status of receptors on the target cells. An excess of drug or endogenous substance (e.g., catecholamines in pheochromocytoma) will lead to a decreased concentration of receptors in the cell membrane (down-regulation), and a decreased pharmacologic effect at the same drug concentration. Tachyphylaxis to exogenous catecholamines may occur for the same reason. Chronic antagonist therapy will lead to the opposite condition, an increase in receptor concentration (up-regulation). This probably explains the rebound seen after abrupt cessation of beta antagonist therapy. The same concentration of endogenous catecholamines, now unopposed by an antagonist, produces an exaggerated response from an increased number of available receptors.

The intrinsic pharmacologic activity of a substance refers to the nature of its interaction with a receptor (agonist, partial agonist, antagonist), the nature of the interacting receptor (histamine receptor, catecholamine receptor), and more precisely, the receptor subtype (H_1 or H_2, α_1, α_2, β_1, β_2, etc.). The intrinsic activity determines the potential pharmacologic effect exerted by the substance (i.e., the efficacy of the drug).

The affinity of a substance for its corresponding receptor determines the concentration of substance necessary to occupy and activate receptor sites. This determines the potency of the drug. Changes in receptor density may also influence the potency of a drug, as described earlier.

DOSE-RESPONSE RELATIONSHIPS

Because all drugs have multiple effects, a single dose-response curve describes only one effect of a drug. A family of dose-response curves, each describing one of the many distinct pharmacologic effects of the drug, must be considered when assessing a drug. A narcotic drug has one curve describing its analgesic properties, another describing its respiratory depressant effect, another its effect on vasodilatation, and so on.

Assuming that a drug exerts its pharmacologic effect by binding reversibly with receptors, and that the effect of a given dose is linearly related to the fraction of receptors occupied, then the effect of a drug concentration [D] can be described by the following equation:

$$\text{fraction of maximum effect} = [D]/(K_D + [D])$$

where: [D] = concentration of free drug
K_D = dissociation constant (k_2/K_1) of the drug receptor complex.

This is the same analysis applied to enzyme substrate interactions described in the Michaelis-Menten equation. The dose plotted against effect results in a rectangular hyperbola (Fig. 7–8). As in the Michaelis-Menten model, when $[D] = 0$, there is no effect; when $[D] = K_D$, half the receptors are occupied and the effect is half maximal; and, as the dose increases, the effect approaches the maximum as the asymptote. Because a wide range of doses are often studied, it is more convenient to display the log dose on the abscissa. This produces

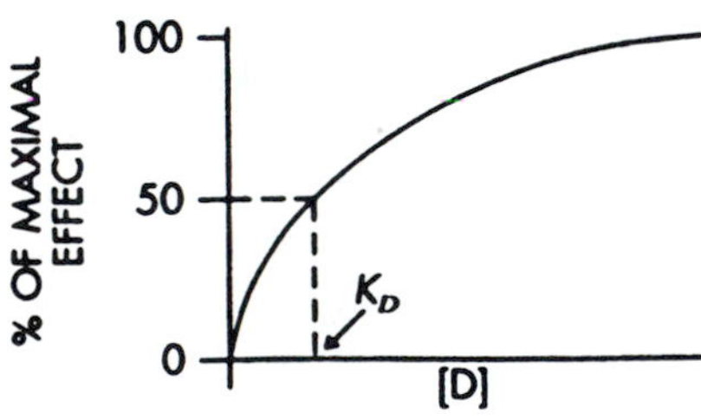

FIGURE 7–8. The relationship of the concentration of a drug and the magnitude of the response to it, with arithmetic abscissa and ordinate.

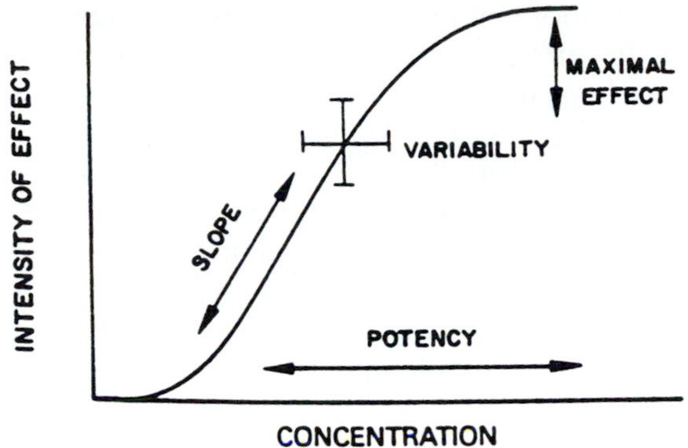

FIGURE 7–9. Plot of the magnitude of a drug effect against the logarithm of the concentration, showing the four characteristics of the dose-response curve: efficacy, or maximum effect; potency, or the amount of drug required to produce the effect; slope, or the rate at which effect changes with respect to dose; and variability.

the familiar sigmoid-shaped dose-response curve seen in Figure 7–9.

Four important parameters are considered when analyzing the dose response curve; potency, slope, efficacy or power, and individual variation (Fig. 7–9).

Potency

Potency is not a description of the magnitude of the pharmacologic effect produced, but merely a statement of how much of the drug is required. Lack of potency becomes a limiting factor only when so much drug is required to produce an effect that it is difficult to administer.

If the potency of a drug is judged from dose-response curves, then pharmacokinetic factors such as absorption, distribution, and elimination affect the results. If concentration response-curves are examined, these confounding effects are eliminated, but there is still considerable interpatient variability. The potencies of two drugs can be compared only if their dose-response curves are parallel. Otherwise, the curves would be closer together on the dose axis (similar potency) at one point, and farther apart (different potency) at another. The curves might even cross. In that case, at a lesser dose one drug is more potent, while at greater dose, the other drug is more potent.

The potency of drugs used in anesthesia is often characterized in terms of the ED_{50}, or median effective dose, which is the dose necessary to produce a specific response in 50 per cent of subjects. When dealing with binary drug effects, such as awake or asleep, the dose is plotted against the percentage of subjects who displayed the specific drug effect being studied. The lethal dose of a drug is often expressed in similar terms: the LD_{50} is the dose of drug that is fatal to 50 per cent of subjects.

An inherently safe drug has an LD_{50} that is much greater than the ED_{50}. The therapeutic index is the ratio of the median lethal to the median effective doses, (LD_{50}/ED_{50}); a large therapeutic index implies a greater margin of safety, but only for a particular pharmacologic effect of the drug. Thus, if the drug effect desired is antiplatelet effect, aspirin has a large therapeutic index; if the effect desired is relief of severe rheumatoid arthritis, the ED_{50} is greater and the therapeutic index correspondingly less. Likewise, the conditions under which the drug is used must be specified to define lethality. In unattended patients, a muscle relaxant would have small LD_{50}; when mechanical ventilation is supplied, the LD_{50} and the therapeutic index are much greater. As compared to safe drugs such as aspirin, the drugs used to produce anesthesia exhibit relatively small therapeutic indices. Lethal alveolar concentrations of potent inhaled anesthetics such as halothane are only a few times those required to produce anesthesia. Because 1.05 atmospheres of nitrous oxide is required to produce surgical anesthesia in half the population, the LD_{50} for this drug (as the result of hypoxia) is actually less than its ED_{50} for surgical anesthesia.

Slope

The slope of the dose-response curve is related to the number of receptors that must be occupied to produce the pharmacologic effect. If a drug must occupy a large fraction of receptors before any effect is seen, the slope will be steep once the effect begins to appear. This is characteristic of nondepolarizing neuromuscular blockers as well as inhaled inhalation anesthetics. A steep slope implies that small increments in dose produce large increases in pharmacologic effect. It is also likely that the difference between therapeutic dose and toxic dose will be small. Drugs with steeply sloped dose-response curves demand careful titration to achieve the desired effect in all patients.

Efficacy

The efficacy of a drug is the maximum pharmacologic effect that the drug can produce. It is unrelated to potency. Efficacy is determined by the intrinsic activity of the drug in its interaction with cell membrane receptors. In practice, the efficacy of a drug may be limited by the appearance of side effects within the dose range needed to produce the desired effect, as the dose-response curves for the desired effect and the undesired side effect overlap.

Individual Variation

Whereas the usual dose-response curves describe the behavior of a population, interpatient variation may make individual patients' responses unpredictable. All the factors described above that influence pharmacokinetics (bioavailability, renal and hepatic function, age) or pharmacodynamics (genetic differences, receptor density) come into play to enhance the variability of patients' responses, along with coexisting diseases and drug interactions. The combination of interpatient variability, steep dose-response curves, and small therapeutic indices make the drugs used in anesthesia particularly dangerous.

These hazards are overcome in several ways. Precise monitoring of the effect of the drug (e.g., nerve stimulators with neuromuscular blockers) or of the amounts of drugs used (e.g., precision vaporizers, mass spectrometers or oximeters) add to safety. Knowledge of the patient factors that alter responses allows the anesthesiologist to adjust doses accordingly and to choose drugs with side effects that are least harmful for a specific patient. Combinations of drugs, each chosen to achieve a specific effect, may produce fewer side effects than a large dose of a single drug to achieve a spectrum of effects. This is the argument in favor of combinations of nitrous oxide, opioids, sedatives, muscle relaxants and sometimes small amounts of inhaled anesthetics (''balanced anesthesia''). Unfortunately, the side effects as well as the therapeutic effects of drugs used in combination summate, too; the technique is not a guarantee of freedom from unwanted anesthetic side effects.

The practice of administering drugs in divided doses and allowing time to assess the effects of one dose before giving the next adds greatly to safety, as does the analogous habit of decreasing at intervals the rate of a drug infusion or the concentration of an inhaled agent to ascertain whether less anesthetic might be needed. Most new anesthetic drugs are introduced not because they produced a novel therapeutic effect, but because they offer the promise of a better therapeutic index. Newer muscle relaxants do not produce more profound muscle relaxation than does curare, but they can be applied more easily to a wider range of patients without producing side effects such as prolonged paralysis, hypotension, or tachycardia. Similar principles apply to the introduction of newer narcotics and even inhalation anesthetics.

REFERENCES

Eger EI II, ed. Anesthetic uptake and action. Baltimore: Williams & Wilkins, 1974.

Gilman AG, Goodman LS, Rall RW, Murad F, eds. The pharmacological basis of therapeutics. 8th ed. New York: MacMillan, 1990.

Stanski DR, Watkins WD. Drug disposition in anesthesia. Orlando: Grune & Stratton, 1982.

CHAPTER EIGHT

THE INHALED ANESTHETICS

Inhalational anesthetics are used widely in modern anesthetic practice, especially because they can be administered and excreted via the lungs, and because the depth of anesthesia can be altered rapidly and measured readily. Measurement of anesthetic concentrations in respiratory gases enhances the precision and safety of inhalational anesthesia, to a greater extent than is possible with any injectable agent.

The inhalation of gases and vapors led to the development of surgical anesthesia, first with diethyl ether by William Morton in 1846, and then with nitrous oxide by Gardner Quincy Colton in 1863. The undesirable features of these and other once popular anesthetics have led to the development of new inhalational anesthetics. Diethyl ether and cyclopropane were flammable; chloroform produced unexplained cardiac arrests and liver failure; trichlorethylene formed the toxic gas phosgene in the presence of soda lime; methoxyflurane caused renal tubular damage because its rapid metabolism released fluoride ions. These varied and subtle problems were recognized only after prolonged clinical use; accordingly, each new anesthetic receives more intense scrutiny than its predecessor.

This chapter discusses the inhalational general anesthetics in current use: nitrous oxide, isoflurane (Forane), enflurane (Ethrane), and halothane (Fluothane). Table 8–1 lists the chemical, physical, and pharmacologic properties of the agents and of two new anesthetics undergoing laboratory and clinical testing, sevoflurane and desflurane. The discussion concerns the four agents in current use, but the scientific basis for the use of these anesthetics applies to all.

CHEMICAL STRUCTURE

The chemical structure of an anesthetic gas determines the stability of the anesthetic molecule and its resistance to degradation by physical variables such as heat, light, and the substances that it contacts in use, and its potential for metabolic breakdown in the body. The chemical structures of the inhaled anesthetics are illustrated in Figure 8–1. Nitrous oxide (N_2O) is a simple linear compound that is stable under the usual physical conditions in which it is used clinically, and is not metabolized in the body. However, nitrous oxide inhibits the enzyme methionine synthetase, and thereby may inhibit DNA synthesis and reduce bone marrow activity. These sequelae have been observed in humans only with prolonged exposure (several weeks), and such use is contraindicated. There is no evidence that this action of N_2O is harmful when used for surgical anesthesia, where exposure times are measured in hours, not days or weeks. Interference with vitamin B_{12} availability by prolonged exposure to N_2O may precipitate peripheral nerve dysfunction, which has been reported among dentists chronically exposed to nitrous oxide. These problems do not occur among

TABLE 8–1. General Properties of Inhalational Anesthetics

	N_2O	Isoflurane	Enflurane	Halothane	Desflurane	Sevoflurane
Molecular weight	44	184.5	184.5	197.4	168	218
Boiling point (°C)	−89	48.5	56.5	50.2	23.5	58.5
Specific gravity at 25°C	1.53*	1.5	1.52	1.86	1.45	1.50
Vapor pressure at 20°C (mm Hg)	Gas	238	172	243	664	160
Partition coefficients at 37°C						
Blood: gas	0.47	1.4	1.8	2.3	0.42	0.59
Brain: blood	1.1	2.6	1.4	2.9	1.3	1.7
Muscle: blood	1.2	4.0	1.7	3.5	2.0	3.1
Fat: blood	2.3	45	36	60	27	48
Rubber: gas	1.2	62	74	120	19	30
MAC (in O_2) per cent	105	1.2	1.6	0.75	4.6–6.0	1.7–2.0
MAC (in 70 per cent N_2O) per cent	0.56	0.57	0.29	0.66	4.5	0.66
Stability						
Alkali	Stable	Stable	Stable	Some instability	Stable	Very unstable
Ultraviolet	Stable	Stable	Stable	Unstable		
Metal	Stable	Stable	Stable	Corrodes	Stable	Stable
Preservative	None	None	None	Thymol	None	None
Per cent recovered as metabolities	0.0†	0.2	2.4	20	N/A	1–2

* Specific gravity for N_2O is for the gas relative to air, but for the other anesthetics, is for the liquid relative to water.
† Trace metabolism by gut flora.

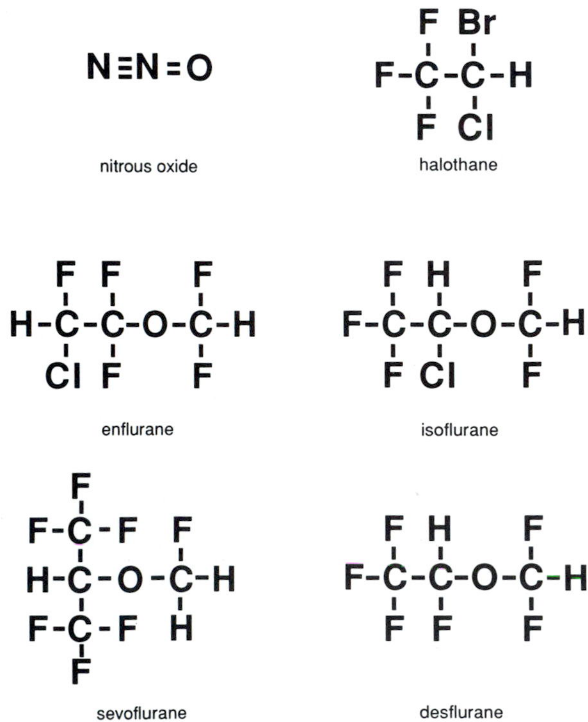

FIGURE 8–1. Chemical structure of the inhaled anesthetics. Note that isoflurane and enflurane are structural isomers.

health care personnel when appropriate scavenging of waste gases is used.

Halothane is a halogen-substituted ethane, superior to earlier ethers and alkanes, with or without halogen substitutions. Following its introduction in the 1950s, halothane rapidly replaced other general anesthetic drugs. However, two problems became evident with halothane that led to a systematic search for a superior drug, based on studies of the structure-activity characteristics of anesthetic molecules. The first was an increased incidence of arrhythmias, particularly in the presence of catecholamines. The introduction of the ether link found in enflurane and isoflurane reduced this tendency markedly. The second problem with halothane involved the metabolism or biotransformation of the drug. As much as 20 per cent of the administered dose may be recovered as nonvolatile products in the urine (mainly bromide ions and trifluoroacetic acid). The mixed function oxidases in the endoplasmic reticulum, primarily of the liver, are responsible. Halothane is also somewhat unstable, as shown in Table 8–1. Alkaline conditions, such as those that occur in the soda lime of carbon dioxide absorbers, and ultraviolet light, tend to cause breakdown of halothane. Prolonged exposure corrodes metal and degrades some plastic parts of the anesthetic circuit.

The principal factor leading to the decreased use of halothane has been the rare (<1:10,000) occurrence of hepatitis, generally beginning a few days after halothane anesthesia. The rarity of the phenomenon and the prevalence of hepatic dysfunction and hepatitis in the surgical population at large have made even the existence of "halothane hepatitis" a subject for debate. The cause of this syndrome also remains uncertain, but a popular view is that metabolic breakdown products of halothane form hapten-protein conjugates, leading to a fulminant, immunologically mediated hepatic necrosis that may be fatal. Usually the severe response occurs after halothane has been administered several times to the same patient, and often a retrospective review reveals fever or mild jaundice following a previous exposure to halothane. However, the severity and random occurrence of this complication has hastened the replacement of halothane by other anesthetics, both inhalational and injectable.

The substitution of fluorine for chlorine or bromine in the anesthetic molecule increases stability, while decreasing potency and solubility. In this way, the properties of enflurane and isoflurane have been improved greatly over those of halothane by the elimination of bromine and the introduction of the ether link. Enflurane and isoflurane are isomers differing only in their structure; they have the same chemical formulae and hence the same molecular weight. The investigational anesthetics sevoflurane and desflurane carry these themes further. The lesser solubilities of both agents are desirable, but come at the expense of decreased potency; the potency of sevoflurane is increased by the bulky propyl side chain.

Physical Properties

The physical properties of anesthetics such as boiling point, vapor pressure, specific gravity, and molecular weight determine the means by which the agents are administered, including the requirements for precision vaporizers.

The boiling point of nitrous oxide is −89°C (Table 8–1); it is therefore a gas at room temperature. However, when compressed to 50 atmospheres (or 745 psig), N_2O is a liquid at room temperature and is supplied in cylindrical steel tanks for clinical use. As the N_2O is used, the liquid vaporizes and the gas pressure remains constant, until the tank is almost empty; the weight of the tank rather than the pressure of its contents is the only reliable guide to how much of the liquid remains. Desflurane poses a similar challenge to practical use. Because its boiling point is near room temperature, evaporative cooling has relatively great effects on vapor pressure and the delivered concentration.

Isoflurane, enflurane, and halothane are colorless liquids at room temperature and are diluted in a carrier gas by a vaporizer, as described in Chapter 5. A vaporizer used with halothane must be cleaned frequently because thymol, added to prevent halothane breakdown, accumulates with time and forms a gummy deposit in the vaporizer. The other volatile agents do not contain stabilizing agents.

Concentrations of inhaled anesthetics may be quantitated by partial pressure (mm Hg) or by fractional concentration (gas concentration in vol per cent). The partial pressure of the anesthetic is the more fundamental measure. Consider a vaporizer calibrated at sea level (760 mm Hg) and set to a 2 per cent concentration of isoflurane, providing a partial pressure of 15 mm Hg [(2/100) × 760]. At 6000 feet above sea level (e.g., in the hills above Denver, Colorado), the barometric pressure is 609 mm Hg, and 2 per cent isoflurane would contain a partial pressure of only 12 mm Hg. The vaporizer delivers neither the expected partial pressure nor the anticipated concentration at this altitude. For a variable bypass vaporizer set to 2 per cent isoflurane, the constants are the saturated vapor pressure of isoflurane and the gas dilution ratio of the vaporizer's bypass valve at a given dial setting (21:1 for the ratio of diluent gas to gas flow entering the anesthetic chamber of an isoflurane vaporizer set to 2 per cent). If the barometric pressure were to be reduced to 609 mm Hg, however, calculation of the actual volumes of gas leaving the vaporizer shows that the final concentration of the isoflurane would be 2.8 per cent instead of the 2 per cent set on the dial, and the partial pressure would be nearer 17 mm Hg instead of the 15 mm Hg obtained at sea level (Fig. 8–2).

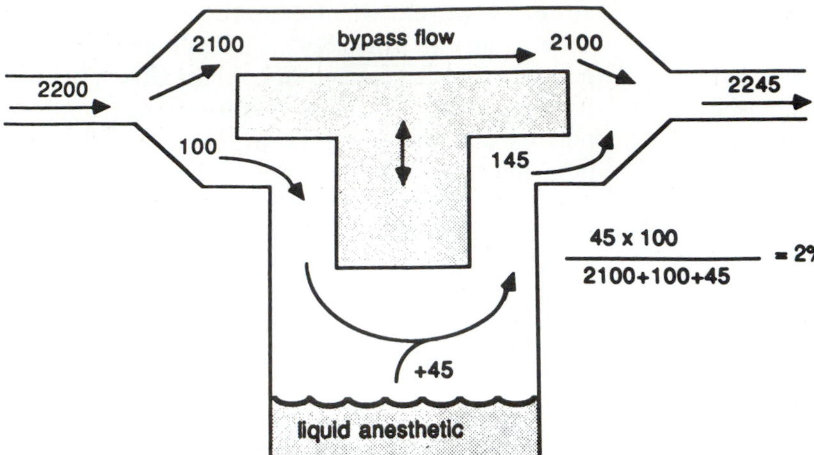

FIGURE 8–2. The gas flows in a variable bypass vaporizer for preparation of a 2 per cent isoflurane gas mixture. The splitting ratio for the gas flows is 21:1 assuming a temperature of 20°C. The gas flows in ml per minute are indicated by the numbers in the figures. (Adapted with permission from Eisenkraft JB. Vaporizers and vaporization. Progress in Anesthesiology. Vol 2, No 24, 1989.)

BIOPHYSICAL PROPERTIES

At induction with an inhaled anesthetic, patients do not lose consciousness immediately, nor do they wake up immediately when the anesthetic is discontinued. The delays that occur between changes in concentration of anesthetics in the inspired gas and those in the brain are due to the solubility of the anesthetics in blood and body tissues, which determines the kinetics of uptake, distribution, and elimination.

Partition Coefficients

The difference in partial pressure of an anesthetic in a gas phase (alveolar gas) and a liquid phase (blood) determines the movement of the anesthetic molecules between the phases. Because more anesthetic is in the gas phase at the beginning of induction, the net direction of movement is from the alveolar gas to the blood. As anesthetic accumulates in the blood, molecules also diffuse back from the blood into the alveolar gas. Eventually the rate of diffusion in both directions is equal and the net exchange of anesthetic is zero. This is the definition of equilibrium; in clinical practice, however, this state is never achieved because the blood also gives up molecules of anesthetic to other tissues.

The partition coefficient describes the ratio of concentrations of anesthetics in two phases at equilibrium. For example, in a volume of blood in equilibrium with 2 per cent enflurane at 37°C and an atmospheric pressure of 760 mm Hg, the partial pressures of enflurane in both gas and liquid phase are 15.2 mm Hg. However, the volume of anesthetic vapor measured in the blood is 3.6 ml of enflurane per 100 ml of blood, or 3.6 vol per cent, whereas the gas phase contains 2 vol per cent. The ratio of these concentrations is expressed as the blood:gas coefficient (3.6/2 = 1.8). Blood:tissue coefficients are measured and expressed similarly. These partition coefficients, which are characteristic of the individual agents, determine the pharmacokinetic properties (called ''uptake and distribution'' for anesthetics) of each agent. The desire for low solubilities and anticipated rapid induction and emergence has driven the search for new agents beyond isoflurane and enflurane.

Several points are critical to the practical use of inhalational anesthetics. First, the net movement of gas molecules always proceeds from the phase with greater partial pressure to that with lesser. Second, the actual quantity or volume of anesthetic vapor that is contained in the liquid or solid phase depends on its partial pressure and its solubility in that particular tissue. Returning to the enflurane example, if the blood equilibrated with gas containing enflurane at 15.2 mm Hg is exposed to brain, muscle, and fat tissue until they too are in equilibrium (in practice this will never be achieved), then the entire system demonstrates no further net exchange between the phases, and the partial pressure throughout is 15.2 mm Hg. Measurement of the concentrations of enflurane in the different tissues shows that the brain, muscle, and fat, respectively, contain 1.4, 1.7, and 36 times greater volumes of enflurane vapor than does the same quantity of blood; these are the values of the brain:blood, muscle:blood, and fat:blood partition coefficients in Table 8–1. Compared to the gas phase, the blood, brain, muscle, and fat therefore contain 1.8, 2.5, 3.1, and 65 times more anesthetic per unit volume, although the partial pressure of enflurane is the same (15.2 mm Hg) throughout. Prior to equilibrium (Fig. 8–3), enflurane moves from gas to blood, then to brain, muscle, and fat in the direction of decreasing partial pressure even though the concentrations in the brain, muscle, and fat soon exceed those in blood and gas.

Uptake, Distribution, and Elimination

When the anesthetic vaporizer dial is set to the required percentage, the fresh gas flowing from machine to breathing circuit almost immediately contains the anesthetic vapor at the selected concentration, but the inspired gas concentration takes some time to approach this value. There are three reasons for this delay. First, the circuit itself contains a volume of gas that must be replaced by the fresh gas. Assuming exponential mixing, the time constant for this process can be calculated by dividing the gas volume of the circuit by the fresh gas inflow rate. For example, with a circle system having a total gas volume of 6 L (reservoir bag = 3 L; carbon dioxide absorber = 2 L; anesthetic hose, connections, and valves = 1 L) and a fresh gas flow of 3 L per minute, the time constant is 2 minutes (6/3). Neglecting losses due to uptake by the patient and the rubber in the system, concentrations increase exponentially, and at 1, 2, and 3 times constants, the anesthetic concentration is 63, 86.5, and 95 per cent, respectively, of the fresh gas

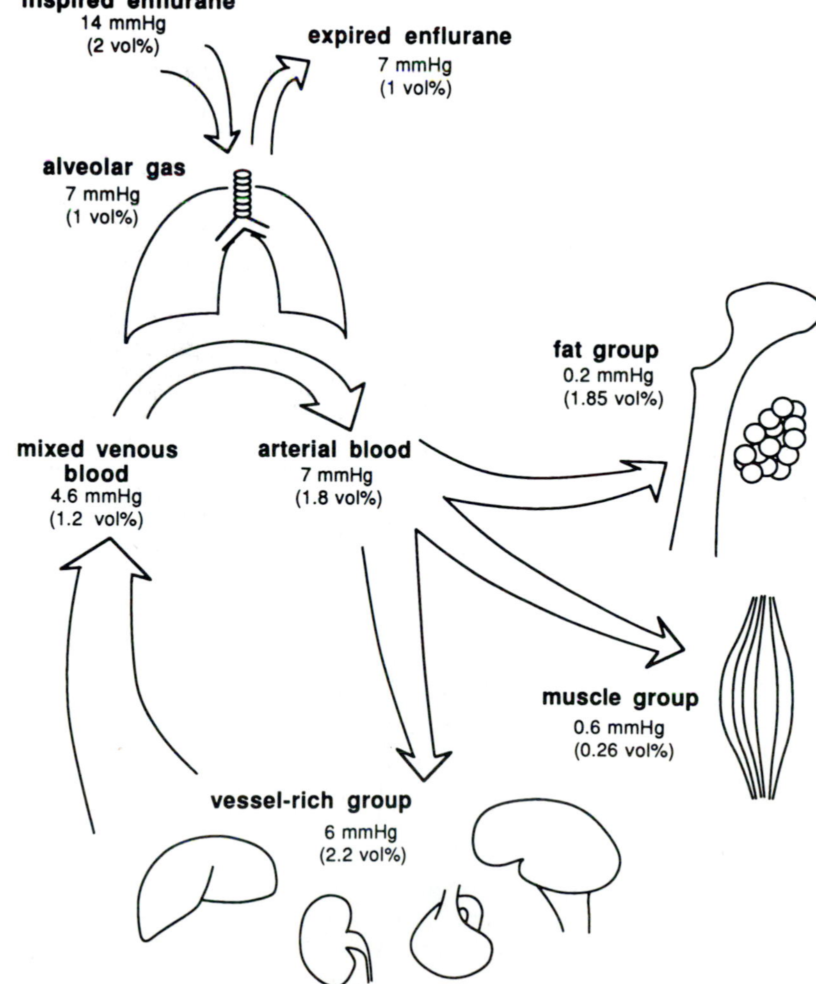

FIGURE 8–3. The distribution of partial pressures (mm Hg) and concentration (vol per cent) for enflurane in the body tissues calculated for 10 minutes after beginning ventilation with 2 per cent enflurane in the inspired gas. The figure illustrates that at this time, the alveolar gas concentration and partial pressure is about half that of the inspired gas. Anesthetic flow is in the direction of decreasing partial pressure, and is indicated quantitatively by the size and direction of the arrows. The vessel-rich group is close to equilibrium, while the partial pressures show that the vessel-rich group of tissues is close to equilibrium while the muscle and fat group are still far from equilibrium. Note that the concentration (vol per cent) of enflurane in the tissues depends on the partition coefficients and that anesthetic uptake continues into the vessel-rich and fat groups, even though the concentration (vol per cent) in the fat group is already greater than that of the blood.

flow value. For a dial setting of 2 per cent enflurane, the concentration in the circle system will be about 1.26, 1.73, and 1.9 per cent at two, four, and six minutes, respectively. The time constant can be reduced by increasing the gas flow rate or reducing the circuit volume by emptying the reservoir bag.

A second factor that delays the rate of increase of the anesthetic concentration in the circuit is the solubility of the anesthetic in some rubber and plastic materials (Table 8–1). Losses due to uptake by rubber are sufficient to reduce initially the inhaled anesthetic concentration in breathing circuits made of rubber.

The third and most important factor delaying the increase in inhaled anesthetic concentration in a circle system is dilution in the functional residual capacity of the lungs, and uptake of anesthetic by the patient. These reduce the anesthetic concentration in the exhaled gas, the rebreathing of which reduces the concentration in the inspired limb. Therefore, the rate of rise of the inspired concentration towards the fresh gas concentration is slower and more complex than accounted for by a single exponential time constant. The precise formulation is not so important as is the realization that the fresh gas, circuit, inspired, and end-tidal (or alveolar) concentrations of the anesthetic differ in a systematic manner; that their relationship changes with time during induction and maintenance; and that concentration gradients are reversed during elimination. In practice, the delay in achieving the desired concentration is anticipated by altering vaporizer settings well before a change in concentration is needed, and by increasing fresh gas flows.

The aim in administering an inhalational anesthetic is to achieve a partial pressure of anesthetic in the brain corresponding to the desired depth of anesthesia. Because the brain is very well perfused, the anesthetic in the arterial blood equilibrates rapidly with the brain. The exchange of anesthetic across the alveolar membranes also is efficient, so that the arterial partial pressure of anesthetic is close to that in the alveolar gas, and the partial pressure of anesthetic in the brain follows closely the alveolar partial pressure. Thus, the anesthesiologist's task of regulating anesthetic partial pressure in the central nervous system is equivalent to fixing the patient's alveolar partial pressure.

The alveolar concentration of anesthetic (F_{A_X}) is determined by the balance of delivery (by ventilation, $\dot{V}_A$) of an inspired concentration (F_{I_X} of anesthetic, and the uptake by the blood ($\dot{V}_X$):

$$\frac{F_{A_X}}{F_{I_X}} = 1 - \frac{\dot{V}_X}{(F_{I_X} \cdot \dot{V}_A)}.$$

At induction, uptake is maximal, $\dot{V}_X$ is equal to delivered anesthetic ($\dot{V}_A \cdot F_{I_X}$), so that F_A/F_I = 0. With long exposure time, uptake is minimal, and F_A/F_I approaches 1.

Uptake by the blood ($\dot{V}_X$) is determined by the blood:gas partition coefficient (γ), cardiac output ($\dot{Q}$), and by the difference of anesthetic partial pressure between alveolar gas and mixed venous blood ($P_{A_X} - P_{\bar{v}_X}$):

$$\dot{V}_X = \gamma \times \dot{Q} \cdot \left(\frac{P_{A_X} - P_{\bar{v}_X}}{P_B}\right)$$

where P_B is the barometric pressure.

The equations combine to the complete expression:

$$\frac{F_{A_X}}{F_{I_X}} = 1 - \gamma \left(\frac{1}{F_{I_X}}\right)\left(\frac{\dot{Q}}{\dot{V}_A}\right)\left(\frac{P_{A_X} - P_{\bar{v}_X}}{P_B}\right)$$

This equation summarizes all of the relationship discussed above that determine the curves of Figure 8–4. This "alveolar: inspired" concentration ratio describes the extent to which the patient has reached equilibrium with the anesthetic to which he is exposed. The approach of the alveolar, and hence the brain, partial pressure to that of the inspired gas is delayed by losses of soluble anesthetics into the blood, increased cardiac output or a large difference between the alveolar and the mixed venous partial pressures, and accelerated by increasing the inspired concentration of anesthetic or by increasing the alveolar ventilation.

Initially during induction, $P_{\bar{v}_X}$ is zero, and uptake will be maximal, and proportional to solubility and cardiac output. As the well-perfused tissues (brain, heart, liver, kidney) take up anesthetic, the venous blood concentration increases, uptake from the alveoli decreases, and alveolar concentration increases. Less well-perfused tissues such as muscle and skin take up anesthetic more slowly, and the venous blood leaving these tissues is lower in concentration than for the well-perfused tissues. Finally, poorly perfused tissues (bone, cartilage, fat) take up small quantities, but do not greatly

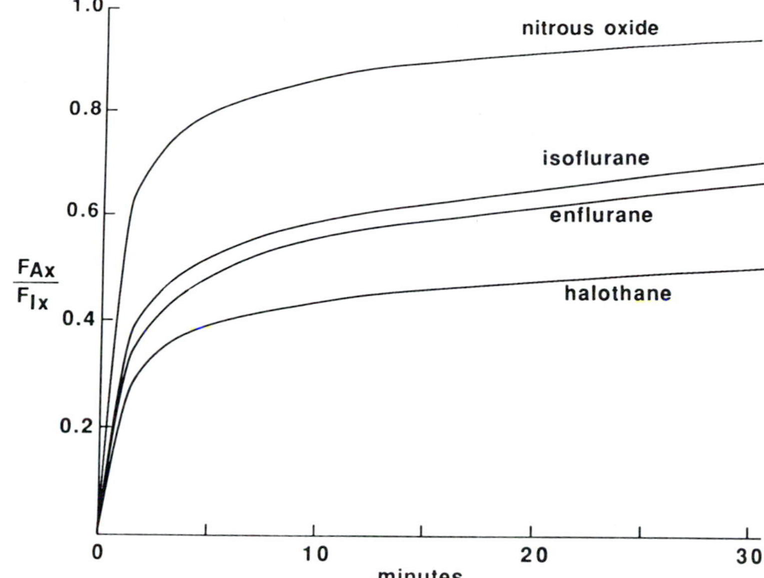

FIGURE 8–4. The increase of the alveolar fractional concentration (F_{AX}) towards that of the inspired concentration (F_{IX}) with time is compared for the different agents. Note the more rapid rise for the less soluble anesthetics. (Modified with permission from Eger EI II. Isoflurane (Forane). 2nd ed. Madison: BOC Inc., 1988.)

affect the initial rise in blood concentrations. Thus, body composition has an effect on the duration of induction, on the dose of anesthetic required to maintain anesthesia, and on the duration of the elimination phase during emergence, mainly by determining the concentration of anesthetic in mixed venous blood.

Clinical Application of Pharmacokinetics

Knowledge of uptake and elimination pharmacokinetics play an essential part in the administration of inhalational agents. The use of gas-measuring devices such as the mass spectrometer to follow the end-expiratory concentrations of the inhaled anesthetics are particularly helpful in understanding these phenomena.

The rate of uptake at the start of an anesthetic is so large that it is usual to increase the concentration of a volatile anesthetic in the inspired gas, as rapidly as the patient will tolerate, to a value several times the desired alveolar concentration. This technique of "over pressure" during the first few minutes compensates for the early rapid uptake, but requires vigilance to avoid overdose.

Neither cardiac output nor total ventilation are constant during induction or maintenance. Surgical pain early in the course of an anesthetic might increase cardiac output, abruptly increasing blood uptake and decreasing alveolar, arterial, and brain concentrations of anesthetic. The patient might become hypertensive or may even move, unless the stimulus has been anticipated by increasing ventilation or inspired anesthetic concentration. Later, when mixed venous concentrations have increased, the effect of a change in cardiac output is less abrupt; a stimulus merely increases uptake slightly. The arousal might then increase only ventilation and thus delivery of anesthetic. Likewise, an increase in inspired anesthetic concentration at this point decreases ventilation, and thus anesthetic delivery, so that blood concentrations increase by only a small amount. This self-regulating behavior slows unwanted deepening of anesthesia, a major advantage of spontaneous ventilation during the maintenance of anesthesia.

Later in the course of anesthesia, if inspired gas concentration is maintained unchanged, the alveolar and total body content of anesthetic will continue to increase, particularly in the muscle and fat tissues. These stores of anesthetic delay awakening and increase metabolism of the anesthetic, as these tissues release their anesthetic back into the blood during postoperative recovery. As uptake proceeds, the inspired concentration of anesthetic is reduced with time so as to maintain the desired brain concentration.

Near the end of operation, the inspired anesthetic concentration is reduced and recovery from anesthesia begins. The elimination of the anesthetic is governed by the same principles as is uptake, but elimination curves are not mirror images of the uptake curves, for two reasons. First, it is not possible to reduce the inspired concentration to less than zero; there is no comparable maneuver during recovery to that of "over pressure" during induction. Second, the first compartments from which the anesthetic is cleared are the vessel-rich tissues in equilibrium with the arterial blood. In contrast, the partition coefficient of fat is so great that the tissue partial pressure of the anesthetic is still less than that of the arterial blood even though the anesthetic has been discontinued. These tissues continue to take up anesthetic from the blood even after the inspired anesthetic has been discontinued. This effect hastens the initial awakening from anesthesia, but also may delay the complete elimination of the drug for days.

When 70 per cent nitrous oxide is used, the volume of anesthetic taken up during the first 10 minutes after induction amounts to several liters; conversely, during recovery, large volumes of N_2O are eliminated. This unusually large volume of exchange alters the concentration of the other gases in the lungs. During induction, the concentrations of oxygen and volatile anesthetics are augmented (second gas effect), thus hastening induction. During recovery the reverse is true. It is usual to follow discontinuance of nitrous oxide with a few minutes of 100 per cent oxygen to prevent the decrease of alveolar oxygen (diffusion hypoxia) that otherwise occurs if N_2O is replaced with air immediately.

Although the blood:gas partition coefficient for N_2O is the least among the inhalational agents, it is still 31 times greater than that of nitrogen. During N_2O administration, any body cavities that contain gaseous nitrogen, not open to the atmosphere, exchange nitrous oxide for nitrogen in proportion to the partial pressure differences for each agent between the gas and the blood phases. However, for an equal change in partial pressure, the blood can carry approximately a 31 times greater volume of N_2O toward the cavity than it can carry nitrogen away per unit of time; therefore the body cavity expands. This phenomenon explains at least in part the distortion of hearing that is observed prior to loss of consciousness as N_2O enters the middle ear. Of greater significance is the potential for complications in patients with gas-filled cavities: bowel obstruction, pneumothorax, pneumopericardium, or air injected for encephalography. The use of N_2O is contraindicated in such conditions; other volatile agents exchange in the same way but the volume of the agents is too small to be of significance.

Pharmacology

Minimum Alveolar Concentration (MAC)

In the early days of anesthesia, a great deal of attention was paid to physical signs that correlated with depth of anesthesia. Particularly with diethyl ether, a combination of respiratory, circulatory, pupillary, and reflex response signs allowed a reasonable prediction of when a patient was sufficiently anesthetized for surgery. The use of premedicants and narcotics often interfere with pupillary signs, and muscle relaxants may abolish respiratory movements, so that circulatory signs and reflex responses are all that remain. Circulatory responses depend on the individual anesthetic properties as well as blood loss and the patient's disease state; therefore, the depth of anesthesia is primarily judged by experience and the patient's responses to surgical stimulation. It is often appropriate for the depth of anesthesia to oscillate between levels that just abolish motor and autonomic responses to surgery. In general, a patient who moves is receiving too little anesthetic, whereas the absence of circulatory responses to stimuli (i.e., no changes in blood pressure or pulse rate) may indicate that anesthetic depth is greater than necessary. No single concentration of anesthetic is appropriate for all patients or for all circumstances; the amount of anesthetic must be tailored to the operative needs and individual characteristics of the patient (age, illness, concomitant drug therapy). Not only is it necessary to reduce progressively the inspired anesthetic concentration with time, as discussed in the preceding section, but it is also appropriate to change the anesthetic depth to match the surgical stimulation. Often, the initial skin incision and final closure are stronger stimuli than the operative procedure itself, and the depth of anesthesia is adjusted to anticipate these changes in stimulation.

The matching of anesthetic administration to the requirements of the patient and the surgical procedure is greatly assisted by knowing the measure of potency called minimum alveolar concentration (MAC). Minimum alveolar concentration is that concentration at which 50 per cent of the patients do not move in response to skin incision (or supramaximal pain stimulus in animal studies). In humans, MAC is established for each anesthetic by maintaining a constant alveolar partial pressure for about 15 minutes to achieve near equilibrium with brain tissue, and then recording whether movement occurs in response to the stimulus. The number of subjects moving in response to the stimulus is then plotted against the end-tidal anesthetic concentration and the 50 per cent response rate is interpolated.

The values for MAC for each of the inhalational agents are listed in Table 8–1. By convention, MAC is expressed in terms of per cent concentration of alveolar gas at1 atmosphere, but minimum alveolar partial pressure (MAP) is also appropriate.

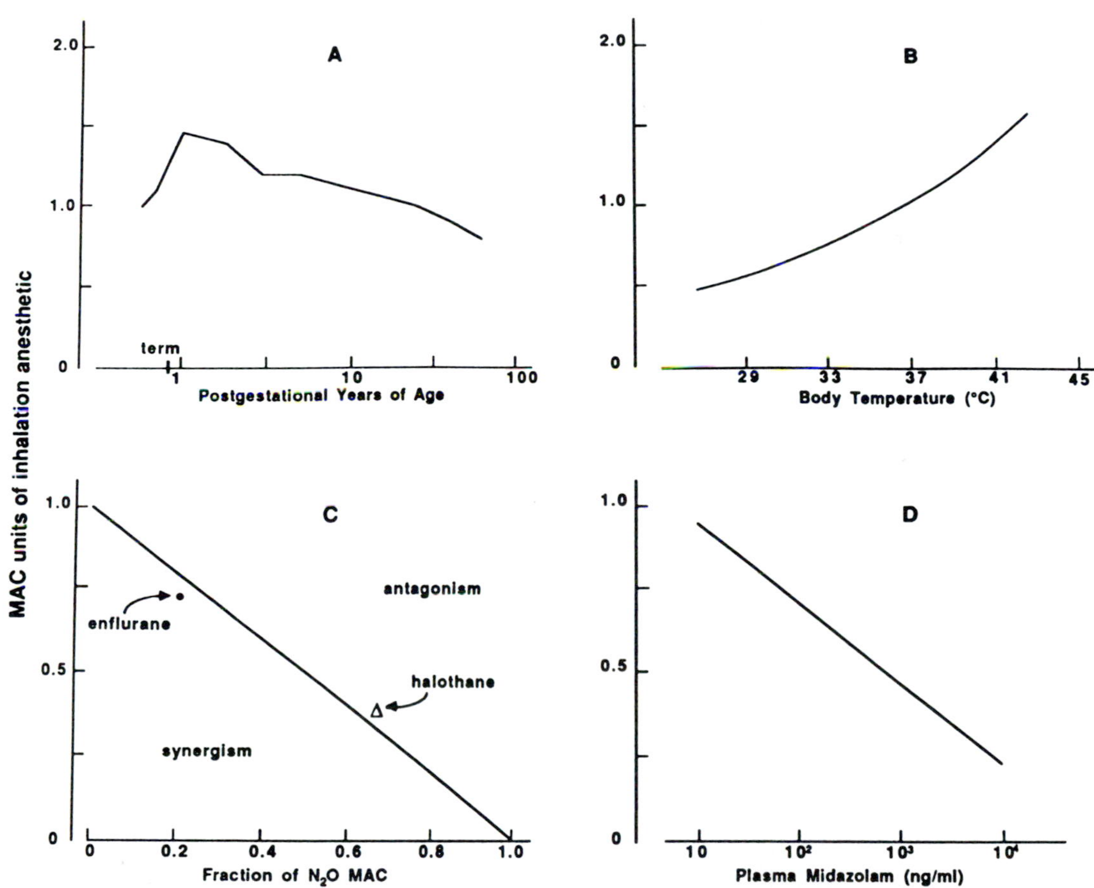

FIGURE 8–5. The influence of age, body temperature, nitrous oxide, and midazolam on MAC.

A, The change in MAC relative to unity in young adults (solid circle) is shown as a function of age in years on a logarithmic scale. (Modified with permission from Le Dez KM, Lerman J. The minimum alveolar concentration (MAC) of isoflurane in preterm neonates. Anesthesiology 1987; 67:301–307.)

B, The normal MAC value at 37°C is increased or decreased as a direct function of the body temperature. (Adapted from Steffey EP, Eger EI. Hyperthermia and halothane MAC in the dog. Anesthesiology 1974; 41:392–396.)

C, The additive effect of halothane or enflurane MAC with the MAC for N_2O is illustrated. Adapted with permission from Torrig G, Damia G, Fabiani ML. Effect of nitrous oxide on the anesthetic requirement of enflurane. Br J Anaesth 1974; 46:468–472.)

D, The influence of increasing doses of midazolam, a common premedicant and anesthetic adjuvant agent, in the MAC for enflurane. The data are for dogs. (Adapted with permission from Hall RZ, Schwieger IM, Hug CC. The anesthetic efficacy of midazolam in the enflurane-anesthetized dog. Anesthesiology 1988; 68:862–866.)

Minimum alveolar concentration is analogous to any other ED_{50} value computed from a pharmacologic dose-response curve. Once the concept was defined for the inhalational anesthetics, it was used to test the influence of many factors that empirical observation suggested influenced anesthesia. The effects of age, body temperature, drugs, and disease states (Fig. 8–5) are important examples. Further, the potencies of different inhalational agents can be compared; so can combinations of the agents. In general, a half MAC of each of two inhalational agents is equivalent in anesthetic potency to one MAC of either; not only does this observation have clinical use, but it also suggests that the fundamental mechanisms by which these agents induce anesthesia are the same.

Because MAC is defined in terms of response to a surgical incision, it is a useful guide in practice. It is not satisfactory to have 50 per cent of patients moving during surgery; usually 1.5 to 2.5 times MAC is required to maintain anesthesia solely with a single inhalational agent, and to suppress cardiovascular response to incision.

The MAC for N_2O is 105 per cent, so that one MAC of N_2O is achievable only under hyperbaric conditions. Because the anesthetic properties of the inhalational agents are additive, N_2O is commonly used as a 70 per cent mixture in oxygen with a volatile agent added to achieve the desired anesthetic effect. So common is this technique that Table 8–1 includes the MAC values for the volatile agents in the presence of 70 per cent N_2O, which are appropriately reduced. Among the advantages of this combination are the reduced quantity of either agent that is required, the speed with which the depth of anesthesia can be changed (owing to the insolubility of N_2O) and the greater blood pressures observed, as compared with the use of a volatile agent alone (particularly halothane).

Effects of Inhalational Anesthetics

All inhalational agents impair respiratory and circulatory function, and in one way or another influence every organ. Some of these actions do not inevitably accompany anesthetic effects, but are side effects that will be reduced further as more specific anesthetics are developed. Anesthetics differ in their side effects, and it is these differences that lead to preferences for one or another agent for a particular patient and operation.

RESPIRATION

Airway irritation is not prominent with the inhalational agents; halothane has a somewhat sweet odor that is tolerated best, whereas enflurane and isoflurane are more pungent. Spontaneous ventilation is progressively impaired by increasing doses of the inhalational agents, as tidal volume decreases more than ventilatory rate increases. The arterial carbon dioxide tension is correspondingly increased, because the reduction of alveolar ventilation is greater than the reduction of carbon dioxide production. These changes are summarized in Figure 8–6, which shows that all the inhalational agents have similar respiratory effects

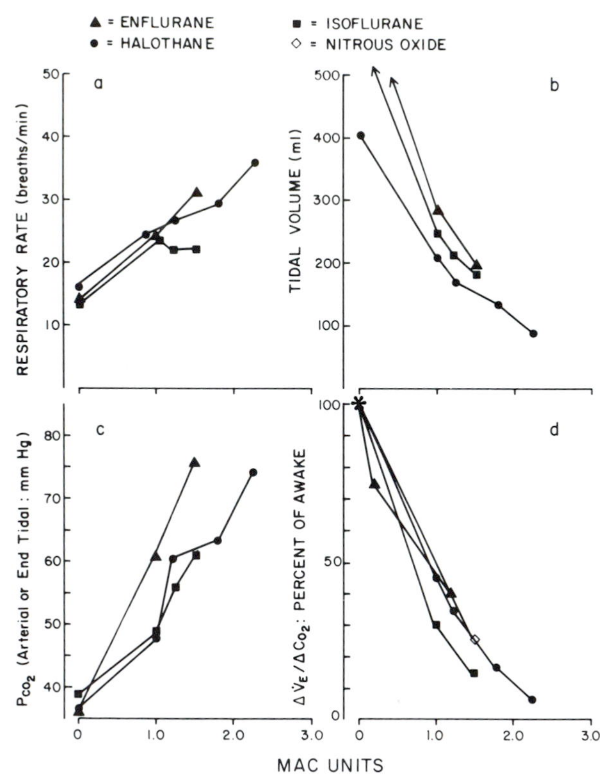

FIGURE 8–6. Inhalational anesthetics and ventilatory control. The changes in respiratory rate (a), tidal volume (b), arterial carbon dioxide tension (c), and ventilatory response to carbon dioxide ($\dot{V}_E/Pa_{CO_2}$) as a per cent of the awake value (d) are shown at different concentrations in MAC units for the volatile anesthetics enflurane, isoflurane, and halothane. Panel d includes nitrous oxide. All inhalational anesthetics have very similar effects, with dose-dependent increases in respiratory rate and Pa_{CO_2}, and decreases in tidal volume and in the ventilatory response to Pa_{CO_2}. (Reproduced with permission from Marshall BE. Pulmonary ventilation. In Marshall BE, Longnecker DE, Barrie Fairley H, eds. Anesthesia for thoracic procedures. Boston: Blackwell Scientific Publications 1988:39–72.)

when compared in terms of MAC units. Even N_2O has the same respiratory depressant property, but this is not noticeable at concentrations normally used. The basis for the respiratory depression is summarized in panel d of Figure 8–6 as a progressive decrease in the slope of the carbon dioxide response to CO_2 with increasing anesthetic depth. Hypoxic ventilatory drive, evident when the arterial oxygen tension is less than 50 mm Hg, is especially sensitive to inhalational agents; it is totally abolished by 1 MAC of the volatile agents and 25 per cent inhibited even by 0.1 MAC.

All of these side effects are readily overcome during anesthesia by assisting or controlling ventilation. However, when spontaneous ventilation is permitted throughout operation, and after returning to spontaneous respiration in the postoperative period, these factors are important in the differential diagnosis of ventilatory inadequacy.

There are a number of changes in the mechanical and gas exchanging properties of the lung that are similar with all the agents when compared at equivalent MAC values. Under anesthesia, the airways are dilated and there is collapse or atelectasis of the most dependent regions of the lung. The atelectasis is most probably due to alterations in the passive distribution of pressure across the diaphragm between the abdominal and thoracic cavities; the consequences are decreases in compliance, functional residual capacity, and efficiency of oxygen exchange.

When atelectasis occurs in an otherwise normal awake subject, hypoxic pulmonary vasoconstriction in small pulmonary arteries diverts blood flow away from the atelectatic area, reducing arterial hypoxemia. This homeostatic response is impaired by all the inhalational agents to a variable extent. Inhalational agents both encourage atelectasis and impair the homeostatic response to atelectasis, increasing the incidence and severity of arterial hypoxemia. Patients with acute and chronic lung disease are particularly sensitive to further impairment of respiratory function during anesthesia, but there is no reason for preferring one anesthetic over another, except that volatile agents permit increased concentrations of oxygen in the inspired gas (see Chapter 22).

CIRCULATION

Changes in circulatory signs are among the best indices of anesthetic depth. Inadequate anesthesia is often manifested as increased pulse and blood pressure in response to a surgical stimulus, whereas circulatory depression results from anesthetic overdose.

All inhalational anesthetics cause circulatory changes which may include myocardial depression, systemic vasodilation, and decreased sympathoadrenal activity. The signs and symptoms of anesthesia-induced circulatory depression may mimic those caused by disease, blood loss, or hypoxemia. When changes are modest and time permits, it is appropriate to establish the etiology of the circulatory depression by systematic evaluation. However, the first response to circulatory collapse is to discontinue inhalational anesthetics and to administer 100 per cent oxygen. It is much easier to reestablish anesthesia than it is to resuscitate after an anesthetic overdose.

The influences of nitrous oxide on the circulation are minor compared to those of the potent volatile agents. Stimulation of the sympathetic nervous system by N_2O may cause small increases in arterial blood pressure and peripheral vascular resistance. However, the hemodynamic improvement that accompanies the addition of N_2O to a potent inhalational anesthetic is brought about by the concomitant reduction in the required dose of the potent agent also. In the patient in shock or with a severely compromised heart, even N_2O alone may cause deterioration of cardiac output and blood pressure.

With increasing concentrations of halothane, the arterial blood pressure is progressively reduced because of direct depression of the myocardium with a decreased cardiac output, and because of inhibition of the normal baroreceptor-mediated tachycardia in response to hypotension. The heart rate is slowed with halothane due to both a relative vagal predominance and direct slowing of the cardiac pacemaker tissues. Slowing of impulse conduction rate, increased refractory period in the conductive tissues, and increased automaticity of myocardial cells all contribute to the occurrence of arrhythmias. Sinus bradycardia, wandering pacemaker, or junctional rhythms are very common, but tachyarrhythmias may occur also. These conduction abnormalities can be minimized by adequate depth of anesthesia (to blunt catecholamine responses), by maintaining normal or moderately less than normal carbon dioxide tensions, and by limiting the dose of epinephrine used for hemostasis. The use of halothane in asthmatics is also complicated by arrhythmias when phosphodiesterase inhibitors are used concurrently. Whereas these arrhythmias are generally benign, they may be functionally significant in the presence of disease, acidosis, hypoxia, or electrolyte abnormalities.

The distribution of blood flow to the organs is altered in the presence of halothane, but the overall vascular resistance is little changed, and the coronary circulation remains responsive to metabolic needs.

In usual clinical concentrations, enflurane decreases the blood pressure in a dose-dependent manner similar to that observed with halothane. Myocardial depression, reduced baroreceptor response, and reduced sympathetic activity are also similar, but there are other differences. The cardiac output is not reduced as much with enflurane, and bradycardia and arrhythmias are not as common, but peripheral vascular dilation is generally greater than with halothane. Deep levels of enflurane (>2.5 MAC) may result in profound hypotension.

The blood pressure also decreases with isoflurane in a dose-dependent manner, but the heart rate and cardiac rhythm are well maintained and the hypotension is due to peripheral vascular dilation, particularly in skin and muscle. Myocardial depression is less obvious with isoflurane, and the coronary circulation is often maximally dilated. The latter two properties are currently the source of controversy because the preservation of myocardial pump function by isoflurane suggests that it is of particular value in patients with myocardial impairment from disease. In contrast, there is evidence that the maximal dilation of normal coronary vessels may draw blood away from vessels that are pathologically narrowed ("coronary steal"), leading to further ischemia. Although clearly demonstrable under some conditions, clinical evidence of significant coronary steal during isoflurane is rare.

CENTRAL NERVOUS SYSTEM

The inhalational agents alter the electroencephalogram (EEG) and may interfere with the interpretation of central nervous system-evoked potential monitoring. As the depth of anesthesia is increased with the inhalational agents, the electrical activity of the cerebral cortex slows, with progressive replacement of fast low-voltage activity by slow waves of greater amplitude. Deep levels of anesthesia produce electrical silence. Because of the complexity and detail of the electroencephalogram, several more concise indices of EEG activity have been developed. These indices correlate well with anesthetic concentrations in controlled experiments, but in clinical circumstances the interpretation is often obscured by hypoxemia, cerebral ischemia, and the effects of other drugs. The EEG is therefore a useful indicator of change, but cannot yet be used alone as a reliable index of anesthetic depth.

A peculiarity associated only with enflurane is that the usual pattern of EEG depression described above may be interrupted by a high-voltage, fast frequency pattern progressing to spike-dome complexes and tonic-clonic muscle activity. This excitatory action of enflurane can be prevented by avoiding deep enflurane anesthesia and hypocarbia; although these effects are not thought to be of special concern, this agent is not recommended for use in patients with seizure foci. This EEG pattern is not seen with isoflurane.

The three potent agents cause dose-dependent cerebral vasodilation, increased cerebral blood flow, and impaired autoregulation of blood flow. There are regional differences in the magnitude of the changes in blood flow and brain metabolism, but there is no evidence of ischemia. However, cerebrospinal fluid pressure is increased and may aggravate pathologic processes accompanied by increased intracranial pressure. Although cerebral blood flow is also increased during isoflurane anesthesia, the cerebral circulation remains more responsive to hypocarbia than during halothane or enflurane anesthesia. The combination of low doses of isoflurane and hyperventilation results in reduction of cerebral flow, metabolism, and intracranial pressure, therefore, it is often preferred for neurosurgery (see Chapter 30).

Recovery from anesthesia is accompanied by a progressive pattern of improving neurologic state with signs and symptoms that can mimic a variety of neuropathologies (including spasticity). The rapidity of the changes distinguishes those due to anesthesia from those due to organic damage. Shivering is also common during the early postoperative period because temperature regulation is impaired during anesthesia and the circumstances of operation favor heat loss. Increased oxygen consumption and cardiac output accom-

shivering and may be deleterious for critically ill patients.

RENAL FUNCTION

Anesthesia with any of the potent agents reduces renal blood flow and glomerular filtration rate in a dose-related manner; healthy anesthetized patients produce only small volumes of concentrated urine. The changes in urine volume are primarily due to circulatory changes and are minimized by preoperative hydration and prevention of hypotension. The effects are rapidly reversed after discontinuing the anesthesia. Although enflurane is metabolized to free fluoride, the amount released is small and not likely to be nephrotoxic except in extraordinary circumstances, such as when large doses are given to obese patients for long operations. None of the agents currently in use is associated with renal failure.

LIVER AND GASTROINTESTINAL TRACT

Nausea and vomiting may occur after administration of inhalational anesthetics, but factors such as age, gender, site, and duration of operation, and the presence of drugs and disease have a greater influence than does the choice of agent.

Splanchnic and hepatic flows are reduced in proportion to the reduction of cardiac output during anesthesia with all these agents. The depression may be less severe with isoflurane, as hepatic blood flow and venous oxygen saturation are greater with this agent than with halothane. Hepatic cellular function and the metabolism of drugs are depressed by inhalational anesthetics. This mild depression of hepatic function is not related to the severe hepatic necrosis that has been reported following halothane (see above).

SKELETAL MUSCLE

The operating conditions for many procedures are improved by adequate relaxation of skeletal muscles; this is true not only for abdominal or thoracic procedures, but even for head, neck, and limb procedures where control of ventilation and prevention of coughing or movement are desirable. The potent inhalational agents produce some modest skeletal muscle relaxation by central depression, but more important is their enhancement of the muscular relaxation induced by nondepolarizing relaxants. In this regard, both enflurane and isoflurane are substantially more effective than halothane, whereas N_2O has no detectable effect. The dose of pancuronium may be halved in the presence of isolfurane, for example.

SELECTION OF INHALATIONAL AGENT

The selection of the anesthetic technique and specific drugs is based on a rational analysis of the patient's condition and the planned operation. The different properties of these anesthetics make one preferable to another in some circumstances. These relative indications and contraindications are summarized in Table 8–2.

The ideal volatile anesthetic is one which is stable in the long term under normal conditions (temperature, humidity, light, alkali) found in the anesthesia apparatus, nonflammable in air, oxygen, or nitrous oxide, and easily handled in liquid or gas form. It must be potent, allowing inspired oxygen concentrations close to 1.0, and poorly soluble in blood and tissue, allowing rapid induction and emergence. It must not irritate the airway. Trace concentrations must not be toxic, even during long exposure, and the agent must not be metabolized.

TABLE 8–2. Clinical Qualities of Inhalational Anesthetics

Agent	Strengths	Weaknesses
Nitrous oxide	Analgesia Rapid uptake and elimination Little cardiac or respiratory depression	Sympathetic stimulation Expansion of closed air spaces Interferes with B_{12} metabolism Limits FIO_2
Halothane	Inexpensive Effective in low concentrations Little airway irritability Uterine relaxation	Chemically less stable Slow uptake and elimination Biodegradable Hepatic necrosis Cardiac depression and arrhythmias
Enflurane	Good muscle relaxation Stable cardiac rate and rhythm	Pungent odor Seizure activity on EKG
Isoflurane	Good muscle relaxation Stable cardiac rate and rhythm Usable in neurosurgery	Pungent odor Expensive

It must have minimal and predictable cardiovascular and respiratory effects, and no adverse interactions with other drugs.

The ideal inhalational anesthetic is not yet at hand. The relative merits and disadvantages of each anesthetic prevent absolute assignment of a single "best" agent. The new agents, desflurane and sevoflurane, approximate the ideal in some ways, and depart from it in others. Both agents have very low gas:blood and blood:tissue partition coefficients, allowing rapid induction and emergence. Desflurane is difficult to handle, will require new vaporizers, and may possibly be limited to closed-circuit administration due to cost; sevoflurane is more like isoflurane in its physical properties. Desflurane is nearly inert under normal conditions, with less metabolic breakdown than isoflurane; sevoflurane is very unstable in alkali, thus preventing use of current CO_2 absorbers, and is metabolized (including fluoride) to a greater degree than isoflurane. Both anesthetics produce cardiovascular and respiratory depression, which are dose-related and similar to that for isoflurane. No specific toxicity for desflurane has been identified; sevoflurane has been reported to cause hepatotoxicity in animals and decreases in measured protein synthesis that were greater than for other anesthetics.

The inhalational anesthetic agents are easily administered, their concentrations can be regulated and measured precisely, their effects are rapidly reversed, and they are relatively inert. Few other classes of drugs can match their record of safety and utility.

REFERENCES

Brown BR. Anesthesia in hepatic and biliary tract disease. Philadelphia: FA Davis Co, 1988.

Eger EI II. Anesthetic uptake and action. Baltimore: Williams & Wilkins, 1974.

Lowenstein E, Reiz S. Effects of inhalation anesthetics on systemic hemodynamics and the coronary circulation. *In* Kaplan JA, ed. Cardiac anesthesia. 2nd ed. Vol 1. New York: Grune and Stratton, 1987: 3–36.

Marshall BE, Longnecker DL. General anesthesia. *In* Gilman AG, Goodman LS, Rall TW, Murad F, eds. The pharmacological basis of therapeutics. 8th ed. New York: MacMillan, 1990.

Nunn JF. Applied respiratory physiology. 3rd ed. Boston: Butterworth's, 1987.

Pavlin EG, Hornbein TR. Anesthesia and the control of ventilation. *In* Cherniak NS, Widdicombe JG, eds. The respiratory system. Vol 2, Part 1. American Physiological Society, 1986: 793–813.

CHAPTER NINE

Nonopioid Intravenous Anesthetics

The components of general anesthesia include analgesia, hypnosis, blunting of reflexes, and muscle relaxation. The nonopioid intravenous anesthetic drugs principally provide hypnosis and blunting of reflexes; narcotics and neuromuscular blockers are used for analgesia and muscle relaxation.

The ideal intravenous anesthetic drug would provide all of these components with rapid, nearly instantaneous onset, without irritating the veins or causing pain on injection. Induction would be smooth, without any signs of muscular twitching or excitement. The drug would be safe and cause minimal perturbation of cardiovascular or respiratory function. The drug would be short acting, allowing the patient to awaken rapidly to full, normal central nervous system (CNS) function. Metabolism to inert substances and excretion would be rapid and complete, so that accumulation would not occur, thereby allowing the drug to be used as a constant infusion over long periods of time. Amnesia for intraoperative events would be complete. These attributes have yet to be attained in a single drug, but are the ideals against which we judge present intravenous drugs.

Barbiturates

Barbituric acid itself (Fig. 9–1) has no intrinsic CNS activity, but substitutions at the number 2 and 5 carbon atoms produce drugs with substantial CNS effects, including loss of consciousness and anticonvulsant activity. For example, at the number 5 carbon, substituting a straight chain produces hypnotic activity, substituting a branched chain produces even greater hypnotic activity; substituting a phenyl group (phenobarbital) produces anticonvulsant activity, whereas a methyl group (methohexital) may actually produce seizure-like muscle movement.

Barbiturates with an oxygen atom on the number 2 carbon are called oxybarbiturates; those with a sulfur atom are thiobarbiturates. Replacement of the oxygen atom with sulfur increases the lipid solubility of the drug, increasing the hypnotic potency and greatly reducing onset time and duration of action. Sulfur substitution at the number 2 carbon of pentobarbital produces thiopental, a potent hypnotic drug characterized by rapid onset and brief duration of effect. The same is true when the ox-

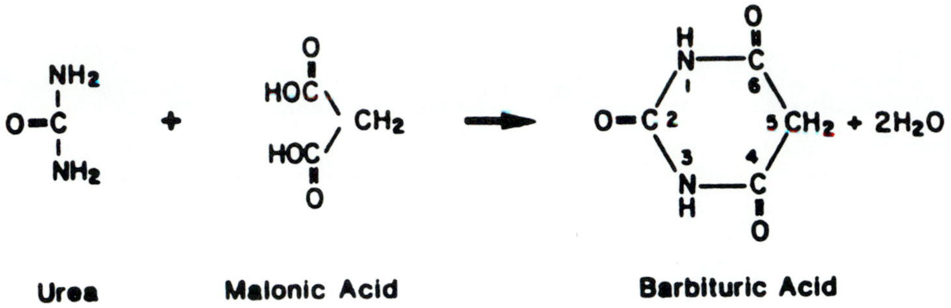

FIGURE 9–1. Barbituric acid.

ygen atom of secobarbital is replaced with sulfur, producing thiamylal.

An oxybarbiturate may be converted to a short-acting drug by adding a methyl group to the nitrogen atom of the barbiturate ring, as with methohexital. The chemical structure of several commonly used barbiturates is depicted in Figure 9–2.

Whereas the exact mechanisms of barbiturate action in the CNS are unknown, many other features are understood. The stereochemistry of barbiturates is clearly important in determining pharmacologic effects: optical isomers can have markedly different CNS effects. This stereospecificity strongly suggests that barbiturates interact with specific membrane sites complementary to their structure, most likely particular synapses in the CNS.

Barbiturates can exert two types of effects at synapses in the CNS: facilitation of inhibitory transmitters, including gamma-aminobutyric acid (GABA); and blockade of excitatory transmitters, such as glutamic acid and acetylcholine. Unlike inhalation anesthetic agents, barbiturates do not block afferent sensory impulses very well. In fact, thiobarbiturates may actually produce an antianalgesic effect, but this is not clinically important as long as the thiobarbiturate is not the sole anesthetic agent used during a painful procedure.

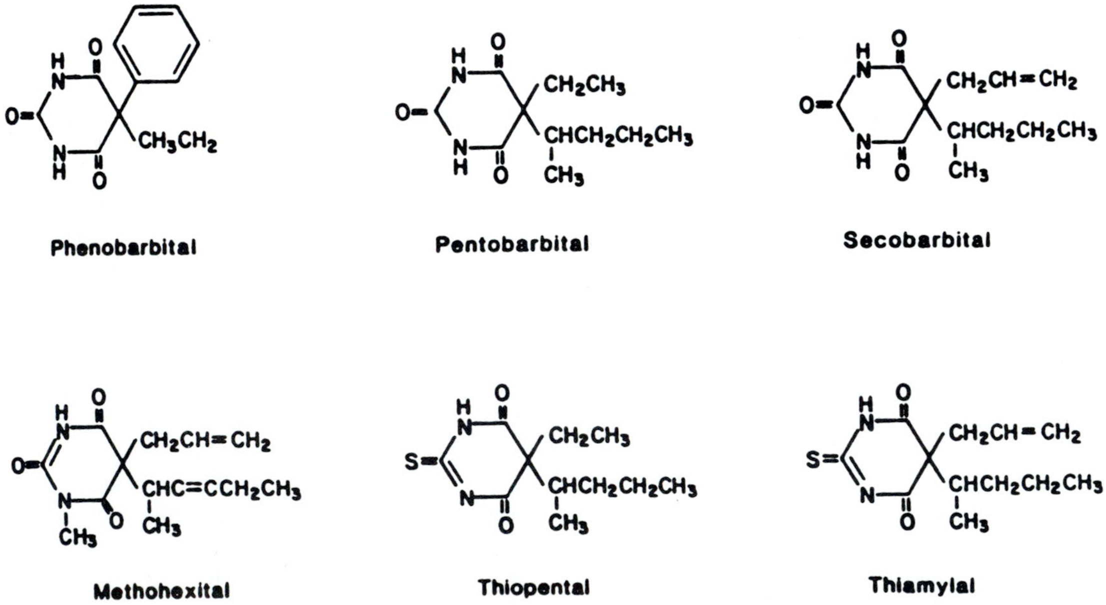

FIGURE 9–2. Structures of useful barbiturate sedative/hypnotics.

TABLE 9–1. Typical Doses of Nonopioid Intravenous Anesthetics*

	Oral Premedication	Intramuscular Premedication	Intravenous Sedation	Intravenous Induction	Intravenous Infusion (Anesthesia)
Thiopental (Thiamylal†)	N/A	N/A	0.5–1.0 mg/kg repeated prn	3–5 mg/kg	Rarely used‡
Midazolam§	0.05–0.1 mg/kg	0.05–0.01 mg/kg	0.5–1.0 mg repeated prn	0.1–0.3 mg/kg	0.001 mg/kg/min
Ketamine	N/A	N/A	0.1–0.3 mg/kg repeated prn	IV: 0.5–2.0 mg/kg (IM: 5 mg/kg)	0.03–0.10 mg/kg/min; the less with N_2O; the greater doses when given alone
Propofol	N/A	N/A	0.025–0.075 mg/kg/min	1–2.5 mg/kg	0.05–0.15 mg/kg/min
Etomidate	N/A	N/A	0.005–0.01 mg/kg/min	0.3 mg/kg	0.01 mg/kg/min with N_2O

* Doses are for healthy 70 kg adults, unless otherwise specified.

† Thiamylal may be used interchangeably with thiopental.

‡ Intravenous infusions of thiopental are rarely used to maintian anesthesia, because the rate must continually be adjusted downward in the first hours of use to avoid relative overdose and prolonged emergence. Infusions ajusted to achieve blood concentrations of 10 to 20 μg/ml can be used. (See Crankshaw DP, Boyd MD, Bjorksten AR. Plasma drug efflux—a new approach to optimization of drug infusion for constant blood concentration of thiopental and methohexital. Anesthesiology 1987;67:32.

§ Of the benzodiazepines, midazolam's water solubility and rapid kinetics make it the most useful in anesthesia practice. Diazepam may be substituted, in two or three times the doses shown for midazolam, but it is not absorbed well after IM injection.

Thiopental

PHYSICAL PROPERTIES

Like all the intravenous barbiturates, thiopental is water-soluble and stable in aqueous solution for weeks. Generally prepared as the sodium salt, thiopental in solution is quite alkaline; a 2.5 per cent solution has a pH of 10.5. This alkalinity makes thiopental incompatible with many other drugs that are acidic (opiates, catecholamines, some neuromuscular blockers). Because extravasation of an alkaline substance such as thiopental is quite painful and may result in skin necrosis, the drug is injected only into a freely flowing intravenous system.

Inadvertent intra-arterial injection is a more serious complication. This usually occurs at the antecubital space, but can occur in any place where vein and artery are in close proximity. Especially in an emergency, it is easy to cannulate by mistake an anomalous radial artery at the wrist. Arterial injection produces severe pain immediately. A chemical endarteritis, which may damage even deep layers of the vessel wall, occurs rapidly, followed by thrombosis. Damage is related to the concentration of drug injected. A 5 per cent solution (contraindicated in current practice) will readily damage vascular tissue, whereas serious injury is much less likely at 2.5 per cent, the standard concentration used in clinical practice. There is no clear treatment of choice after intra-arterial injection, but several reasonable measures may be applied. If the needle is still in place, 10 ml of 0.5 per cent lidocaine may be injected to decrease the effects of alkaline extravasation. Because the mechanism of injury appears to be vasospasm, the injection of an alpha-adrenergic blocker such as phentolamine has been suggested. Heparin has also been suggested, because thrombosis is common. A subsequent stellate ganglion block might also promote vasodilatation.

PHARMACOLOGY

The physicochemical properties of thiopental determine its pharmacokinetics. Given as an intravenous bolus of 3 to 5 mg per kg, thiopental rapidly reaches its peak concentration in the central circulation. With a pKa of 7.6, approximately 60 per cent of the drug exists in the un-ionized form at physiologic pH of 7.4, and the drug is lipid-soluble. For these reasons, there is rapid diffusion of thiopental into the "vessel-rich group" (VRG) of organs (VRG), namely heart, lungs, brain, and kidneys (Fig. 9–3). The brain concentration of thiopental increases quickly and unconsciousness ensues within 10 to 15 seconds.

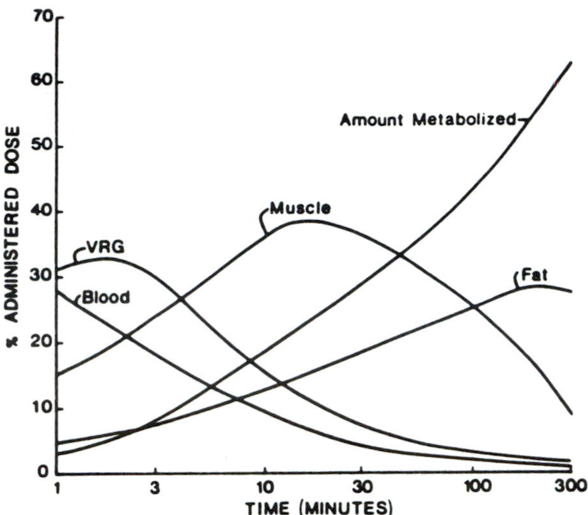

FIGURE 9–3. After a bolus of thiopental is given intravenously at time 0, the blood level decreases steadily from its maximum value as the drug is redistributed. After the first three minutes, the thiopental levels in the vessel-rich group (VRG) (including the brain) decrease as well. The less well-perfused muscle does not experience the maximum thiopental level until 15 to 30 minutes after the injection and the even less well-perfused fat reaches the maximum thiopental level hours later. (Reproduced with permission from Saidman LJ. Uptake, distribution and elimination of barbiturates. In Eger EI, ed. Anesthetic uptake and action. Baltimore: Williams & Wilkins, 1974.)

The peak concentration of drug achieved after intravenous bolus is a function of the initial volume of distribution for thiopental, which decreases with the patient's age (Fig. 9–4). Because of this, thiopental dose requirements decrease with the patient's age also.

When first introduced, the short duration of action of thiopental was thought to result from rapid metabolism; it is now clear that the short duration of action is due to rapid redistribution of the drug (see Chapter 7). Although body fat is an important reservoir of lipid-soluble drugs like thiopental (fat:blood partition coefficient = 11), the blood supply to fat is meager compared to other organs, so that entry of thiopental into fat is a slow process. Accumulation in fat occurs only after hours and release back into the circulation is similarly delayed. In clinical practice, this reservoir phenomenon is only important after very large doses, generally given by long-term constant infusion.

The degree of plasma protein binding and tissue binding of barbiturates parallels their lipid solubility. From 70 to 85 per cent of an injected dose of thiopental is bound to albumin, leaving only 15 to 30 per cent free as the active substance capable of producing tissue levels. The degree of protein binding may be reduced in disease states such as cirrhosis (decreased protein levels) or if other substances compete with thiopental and occupy some binding sites (phenylbutazone, some sulfonamides, nonsteroidal anti-inflammatory drugs including aspirin, or urea in patients with renal failure). With fewer binding sites available, more free drug enters tissue and exerts a pharmacologic effect. Acidosis also reduces protein binding. In any of these clinical situations of reduced protein binding, the dose of thiopental must be reduced.

Elimination of thiopental depends on metabolism, because less than 1 per cent is excreted unchanged in the urine. All thiobarbiturates undergo a small amount of metabolism in brain and kidneys, but for practical purposes the liver is the site of drug biotransformation. Oxybarbiturates are metabolized exclusively in the liver. In the liver, barbiturates are converted to inactive compounds with increased water solubility to facilitate urinary excretion. Thiopental is metabolized at the rate of about 10 to 14 per cent per hour, chiefly by oxidation of side chains at the number 5 carbon, desulfuration of the number 2 carbon atom, and hydrolysis of the barbituric acid ring. Thiopental has a hepatic extraction ratio of 0.1 to 0.2, implying capacity-dependent elimination (see Chapter 7).

The impact of hepatic clearance rates on elim-

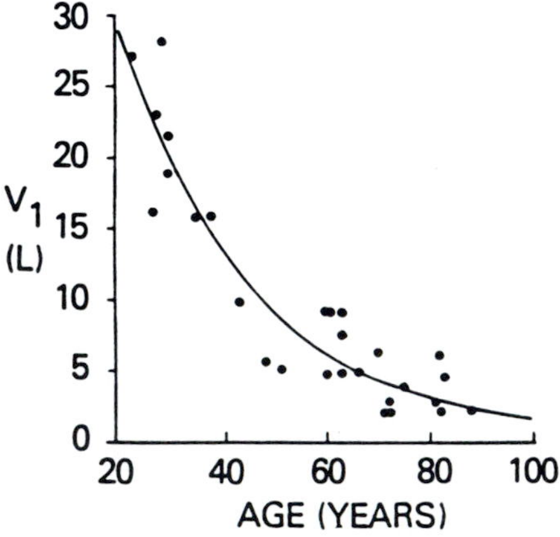

FIGURE 9–4. The initial volume of distribution of thiopental decreases markedly with age. (Reproduced with permission from Homer TD, Stanski DR. The effect of increasing age on thiopental disposition and anesthetic requirement. Anesthesiology 1985; 62:714.)

ination is clearly demonstrated when thiopental and methohexital are compared. Both these drugs have similar volumes of distribution and distribution half-times, but methohexital is cleared more rapidly, owing to its greater hepatic clearance (hepatic extraction ratio of 0.5 to 0.6).

Protein binding limits the glomerular filtration of thiopental, and its lipid solubility favors tubular reabsorption. Consequently, less than 1 per cent of a thiopental dose is excreted unchanged in the urine. Of all the barbiturates, only phenobarbital, which is not greatly protein bound, is excreted in the urine in significant amounts.

For reasons that are not well understood, patients may develop acute tolerance to thiopental. Even during the course of a brief anesthetic, the dose requirement may increase.

CLINICAL EFFECTS

For rapid induction of general anesthesia, thiopental has received wide acceptance among patients and clinicians alike. It is also used as an adjunct to general anesthesia. Its antianalgesic property limits its usefulness as a solitary anesthetic agent, except for brief procedures that are not painful.

As an induction agent, thiamylal is indistinguishable from thiopental. Methohexital also rapidly induces sleep, and recovery is usually quicker than with thiopental; involuntary muscle activity limits its application. Methohexital is most useful in very brief procedures such as cardioversion or electroconvulsive therapy.

The CNS effects of thiopental go beyond producing unconsciousness. Adequate levels of thiopental depress cortical brain activity measured on the electroencephalogram (EEG) to the point of electrical silence. Correlated with this EEG suppression is decreased brain metabolism, evidenced by decreased cerebral oxygen consumption, and a corresponding decrease in cerebral blood flow. Once enough thiopental has been given to produce electrical silence in the EEG, additional doses of thiopental produce no further reduction in brain metabolism, suggesting that the reduction in metabolism is related to the specialized electrochemical functions of neuronal tissue. The metabolism present when the EEG is flat presumably represents the basal metabolic requirements of cell function (e.g., maintaining cell membrane integrity). Further reductions in brain metabolism can be achieved if the body temperature is reduced.

In patients with severe brain injury and increased intracranial pressure, an induction dose of thiopental reduces pressure in most cases. When used for this purpose, thiopental must be given carefully, so as not to reduce arterial blood pressure and decrease the net cerebral perfusion pressure (see Chapter 30).

Thiopental may have profound impact on the cardiovascular system in some patients and virtually no effect in others. Healthy patients given typical doses of 3 to 5 mg per kg may experience a transient decrease in arterial blood pressure that usually elicits a mild compensatory tachycardia and return of blood pressure toward normal. In this situation, there is little cardiac depression. Presumably, the initial decrease in pressure is due to increased venous capacitance and subsequent decreased venous return secondary to depression of the medullary vasomotor center and depression of central sympathetic nervous system activity. This is followed by a baroreceptor-mediated increase in sympathetic nervous activity, increasing contractility, heart rate, and venous return.

In isolated heart muscle preparations, thiopental clearly has a negative inotropic effect. Large doses in otherwise healthy patients, or standard doses in patients with limited ability to activate a baroreceptor reflex response, produce the clinical picture of myocardial depression. Patients taking beta-adrenergic antagonists or certain antihypertensive drugs may have impaired baroreceptor compensatory ability. Hypovolemic patients are particularly likely to become hypotensive after the usual doses of thiopental, because they are dependent on intrinsic catecholamine stimulation to maintain blood pressure. Following a standard dose of thiopental, normal compensatory reflexes will be blunted and the hypovolemic patient will be less able to compensate for venous pooling. Adequate volume repletion, slow incremental dosing (beginning with doses of 0.5 to 1.0 mg per kg), and sympathomimetic drugs all play a role in preventing and treating thiopental-induced hypotension in these patients.

Thiopental produces a dose-dependent depression of medullary and pontine respiratory centers. Following an induction dose, the patient typically takes a large breath, then becomes apneic for a short period. Carbon dioxide responsiveness is blunted in a dose-dependent fashion, with virtually no response at deep levels of anesthesia. Ventilatory responses to hypoxia are also blunted. As the drug redistributes, the patient resumes breathing with small tidal volumes and increased respiratory rate, resulting in a modest decrease in minute ventilation.

Apnea following induction of anesthesia is managed by administering oxygen before giving thiopental (denitrogenation, described in Chapter 13) and by manual ventilation, if necessary. Aggressive positive pressure ventilation may lead to coughing, hiccups, or laryngospasm. It is not clear that thiopental increases airway irritability; this may result from manipulation of the airway in any lightly anesthetized patient. Thiopental is not contraindicated in asthmatic patients, but the dose of thiopental must be adequate and the airway must not be manipulated until the patient is adequately anesthetized (often with a potent vapor).

Although the recommended dose of thiopental for induction of anesthesia is 3 to 5 mg per kg, this varies among patients, mostly because of the additive effects of premedications or other drugs, but also because of intercurrent disease (such as hypovolemia, cardiac disease) or old age. In addition to these anticipated instances, there remain patients who unexpectedly require less than 2.5 mg per kg or more than 6 mg per kg for induction. The first group is at risk of overdose. Some anesthesiologists routinely administer a small dose of thiopental (25 to 50 mg, the "test dose") to verify that the drug does not escape into the subcutaneous tissue and to assess the patient's response before giving additional drug; this precaution is prudent for any patient who might be sensitive to barbiturates for any reason.

BENZODIAZEPINES

The benzodiazepines are commonly used as premedicants or adjuncts to regional or general anesthesia, and only in certain clinical situations as induction agents. In some ways, these drugs are preferable to the barbiturates: they often produce amnesia; the therapeutic index is usually greater; there is less cardiovascular and respiratory depression; tolerance is rare. However, large doses are usually required to produce unconsciousness, and the duration of effect is longer than that of the ultra–short-acting barbiturates. The commonest benzodiazepines in anesthetic practice are diazepam, lorazepam, and midazolam.

Benzodiazepines are made up of a benzene ring and a seven-member diazepine ring. All the clinically useful benzodiazepines also contain a 5-aryl substituent ring at number 5 carbon. Lorazepam and diazepam are similar in structure, whereas midazolam incorporates an imidazole ring structure also.

Mechanisms of Action

The benzodiazepines exert their action at specific receptor sites, mostly on postsynaptic nerve endings in the CNS, producing very little pharmacologic effect outside the CNS. Sedation by benzodiazepines results from facilitation of the inhibitory neurotransmitter gamma-aminobutyric acid (GABA). The benzodiazepine receptors and the GABA receptors are separate, but closely linked. When a benzodiazepine drug occupies its own site on a subunit of the GABA receptor site, the affinity of GABA and its receptor sites is increased; inhibition of nerve conduction and sedation follow. If the benzodiazepine receptor is occupied by an antagonist, GABA-mediated transmission is blocked and the sedative effects of benzodiazepines are prevented.

Flumazenil, an imidazobenzodiazepine, binds to benzodiazepine receptors, where it competitively inhibits binding and allosteric effects of the therapeutic benzodiazepines. It is the first of the specific benzodiazepine antagonists subjected to clinical trial. Flumazenil may be useful in reversing the sedative effects of long-acting benzodiazepines or to treat drug overdose. Interestingly, flumazenil may also ameliorate some of the neurologic sequelae of hepatic encephalopathy that are presumably related to accumulation of endogenous benzodiazepine-like substances. Aminophylline may also antagonize benzodiazepines.

Diazepam

Relatively insoluble in water, diazepam is dissolved in propylene glycol and sodium benzoate for parenteral use. These organic solvents make parenteral injection painful and absorption after intramuscular (IM) injection unreliable; the IM route is not recommended. Diazepam is rapidly absorbed from the gastrointestinal tract, especially in children.

Although lipid soluble and rapidly taken up in CNS tissue, the onset of action of diazepam is not rapid. The reason for this delayed onset is unclear and may relate either to the pharmacokinetics or pharmacodynamics of the drug. Like thiopental, this lipid-soluble drug distributes rapidly into well-perfused organs, then redistributes, decreasing the plasma concentration and enhancing recovery.

Lipid solubility of benzodiazepines corresponds to protein binding; thus, diazepam is extensively bound. The free fraction of diazepam is blood is only about 1 to 2 per cent of the total; the rest tightly binds to albumin. Anything that affects protein binding influences the amount of free drug available. Large increases in the free fraction of drug may occur in hepatic and renal disease, markedly increasing sensitivity to the drug. In hepatic disease, the increased volume of distribution and reduced drug metabolism may double the elimination half-life. In renal disease, drug metabolism is maintained, so the increased fraction of free drug leads to a two- to threefold increase in hepatic metabolism and reduces the elimination half-life. Elimination is prolonged in the elderly due to increased volume of distribution and decreased protein binding, rather than changes in hepatic clearance.

The duration of action of diazepam is not as short as that of thiopental, partly because of the way diazepam is metabolized. Metabolism occurs principally in the liver where oxidative metabolism produces several active metabolites including desmethyldiazepam, 3-hydroxydiazepam, and oxazepam (itself a commercially available sedative). These active metabolites produce their own benzodiazepine effect, prolonging CNS depression, especially after multiple doses of diazepam. In addition, enterohepatic circulation may also contribute to the prolonged CNS effects of diazepam. Oxidative metabolism of diazepam may be reduced by other drugs, such as cimetidine. The lipid-soluble oxidative metabolites of diazepam are conjugated in the liver to water-soluble glucuronides, then excreted in the urine. The relatively large volume of distribution (1 to 1.5 L per kg), small clearance (0.2 to 0.5 ml per kg per minute), and small hepatic extraction ratio (0.01 to 0.025), imply a terminal elimination half-life of 20 to 40 hours.

CLINICAL USES

The principal clinical uses of diazepam are as an oral premedicant (0.1 to 0.2 mg per kg), an intravenous sedating agent during regional anesthesia (0.03 to 0.07 mg per kg doses repeated as needed), and rarely as an induction agent (0.5 mg per kg). The benzodiazepines have no analgesic properties. Diazepam reduces the minimum alveolar concentration (MAC) of inhalation anesthetics; a premedication dose of 0.2 mg per kg reduces the halothane requirement by nearly 30 per cent.

Although an intravenous bolus of diazepam, 10 mg, can occasionally produce apnea, an increase in Pa_{CO_2} usually is not seen until the intravenous dose reaches 0.2 mg per kg. Tidal volume is decreased. In the dose range 0.2 to 0.4 mg per kg, respiratory depression is seen within minutes after intravenous administration and typically persists for 30 minutes or more. Depression of mental status tends to correlate with the degree of respiratory depression. Diazepam, in combination with other respiratory depressant drugs or chronic lung disease, may produce substantial and prolonged respiratory depression.

Large doses of diazepam are occasionally used to induce general anesthesia for long operations, although most anesthesiologists prefer midazolam for this purpose because intravenous diazepam causes pain and subsequent phlebitis. Induction is much slower than with thiopental. At doses of 0.5 to 1.0 mg per kg, diazepam produces only a modest decrease in blood pressure, cardiac output, and vascular resistance. Because baroreceptor reflexes are blunted, compensatory tachycardia is generally not seen. Inhibition of compensatory reflexes is less with diazepam than with barbiturates and inhalation agents, but may cause significant decrease in blood pressure in hypovolemic patients. Following diazepam induction, nitrous oxide does not lead to myocardial depression as it does in the presence of narcotics.

Lorazepam

Lorazepam is five to ten times as potent as diazepam, but resembles it in its clinical effects on the cardiovascular and respiratory systems. Lorazepam reliably produces anterograde amnesia.

Like diazepam, lorazepam is insoluble in water, so it must be dissolved in propylene glycol (or polyethylene glycol). However, it is less painful on injection than diazepam and causes less phlebitis. Unlike diazepam, intramuscular injections as well as oral doses are reliably absorbed. Following absorption, onset of action is quite slow. Peak plasma levels after oral administration are achieved in two to four hours, and effects persist for up to 24 to 48 hours.

Lorazepam has a smaller volume of distribution (0.8 to 1.3 L per kg) and greater clearance (0.75 to 1.0 ml per kg per minute) than diazepam. The elimination half-life is 10 to 20 hours. Elimination is unaffected by renal disease but is prolonged in cirrhosis.

The usual dose of lorazepam as for oral premedication is 50 μg per kg to a maximum dose of 4 mg. This usually produces amnesia without excessive sedation. The slow onset and long duration of lorazepam make it unsuitable for outpatients. Drugs with shorter onset and shorter duration are favored as adjuncts to regional anesthesia.

Midazolam

Midazolam is two to three times as potent as diazepam. Unlike other benzodiazepines, midazolam incorporates an imidazole ring that makes it stable in aqueous solutions. The drug is prepared in solutions buffered to a pH of 3.5; the open imidazole ring makes the drug water soluble and painless on injection, because solubilizing agents are unnecessary. Absorption after intramuscular injection is rapid and dependable. Above pH 4 (at physiologic pH), the imidazole ring closes, making the molecule lipid soluble. Midazolam is bound to plasma albumin (95 per cent).

The drug may be given orally. Absorption from the gastrointestinal tract is rapid, but a substantial first pass effect allows only half the drug to reach the systemic circulation. After intravenous injection, peak effect is reached in three to five minutes. Peak effect after intramuscular injection occurs in 15 to 30 minutes. To a great extent, the brief action of midazolam is due to tissue redistribution of the lipid-soluble molecule. Metabolism occurs in the liver by oxidation to metabolites that are then conjugated and excreted in the urine. Some metabolites, such as 1-hydroxymethylmidazolam, are active and contribute to the CNS effects. The volume of distribution of midazolam is similar to that of diazepam (1 to 1.5 L per kg), but the clearance is nearly ten times greater (4 to 8 ml per kg per minute) due to increased hepatic metabolism (hepatic extraction ratio 0.2 to 0.4). The elimination half-life of a midazolam is two to four hours, substantially less than that of other benzodiazepines. The kinetics do not appear to be affected by advancing age. Because the drug is almost totally metabolized, elimination is not affected by renal disease.

Midazolam decreases cerebral blood flow and metabolism, and does not worsen diminished intracranial compliance. Respiratory depression is similar to that produced by diazepam in equipotent doses. An induction dose of midazolam (0.2 mg per kg) induces cardiovascular changes similar to those seen during thiopental induction (3 to 4 mg per kg): a decrease in blood pressure and compensatory increase in heart rate. The decrease in blood pressure is exaggerated in hypovolemic patients.

Midazolam is an anxiolytic, sedative, and amnestic drug. Amnesia is dose related and, like respiratory depression, tends to parallel the sedative effect. An intravenous dose of 5 mg produces 20 to 30 minutes of amnesia. Intramuscular injection often produces amnesia of even longer duration. Midazolam 0.05 to 0.1 mg per kg orally or intramuscularly is an effective premedication.

One of the most popular clinical applications of midazolam is sedation during regional anesthesia or during diagnostic or therapeutic procedures. Intravenous doses of 0.5 to 2 mg (up to 0.1 mg per kg) are titrated to effect. Patients have less postoperative sedation than after diazepam, but time to complete recovery is unchanged. Like other benzodiazepines, midazolam has no analgesic properties.

Midazolam can be used to induce anesthesia, in doses of 0.1 to 0.3 mg per kg given intravenously over 30 to 60 seconds. Because induction time is considerably shorter with thiopental, midazolam is not a popular drug for induction of anesthesia. It can also be used as an infusion to supplement nitrous oxide/narcotic-relaxant anesthesia, in doses of approximately 1 μg per kg per minute.

KETAMINE

An arylcyclohexylamine related to phencyclidine (PCP), ketamine produces a unique state often called "dissociative anesthesia," reminiscent of a cataleptic condition, as well as profound analgesia. Patients given ketamine may appear to be awake: the eyes often remain open, a slow nystagmus creates the illusion that the patient is gazing about and muscular activity that appears purposeful all contribute to the illusion. In fact, the patient is unaware and has no recollection of events under ketamine anesthesia.

Ketamine is a water-soluble molecule with an asymmetric carbon. Its optical isomers have quite different pharmacologic effects (the positive isomer is a better analgesic and produces less delirium), suggesting specific receptor site interaction. Commercial preparations are racemic mixtures of equal amounts of each isomer. The exact mechanism of action is not known, but analgesia is thought to result from lamina-specific suppression of spinal cord activity that interrupts transmission of the affective component of pain signals to the brain.

Following intramuscular injection, bioavailability is 90 per cent, and peak blood levels are achieved within 15 minutes. Like thiopental, its lipid solubility (5 to 10 times that of thiopental) contributes to rapid onset of the drug. About 45 to 50 per cent of ketamine is bound to plasma proteins, principally alpha 1-acid glycoprotein; therefore, more free drug is available for action compared to thiopental. Neither renal failure nor hepatic enzyme induction influence the duration of the drug's effect, suggesting that redistribution plays the major role in the short duration of action of ketamine (distribution half-life is approximately 7 to 17 minutes).

Because only 5 per cent of the dose is recovered unchanged in the urine, metabolism is the important route of clearance. Hepatic clearance is 18 ml per kg per minute, with a hepatic extraction ratio of 0.9. Volume of distribution is also rather large—3 L per kg—resulting in an elimination half-life of two to three hours. Hepatic metabolism of ketamine, mostly oxidative, is complex and produces at least eight metabolites. One of these, formed via demethylation by cytochrome P-450 enzymes, is norketamine, an active metabolite with about one-third the potency of ketamine. This substance may be responsible for prolonging the CNS effects of ketamine. Prolonged use of ketamine induces hepatic metabolic enzymes, and tolerance eventually develops.

Respiratory depression is also related to dose, but at typical anesthetic doses of 2 mg per kg only modest depression is seen. Upper airway skeletal muscle tone is well maintained with ketamine, and airway reflexes are less blunted than with the usual doses of other induction agents, but the risk of aspiration and airway obstruction is still present. Ketamine relaxes bronchial smooth muscle and is a useful drug for induction of anesthesia in patients with asthma. Stimulation of oral secretions can be a problem with ketamine; these are best handled with an antisialagogue such as glycopyrrolate.

Emergence delirium occurs in 5 to 30 per cent of patients—especially in women over age 16 and in patients with personality disorders—with doses greater than 2 mg per kg. Patients experience visual and auditory illusions and a confused state that may progress to true delirium. Vivid, unpleasant dreams, often with morbid content, may occur up to 24 hours later. Premedication with benzodiazepines helps prevent delirium, but not some of the proprioceptive illusions (a ''floating'' sensation) or dreaming in the postoperative period. Thiopental and inhalation agents also decrease the incidence of delirium. Atropine and droperidol increase the incidence of postoperative delirium and are avoided if ketamine is to be used. In some hospitals, patients emerging from ketamine anesthesia are kept in a quiet area, but there is no evidence that this reduces the incidence or severity of emergence delirium.

Ketamine indirectly produces a dose-related increase in heart rate and arterial blood pressure, secondary to central CNS stimulation. This indirect cardiovascular stimulation makes ketamine useful in patients who require rapid sequence induction of anesthesia but who might become hypotensive with thiopental; these include trauma patients with partially corrected hypovolemia and patients with restrictive pericarditis or tamponade. The use of ketamine does not eliminate the need for appropriate monitoring and treatment with volume expansion for these patients, especially because the autonomic compensatory reflexes may be at maximum capacity already, allowing the direct depressant effects of the drug to predominate. Ketamine is not usually chosen for patients with hypertension or coronary artery disease, in whom hypertension or tachycardia are undesirable.

Ketamine increases cerebral blood flow and may cause a dangerous increase in intracranial pressure in patients with reduced intracranial compliance, making it unsuitable for patients with a suspected mass lesion in the brain.

The usual dose for induction of anesthesia is 0.5 to 2 mg per kg given intravenously; it can be continued as an infusion by itself to maintain ketamine anesthesia (50 to 100 μg per kg per minute) or in lesser doses (40 μg per kg per minute or less) as a supplement to nitrous oxide and narcotics in a balanced technique. Ketamine acts rapidly when given via the intramuscular route (5 mg per kg), making it useful when there is no intravenous access. Given in small intravenous increments (0.1 to 0.3 mg per kg), ketamine can provide analgesia without loss of consciousness; it is occasionally used in this manner to produce brief periods of analgesia for burn dressing changes or vaginal delivery.

PROPOFOL

Propofol is a new intravenous anesthetic agent, similar in action to thiopental. It is a sedative/hypnotic, and a rapid-acting induction agent that can be used to maintain anesthesia by constant infusion. Formerly known as disoprofol, it is an alkyl phenol that is insoluble in water. Initially, it was dissolved in Cremophore EL, a substance that led to anaphylactic reactions. Propofol was withdrawn from clinical use, then reformulated as an aqueous emulsion of soy bean oil, glycerol, and egg phosphatide. The emulsion may produce pain on intravenous injection, especially into a small vein, but the formulation is greatly improved overall.

Unconsciousness usually follows in less than a minute after an intravenous induction dose of 2 to 2.5 mg per kg. With a three-compartment model, elimination half-life from well-perfused tissues ($t1/2\beta$) is 0.5 to 1.0 hours, and terminal elimination has a half-life of three to six hours. This suggests slow return of propofol from poorly perfused tissue such as fat, especially after prolonged infusion. Clearance of propofol is reduced in the elderly, but not significantly lessened by renal or hepatic disease. In the liver, the drug is metabolized to water-soluble glucuronide and sulfate conjugates, and then excreted in the urine. Total clearance of propofol (30 to 60 ml per kg per minute) exceeds hepatic blood flow, implying extrahepatic sites of metabolism. Metabolites are inactive.

An induction dose of propofol reduces arterial blood pressure by about 30 per cent without much effect on heart rate. This appears to result from reduced systemic vascular resistance rather than reduction of stroke volume or cardiac output. Compared to thiopental, propofol is associated with greater reductions in blood pressure but smaller changes in heart rate.

Compared to thiopental, the incidence of apnea on induction with propofol is similar, but the duration of apnea may be greater. A 2 to 2.5 mg per kg intravenous bolus of propofol produces 30 to 90 seconds of apnea in 60 per cent of unpremedicated patients. After narcotic premedication, essentially all patients become apneic on induction with propofol. During infusion of propofol, respiratory rate may increase, but minute ventilation is reduced. Narcotics further reduce respiratory drive.

The major advantage of propofol over other induction agents is its rapid clearance and the fact that so few residual effects are seen on awakening. After short procedures under propofol anesthesia, patients awaken quickly. This has made the drug particularly useful for outpatients.

Propofol is used as an induction agent followed by other general anesthetic agents, as a supplement to general anesthesia, or as a total intravenous anesthetic. Given at the rate of about 40 mg every 10 seconds to a total dose of 1 to 2.5 mg per kg, induction is rapid, occasionally accompanied by hiccups (15 per cent) or spontaneous muscle activity (25 per cent). Infusion rates of 0.05 to 0.2 mg per kg per minute, given by automated infusion pump, can be adjusted to maintain anesthesia as a supplement to nitrous oxide; infusions at half these rates suffice for sedation.

ETOMIDATE

Like midazolam, etomidate contains a imidazole ring that makes it water-soluble to acid pH and lipid-soluble at physiologic pH. An induction dose of 0.3 mg per kg rapidly produces unconsciousness, followed by awakening in 3 to 12 minutes. Awakening is more rapid than with thiopental, and there is less grogginess. Etomidate has no analgesic properties.

The volume of distribution is large, consistent with substantial tissue uptake. Approximately 75 per cent of etomidate is bound to albumin. Both hepatic enzymes and plasma esterases are responsible for the hydrolysis of etomidate to its carboxylic acid ester, an inactive substance. Nearly 85 per cent of an administered dose is metabolized to this ester and excreted in the urine; another 10 to 13 per cent appears in bile. The total clearance rate of etomidate is about five times the clearance of thiopental; its elimination half-life is two to five hours. Dose requirements are reduced in the elderly due to a reduced volume of distribution.

Like thiopental, etomidate reduces cerebral blood flow, cerebral metabolism, and intracranial pressure. Etomidate also decreases intraocular pressure. Like methohexital, it may also stimulate seizure activity. About one third of patients will manifest myoclonic muscle movements during induction. This is presumably caused by subcortical disinhibition of normally suppressed extrapyramidal tract motor activity. Premedication with a narcotic or benzodiazepine reduces the incidence of myoclonus.

One of the major advantages of etomidate is its minimal impact on hemodynamics. Following an induction dose of 0.3 mg per kg, there is little change in heart rate, stroke volume, or cardiac output. Arterial blood pressure may decrease 10 to 15 per cent owing to a corresponding decrease in peripheral vascular resistance.

An induction dose of etomidate given rapidly may produce transient apnea, but there is generally little effect on minute ventilation once respiration resumes. In the presence of narcotics, respiratory depression may be substantial, especially if etomidate is given by infusion.

Adrenocortical suppression by etomidate was first noted in critically ill patients receiving continuous infusions of the drug. The phenomenon has been documented after a single dose, producing decreased plasma cortisol levels and impaired responsiveness to ACTH lasting four to eight hours after the single bolus. Adrenocortical suppression could limit the normal physiologic response to stress in a critically ill patient given etomidate, although the clinical significance of this effect remains undocumented.

Induction with etomidate is associated with an increased incidence of postoperative nausea and vomiting compared to thiopental. This may be reduced with droperidol premedication.

Although myoclonic movements, adrenocortical suppression, and an increased incidence of nausea and vomiting limit its usefulness, etomidate may be a good alternative to thiopental in the patient with unstable cardiac disease. It may also be used for brief outpatient procedures, although either propofol or a short acting barbiturate seem more appropriate. Intravenous induction requires 0.3 mg per kg; to maintain anesthesia with nitrous oxide requires about 0.01 mg per kg per minute; brief intravenous sedation can be provided with infusions at half this rate.

REFERENCES

Dundee JW, Wyant GM. Intravenous anaesthesia. 2nd ed. New York: Churchill Livingstone, 1988.

Fragen RJ, Shanks CA, Moltgeni A, Avram MJ. Effects of etomidate on hormonal response to surgical stress. Anesthesiology 1984; 60:652.

Hudson RJ, Stanski DR, Burch PG. Pharmacokinetics of methohexital and thiopental in surgical patients. Anesthesiology 1983; 59:215.

CHAPTER TEN

OPIOIDS IN ANESTHESIA PRACTICE

The opiates come from the juice of the poppy, *Papaver somniferum*. Crude opium has been in use for its analgesic actions for more than 2000 years. During the United States Civil War, morphine given by injection was first used widely for treating wounded soldiers. *Opiates* occur naturally, while *opioids* are synthetic or semisynthetic compounds. The term *opioid* is also used generally to describe any compound that binds to the opiate receptor. Most of the semisynthetic compounds are chemical modifications of morphine.

Anesthesiologists administer opioids as premedicants, analgesics, and anesthetics via the intramuscular, intravenous, oral, epidural, subarachnoid, and transcutaneous routes. Although there are significant differences among the opioids, they have many physiologic effects in common. Some of these can be predicted from opiate receptor pharmacology; others, especially interactions with anesthetics, are not fully understood (Table 10–1).

OPIATE RECEPTORS

Specific receptors for opioids have been identified and subclassified, along with endogenous compounds having opioid activity. To date, these compounds include the enkephalins, endorphins, and dynorphins. The physiologic roles of these compounds are not entirely clear, but their identification has aided understanding the locations and specificities of opioid receptors. Specific peptide binding studies have led to classification of the receptors into types: mu, kappa, delta and sigma. The mu, kappa, and delta receptors mediate analgesia. Sigma receptors are responsible for dysphoric effects. Delta receptors are also thought to affect behavior in response to pain. The combined actions of different receptor types may act together to produce analgesia (Table 10–2).

Some opioids have agonist, some antagonist, and others mixed effects on opiate receptors. Morphine is a typical agonist, with its major actions mediated by the mu receptor. Antagonists have no effect on normal patients, but reverse the effects of administered agonists by inhibiting mu effects. They also precipitate withdrawal in opiate-addicted patients. Agonist/antagonists produce significant analgesia and generally less sedation than pure agonists, but their greater sigma receptor activity often produces dysphoria.

All the effects of opioids cannot be explained by what is now known about receptor pharmacology. However, mu receptor activity decreases spontaneous neuronal activity in the central nervous system (CNS) and gastrointestinal (GI) tract, and inhibits excitatory inputs to the dorsal horn areas of the spinal cord as well. These CNS and GI actions may explain such actions of opioids as nausea, respiratory depression, and somnolence; the spinal cord effects may modulate pain perception.

TABLE 10–1. Clinical Uses of Opioids in Anesthesia

Use	Advantages	Disadvantages
Premedication	Analgesia for preoperative pain, as with fractures Reduced doses of induction agents	Respiratory depression before the patient reaches the OR Intraoperative respiratory depression Nausea
Adjunct to induction	Reduced cough Reduced doses of induction agents Reduced hypertension or tachycardia with intubation	Prolonged apnea after IV induction Hypotension or bradycardia
High-dose narcotic anesthesia	Minimal cardiac depression Reduced hypertension and tachycardia	Prolonged apnea postoperatively Awareness Hypotension Postoperative mechanical ventilation required
Component of mixed or balanced anesthesia	Analgesia: reduced catechol secretion Decreases MAC, reduces dose of other agents	May slow emergence Postoperative respiratory depression

ACTIONS OF OPIOIDS

The various opioids are more alike than different in their major effects.

Analgesia

Opioids both diminish the sensations of pain and alter patients' responses to pain. After receiving opioids, patients may report the presence of pain, but they are indifferent to it. This effect of opioids is specific for pain sensations; other sensory modalities remain relatively intact. Analgesic doses of opioids variably produce sedation and changes in mood as well.

Acting in the dorsal horn, intrathecal or epidural opioids initially produce segmental spinal analgesia. More central effects such as respiratory depression follow, because of the rostral spread of the drug in the spinal fluid.

TABLE 10–2. Opiate Receptor Types*

	Receptor Type			
	mu	*kappa*	*sigma*	*delta*
Agonist	*Morphine*	*Ketocyclazocine*	*SKF 10047*	*d-ala,d-leuenkephalin*
Pain	Analgesia	Analgesia	—	Weak analgesia
Pupil	Miosis	Miosis	Mydriasis	—
Respiration	Depression	—	Stimulation	Depression
Heart rate	Bradycardia	—	Tachycardia	—
Temperature	Decreased	—	—	—
Affect/mood	Indifference	Sedation	Delirium	—
Drugs				
Morphine and all analgesics	+ +	+	+	0
Naloxone	–	–	–	–
Buprenorphine	P	0	–	0
Nalbuphine	–	0	+ +	0
Nalorphine	–	0	+	0
Pentazocine	–	0	+ +	0
Butorphanol	–	0	+ +	0

* Modified from Martin WR. Multiple opioid receptors. Life Sci 1981;28:1547–1554. *Symbols*: + +, + = agonist; P = partial agonist; – = antagonist; 0 = no effect or unknown.

Pupil

Opioids cause pupillary constriction by altering the usual inhibition by the Edinger-Westphal nucleus in the brain. This sign may be an indicator of opioid effects, but it is nonspecific because other drugs and physiologic factors affect pupil size as well.

Respiratory Depression

Opioids depress breathing via a specific dose-related effect on the brainstem response to carbon dioxide. Slow, deep respirations distinguish opioid-induced depression from that of inhalation anesthetics, which is characterized by rapid, shallow breathing. The degree of depression varies from imperceptible to profound, depending on several factors. Greater doses produce greater depression, although there is significant interpatient variation. A patient who receives opioids and remains awake may have little apparent respiratory depression, but may develop profound hypoventilation or apnea after losing consciousness. Stimuli such as pain, noise, movement, or touch antagonize respiratory depression due to opioids.

The effects of the level of consciousness on respiratory depression are especially important in evaluating patients in the recovery room who have received opioids. The stimulation of being moved to the recovery room may arouse a patient who later falls asleep and becomes apneic after being left alone. Other factors, such as recirculation of opioids or clearance of a previous dose of an antagonist such as naloxone, may also contribute. Close observation of respiration and oxygenation must continue until it is clear that a somnolent patient who has received opioids breathes adequately.

Opioids also depress the cough reflex. This facilitates awake intubation of the trachea, or makes smoother a stormy induction or emergence, especially for patients with reactive airways.

Gastrointestinal

Opioids commonly cause nausea and vomiting by stimulating the chemoreceptor trigger zone in the medulla. Phenothiazines, scopolamine, or droperidol counteract this response. One droperidol-fentanyl combination, Innovar, is available for a "balanced" anesthetic technique, but the long action of droperidol in this combination can produce excessive postoperative sedation, and most anesthesiologists prefer to give these drugs separately rather than use them in a fixed dosage ratio.

Opioids also impair gastric motility and reduce secretion of gastric acid and pancreatic and biliary fluids. Paradoxically, biliary tract pressure increases, due to spasm of the sphincter of Oddi in some patients. To avoid this, opioids are often withheld from patients undergoing common bile duct exploration for stones. Preoperatively, biliary spasm may worsen pain from cholelithiasis, or mimic angina pectoris. Intraoperatively, biliary spasm may interfere with cholangiography or bile duct pressure measurements.

Other CNS Effects

There are CNS effects of opioids other than analgesia, sedation, and dysphoria. Pruritus probably represents a direct action of opioids on the CNS; the antagonist naloxone reverses the effect.

In large doses, morphine and other opioids may cause seizures, through excitation of pyramidal cells in the hippocampus. Anticonvulsant medication may not halt the seizures, but naloxone does. Without a convulsion, opioids reduce slightly the cerebral metabolic rate for oxygen, decrease cerebrospinal fluid production and slow the electroencephalogram in a dose-dependent fashion. Direct effects on cerebral circulation are minimal as long as normocarbia and normotension are maintained. If arterial P_{CO_2} increases after opioid administration, cerebral vasodilation and increased intracranial pressure may result.

Cardiovascular Effects

Direct cardiovascular effects of opioids include moderate peripheral vasodilation, but hypotension and decreased cardiac output may result from indirect mechanisms as well. Some opioids, notably morphine, provoke histamine release that in turn causes vasodilation. The combination of pain relief (which decreases sympathetic tone) with peripheral vasodilation may result in hypotension, especially if the blood volume is decreased or the patient is tilted head-up.

Opioids often slow cardiac rate by depression of the central vagal nucleus in the medulla, especially following the rapid administration of large doses, as in the induction of anesthesia. This effect is overcome by the simultaneous administration of an anticholinergic, or by using a muscle relaxant like pancuronium, which has vagolytic properties of its own. However, even large doses of opioids rarely alter cardiac rhythm or myocardial contractility.

Because opioids have so little direct depressant effect on the cardiovascular system, and because adequate doses of narcotics blunt the sympathetic responses to operation, general anesthesia based on large doses of opioids is often used for patients with impaired myocardial function or myocardial ischemia. Nevertheless, the choice of a narcotic-based anesthetic is not a panacea for the critically ill patient, as the indirect mechanisms described above can produce catastrophic hypotension, especially if the drugs are given too rapidly or in excessive amounts.

Tolerance, Addiction, and Dependence

All opioids produce tolerance and physical dependence with prolonged use. *Tolerance* represents decreased physiologic effect from a given dose of drug; the dose-response curve is shifted to the right. It probably results from both down-regulation of receptor numbers and uncoupling between receptors and their second messengers. *Addiction* is a behavior pattern of compulsive drug use and drug-seeking behavior. Physical *dependence* is a physiologic need for a drug, which may not include addictive behavior.

Tolerance can be expected but need not be feared by anesthesiologists and their patients. Patients who require opioids for long periods of time because of extensive trauma or chronic cancer pain become tolerant to opioids, requiring increasing doses to maintain pain relief, but these patients are not addicted to narcotics. This effect is often due not only to tolerance, but to progression of the disease. Patients in pain are sometimes afraid to ask for adequate analgesia or denied it because they or their physicians needlessly fear addiction.

Pain relief for postoperative patients has been improved recently by a willingness to prescribe adequate doses of opioids, and by more effective delivery methods such as long-acting oral preparations, epidural and spinal opioids, and patient-controlled analgesia (PCA). Narcotic addicts undergoing operation require opioids to prevent acute withdrawal (e.g., methadone) and to treat pain. Opioids required to treat pain must not be withheld because of the concomitant problem of addiction.

Routes of Administration

Opioids can be given orally. They undergo significant first-pass metabolism by the liver; larger oral doses than parenteral are required to produce clinical effects. For cancer pain, a common rule is that the equivalent intramuscular dose is one-half to two-thirds the oral dose.

The time of onset of an opioid's effect, especially when it is given intramuscularly, intrathecally, or epidurally, is related to its lipid solubility. Lipophilic drugs such as fentanyl act quickly because of rapid passage across the blood-brain barrier. Morphine is the least lipophilic of the opioids in clinical use. Because morphine is poorly absorbed by the spinal cord, it has the slowest onset and is most likely to cause delayed respiratory depression when given intrathecally or epidurally, as more of the administered dose is available to migrate to the brain (see Chapter 36).

Interpatient Variation

Opioid dose-response curves vary from patient to patient because of age, weight, concurrent disease, acquired tolerance, and the additive effects of anesthetics and sedatives. Elderly and debilitated patients may prove especially susceptible to narcotics. Patients with significant renal or hepatic disease may experience prolonged effects because of decreased clearance.

Other Effects

Rarely are patients truly allergic to opioids, although patients report as allergic responses side effects such as nausea. In particular, morphine and meperidine, which release histamine, can cause anaphylactoid reactions.

Opioids given to the mother move easily across the placenta and cause respiratory depression and behavioral changes in the neonate (see Chapter 26).

SPECIFIC OPIOIDS

Morphine

In addition to the general effects already listed (most of which were first described for morphine), the major distinguishing feature of morphine is its tendency to release histamine (Table 10–3). This causes peripheral vasodilation, hypotension, reflex tachycardia, and cutaneous flushing. These adverse consequences are most effectively avoided by administering morphine slowly or in divided doses. This not only allows time to respond to the drug's cardiovascular effects, but minimizes histamine release. H_1 and H_2 blockers blunt the histamine-mediated cardiovascular effects of morphine. Histamine release may also contribute to the pruritus experienced by some patients with morphine, although pruritus is a direct opioid effect as well.

The most water-soluble of the opioids in common use, morphine is 30 percent protein bound in plasma. The half-life of morphine in plasma is approximately three hours, the interval between intramuscular doses. Most of the morphine given is cleared by the liver as morphine-glucuronide; its hepatic extraction accounts for the decreased potency of orally administered morphine. About 10 per cent of morphine appears unchanged in the urine.

Fentanyl

Fentanyl is the most commonly used opioid in contemporary anesthesia practice. Lipid soluble and more potent than morphine, small intravenous doses of fentanyl (1 to 4 μg per kg) can be given to produce the rapid onset of narcotic effects, with rapid offset due to redistribution. In larger doses (10 to 50 μg per kg), it provides profound degrees of narcotic effect that require only minimal supplementation with sedatives or small concentrations of inhaled anesthetics to produce satisfactory general anesthesia.

Patients do not recover rapidly from these larger doses, because metabolic elimination instead of simple redistribution is required to reduce plasma levels below the safe threshold for spontaneous ventilation. After large doses of fentanyl, some patients experience what appears to be reoccurrence of narcotization after initial recovery. Recirculation of fentanyl from gastric pools has been demonstrated, but other factors such as lack of stimulation, the use of other sedative drugs, and the residual effects of general anesthetics undoubtedly play a part also.

Large doses of fentanyl are better tolerated than large doses of morphine, because fentanyl causes little or no histamine release. Direct cardiovascular depressant effects are minimal, and the only cardiovascular depression to be expected is that resulting from bradycardia or release from increased sympathetic tone. Although newer agents exhibit more rapid kinetics, fentanyl remains the most useful drug for opioid-based anesthesia for patients undergoing major operations.

Rapidly administered opioids sometimes cause skeletal muscle rigidity, severe enough in the chest

TABLE 10–3. Properties of Specific Opioids*

Opioid	Potency	Protein Binding (%)	t (α) (min)	t (β) (hr)	V_D (L/kg)	Cl (ml/min)	Octanol/H_2O Part Coeff
Morphine†	1	30	1.7	2–4	3–5	10–20	1.4
Meperidine†	0.1	70	4–11	3–5	3–5	8–18	39
Fentanyl	100	84	13	2–4	3–5	10–20	813
Alfentanil‡	25	92	12	1–2	0.5–1	3–8	145
Sufentanil	500–1000	93	18	2–3	2.5	10–12	1778

* Modified from Hug CC. *In* Estafanous FG. ed. Opioids in anesthesia. Stoneham, Butterworth's, 1984.

† Indicates significant histamine release: expect some vasodilation, are hypotension, reflex tachycardia, cutaneous flushing. Effects are more profound with large doses, or in hypovolemic patients.

‡ Much of offset of effect due to redistribution. Therefore, this drug is commonly used by infusion. Some clinical reports of relapse of patients in recovery room recently published.

Note: The relative potencies listed for these drugs can be deceptive if pharmacokinetic differences between drugs are ignored. For example, in single intravenous doses, 5 mg of morphine or 50 μg of fentanyl produce similar short term effects (potency ratio = 100), but for a procedure lasting an hour, appropriate doses of these drugs might be 10 mg of morphine and 500 μg of fentanyl (ratio = 20).

wall muscles to make it impossible to ventilate the patient without giving muscle relaxants. Although the phenomenon probably occurs with all opioids, it has most often been reported with fentanyl, perhaps because its lipid solubility allows prompt uptake into skeletal muscle.

Sufentanil

Sufentanil is an extremely potent (500 to 1000 times as potent as morphine) synthetic opioid prescribed almost exclusively by anesthesiologists. Sufentanil, like fentanyl, provokes no histamine release, and even in large doses does not impair cardiovascular function directly. In addition, sufentanil has less potential for producing convulsions when given in large doses than does fentanyl. Like fentanyl, it also causes some bradycardia. The half-life of sufentanil is 148 minutes, slightly less than that of fentanyl. Like fentanyl, sufentanil is cleared by the liver.

Alfentanil

Alfentanil is a very short-acting synthetic opioid, approximately one fourth as potent as fentanyl. Alfentanil's plasma half-life is 1.5 hours, and the distribution half-life is 20 to 30 minutes. The offset of effect owing to redistribution is so rapid that alfentanil is best given by infusion. Common clinical practice is to administer a loading dose and then adjust an infusion to just abolish signs of light anesthesia, giving additional small doses in anticipation of or in response to surgical stress. This technique minimizes the possibility of overdose of the drug and promotes prompt patient awakening and the return of spontaneous ventilation.

As with fentanyl, there have been recent reports of delayed respiratory depression (rebound) following alfentanil anesthesia. It is not clear whether these episodes were due to redistribution of the drug. Alfentanil is most useful for brief procedures after which the patient must awaken quickly. Alfentanil appears to be associated more frequently with postoperative nausea and vomiting than are other synthetic opioids.

Meperidine

Meperidine (Demerol) is a synthetic opioid of entirely different structure than morphine. It is approximately one tenth as potent as morphine and has a half-life of approximately three hours, like morphine. It is hydrolyzed, then conjugated, or N-demethylated and conjugated, in the liver. The N-demethylated metabolite, normeperidine, has a half-life of 15 to 20 hours and causes seizures if it accumulates in large doses.

When meperidine is given to patients taking monoamine oxidase inhibitors (MAOI), a severe, possibly fatal excitatory state results, with hypertension, tachycardia, delirium, seizures, and hyperpyrexia. This interaction seems to be specific for meperidine; other opioids appear to be safe. Meperidine also controls shivering after general anesthesia, although the mechanism is unclear.

Heroin (Diacetylmorphine)

Heroin, a semisynthetic agonist, is used only illegally in the United States, but in England and other countries is prescribed for treatment of chronic cancer pain. Heroin is twice as potent as morphine, is metabolized to morphine, and is more transient in its effect. There appear to be no major advantages to the use of heroin over morphine for pain control.

Methadone

In the chronic maintenance of addicts, methadone replaces heroin, as it has a long duration of action and can be taken orally. Methadone reaches peak effects four hours after oral administration and one to two hours after subcutaneous or intramuscular administration. It is used for treatment of chronic cancer pain and occasionally as an adjunct to general anesthesia.

Agonist/Antagonists

Nalorphine was one of the first narcotic antagonists to be recognized as having agonist activity as well. Nalorphine is an antagonist at the mu receptor, and an agonist at kappa and sigma sites. It produces minimal analgesia, with some psychic side effects.

Attempts to produce desirable analgesia without such undesirable opioid effects as respiratory depression, nausea, or addiction led to the development of other opioid agonist/antagonist drugs. Pentazocine (Talwin) is an agonist/antagonist that produces analgesia, respiratory depression, and sedation in small doses, but dysphoria in greater doses. This drug causes less biliary spasm than the pure agonists. It also causes an increase in catecholamine release with increased heart rate and cardiac work, which limits its application in anesthesia.

Commonly used agonist/antagonist drugs in anesthetic practice include butorphanol (Stadol), nalbuphine (Nubain), and buprenorphine (Buprenex). The effects of butorphanol are similar to those of pentazocine, but it has fewer dysphoric effects and similar cardiac-stimulating actions. Nalbuphine (Nubain) produces no hemodynamic side effects, but does antagonize pure agonists given concomitantly. Buprenorphine is different from the other agonist/antagonists because of its slow onset and long duration, agonist and antagonist properties at the mu receptor, withdrawal effects after chronic use, and lack of CNS side effects. It has been used for treatment of chronic pain and intravenously as the narcotic in N_2O-opioid anesthetic techniques. In general, because the agonist/antagonists have mixed effects and significant deficiencies, none have replaced agonists for use in anesthetic practice.

Pure Antagonists

Naloxone is the opioid antagonist in common clinical use. Unlike the partial agonists described above, it is antagonistic at the mu, kappa, delta, and sigma receptors. Naloxone is used to reverse opioid toxicity or opioid overdose during anesthesia, and to counteract some of the side effects (nausea, pruritus) of spinal opioids.

Naloxone is best given intravenously in small increments (0.1 mg) or by infusion, to avoid the abrupt reversal of narcotic effects, a dangerous syndrome that may be simply unpleasant or may include severe pain, excitation, cardiovascular stimulation, pulmonary edema, or death. Naloxone is not given to opioid addicts except to treat overdose, as it precipitates severe withdrawal and suffering. The half-life of naloxone is one hour, less than that of many opioids. Therefore, naloxone is often infused continuously to treat opioid overdose, and patients are observed closely for signs of returning opioid effects as naloxone is metabolized.

CLINICAL USES OF OPIOIDS IN ANESTHESIA

Opioids as Anesthetics

In 1969, Lowenstein described the use of morphine in large doses to provide anesthesia for patients undergoing open heart operations. The major benefit of this technique was hemodynamic stability for patients with severe cardiovascular disease. Cardiac output was preserved with minimal changes in heart rate, blood pressure, or peripheral resistance. Newer opioids such as fentanyl have largely replaced morphine for opioid-based anesthesia because of the hypotensive effects of histamine release and the prolonged respiratory depression following morphine.

For noncardiac anesthetics and shorter procedures, opioid-based techniques are used with smaller doses of narcotic in combination with other intravenous agents, nitrous oxide, or very small doses of inhalation anesthetics. These "balanced" techniques seek to minimize the doses and side effects of each drug by giving synergistic combinations of agents, each chosen for a specific effect. However, adding nitrous oxide, volatile anesthetics, or intravenous agents to opioids may provoke cardiovascular depression not seen when opioids are used alone.

Opioid-based anesthetics are associated with predictable effects, including bradycardia, ventilatory depression, nausea and vomiting, and chest wall rigidity. The anesthetic depth is often light, so that painful surgical stimulation may provoke hypertension, especially in patients with pre-existing hypertension. The doses of fentanyl, sufentanil, and alfentanil used for major operations suppress the stress response to some extent; "stress-free" anesthesia cannot be guaranteed for all patients.

Muscle relaxants are usually used with narcotic anesthesia techniques to guarantee immobility during the operation. The light anesthesia may leave the patient aware of intraoperative events, yet the muscle relaxant may keep the patient from making his plight known. Some clinicians intermittently allow muscle relaxation to lapse, so as to allow the patient to respond to command or to pain. Other signs of light anesthesia such as tachycardia, hypertension, or tearing may be absent, even though the patient is aware of what is hap-

TABLE 10–4. Intravenous Doses of Opioids for Anesthesia*

Drug	Concentration	Sedation/Pain	N_2O/Opioid Anesthesia	Repeat Dose	Cardiac Anesthesia
Fentanyl	50 μg/ml	0.5–1.0 μg/kg	5–15 μg/kg	0.5–1 μg/kg	20–50 μg/kg
Morphine	1–10 mg/ml	0.02–0.1 mg/kg	0.2–0.5 mg/kg	0.2–0.1 mg/kg	1–2 mg/kg
Sufentanil	50 μg/ml	Not recommended	1 μg/kg/hr	0.1–0.3 μg/kg	5–20 μg/kg
Alfentanil	500 μg/ml	10–20 μg/kg	50–75 μg/kg + 0.5–2 μg/kg/min	10–25 μg/kg	—
Nalbuphine	10 mg/ml	0.1–0.15 mg/kg	0.3–3 mg/kg	0.25–0.5 mg/kg	—

* These intravenous doses are for healthy adults and are given slowly or in divided doses. Other patients require smaller doses, given more slowly. A few tolerant patients require more.

pening. Adequate doses of agents such as nitrous oxide, benzodiazepines, droperidol, scopolamine, or small doses of inhalation agents help prevent recall. Even if every effort is made to ensure adequate anesthesia, a rare patient will remember intraoperative conversations and events during light narcotic-based anesthesia.

Opioids also are used as adjuncts to inhalation anesthesia: to relieve pain and decrease minimum alveolar concentration (MAC), to obtund airway reflexes at induction or emergence, to prevent tachycardia, and to slow and deepen spontaneous ventilation during inhalation anesthesia (Table 10–4). For patients who might be sensitive to the hypotensive effects of potent inhalation agents, small doses of opioids may permit the use of lesser anesthetic concentrations, minimizing decreases in myocardial contractility and systemic vascular resistance.

Spinal Opioids and Patient-Controlled Analgesia

The slow absorption of opioids from intramuscular injection sites, combined with marked interpatient variability, make pain relief with intermittent intramuscular opioids unsatisfactory for many patients. Allowing the patient to obtain small in- analgesia'' [PCA]), or delivery of the drugs via the epidural or subarachnoid space has provided greatly improved treatment of postoperative pain (see Chapter 36).

CONCLUSION

Opioids are used in every phase of anesthesia practice. Although deaths have resulted from their respiratory depressant effects, safety can be assured by giving minimal effective doses for individual patients, by anticipating drug interactions, and by observing the effects produced in each patient.

REFERENCES

Hug CC Jr, Longnecker DR. Narcotics and narcotic antagonists. *In*, Smith NT, Corbascio A, eds. Drug interactions in anesthesia. 2nd ed. Philadelphia: Lea and Febiger, 1986: 321–339.

Philbin DM, et al. Fentanyl and sufentanil anesthesia revisited: how much is enough? Anesthesiology 1990; 73:5–11.

Stanski DR, Hug CC Jr. Alfentanil—a kinetically predictable narcotic analgesic (editorial). Anesthesiology 1982; 57:435–438.

Thorpe DH. Opiate structure and activity—a guide to understanding the receptor. Anesth Analg 1984; 63:143–151.

CHAPTER ELEVEN

MUSCLE RELAXANTS

Muscle relaxants form an important part of the armamentarium of the anesthesiologist. Whereas older anesthetic agents such as ether produced excellent skeletal muscle relaxation, current anesthetics, including both intravenous and inhaled agents, often depend on muscle relaxants to provide adequate operating conditions. Since its introduction in the 1940s, d-tubocurarine has declined in use, replaced initially by metocurine and pancuronium, and more recently by atracurium and vecuronium. The development of muscle relaxants with more rapid onsets, shorter and predictable durations, and minimal side effects continues.

This chapter reviews the basic physiology of the neuromuscular junction, the clinical pharmacology of relaxants and their antagonists, the techniques for monitoring neuromuscular blockade, and the uses of these drugs in anesthesia.

NEUROMUSCULAR PHARMACOLOGY AND PHYSIOLOGY

Muscle relaxants produce their desired effect at the neuromuscular junction, but also have nonspecific effects at many other sites. A brief review of the physiology of neuromuscular transmission aids understanding of the actions of muscle relaxants.

Neuromuscular Transmission

The neuromuscular junction (Fig. 11–1) consists of the terminus of the axon of a nerve, the motor end-plate of a muscle, and the area between these, the synaptic cleft. In the nerve terminal of the axon are vesicles, each containing approximately 10,000 molecules of acetylcholine. The surface of the motor end-plate contains invaginations called synaptic folds. Along the surface of the motor end-plate are the nicotinic receptors, large proteins consisting of five subunits arranged in a ring to form an ion channel; the concentration of these receptors is highest at the shoulder of each synaptic fold. Molecules of the enzyme acetylcholinesterase dangle on stalks from the surface of the motor end-plate, protruding into the synaptic cleft and the synaptic folds.

Normal neuromuscular transmission begins in the nerve. At rest, an active transport mechanism, the Na^+/K^+ pump, maintains a high concentration of Na^+ ions outside and K^+ ions inside the axon, producing a transmembrane potential of approximately −90 mV. When the nerve is stimulated, Na^+ channels open, permitting Na^+ ions to cross the membrane. As the transmembrane potential becomes less negative, the threshold for depolarization is reached and an action potential is generated. This, in turn, generates local currents along the nerve surface, opening adjacent Na^+ channels and propagating the action potential along the

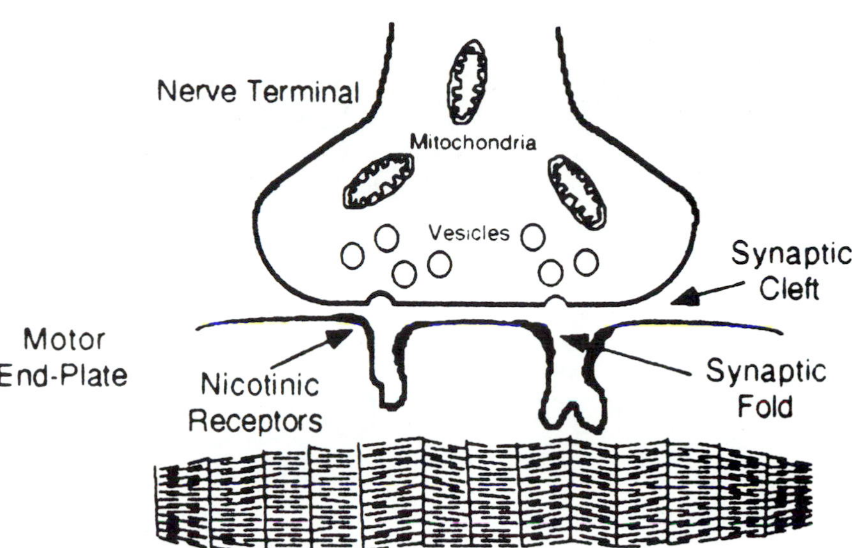

FIGURE 11–1. The neuromuscular junction consists of an axon of a nerve and the motor end-plate, separated by the synaptic cleft. Vesicles containing acetylcholine are located in the nerve terminal. Nicotinic receptors, large proteins consisting of five subunits arranged in a ring to form an ion channel, are located in the motor end-plate, near the junction of the synaptic cleft and the synaptic field.

nerve. As the action potential reaches the nerve terminal, entry of calcium into the nerve causes vesicles to move to, and fuse with, the cell membrane, thereby releasing acetylcholine into the synaptic cleft. These acetylcholine molecules traverse the narrow width of the synaptic cleft (50 nm), binding to one or both alpha subunits of the nicotine receptor and changing its conformation. If both alpha subunits are occupied by acetylcholine, the channel opens, permitting rapid entry of NA^+ ions and depolarizing the motor end-plate. Acetylcholine is not tightly bound to the receptor and moves on and off the receptor rapidly. Within nanoseconds, unbound acetylcholine is metabolized by the enzyme acetylcholinesterase found in the junctional cleft. The products of this enzymatic reaction, choline and acetate, return to the nerve terminal where they are used to synthesize new acetylcholine.

When the nerve is stimulated electrically, the resulting muscle contraction is known as a twitch. When neuromuscular transmission is normal, the amplitude of this twitch is similar whether the electrical stimulus occurs once or repeatedly.

Neuromuscular Blockade

Neuromuscular blockade occurs when the normal events in neuromuscular transmission are disrupted at one or more sites. Succinylcholine (Fig. 11–2), whose molecular structure resembles two acetylcholine molecules attached end-to-end, enters the synaptic cleft, attaches to the receptor, and depolarizes the neuromuscular junction; thus it is a depolarizing muscle relaxant. Unlike acetylcholine, whose effect is terminated rapidly by the action of acetylcholinesterase, succinylcholine is not metabolized locally at the neuromuscular junction. Consequently, the depolarizing action of succinylcholine persists longer than that of acetylcholine, and the motor end-plate remains depolarized and refractory to the effects of acetylcholine. This is known as Phase I neuromuscular blockade. With electrical stimulation, twitch is decreased from baseline and repeated stimuli evoke no further decrease (Fig. 11–3). Continued exposure of the motor end-plate to succinylcholine decreases the neuromuscular junction's sensitivity to succinylcholine's effects. Although relatively little is known about this type of neuromuscular blockade, known as Phase II, the response to nerve stimulation has a consistent pattern—a decrease in twitch (as with Phase I blockade) and fade with repeated stimuli (unlike Phase I blockade).

The neuromuscular effects of nondepolarizing muscle relaxants differ greatly from those of succinylcholine: stimulation of the nerve evokes twitches which are decreased from baseline, but repeated stimuli elicit progressively smaller twitches (Fig. 11–3). Although these drugs act principally by binding to the same sites in the receptor as do acetylcholine and succinylcholine (a result of their similar molecular structure, see Fig. 11–2), the nondepolarizing muscle relaxants do not depolarize the motor end-plate. They interfere with neuromuscular transmission by three mech-

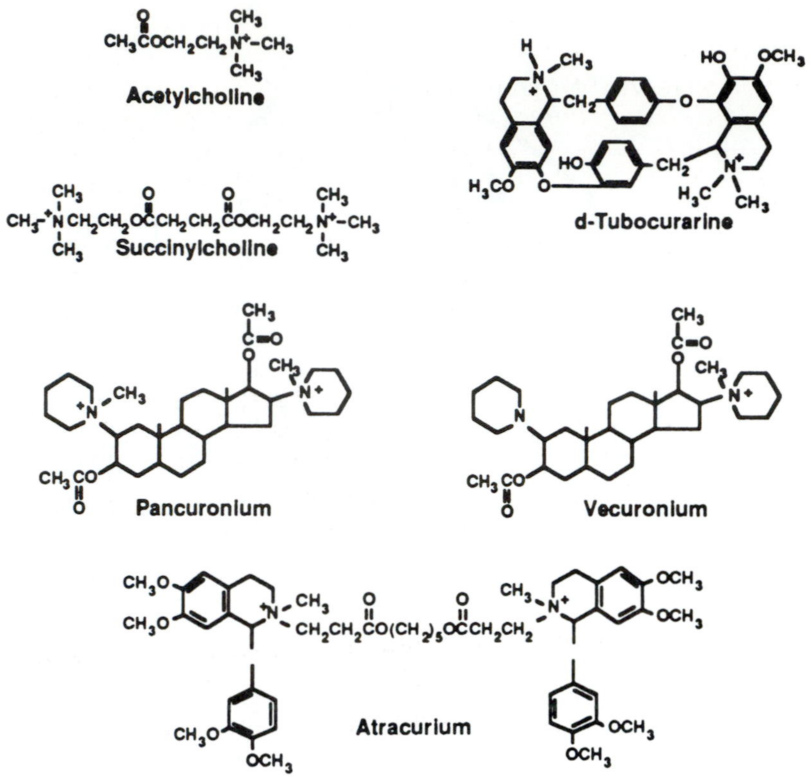

Acetylcholine

d-Tubocurarine

Succinylcholine

Pancuronium

Vecuronium

Atracurium

FIGURE 11–2. The molecular structures of acetylcholine, succinylcholine, and four nondepolarizing muscle relaxants are shown. Succinylcholine consists of two molecules of acetylcholine; the nondepolarizing muscle relaxants each contain some portion of the acetylcholine molecule.

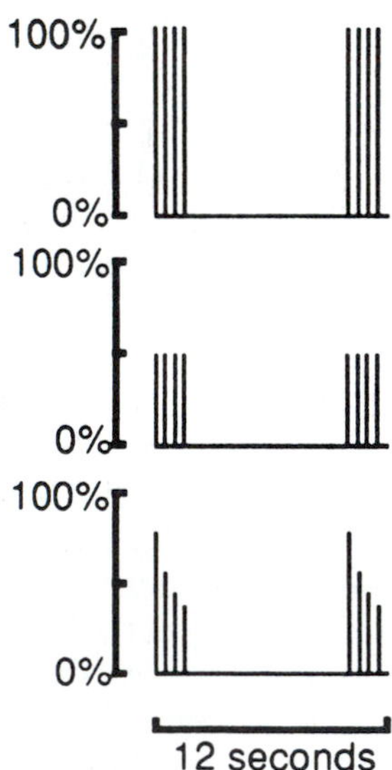

FIGURE 11–3. The motor response (twitch) in response to a 2-Hz stimulus is shown in three different circumstances. In the absence of muscle relaxants (top), all responses are similar in amplitude. After a subparalyzing dose of succinylcholine, all responses are similar in amplitude but smaller than the baseline value (middle). After a subparalyzing dose of a nondepolarizing muscle relaxant, the first response is smaller than baseline, and subsequent responses demonstrate fade (bottom); a similar response is seen during succinylcholine-induced Phase II block.

anisms. First, they prevent acetylcholine from binding normally to the receptor, thereby preventing depolarization of the motor end-plate. Second, if the concentration of a nondepolarizing muscle relaxant is excessive, molecules of the muscle relaxant may enter the channel of the receptor, causing channel blockade. Finally, nondepolarizing muscle relaxants act at presynaptic sites, blocking Na^+ channels and preventing movement of acetylcholine from synthesis sites to release sites, although the clinical importance of this mechanism has been questioned.

Because the motor end-plate is depolarized only when both alpha subunits of the receptor are occupied by acetylcholine, and neither acetylcholine nor muscle relaxants in clinical use are tightly bound to the alpha subunits, the neuromuscular response to nondepolarizing muscle relaxants depends on the relative concentrations of acetylcholine and muscle relaxant at the receptor ("competitive inhibition"). If the concentration of muscle relaxant is high relative to that of acetylcholine, it is unlikely that acetylcholine will occupy both alpha subunits, and thus neuromuscular transmission will be compromised. As the ratio of nondepolarizing muscle relaxant to acetylcholine decreases, it is more likely that both alpha subunits will be occupied by acetylcholine and that neuromuscular transmission will be normal. This competitive relationship is exploited to speed recovery from nondepolarizing muscle relaxants. Drugs such as neostigmine increase the local concentration of acetylcholine in the synaptic cleft (either by slowing normal destruction of acetylcholine or by increasing its release from the nerve terminal) and increase the ratio of acetylcholine to that of the nondepolarizing muscle relaxant, favoring normal neuromuscular transmission. Although the physiology is not well understood, increasing the local concentration of acetylcholine also improves neuromuscular transmission when succinylcholine-induced Phase II blockade has occurred; succinylcholine-induced Phase I blockade is not antagonized by this mechanism.

Blood flow to a muscle also influences its response to muscle relaxants. Following administration of bolus doses of muscle relaxants, muscles having high blood flow (e.g., diaphragm) may develop neuromuscular blockade before muscles with lower blood flow (e.g., hand). Additionally, various muscles respond differently to muscle relaxants. For example, the diaphragm is resistant to the effects of nondepolarizing muscle relaxants compared to intercostal and abdominal muscles or the adductor pollicis (the muscle typically monitored during clinical anesthesia).

Clinical Pharmacology of Depolarizing and Nondepolarizing Relaxants

Depolarizing Relaxants—Succinylcholine

Although it has many disadvantages, succinylcholine remains popular because of its unique pharmacokinetics. Its onset is faster than that of any of the nondepolarizing relaxants, yet its duration of action is the briefest of all muscle relaxants, particularly important if airway problems prevent intubation and require that the patient breathe spontaneously within several minutes of drug administration.

PHARMACOKINETICS

Succinylcholine differs from most drugs administered by anesthesiologists in that the acute offset of its effects is not due to redistribution of the drug but to metabolism by pseudocholinesterase. Because pseudocholinesterase exists in plasma but not at the neuromuscular junction (unlike acetylcholinesterase, the enzyme that degrades acetylcholine), succinylcholine is not metabolized at the neuromuscular junction. Thus, succinylcholine's effect terminates as its plasma concentration decreases and it diffuses from the neuromuscular junction into plasma.

This process of enzymatic destruction provides for succinylcholine a much more rapid offset of effect than does the redistribution, hepatic metabolism, and renal excretion typical of other muscle relaxants. This unique rapid recovery is especially advantageous if airway or intubation difficulties make it important for a patient to regain strength as soon as possible. Likewise, the rapid destruction of succinylcholine permits the use of very large doses, accounting for its rapid onset (30 to 60 seconds from intravenous administration to adequate relaxation for intubation), faster than the onset of the nondepolarizers. Although similar overdoses (20-fold) of nondepolarizing drugs likely produce similarly rapid onsets, the prolonged recovery from large doses of nondepolarizing relaxants limits the utility of this technique.

Recovery from succinylcholine-induced neuromuscular blockade (as demonstrated by respiratory effort) occurs in most patients within five to ten minutes, but may be prolonged in those who have decreased cholinesterase activity, often drug-induced or associated with liver disease or pregnancy. More significant prolongation results from genetically abnormal cholinesterase, most commonly atypical cholinesterase. Patients who are heterozygous for atypical cholinesterase (one in 480) have slightly prolonged blockade (recovery to 90 per cent of baseline twitch in 15 minutes following succinylcholine, 1 mg per kg), whereas homozygous patients (one in 3200) show marked prolongation (160 minutes to 90 per cent twitch). A history of prolonged blockade following succinylcholine in the patient or his family suggests this enzymatic abnormality. Laboratory evaluation includes measurement of both cholinesterase activity and the dibucaine number (dibucaine is a local anesthetic that inhibits activity of the normal enzyme 80 per cent and of the atypical enzyme only 20 per cent).

SIDE EFFECTS

Malignant Hyperthermia. The massive, sustained depolarization of the muscle membrane caused by succinylcholine probably accounts for the fact that the drug readily precipitates malignant hyperthermia syndrome (see Chapter 33). The drug is too dangerous to use in patients susceptible to this syndrome.

Masseter Spasm. On occasion, after succinylcholine has been administered for tracheal intubation, the jaw muscles become rigid rather than relaxed, limiting (but usually not preventing) tracheal intubation. This spasm of the masseter muscles sometimes progresses to malignant hyperthermia, although increased jaw tone and decreased mouth opening occur far more frequently after succinylcholine than does malignant hyperthermia. Thus, when the patient develops masseter spasm, the clinician must assess its significance: is the episode benign or a harbinger of malignant hyperthermia? If surgery is elective, it seems reasonable to discontinue anesthesia and monitor the patient closely for 24 hours, treating with dantrolene if needed, even though the expected incidence of malignant hyperthermia remains small. If no unequivocal evidence of malignant hyperthermia appears, muscle biopsies obtained for caffeine/halothane contracture tests are appropriate.

Cardiovascular. Succinylcholine, because of its similarity to acetylcholine, exerts many effects on the cardiovascular system. Ganglionic stimulation may either increase or decrease both heart rate and blood pressure, depending on the prior state of the patient's autonomic nervous system. Cardiac slowing occurs more frequently following a second dose (particularly if atropine has not been administered) and more frequently in children than in adults. Rarely, asystole may occur, even following single doses or brief infusions.

Hyperkalemia. Serum potassium concentration routinely increases 0.5 to 1.0 mEq per L following succinylcholine but extreme elevations, exceeding 5 mEq per L, occur rarely. Risk factors for massive hyperkalemia include acute upper motor neuron lesions or spinal cord injury, large burns, and massive trauma, including closed head injury. The period of vulnerability, although variable for each of these risk factors, appears to begin a few days after the insult and to persist for three to six months or longer. Such patients may suffer lethal hyperkalemia if given succinylcholine.

Myalgias. After succinylcholine, many patients report postoperative muscle pain, typically worse in the shoulders and back, sometimes exceeding the discomfort produced by the operation. Muscle pain is most likely to occur in young, muscular men and least likely to occur in infants, children, and the elderly. It also is more likely to occur in patients who are ambulatory after operation, such as those having minimal surgical procedures. Assuming this pain to be related to fasciculations (although this assumption has been challenged), efforts to prevent pain have focused on minimizing fasciculations (described below).

Increased Intraocular, Intragastric, and Intracranial Pressure. Because succinylcholine depolarizes muscles before relaxing them, its initial effect is to increase the tone of various muscles. This probably explains succinylcholine-induced increases in intraocular and intragastric pressure; the etiology of increased intracranial pressure is less well understood. These pressure increases are of clinical concern: increased intraocular pressure might force vitreous from a ruptured globe; increased intragastric pressure might cause a patient with residual gastric contents to regurgitate; and increased intracranial pressure might compromise the patient with central nervous system disease. Whether to avoid succinylcholine because of these increases in pressure is controversial. In one study, patients with ruptured globes given succinylcholine did not extrude vitreous. Although intragastric pressure increases after succinylcholine, distal esophageal pressure increases, maintaining the normal gradient. It seems likely that the magnitude of the clinical problem depends on the occurrence of fasciculations (as well as predisposing factors such as hiatal hernia); maneuvers that decrease the incidence and magnitude of fasciculations likely minimize increases in pressure and resulting complications.

CLINICAL USE

Bolus Administration. The most common use of succinylcholine is to facilitate tracheal intubation, particularly if rapid control of the airway is necessary, as in the patient at risk for aspiration.

The onset of relaxation is sufficiently fast (60 seconds in adults given 1.5 mg per kg) that most patients can be left apneic from the time succinylcholine is administered until intubation is completed. Additional relaxation for the remainder of the operation is provided by additional (typically small) doses of succinylcholine or nondepolarizing relaxants.

Defasciculation. The most popular technique to prevent fasciculations is to administer a small dose of a nondepolarizing muscle relaxant several minutes before succinylcholine. Presumably, the nondepolarizing relaxant occupies some fraction of the receptors at the neuromuscular junction so that succinylcholine does not produce the usual sustained depolarization, but is able to produce muscle relaxation. Usually, such "defasciculating doses" are approximately one tenth the dose required for intubation. Because some receptors are occupied by the defasciculating drug, the dose of succinylcholine usually is increased 50 per cent to assure adequate paralysis. Attempts also have been made to prevent fasciculations by administering small doses of succinylcholine, for example, 10 mg per 70 kg (*not* in awake patients), followed three to five minutes later by a usual dose. This technique, known as "self-taming," was briefly popular; however, the incidence of fasciculations appears to be similar to that without self-taming. Because of biological variation, a small number of patients (1 to 5 per cent) may experience significant weakness after defasciculating doses of any of these drugs, in which case prompt induction of anesthesia and controlled ventilation are required. This constitutes the chief hazard of this technique.

Continuous Infusion. Rapid elimination by pseudocholinesterase makes succinylcholine an ideal candidate for administration by infusion. However, with repeated succinylcholine administration, neuromuscular blockade changes from Phase I to Phase II blockade, accompanied by increases in dose requirement (tachyphylaxis) and fade with repeated stimuli: some signs of Phase II blockade (e.g., fade) may be apparent following a single dose. The occurrence of Phase II blockade has limited the popularity of continuous infusions.

Antagonism of Phase II Blockade. Recovery from Phase I succinylcholine-induced neuromuscular blockade typically is quite rapid and not hastened by drugs such as neostigmine or edrophonium. In contrast, recovery from Phase II blockade frequently is prolonged. As one might expect, cholinesterase inhibitors such as neostigmine speed recovery from Phase II block owing to succinylcholine. However, if any free succinylcholine remains in plasma, inhibition of plasma pseudocholinesterase by the neostigmine will retard clearance of the drug and impede the patient's recovery. This risk makes it advisable to withhold neostigmine in most cases of slow recovery from Phase II block and to await spontaneous recovery, usually a matter of 20 to 30 minutes.

Nondepolarizing Relaxants

At present, at least six nondepolarizing relaxants are available and used clinically. These muscle relaxants are classified as having intermediate duration (atracurium and vecuronium) and long duration (d-tubocurarine, metocurine, pancuronium, and pipecuronium). One additional relaxant, gallamine, is no longer in common use because of pronounced tachycardia associated with its use.

PHARMACOKINETICS AND PHARMACODYNAMICS

Because nondepolarizing muscle relaxants are polar, charged molecules, they do not penetrate cell membranes well. Consequently, the volume of distribution at steady state for all muscle relaxants is approximately the volume of the extracellular fluid space. All muscle relaxants require minimal time to move on and off the receptor; consequently, the factors limiting onset and recovery from neuromuscular blockade for each muscle are blood flow to the muscle and changes in the plasma concentration of the muscle relaxant.

These pharmacokinetic and pharmacodynamic characteristics have important implications for the onset of paralysis. Time to peak effect for doses of nondepolarizing muscle relaxants producing less than 90 per cent blockade in adults generally is similar, approximately four to six minutes. However, following administration of commonly used clinical doses (i.e., those producing greater than 99 per cent blockade), twitch decreases to less than one per cent of baseline in as little as two minutes. Although twitch continues to decrease until four to six minutes after administration of the muscle relaxant, measurement techniques are inadequate to differentiate profound degrees of neuromuscular blockade (e.g., 99.5 per cent versus 99.9 percent).

Pharmacokinetic and pharmacodynamic characteristics also influence the recovery of neuromuscular function. Following single clinical doses, neuromuscular recovery typically begins during redistribution of the drug, whereas recovery from repeated doses depends on elimination of the muscle relaxant. Thus, recovery from initial doses is rapid compared to that from subsequent doses, a phenomenon known as cumulation. In addition, even when failure of the metabolizing organ results in almost no elimination of the muscle relaxant, neuromuscular function might recover after a single dose, based on distribution alone. However, with repeated doses, the decline in plasma concentration of the muscle relaxant is slowed by organ failure and cumulation is pronounced. Most nondepolarizing relaxants are eliminated by the kidney (d-tubocurarine, pancuronium, metocurine, and gallamine) or the liver (vecuronium, d-tubocurarine). While it is wise to select muscle relaxants for patients with liver or kidney failure accordingly, the effects of even marked degrees of organ failure on the pharmacokinetics of muscle relaxants are, to a degree, unpredictable in the individual patient.

Atracurium was synthesized specifically to undergo Hofmann elimination (spontaneous degradation at physiologic pH and temperature); it also undergoes ester hydrolysis. Since its elimination does not depend exclusively on organ function, it is a good choice for patients with renal or hepatic failure.

Pediatric Patients. Volume of distribution at steady state of nondepolarizing muscle relaxants changes in a manner similar to maturational changes in volume of the extracellular fluid space, being greatest at birth and decreasing during the first year of life. Plasma clearance of muscle relaxants also changes with age. For example, clearance of d-tubocurarine changes in a manner parallel to that of the maturation of glomerular filtration (i.e., increasing during the first year of life before reaching adult values). However, compared to the changes in volume of distribution, age-related changes in clearance are minimal. The consequence of a larger volume of distribution in younger patients generally is a longer pharmacologic half-life, resulting in a slower recovery of neuromuscular function in younger patients (observed in many, but not all, studies). Although atracurium is similar to other nondepolarizing muscle relaxants in having a larger volume of distribution in young patients, its unusual metabolic pathways counterbalance age-related changes in volume of distribution, resulting in minimal changes in duration of action with age. One other factor that changes with maturation is sensitivity to the nondepolarizing muscle relaxants. For both d-tubocurarine and vecuronium, neuromuscular blockade occurs at lower concentrations in neonates and infants than in children and adults. Age-related changes in neuromuscular junction sensitivity to atracurium appear to be minimal.

Elderly Patients. The durations of action of d-tubocurarine, metocurine, pancuronium, and vecuronium (but not atracurium) are prolonged in the elderly. The prolonged action of the former drugs likely results from pharmacokinetic changes associated with aging, particularly decreased hepatic and renal function, rather than from changes in neuromuscular junction sensitivity. The absence of age-related changes for atracurium may result from its multiple elimination pathways.

DRUG INTERACTIONS

The intensity and time course of neuromuscular blockade of the nondepolarizing muscle relaxants depends not only on the muscle relaxants, but also on other drugs administered to the patient, including inhaled anesthetics and antibiotics.

Inhaled Anesthetics. Although most inhaled anesthetics do not produce measurable decreases in twitch, they depress the response of the motor end-plate to acetylcholine, thereby potentiating the effects of nondepolarizing muscle relaxants. The degree of potentiation varies for each inhaled agent and each muscle relaxant. For example, atracurium is least affected by inhaled anesthetics, whereas both d-tubocurarine and pancuronium are potentiated markedly by both isoflurane and enflurane.

Magnesium. Magnesium decreases the release of acetylcholine from the nerve terminal, presumably by competing with calcium. Magnesium also decreases the depolarizing action of acetylcholine on the motor end-plate and the excitability of muscle fibers, but these effects probably are less important than the decrease of acetylcholine release. When magnesium sulfate is used to treat preeclampsia and eclampsia, serum magnesium concentrations are sufficient to potentiate neuromuscular blockade caused by both succinylcholine and nondepolarizing muscle relaxants. Although calcium enhances release of acetylcholine from the nerve terminal and should antagonize magnesium's effects, calcium also stabilizes the postjunctional membrane, which may explain why calcium only partially antagonizes a combined magnesium-nondepolarizing muscle relaxant blockade and may augment combined magnesium-succinylcholine blockade.

Antibiotics. Numerous antibiotics potentiate muscle relaxants, acting at both prejunctional and postjunctional sites. The prejunctional mechanism appears to be similar to that of magnesium. The relative prejunctional and postjunctional effects vary for each antibiotic: for example, streptomycin acts primarily on the nerve terminal, but clindamycin has mixed effects. Neostigmine antagonizes the increased blockade produced by many antibiotics, while calcium may be beneficial for some, but not all. However, administration of calcium probably should be avoided because it may antagonize the antibacterial effect of some antibiotics.

Other Drugs. Numerous drugs potentiate or antagonize the neuromuscular effects of nondepolarizing muscle relaxants. Those that potentiate include furosemide, local anesthetics, quinidine, and calcium channel blockers, while phenytoin, carbamazepine, and theophylline appear to antagonize neuromuscular blockade.

SIDE EFFECTS

The side effects of nondepolarizing muscle relaxants are generally of less consequence than those of succinylcholine.

Cardiovascular. Several muscle relaxants release histamine, resulting in a decrease in blood pressure and an increase in heart rate. d-Tubocurarine was known for this property; atracurium also releases histamine, but rarely results in significant hypotension and tachycardia. With either drug, administering the drug in divided doses over several minutes substantially eliminates the risk of histamine release.

In contrast, pancuronium produces hypertension and tachycardia, presumably owing to the release of norepinephrine and blockade of cardiac vagal receptors; these effects are dose-dependent and can be minimized by slow administration of pancuronium (e.g., over one to two minutes). Metocurine has few cardiovascular effects but is now rarely used. Vecuronium has minimal cardiovascular effects, even with extremely large doses, making it a most practical muscle relaxant when cardiovascular changes must be avoided.

Pulmonary. Some nondepolarizing muscle relaxants produce wheezing in susceptible patients. This problem has been well documented for d-tubocurarine. Although atracurium releases histamine, wheezing rarely has been reported.

TIME COURSE OF NONDEPOLARIZING MUSCLE RELAXANTS

One major factor influencing the usefulness of muscle relaxants is their time course (i.e., both onset and duration of neuromuscular blockade).

Onset of Neuromuscular Blockade. Time to peak neuromuscular depression depends primarily on the time it takes a muscle relaxant to reach the neuromuscular junction, and the magnitude of the dose administered. The role of circulation time to the junction is illustrated by comparing onset time for equipotent doses in infants and adults: invariably the onset is faster in younger patients, presumably because of their higher cardiac outputs and more rapid circulation times. The role of dose is revealed by comparing onset time for different doses. As larger doses of vecuronium are administered, onset time (defined as time for disappearance of all components of a "train-of-four" stimulus) becomes shorter (Fig. 11–4). Some muscle

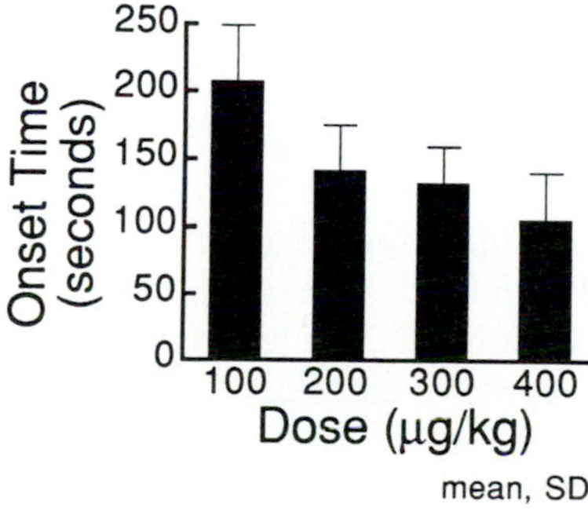

FIGURE 11–4. Onset time (defined as time from administration of vecuronium to disappearance of all four responses to a train-of-four stimulus) following varying doses of vecuronium in adults. As the dose increases, onset time decreases. (Redrawn with permission from Ginsberg B, Glass PS, Quill T, Shafron D, Ossey KD. Onset and duration of neuromuscular blockade following high-dose vecuronium administration. Anesthesiology 1989; 71:201–205.)

TABLE 11–1. Pharmacokinetics of Neuromuscular Blockers*

Relaxant	Plasma Clearance (ml/kg/min)	Steady State Volume of Distribution (ml/kg)	Elimination Half-Life (min)	Maintenance Infusion (μg/kg/min)
Succinylcholine	Unknown	Unknown	Unknown	100
d-Tubocurarine	3	300	90	3
Pancuronium	2	250	140	0.3
Vecuronium	5	270	70	1
Atracurium	5	100	16	10

* These figures are rounded to aid calculation; variation among patients exceeds the rounding errors. To administer these drugs by infusion, give an initial dose from Table 11–2 and begin the infusion when the twitch response recovers to the desired level.

relaxants do not demonstrate a faster onset with larger doses; most likely, cardiovascular changes produced by these muscle relaxants delay their delivery to the neuromuscular junction.

Duration of Neuromuscular Blockade. Because nondepolarizing muscle relaxants are not metabolized at the neuromuscular junction, their effect terminates as the plasma concentration decreases, causing the muscle relaxant to diffuse from neuromuscular junction to plasma. Consequently, duration of action of nondepolarizing muscle relaxants is influenced predominantly by factors affecting the plasma concentration of the drug. With usual single doses of a nondepolarizing muscle relaxant, recovery occurs late in distribution or early in the elimination phase. As a result, differences in duration of action of the nondepolarizing muscle relaxants do not correlate well with their elimination half-lives. For example, atracurium's elimination half-life averages 16 minutes, while vecuronium's averages 71 minutes. Despite this marked difference between the two drugs, the time course following doses used for tracheal intubation is similar. A better predictor of the duration of action of muscle relaxants may be apparent plasma clearance (Table 11–1). For example, clearances of d-tubocurarine and pancuronium are similar, as are their durations of action; atracurium and vecuronium have similar, higher clearances and correspondingly shorter, similar durations of action.

Cumulative Effects. With repeated administration, the duration of action of certain muscle relaxants, particularly pancuronium, increases. Similarly, the time for twitch to recovery from 25 per cent to 75 per cent of baseline increases as the size of the dose increases. These changes, known as cumulative effects, can be explained by the pharmacokinetics of the muscle relaxants rather than changes in pharmacodynamics. Although recovery of neuromuscular function following initial doses is largely a function of distribution rather than elimination, repeated or larger initial doses shift recovery to a later, less steep, portion of the plasma concentration versus time curve. For pancuronium (and other older nondepolarizing relaxants), recovery shifts from the early steep distribution phase to the slower elimination phase. Recovery from larger or repeated doses of vecuronium similarly shifts from distribution to the later elimination phase; however, the elimination half-life of vecuronium is markedly shorter than that of pancuronium so that cumulative effects, although present, are much less marked than those of pancuronium. Atracurium does not appear to be affected by this phenomenon—it has a very brief distribution phase and enters its elimination phase earlier than other muscle relaxants, a result of its multiple elimination pathways (particularly those that result in elimination from both plasma and tissues, e.g., Hofmann elimination). Consequently, recovery from single or repeated doses of atracurium occurs during elimination rather than during distribution, and atracurium has no obvious cumulative effect.

The problem of cumulation, the significant interpatient variability in response to these drugs, the potentiating effects of anesthetics and other medications, and the inconsistent effects of organ failure, make it impractical to give muscle relaxants according to a fixed dosage schedule. Although suggested doses are given in Table 11–2, successive doses must be judged according to the patient's response. Infusion rates, the size of bolus doses, or the intervals between doses must be adjusted to just give the desired effect for any given segment of the operation and the anesthetic. This scheme of titration to effect allows even patients with severely compromised organ function or those with unusual sensitivity to the drugs to be managed without unwanted postoperative weakness. When extreme prolongation of relaxant effect is anticipated, atracurium is a rational choice because of its rapid metabolism and freedom from cumulative effects.

MODES OF ADMINISTRATION

Bolus Administration. The initial dose of a nondepolarizing muscle relaxant depends on whether succinylcholine has been administered for tracheal intubation. If the nondepolarizing muscle relaxant is used for tracheal intubation, then a large dose, twice the ED_{95}, typically is given to hasten the onset of relaxation. If succinylcholine has been used for tracheal intubation, then the dose of the nondepolarizing muscle relaxant, given as neuromuscular function recovers, can vary from small (e.g., a dose approximating the ED_{50}) to large (e.g., twice the ED_{95}). If the smaller dose is administered (additional doses usually are required to produce the desired degree of relaxation), and their magnitude can be estimated by the response to the initial dose, additional relaxation often is required; if so, additional doses of muscle relaxant usually are administered.

Priming Doses. The slow onset of nondepolarizing muscle relaxants compared to succinylcholine has limited their use for rapid tracheal intubation. One means to speed the onset of neuromuscular blockade has been to administer a small dose of the muscle relaxant, a "priming dose," several minutes before the usual dose. The initial small dose, approximately 10 to 20 per cent of a dose given to facilitate tracheal intubation, occupies many of the receptors at the neuromuscular junction but, ideally, does not produce clinical evidence of weakness: the patient should be able to breathe spontaneously, maintain a patent airway, and avoid aspiration. Following an interval of about four minutes, administration of a large bolus of the muscle relaxant results in paralysis markedly faster than would occur if the two doses were administered together.

Administration of priming doses decreases the time to 100 per cent neuromuscular blockade from three to five minutes to 70 to 100 seconds (compared to 60 seconds for succinylcholine). This technique is of limited value in clinical practice, because some patients become profoundly weak following the initial small dose, and the benefits of priming vary from patient to patient.

Continuous Infusions. Small volume of distribution, high clearance, and rapid equilibration between plasma and the neuromuscular junction make atracurium and vecuronium well suited for administration by infusion (Table 11–1).

TABLE 11–2. Suggested Doses of Neuromuscular Blockers*

Relaxant	Initial Dose for Intubation (mg/kg)	Initial Dose, Following Intubation (mg/kg)	Supplemental Dose (mg/kg)	Dosing Interval (min)
Succinylcholine	1.0	0.3	0.3	5
d-Tubocurarine	0.6	0.3	0.1	30
Metocurine	0.4	0.2	0.1	30
Pancuronium	0.1	0.05	0.015	40
Vecuronium	0.1	0.05	0.015	30
Atracurium	0.5	0.3	0.1	20

* These doses are for healthy adults and children, but not infants, and are rounded to make them easier to use. Supplemental doses are administratered according to signs such as recovery of twitch response, rather than by a fixed schedule. In case of doubt, it is often best to give doses less than those shown, adding additional relaxant depending on the response to the initial dose. For rapid sequence induction, doses twice those shown for intubation speed onset but worsen side effects and prolong neuromuscular blockade.

TABLE 11–3. **New Nondepolarizing Muscle Relaxants***

Relaxant	Onset	Duration	Features
Doxacurium (Burroughs Wellcome)	Slow	Similar to pancuronium	Minimal cardiovascular effect
Mivacurium (Burroughs Wellcome)	Fast, but slower than succinylcholine	Brief, but longer than succinylcholine	Time course closest to that of succinylcholine
Pipecuronium (Organon)	Similar to pancuronium	Similar to pancuronium	Lacks cardiovascular effects
Rocuronium (Organon)	Fast, but slower than succinylcholine	Similar to vecuronium	Fast-acting nondepolarizer

* Only doxacurium and pipecuronium have been released for approval as of July 1991. This information is based on clinical trials published prior to that date.

With continuous monitoring of neuromuscular function, neuromuscular blockade can be titrated to a constant intensity.

Combinations of Muscle Relaxants. Combinations of pancuronium with either d-tubocurarine or metocurine appear to be synergistic; that is, simultaneous administration of one half of the ED_{50} of each drug results in more than 50 per cent neuromuscular blockade. The mechanism of synergy is not known, but has been attributed to combined prejunctional and postjunctional effects specific to each drug or to their different affinities to the alpha subunit of the postjunctional receptor; either of these mechanisms would explain why other combinations of muscle relaxants (e.g., metocurine with d-tubocurarine or pancuronium with vecuronium) are not synergistic. One advantage of combining muscle relaxants is that cardiovascular effects are minimized compared to the effects when the drugs are used individually. The development of muscle relaxants having minimal cardiovascular effects when administered alone (e.g., vecuronium) has diminished this advantage.

CHOICE OF NONDEPOLARIZING RELAXANT

Many factors influence the choice of muscle relaxant for a given patient. First, consider that patients with liver or kidney failure may suffer prolonged paralysis if given neuromuscular blockers which are metabolized primarily by the diseased organ. Second, consider the operation. For brief procedures, administration of a long-acting muscle relaxant may result in postoperative paralysis. However, when operations last several hours, repeated administration of an intermediate-duration muscle relaxant may result in fluctuating levels of neuromuscular blockade. Third, consider cardiovascular effects of the muscle relaxants. For example, pancuronium may produce undesirable tachycardia in an elderly patient with heart disease, but for pediatric patients in whom tachycardia often is desirable, one might administer pancuronium rather than vecuronium and atropine. Fourth, patients with histories of asthma or diseases that may be exacerbated by histamine release may not be given d-tubocurarine or atracurium. A final consideration is cost: muscle relaxants available as generic drugs are less expensive than those still under patent. A single dose of vecuronium or atracurium costs three times as much as an equivalent dose of pancuronium. Because the newer, more expensive drugs are shorter acting as well, the cost of using them as compared to pancuronium or curare is even greater for longer cases.

NEW NONDEPOLARIZING MUSCLE RELAXANTS

None of the available nondepolarizing muscle relaxants has a time profile identical to that of succinylcholine. Although large doses of nondepolarizing relaxants may produce rapid onset of neuromuscular blockade, these doses also result in markedly longer blockade than does succinylcholine. In addition, no nondepolarizing muscle relaxant has a duration as short as that of succinylcholine. Assuming that many of succinylcholine's side effects are related to its depolarizing action, several pharmaceutical companies are developing nondepolarizing muscle relaxants that offer the advantages of succinylcholine without its disadvantages, but none yet match succinylcholine's rapidity of onset (see Table 11–3).

Antagonism of Neuromuscular Blockade

When a nondepolarizing muscle relaxant is given, neuromuscular function recovers spontaneously provided that sufficient time passes after drug administration. However, waiting for spontaneous recovery is usually impractical, even if the newer intermediate-duration relaxants have been used; this is particularly true if paralysis has been required at the end of surgery, as during peritoneal closure. Therefore, recovery of neuromuscular function following administration of nondepolarizing neuromuscular relaxants typically is promoted by administering antagonist drugs, which increase the concentration of acetylcholine in the synaptic cleft. This is accomplished by inhibiting destruction of acetylcholine in the synaptic cleft, or by increasing its release from the nerve terminal. The first of these mechanisms typically is used clinically: drugs such as neostigmine, pyridostigmine, and edrophonium inhibit acetylcholinesterase, thereby increasing the local concentration of acetylcholine and antagonizing neuromuscular blockade. 4-Aminopyridine antagonizes neuromuscular blockade by increasing acetylcholine release from the nerve terminal; however, undesirable side effects have limited its clinical use.

The commonly used cholinesterase antagonists share one problem: because the increase in acetylcholine concentration is not limited to the neuromuscular junction, these drugs produce multiple side effects including profound cardiac slowing, nodal rhythms, increased intestinal tone, and oral secretions. These effects can be minimized or prevented by an anticholinergic drug, typically atropine or glycopyrrolate (Table 11–4).

Several factors are considered in selecting among edrophonium, neostigmine, or pyridostigmine. The greatest difference relates to onset time, edrophonium being the fastest acting of these and pyridostigmine the slowest. Although early studies using small doses of edrophonium suggested that its duration of action was inadequate for clinical purposes, the durations of action of edrophonium and neostigmine are similar; pyridostigmine is slightly longer acting. One potential difference among antagonists arises in antagonizing profound neuromuscular blockade, such as 95 to 99 per cent twitch depression. Usual doses of edrophonium, 0.5 mg per kg, do not adequately antagonize profound blockade, although larger doses, such as 1.0 mg per kg, reportedly are effective; neostigmine is the preferred antagonist in this setting. The cardiovascular effects of the antagonists differ markedly. When given without an anticholinergic, edrophonium produces a rapid and profound decrease in heart rate, whereas the bradycardia induced by neostigmine and pyridostigmine is slower in onset. If neostigmine or pyridostigmine are administered as antagonists, either atropine or glycopyrrolate can be given as the anticholinergic; however, edrophonium-induced bradycardia occurs faster and is more profound than glycopyrrolate-induced tachycardia, making this combination of drugs undesirable.

Table 11–4. Drugs for Antagonizing Nondepolarizing Neuromuscular Blockade*

	Anticholinesterases	
	Drug *Time to Peak Effect*	*Dose*
Edrophonium	1–2 min	0.5–1.0 mg/kg
Neostigmine	3–5 min	0.04–0.07 mg/kg
Pyridostigmine	10–20 min	0.2–0.3 mg/kg
	Anticholinergics	
	Drug *Dose*	*Use With*
Glycopyrrolate	0.008 mg/kg (0.5–0.6 mg/70 kg)	Neostigmine Pyridostigmine
Atropine	.007–0.02 mg/kg (0.5–1.5 mg/70 kg)	Edrophonium Neostigmine

* For reliable results in reversing the effects of nondepolarizing muscle relaxants, administration of anticholinesterases is delayed until spontaneous recovery permits three out of four responses to a train-of-four stimuli. For patients with more profound blockade, larger amounts of anticholinesterase may be required, but doses of neostigmine greater than 0.14 mg per kg are unlikely to produce additional improvement.

Monitoring Neuromuscular Function

Decades of clinical experience with muscle relaxants has demonstrated their effectiveness, the risks associated with their administration, and patients' variability in dose-response relationship and duration of action. Accordingly, monitoring of neuromuscular function, both during and after administration of relaxants, has become the standard of practice. Monitoring serves two purposes: to demonstrate adequacy of blockade during operation so that additional doses of relaxants can be administered as clinically indicated, and to demonstrate adequacy of neuromuscular function during recovery to assure patient safety.

During anesthesia and operation, the desired degree of neuromuscular blockade varies as a function of various clinical needs. For example, during tracheal intubation, optimal conditions include complete paralysis of the diaphragm; however, if a self-retaining retractor is used during surgery, less intensive blockade is adequate. Immediately after operation, the patient must regain full strength promptly.

The intensity of neuromuscular blockade is estimated by assessing the evoked response of various muscles. The standard for neuromuscular research is to stimulate the ulnar nerve, either at the wrist or the elbow, and quantify strength of contraction of the adductor pollicis muscle that bends the thumb, a muscle supplied solely by the ulnar nerve. In the laboratory, the peroneal nerve frequently is used. When access to an extremity is limited, the facial nerve can be stimulated; however, the relationship between facial muscle twitch and ventilatory function has not been well investigated. Inadvertent direct muscle stimulation (stimulating the muscle directly rather than its nerve) must be avoided because it bypasses the neuromuscular junction and fade is obscured. Thus, when fade is expected (when a nondepolarizing muscle relaxant has been administered) but not present, direct muscle stimulation should be suspected. More confusing is the situation in which both direct and indirect muscle stimulation occur: fade may be present initially but absent with more intense blockade. Direct muscle stimulation is more common when the facial nerve is used, probably because of the superficial position of the facial muscles.

The stimulus to the nerve must be supramaximal (i.e., further increases in stimulus strength produce no increase in response) so that the intensity of neuromuscular blockade will not be underestimated. A square-wave pulse is administered for 0.1 to 0.3 ms through either surface electrodes or needles placed subcutaneously near the nerve, and strength of contraction is quantified using either a mechanical strain gauge or an electromyogram (EMG). A less rigorous but acceptable method for clinical practice is to feel the strength of thumb contraction; to observe, but not feel, thumb movement is less accurate (visual observation tends to underestimate intensity of neuromuscular blockade).

Traditionally, single stimuli are administered no more frequently than every ten seconds (faster stimulation results in smaller evoked responses) and each evoked response is compared to the initial response preceding paralysis (i.e., control or baseline). This method may be impractical in the operating room because it requires measuring neuromuscular response before drug administration, which is not always feasible. Alternatively, stimuli can be administered rapidly, at 50 to 100 Hz. This rapid tetanic stimulation demonstrates exhaustion of acetylcholine reserves, valuable for detecting subtle degrees of neuromuscular blockade during recovery.

A third approach, train-of-four stimulation (four stimuli at 2 Hz every 10 to 15 seconds), resulted from the observation that the response to 2-Hz stimuli declined maximally by the fourth twitch and that the ratio of the fourth to the first twitches (the train-of-four ratio) was similar to the ratio of the first to the baseline response. Thus, the train-of-four ratio could be used to estimate neuromuscular blockade without obtaining a baseline value. This similarity of train-of-four and first-to-baseline response ratio is valid only during recovery; during onset, train-of-four ratio is not depressed as much as is the first-to-baseline ratio. A final form of stimulation, specifically designed to assess profound neuromuscular blockade when there is no response to the modes of stimulation described previously, is to administer a 50-Hz tetanic stimulus for five seconds, wait three seconds, then administer single stimuli at 1 Hz; the number of twitches present is known as the post-tetanic count. During the tetanus, all available acetylcholine is recruited from storage sites in the nerve terminal to the vesicles. With profound neuromuscular blockade, vesicular reserves of acetylcholine are insufficient to produce neuromuscular transmission in response to the tetanus; however, when stimulation decreases to 1 Hz, newly recruited acetylcholine will produce evidence of neuromuscular function. This is known as post-tetanic facilitation.

Many nerve stimulators are available commercially. Although they differ in appearance and certain characteristics, the devices generally offer single, train-of-four, and tetanic stimuli (50 or 100 Hz). The output of these devices, whether constant voltage or constant current, can be adjusted to assure supramaximal stimuli.

In addition to monitoring neuromuscular function with nerve stimulation, numerous clinical signs, associated with various degrees of neuromuscular recovery, are available to assess recovery of neuromuscular function. The ability of the intubated patient to breathe spontaneously provides little assurance of adequate recovery: because the diaphragm is resistant to the effects of muscle relaxants, a patient may be able to breathe spontaneously, yet may develop airway obstruction when extubated. The ability of an adult to sustain head-lift or a child to sustain leg-lift are considered signs of adequate recovery. Another well-accepted standard has been a patient's ability to generate inspiratory airway pressures exceeding -25 cm H_2O (the endotracheal tube is occluded and the maximal inspiratory pressure is measured). Recent evidence suggests that a value of -40 cm H_2O is more appropriate. This maneuver may carry the risk of pulmonary edema with sustained negative intrathoracic pressure. Table 11–5 describes the depths of neuromuscular blockade as measured by nerve stimulator and as observed in the patient.

The rapid spontaneous recovery of function possible with modern intermediate-acting relaxants such as vecuronium and atracurium suggests the possibility that anticholinesterases might be avoided. However, even patients who appear strong may have up to half of their neuromuscular cholinergic receptors occupied by neuromuscular blockers (Table 11–5); studies show that patients often have residual weakness after neuromuscular blockade, despite passing superficial tests of strength. These facts suggest that anticholinesterases are appropriate for almost any patient who has received neuromuscular blockers, especially when extubation of the trachea is planned.

Despite the availability of information about proper dosing of muscle relaxants, antagonists, and the use of nerve stimulators, patients often arrive in the recovery room with significant residual neuromuscular blockade (less commonly following atracurium and vecuronium than after longer acting drugs such as pancuronium). The potentially devastating consequences of persistent neuromuscular blockade, airway obstruction, and hypoventilation make it mandatory that clinicians demonstrate and document the presence of adequate neuromuscular function in their patients at the end of the anesthetic, unless postoperative mechanical ventilation is planned.

To demonstrate full recovery of the patient's strength at the end of the procedure, one may use any of the more stringent tests such as leg-lift,

TABLE 11–5. Hierarchy of Neuromuscular Blockade*

Approximate Fraction of Receptors Occupied by Nondepolarizing Relaxant (%)	Response to Nerve Stimualtor	Whole Body Signs
99–100	No response even with post-tetanic facilitation (PTF)	Flaccid: extreme relaxation needed only rarely to guarantee immobility during neurosurgery, etc.
95	PTF present	Diaphragm moves; hiccup
90	5% One of four twitch height responses to TOF present	Abdominal relaxation adequate to most surgeons' needs
75	Twitch height 100 % Four twitches of TOF present TOF ratio 0.7 50-Hz tetanus sustained	Tidal volume normal, vital capacity normal
50	100-Hz tetanus sustained	Passes inspiratory pressure test
30	200-Hz tetanus sustained	Sustains head-lift and hand-grip

* Receptor occupancies are approximate; there are some differences in results among various studies. Note that while much of normal function returns between 90 per cent and 70 per cent occupancy, subtle but important weakness persists until fewer than half of the receptors are occupied by relaxant molecules. TOF: train of four stimuli.

head-lift, sustained negative inspiratory pressure, or response to tetanic nerve stimuli, *provided the test is sustained for a period of five seconds*. This approach tests the adequacy of acetylcholine reserves relative to the degree of residual blockade and often reveals weakness not demonstrated by briefer challenges. When the patient's strength seems inadequate, or the result of the testing is equivocal, a few minutes' delay or additional antagonist followed by retesting is best.

DISEASES ALTERING THE RESPONSE TO MUSCLE RELAXANTS

Many systemic diseases alter the response to muscle relaxants. Kidney and liver failure have already been mentioned. The effects of neuromuscular diseases are described in Chapter 30.

REFERENCES

Fisher DM, Rosen JI. A pharmacokinetic explanation for increasing recovery time following larger or repeated doses of nondepolarizing muscle relaxants. Anesthesiology 1986; 65:286–291.

Pavlin EG, Holle RH, Schoene RB. Recovery of airway protection compared with ventilation in humans after paralysis with curare. Anesthesiology 1989; 70:381–285.

Viby-Morgensen J. Correlation of succinylcholine duration of action with plasma cholinesterase activity in subjects with the genotypically normal enzyme. Anesthesiology 1980; 53:517–520.

Viby-Morgensen J, Jorgensen BC, Ording H. Residual curarization in the recovery room. Anesthesiology 1979; 50:539–541.

CHAPTER TWELVE

THE MEDICAL GASES

This chapter concerns the simple gases that are important for medical practice, including oxygen, carbon dioxide, carbon monoxide, nitrogen, helium, and water vapor. Anesthesia gases and vapors, and respiratory pathophysiology are covered in other chapters (see especially Chapters 8 and 22).

OXYGEN

Gaseous oxygen derives from hydrolysis by photosynthetic organisms. The production of medical oxygen begins with air, compressed and cooled to a liquid, and then distilled into its major fractions: nitrogen (78 per cent), oxygen (21 per cent) and argon (1 per cent) (Table 12–1). Oxygen in large quantities is supplied as the liquid, the safest and most economical form, requiring only low-pressure insulated flasks (Dewars), and a minimum of space: 1 L of liquid oxygen yields about 850 L of oxygen gas at standard temperature and pressure. Compressed gaseous oxygen needs no insulated containers, but at 2250 psi yields only 150 L of gas per L of storage space. Further, compressed gas is more dangerous to store than the liquid form. Oxygen gas containers and piping are color-coded green in the United States and white in the United Kingdom. (See also Table 12–3.)

Oxygen analyzers can measure either partial pressure (activity, tension) or fraction (concentration, percentage) of oxygen in a gas mixture. Most operating room oxygen analyzers (fuel cell, paramagnetic, polarographic) measure oxygen partial pressure (P_{O_2}) and not percentage, despite the fractional unit scale; the calibration scale assumes one atmosphere ambient pressure. For example, a typical operating room oxygen analyzer calibrated for sea level operation reads 42 per cent, not 21 per cent, when exposed to air at 2 atmospheres. Mass spectrometry measures true fractional concentrations. Although fractional units (F_{IO_2}) are convenient, partial pressure is the biologically important unit. Oxygen toxicity can ensue at an F_{IO_2} of 0.2 and hypoxia at an F_{IO_2} of 1.0, depending on the barometric pressure (P_B). Thus, it is necessary to convert fractional concentration to partial pressure by multiplying by P_B. Variations in P_B can be a significant source of error in calculations of arterial-alveolar oxygen gradients if ignored.

Oxygen is administered by inhalation, except when extracorporeal oxygenators dissolve it directly in the exteriorized blood. Oxygen inhalational devices include nasal cannulae, masks, tents or hoods, and tracheal tubes.

Nasal Cannulae

Plastic tubing is used to deliver 2 to 5 L per minute of humidified oxygen into one or both nostrils. The nasopharynx serves as an oxygen reservoir, the contents of which are diluted with room air during inhalation. The resulting inspired oxygen concentration of less than 35 per cent is un-

TABLE 12–1. **Composition of Air (by Volume)**

Component	Per cent
Nitrogen	78.08
Oxygen	20.95
Argon	0.93
Water vapor*	0–7.0
Carbon dioxide	0.03
Neon	0.002
Helium	0.0005

* Depending on temperature and relative humidity.

predictable and depends on the patient's ventilatory pattern.

Face Masks

A wide variety of masks that cover both the mouth and nose are available for oxygen administration. Masks supplied with flow rates insufficient to meet peak inspiratory demand either entrain room air through ports, or include reservoir bags that fill with fresh gas during exhalation. One-way valves in the bag and sides of the mask encourage escape of exhaled gas, but a small amount of rebreathing occurs. Such masks require a close fit to the face and must be monitored for proper operation of the valves and reservoir bag. Oxygen flow rates must be sufficient to prevent bag collapse during inhalation.

Demand valve masks sense negative pressure during inspiration to trigger oxygen flow, making it mandatory that the mask fit tightly. These demand-type masks can deliver the greatest oxygen concentration, but they are probably the least comfortable for extended use. A tight-fitting seal to the face and valves is less important for masks that deliver gas flows that are sufficient to meet peak inspiratory demands, such as masks using venturi orifices. However, because these masks provide adequate inspiratory rates by diluting oxygen with room air, oxygen concentrations are limited to 50 per cent or less.

Hoods, Tents

Consistent oxygen concentrations can be administered by enlarging the inspiratory reservoir to encompass the entire head (hood), or body (tent) of the patient. These comfortable devices require little cooperation from the patient, but they are not suitable during anesthesia or critical care. Fresh gas flow rates must be adequate to prevent carbon dioxide accumulation.

Tracheal Tubes

Used during anesthesia or in the care of the critically ill, a cuffed tracheal tube reliably delivers to the lungs gas mixtures of known oxygen concentration, often accompanied by mechanical ventilation. Further details are in the chapters on airway management (see Chapter 13) and critical care (see Chapter 37).

OXYGEN UPTAKE AND DISTRIBUTION

Oxygen Uptake

Oxygen moves down a partial pressure gradient from the inspired air to the mitochondria (Fig. 12–1). Oxygen partial pressure decreases as the air is delivered to the distal airways and alveoli by inspiration, because of dilution with carbon dioxide and water vapor and oxygen uptake into the blood. Assuming homogeneity of ventilation and perfusion (see Chapter 22), the partial pressure of oxygen in the alveoli can be calculated to be approximately 110 mm Hg. Diffusion of oxygen into the pulmonary capillary blood is driven by the gradient between the alveolar gas and the mixed venous blood. Because of the extremely thin diffusion barrier between the alveolar space and pulmonary capillary blood, the Po_2 of end-capillary blood is normally within a few mm Hg of that in the local alveoli. Inhomogeneity of ventilation and perfusion influence the size of this gradient, and thus the rate of equilibration and end-capillary Po_2.

The partial pressure of oxygen in arterial blood (Pao_2) is less than that of mixed pulmonary capillary blood because of the addition of a small fraction of venous blood (shunt fraction). Together, the diffusional barrier, ventilation/perfusion inhomogeneity, and shunt fraction are the major components of the alveolar to arterial oxygen gradient (A-a gradient), normally 10 to 12 mm Hg when breathing air and 30 to 50 mm Hg when breathing 100 per cent oxygen.

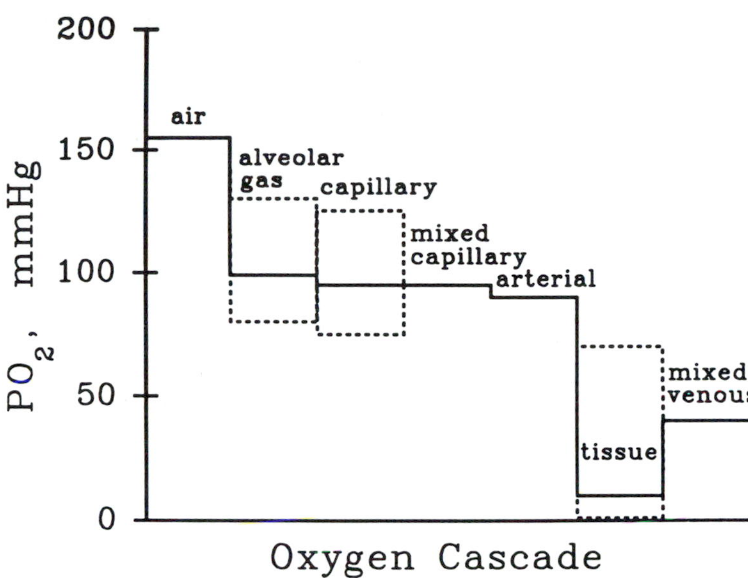

FIGURE 12–1. Normal partial pressure cascade for oxygen as it traverses from the inspired air to the tissues and venous blood. The steps are created by normal physiologic processes, such as ventilation/perfusion inequality, shunt, and metabolic use. Ultimately, metabolic consumption of oxygen is the driving force for oxygen movement through this cascade. The boxes indicate regions where a range of oxygen partial pressures are normally encountered, and the size of the box is an estimation of this range under normal conditions.

At the tissue capillary beds, oxygen again follows a gradient out of the blood into the cells and ultimately to mitochondria. As a result of the loss to the tissues, the PO_2 of mixed venous blood is less than that of arterial blood by about 40 mm Hg. Mean tissue PO_2 is even less than the mixed venous value, because of diffusional barriers and oxygen consumption in the tissues. At rest, approximately 3 ml oxygen are consumed per kg of body weight per minute.

Blood Oxygen Content

The majority of blood oxygen is carried in chemical combination with hemoglobin; lesser amounts are dissolved directly in plasma. The relationship between hemoglobin oxygen content and PO_2 is described by the sigmoid-shaped oxyhemoglobin dissociation curve (Fig. 12–2). When fully saturated, each gram of hemoglobin binds 1.31 ml of oxygen. In healthy subjects breathing air, hemoglobin is about 98 per cent saturated; further increases in PO_2 produced by breathing oxygen increase blood oxygen content by increasing the amount in plasma. The solubility of oxygen in plasma is only 0.003 ml per dl per mm Hg. Even in a healthy patient who achieves an arterial PO_2 of 500 mmHg by breathing 100 per cent oxygen, each 100 ml of plasma carries but 1.5 ml of oxygen in solution, the amount carried by little more than 1 gm of saturated hemoglobin.

The oxygen content of mixed venous blood is less than that of arterial blood by the amount required for metabolic needs, 5 to 6 ml per dl under normal conditions. In subjects breathing air, venous hemoglobin is 70 per cent saturated with oxygen, but this increases to 100 per cent when the inspired oxygen is increased to 3.0 atmospheres.

Oxygen is administered primarily to correct for its deficiency in the blood (hypoxemia) or tissues (tissue hypoxia). It is also used to dilute other gases, to enhance the elimination of an inert gas, and in hyperbaric chambers to treat specific diseases or intoxications.

Treatment of Hypoxia

Hypoxemia or tissue hypoxia are rarely due to a primary deficiency of oxygen in the inspired gas, but usually reflect underlying pathophysiology for which oxygen is a temporizing therapy. In the practice of anesthesiology and critical care medicine, the goals are to reduce the patient's need for supplemental oxygen by treating the pathophysiology responsible for the hypoxia, and to ensure that blood flow is adequate to supply the various tissues.

Oxygen as a Diluent

Oxygen is used as a carrier gas for the administration of other vapors and gases, such as inhaled

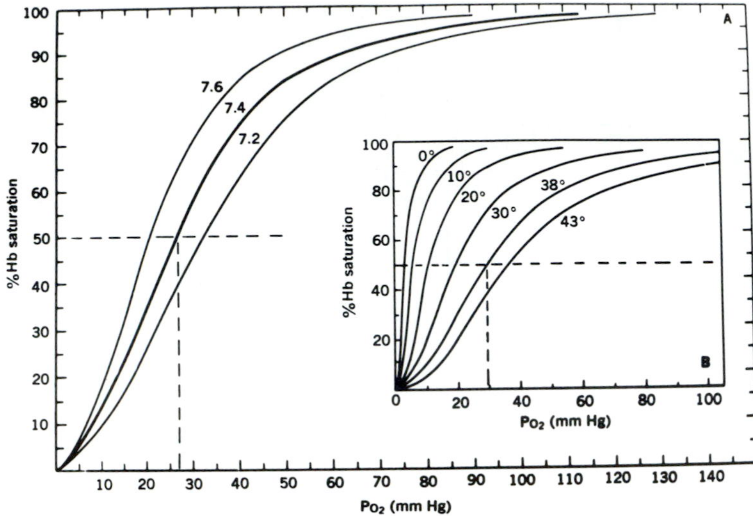

FIGURE 12–2. Oxyhemoglobin dissociation curves for whole blood. Large curve demonstrates the influence of hydrogen ion concentration on hemoglobin affinity for oxygen; the inset shows the effect of temperature on this affinity. In a working muscle, the increase in carbon dioxide and metabolic acid, combined with the increase in temperature, cooperate to increase oxygen unloading from hemoglobin. (With permission from Lambertsen CT. Transport of oxygen, carbon dioxide and inert gases by the blood. In Montcastle VB, ed. Medical physiology. 14th ed. Vol 2. St. Louis: CV Mosby, 1980.)

anesthetics. Oxygen serves a twofold purpose, because patients undergoing operation and anesthesia usually require oxygen supplementation to prevent hypoxemia.

Oxygen to Reduce Inert Gas Partial Pressure

The predominant gas in the body is nitrogen. Because nitrogen is relatively insoluble, reducing the inspired nitrogen concentration by oxygen inhalation rapidly decreases the blood and tissue nitrogen tension, speeding the removal of nitrogen from gas spaces. Closed spaces with free gas include the middle ear, sinuses, and bowel—especially obstructed or atonic bowel. Acquired gas spaces include pneumothorax, and pneumomediastinum, or result from pneumoencephalography, air embolism, or microembolism (decompression sickness).

Hyperbaric Oxygen Therapy (HBO)

Hyperbaric oxygen therapy has two inseparable components: increased hydrostatic pressure and increased oxygen tension. For gas bubble disease (decompression sickness, air embolism) both factors are therapeutic; hydrostatic pressure reduces bubble volume, and oxygen increases the gradient for nitrogen elimination while reducing hypoxia in downstream tissues. Increased tissue oxygen tension is the therapeutic goal for most other indications for HBO. For example, even a small increase in Po_2 in previously ischemic areas may permit leukocyte bactericidal activity, fibroblast function, and angiogenesis. Thus, HBO is a useful adjunct in chronic osteomyelitis, osteoradionecrosis, crush injury, or compromised skin/tissue grafts or flaps. Further, increased oxygen tension alone can be bacteriostatic; spread of organisms and toxin production by *Clostridia* are slowed by tissue oxygen tensions greater than about 250 mm Hg, justifying the early use of HBO in clostridial myonecrosis (gas gangrene).

Hyperbaric oxygen therapy has also found use in selected instances of generalized hypoxia. Carbon monoxide (see later) and cyanide intoxication both produce defects in oxygen utilization that are partially reversible by increased oxygen partial pressures. Hyperbaric oxygen therapy may also be useful in severe acute anemia, because sufficient oxygen can be dissolved in plasma at 3 atmosphere to meet metabolic needs.

Oxygen Toxicity

Temporizing oxygen therapy is limited by pulmonary oxygen toxicity resulting from an increased Po_2 even though oxygen *content* is normal or below normal.

Defenses against oxidative injury evolved along with mechanisms for using oxygen in energy production. These defenses consist of enzymes (superoxide dismutase, glutathione peroxidase, catalase) and reducing agents (glutathione, ascorbate, iron), as well as systems designed to eliminate damaged cellular constituents. Evolved in an atmosphere of less than 150 mm Hg oxygen, these defenses fail at increased oxygen tensions. Oxidative injury is likely initiated by an increased production of reactive species such as superoxide anion, singlet oxygen, hydroxyl radical, and hydrogen peroxide. The damage can be propagated and exaggerated by lipid peroxidation to finally involve the whole cell. Although toxic to all tissues, hyperoxia has different effects in different tissues, owing both to inherent tissue factors and to the Po_2 prevailing in the tissue.

Pulmonary Oxygen Toxicity

The lungs are continuously exposed to the greatest Po_2 of any organ system, and they are the first to demonstrate oxygen toxicity at 1 atmosphere. Oxygen inhalation for as little as six to eight hours decreases tracheal mucous velocity, and symptoms of tracheobronchial irritation and chest tightness begin in as little as 12 hours in normal subjects. Changes in pulmonary function begin after 12 to 24 hours of exposure. Nausea, vomiting, anorexia, and occasionally orthostasis are prominent symptoms with exposure for greater than 24 hours. The development of pulmonary oxygen toxicity is directly related to the PIo_2, so that substantial signs and symptoms are apparent after three to six hours of exposure to 2.0 atmospheres of oxygen. Survival time of otherwise normal primates in 100 per cent oxygen is in excess of a week, with death the result of pulmonary edema and, ironically, hypoxia.

The influence of concurrent disease on oxygen tolerance is poorly understood and unpredictable, and individual susceptibility to oxygen toxicity varies substantially. The maximum nontoxic PIo_2 has not been established, but prolonged exposure to 0.5 atmospheres produces few symptoms in normal subjects, and even allows recovery from acute lung injury in animals and humans. Absorption atelectasis is not an important contributor to pulmonary oxygen toxicity.

The therapy for oxygen toxicity relies on decreasing the PIo_2 and providing supportive measures. There are no specific pharmacologic approaches to therapy. Some amelioration in animals has been obtained by the parenteral administration of antioxidant enzymes in forms designed to gain access to the intracellular space. Dramatic improvements in oxygen tolerance have been produced with prior exposure to sublethal hyperoxia in some species; paradoxically, hypoxic exposure can also result in increased resistance to pulmonary oxygen toxicity. Similarly, human oxygen tolerance has been shown to increase significantly with brief interruptions of oxygen inhalation, a technique commonly employed in hyperbaric oxygen therapy. In animals, adaptation is associated with increased cellular antioxidant enzyme levels, proliferation of alveolar Type II cells, and increased alveolar surfactant levels.

Central Nervous System Oxygen Toxicity

Central nervous system oxygen toxicity is not usually seen at less than 2.0 atmospheres PIo_2. It usually occurs before pulmonary toxicity at pressures above 3.0 atmospheres, and, as with pulmonary toxicity, there is wide variation in individual sensitivity. The major manifestations of toxicity are convulsions, which may be preceded by visual symptoms or muscular twitching. Exercise and hypercarbia speed the onset of symptoms, probably owing to cerebral vasodilatation and increased delivery of oxygen to the brain. Central nervous system oxygen toxicity is rapidly reversed with decreases in the PIo_2, and sequelae have not been reported.

Retinal Oxygen Toxicity

Exposure of infants younger than 44 weeks gestation to increased alveolar oxygen tensions may be associated with retrolental fibroplasia, thought to be the result of aberrant angiogenesis in the developing eye. The fibroplastic changes may regress, or may progress to blindness. The syndrome may be largely prevented by titration of oxygen therapy to achieve defined hemoglobin saturation levels as detected by oximetry. Oxygen-induced retinopathy in adults is rare, even in hyperbaric exposures. Hyperbaric oxygen has been associated with reversible alterations in vision owing to a poorly understood effect on corneal shape.

CARBON DIOXIDE

Carbon dioxide (CO_2) is a product of oxidative respiration. The concentration in air is less than 0.1 per cent. At rest, normal human metabolic processes produce about 2.5 ml per kg body weight of carbon dioxide per minute. Carbon dioxide, having a diffusion coefficient 20 times higher than oxygen, readily diffuses out of mitochondria and cells with only a small gradient. It is then carried in the blood in three forms: dissolved carbon dioxide, carbamino compounds, and bicarbonate. The bicarbonate form predominates, while the dissolved form is the second largest pool in plasma. In red blood cells, carbamino forms constitute the second largest carbon dioxide pool because of the large concentration of amino groups in deoxygenated hemoglobin (Table 12–2).

Blood carbon dioxide content is substantially greater than blood oxygen content, and (in contrast to oxygen) changes little across the lungs. The arterial: alveolar carbon dioxide gradient is normally close to zero and occasionally negative. This small arterial-venous carbon dioxide content change minimizes pH fluctuations at the tissue and cellular level. The relationship between alveolar minute ventilation and the alveolar CO_2 is described in Chapter 2.

Carbon dioxide is stored in compressed gas cylinders for medical use, and in the solid form (dry ice) for refrigeration. Like nitrous oxide, carbon dioxide in cylinders at room temperature has a liquid phase. The room temperature vapor pressure is about 900 psi.

Carbon dioxide has few therapeutic applications, the most common being to stimulate ventilation. At an inspired carbon dioxide concentration of 10 per cent, total ventilation in a normal individual may be increased tenfold. Administered to a spontaneously breathing patient in 5 to 7 per cent concentration from an anesthesia machine, carbon dioxide markedly increases minute ventilation, thereby decreasing the time constants of volatile anesthetic uptake or elimination from the lung. This kinetic benefit to anesthetic uptake and elimination is further aided by the increase in cerebral blood flow produced by carbon dioxide inhalation. Anesthetics and narcotics depress the CO_2 ventilatory response. Because of this, and because of the effects of neuromuscular blockers, anesthetized patients may not respond to CO_2 inhalation with increased minute ventilation. The unwanted respiratory acidosis that can result is a hazard of this technique. The use of carbon dioxide to stimulate ventilation in cases of ventilatory depression is rarely indicated owing to the possibility of further CNS depression and acidosis.

TABLE 12–2. Distribution of Carbon Dioxide Content in Blood

1 L Blood	Arterial	Venous	A-V
P_{CO_2} (mm Hg)	41.0	46.0	5.0
pH	7.40	7.37	
Plasma carbon dioxide (ml)			
Dissolved	0.7	0.8	0.1
Bicarbonate	13.8	14.7	0.9
Carbamino compounds	0.2	0.2	0.0
RBC carbon dioxide (ml)			
Dissolved	0.5	0.5	0.0
Bicarbonate	6.0	6.4	0.4
Carbamino compounds	0.8	1.2	0.4
Total carbon dioxide (ml)	22.0	23.9	1.9

Although carbon dioxide inhalation has been suggested for the treatment of carbon monoxide intoxication, the possibility of further CNS depression and acidosis make it less desirable than the current standard of care, hyperbaric oxygenation. Because it is absorbed rapidly, does not burn or support combustion, and conducts heat poorly, carbon dioxide is also used to expand the abdomen during endoscopic procedures requiring electrocautery.

Inspired carbon dioxide concentrations above 7 per cent produce dyspnea, as well as headache owing to increased cerebral blood flow. Concentrations of 10 to 20 per cent can cause significant CNS depression, while slightly higher concentrations (25 to 30 per cent) can produce CNS excitability and convulsions. Even greater concentrations produce an anesthetic-like CNS depression once again. These concentrations are accompanied by significant acidosis.

Carbon dioxide has opposing direct and indirect cardiovascular effects. Inhalation of moderate concentrations (7 to 10 per cent) produces activation of the sympathetic nervous system and marked increases in circulating catecholamine concentrations. These effects are offset somewhat by a direct depressant effect on cardiac and vascular muscle. Cerebral vessels, having no important sympathetic innervation, dilate at increased carbon dioxide tensions. Carbon dioxide is also a coronary vasodilator, but has little effect on the renal or splanchnic circulations. The thresholds for convulsions are increased by CO_2. Arrhythmias during hypercarbia may be due in part to a decreased threshold for catechol-induced arrhythmias. Conversely, hyperventilation-induced hypocarbia is associated with hypokalemia, an important cause of arrhythmias.

Carbon Monoxide

An intermediate product of the combustion of hydrocarbons, carbon monoxide (CO) is a toxic gas that plays a small role in respiratory diagnostics. It is found in the smoke or exhaust of almost any combustion (fires, internal combustion engines, cigarettes), and may reach levels of 50 parts per million (ppm) in the atmosphere (in cities). It has no therapeutic indications, but is stored for diagnostic use in a premixed form (0.3 per cent) with oxygen and helium in compressed gas cylinders.

Carbon monoxide can be readily detected by infrared absorption, but because the concentration is usually small, and because it is toxic in very small amounts, detectors must be very sensitive. Carbon monoxide concentration in inspired gas is generally only monitored in specific high-risk industrial situations.

Normal persons have carboxyhemoglobin levels (Hbco) of from 1 to 2 per cent, owing to endogenously generated carbon monoxide and the small amounts normally present in the atmosphere. Because cigarette smoke contains 1 to 5 per cent carbon monoxide, smokers have Hbco levels of 5 to 12 per cent, with no significant symptoms. Continuous inhalation of only 0.1 per cent (1000 ppm) carbon monoxide produces Hbco levels in excess of 40 per cent and severe symptoms. Although the concentration of carboxyhemoglobin correlates poorly with symptoms and prognosis it remains the most useful practical measure of CO exposure.

Highly toxic, carbon monoxide is a leading cause of poisoning deaths in the United States. It interferes with oxygen delivery and utilization because of the leftward shift of the oxyhemoglobin dissociation curve, its affinity for hemoglobin, and its interaction with cytochrome oxidase, especially under hypoxic conditions. The result is tissue hypoxia is manifest usually as neurological depression, coma, and perhaps hemodynamic instability, rhabdomyolysis, and myoglobin-induced renal failure. Patients who recover from significant CO exposures are at risk for delayed (2 to 20 days) neurological symptoms: confusion, ataxia, and depression.

The treatment of acute CO poisoning relies on administering 100 per cent oxygen, or hyperbaric oxygen (HBO). The greater number of oxygen molecules achieved with HBO compete with the CO molecules for binding sites on hemoglobin and other proteins, speeding the elimination of CO. For patients with a history of unconsciousness, hemodynamic instability, or who are at the extremes of age, evidence suggests that hyperbaric oxygen given up to six hours after exposure, regardless of Hbco levels, reduces the incidence of delayed neurologic sequelae.

The medical use of carbon monoxide is as a tracer gas for the measurement of pulmonary diffusing capacity. Its affinity for hemoglobin (200 times that of oxygen) is the basis for this use of carbon monoxide; the carbon monoxide tension in the capillary blood remains negligible, which simplifies the calculations necessary to derive diffusing capacity. The diffusing capacity for oxygen is calculated as 1.23 times that for carbon monoxide.

Minimizing the Hbco level by not smoking cigarettes before anesthesia and operation increases oxygen delivery. Cessation of cigarette smoking for four weeks has also been shown to improve lung function and decrease pulmonary symptoms. A transient increase in airway secretions and cough may occur a few days after stopping cigarette smoking owing to recovery of mucociliary function, but this does not outweigh the benefits gained.

Helium

Although the second most common element in the universe, helium is uncommon on earth, constituting only about 0.003 per cent of the atmosphere. Primarily the product of radioactive decay, it is obtained in limited quantities from underground wells in the Midwest. It is stored as high-pressure gas in cylinders, or in the liquid form (a few degrees above absolute zero). The low density, insolubility, and thermal conductivity of helium form the basis for its medical and diagnostic applications.

Although mass spectrometry can be used to measure helium, monitoring normally consists of measuring other inspired gases (usually oxygen) and subtracting from the ambient pressure. Helium is mixed with the desired concentration of oxygen and administered by mask, mouthpiece, or tracheal tube. In certain hyperbaric applications, the entire surrounding atmosphere consists of a helium-oxygen or helium-nitrogen-oxygen mixture.

Pulmonary Function Testing.

Determination of residual lung volume, functional residual capacity, and derived measures requires a highly diffusible gas carried away by the pulmonary circulation only in negligible amounts, so that dilution into the lung gas can be measured. Of the inert gases, helium bests meets these criteria. In practice, a single large breath of known helium concentration is administered, and the concentration of helium is then measured in the mixed expired gas; lung volumes are then derived by appropriate calculations.

Respiratory Obstruction

Most gas flow in the lungs is laminar, especially in the distal airways. However, increased flow rates or airways obstruction increase the proportion of flow that is turbulent. Resistance to turbulent flow is proportional to gas density. Because the density of helium is substantially less than that of air, helium-oxygen mixtures may be useful in cases of respiratory obstruction. Three factors reduce the practicality of this approach. First, oxygenation is the principal concern in airways obstruction, and the increase in flow rates with helium-oxygen mixtures may not improve oxygenation as well as 100 per cent oxygen would. Second, the addition of oxygen to helium increases the density of the mixture. Third, the viscosity of helium exceeds that of air, which reduces gas flow in regions where laminar flow predominates (small airways). One predicts that helium breathing may be most helpful with large airways obstruction and perhaps even detrimental in asthma, where small airway obstruction is the primary problem.

LASER AIRWAY SURGERY

Helium neither burns nor supports combustion, making it valuable during laser operations on the airway. It conducts heat well, minimizing not only the spread of tissue damage but the chance of igniting flammable materials in the airway. Helium also improves the flow rate of gas through the small endotracheal tubes commonly used for such operations.

Although the thermal conductivity of helium is known to increase heat loss in subjects surrounded by a helium atmosphere in a hyperbaric chamber or diving suit, the respiratory component of heat loss is not increased with helium as compared to air or oxygen. This is because respiratory gas is fully equilibrated with body temperature by the time of exhalation, regardless of composition; thus, the heat *capacity*—not its *conductivity*— is the relevant property. The heat capacity of helium per unit volume is less than that of air, so helium-oxygen mixtures may actually reduce the respiratory component of overall heat loss.

TABLE 12–3. Physical Constants for Medical Gases

Gas	MW (g/mol)	Density* (g/L)	Viscosity* (Micropoise)	Solubility* (Blood/Gas)	Thermal Conductivity* (cal/sec cm °C)	Specific Heat (cal/gm °C)
Oxygen	32	1.43	202	0.024†	64	0.22
Nitrogen	28	1.25	175	0.013	62	0.25
Nitrous Oxide	44	1.98	145	0.45	41	
Argon	40	1.78	222	0.026	43	0.12
Carbon Dioxide	44	1.98	148	0.60	40	
Helium	4	0.18	194	0.008	360	1.24

* Density and visosity at about 20°C. and conductivity at 27°C; solubility in ml gas/ml solvent with 100 per cent gas and at 37°C.
† Not including that bound to hemoglobin.

Hyperbaric Applications

Depth and duration of diving or hyperbaric chamber activity is limited by oxygen toxicity, by nitrogen narcosis, and by tissue inert gas content on decompression (occasionally producing decompression sickness, or the "bends"). Oxygen toxicity is apparent with prolonged exposures to compressed air at 5 atmospheres or more, a problem that can be decreased by diluting the oxygen concentration with inert gas. The use of helium as a diluent inert gas for diving is based on its near-complete lack of narcotic potential, and its insolubility in body tissues and fluids, which reduces the volume of dissolved helium. This reduces decompression time and the risk of microembolism (bubbles) after decompression. The low density of helium also reduces the work of breathing in otherwise dense hyperbaric atmospheres.

There is no specific toxicity of helium at atmospheric pressure. Under hyperbaric conditions, its thermal conductivity can result in hypothermia, and the absence of any narcotic potential unmasks the direct CNS-excitatory effect of hydrostatic pressure (high pressure neurological syndrome). The voice distortion that occurs can result in communication difficulties.

WATER VAPOR

Water requires a great deal of heat to vaporize and has a relatively great specific heat as well. Although inspired gas is humidified by the conducting airways, at times supplemental administration of water vapor is needed.

Normal biological humidification of inspired gases maintains a moist and mobile mucociliary blanket, as well as a liquid layer in the respiratory regions that provides elasticity at larger lung volumes, permits a substrate layer on which pulmonary surfactant can function, and generally promotes effective gas exchange. The administration of inspired gases other than atmospheric air is the principal indication for supplementary humidification, especially when a tracheal tube is in place, or in patients at increased risk of hypothermia (infants) or pulmonary complications.

The fully humidified air in the alveoli at 37° C contains 50 mg of water per L, of which the person at rest contributes about half, or approximately 200 ml per day, under normal environmental conditions (60 to 70 per cent relative humidity). Dry inspired gas mixtures increase this requirement, and placement of a tracheal tube shifts the humidification site into the tracheobronchial tree. Although usually tolerable, this increased demand for water and the more distal site increase the heat lost to vaporization, and decreased mobility of the mucociliary blanket results. External warming and humidification of the inspired gas slightly decreases respiratory heat loss and promotes mucociliary mobility.

Supplemental water vapor can be delivered through any of the devices listed previously for inhalation of oxygen or by bubbling the inhaled gas through water that is heated to increase its vapor pressure. Alternatively, water or saline solution may be nebulized ultrasonically to deliver both water vapor and water droplets, which may be used to deliver bronchodilators, mucolytic drugs, or steroids to the respiratory system.

Adverse effects from simple humidification of inspired gases are rare. Adverse reactions to aerosols include infection, airway irritation, bronchospasm, overhydration, and thermal injury.

NITROGEN

Nitrogen is the most common gas in our atmosphere. Its principal medical use is as a diluent for oxygen, to avoid oxygen toxicity. It is provided in either compressed or liquid form.

Nitrogen is a weak anesthetic (minimal alveolar concentration about 10 atmospheres). Although a few studies have purported to demonstrate this effect under normobaric conditions (suggesting that we are all slightly anesthetized!), the effect is only significant at increased atmospheric pressure—above three atmospheres. This has implications for undersea divers, caisson workers, and for workers in hyperbaric chambers. The anesthetic effect is reduced by diluting the inspired gas with other inert gases, such as helium.

Although nitrogen is not extremely soluble, sufficient amounts can be dissolved in blood and tissue at increased pressure so that on decompression, it is released in the form of nitrogen bubbles. This is the etiology of the decompression sickness syndromes, which range in severity from pruritus to paraplegia to death. These syndromes are prevented by gradual decompression or by increasing the gradient for nitrogen elimination by breathing oxygen prior to or during decompression. The treatment for decompression sickness relies on hyperbaric oxygen, as discussed earlier.

REFERENCES

Deneke SM, Fanburg BL. Normobaric oxygen toxicity of the lung. N Engl J Med 1980; 303:76–86.

Eckenhoff RG, Longnecker DE. The therapeutic gases: oxygen, carbon dioxide, helium and water vapor (Chapter 16). *in* Gilman AG, Rall TW, Nies AS, Taylor P, eds. The pharmacologic basis of therapeutics. 8th ed. New York: Pergamon Press, 1990: 332–334.

Klocke RA. Carbon dioxide transport. *In* Handbook of physiology. Sect. 3, Vol 4. Bethesda: American Physiologic Society, 1987; 173–198.

Nunn, JF. Applied respiratory physiology. 3rd ed. Boston: Butterworth's, 1987.

Thom SR. Hyperbaric oxygen therapy. J Intensive Care Med 1989; 4:58–74.

Thom SR, Kiem LW. Carbon monoxide poisoning: a review. Epidemiology, pathophysiology, clinical findings and treatment options including hyperbaric oxygen therapy. Clin Toxicol 1989; 27:141–156.

Weibel ER. The pathway for oxygen. Cambridge: Harvard University Press, 1984.

SECTION 4

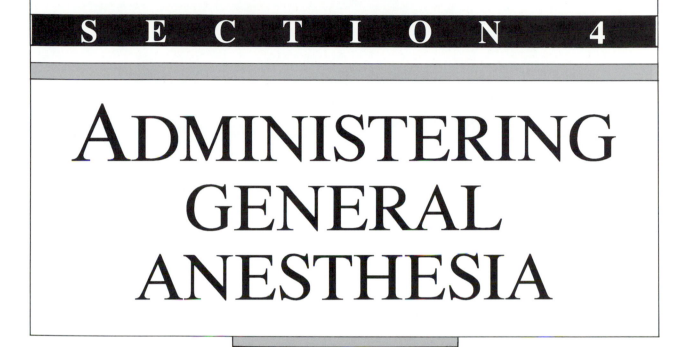

ADMINISTERING GENERAL ANESTHESIA

CHAPTER THIRTEEN

Airway Management

Airway obstruction occurs frequently in unconscious patients. Most serious mishaps in the perioperative period are related to inadequate ventilation and an obstructed airway. Careful attention to airway management is an important part of the care of all surgical patients, whether in the operating room, the postanesthesia recovery room or the intensive care unit.

Applied Anatomy of the Airway

The tongue, mobile despite its attachments to the mandible, hyoid bone, and epiglottis, is the major cause of airway obstruction in anesthetized patients. The nose provides a second route for breathing and a more stable site for endotracheal tubes, although the nasal passages may be blocked by polyps or a septal deformity. Three bony turbinates project from the lateral wall of the nasal cavity. Their mucosal coverings are easily damaged, causing epistaxis during nasotracheal intubation.

The pharynx extends from the base of the skull to join the esophagus at the level of the cricoid cartilage. There, a sphincter is formed by the lower portion of the inferior constrictor muscle that originates from the cricoid cartilage, the cricopharyngeus muscle. The pharynx communicates anteriorly with the nasal cavity, the oral cavity, and the larynx (Fig. 13–1).

The soft palate separates the nasopharynx from the oropharynx. During anesthesia, it can move passively to prevent exhalation through the nose. Largest during childhood, the nasopharyngeal tonsil (or adenoids) may produce obstruction or hemorrhage during nasotracheal intubation. Beneath the nasopharynx, at the level of the second and third cervical vertebrae, is the oropharynx. If excessive negative airway pressure develops during the increased inspiratory efforts associated with partial airway obstruction, the oropharyngeal walls may collapse. At the level of the fourth to the sixth cervical vertebrae, the hypopharynx provides access to the glottis and esophagus, and laterally includes the two pyriform sinuses.

Three single cartilages (thyroid, cricoid, and epiglottic) and three paired cartilages (arytenoid, corniculate, and cuneiform) form the larynx (Fig. 13–2). Abduction of the normally functioning vocal cords during inspiration gives a triangular shape to the glottic opening (rima glottidis), which is the narrowest part of the adult airway (Fig. 13–3). In children, the cricoid cartilage forms a complete ring and is the narrowest portion of the child's airway. Pressing the cricoid ring against the vertebral bodies while the neck is extended (Sellick's maneuver) occludes the esophagus, impeding gastroesophageal regurgitation.

The true and false vocal cords insert anteriorly on the thyroid cartilage and posteriorly on the arytenoid cartilages. The pyramid-shaped arytenoids articulate with the posterosuperior aspect of the cricoid cartilage; movement of the cricoid and arytenoids controls the position and tension of the

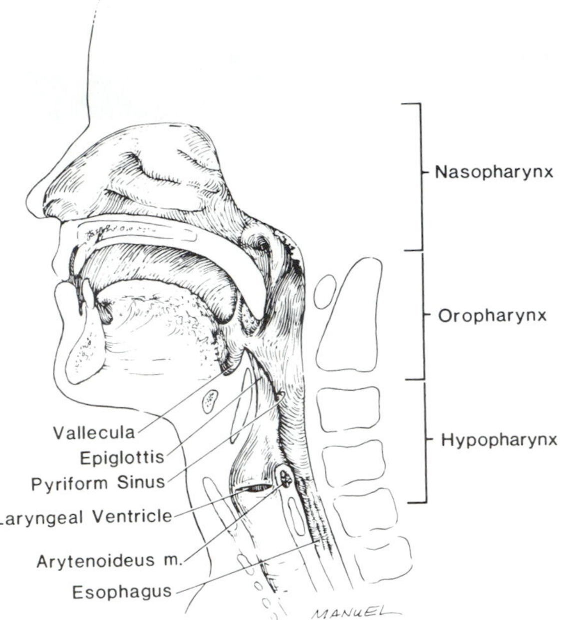

FIGURE 13–1. A sagittal section of the pharynx showing three subdivisions of the pharynx. (Reproduced with permission from Ovassapian A. Fiberoptic airway endoscopy in anesthesia and critical care. New York: Raven Press, 1990.)

vocal cords. Atop the arytenoids and embedded in the aryepiglottic folds, the corniculate and cuneiform cartilages form medial and lateal prominences that provide landmarks for the passage of a tracheal tube during difficult tracheal intubation.

The adult epiglottis has a crescent-shaped cross section; however, in a few adults and most infants, the epiglottic cross section assumes more of a "U" shape, which, in combination with a greater length, makes glottic exposure difficult. The valleculae are depressions between a median and two lateral glossoepiglottic ligaments. These ligaments permit indirect elevation of the epiglottis with the curved laryngoscope.

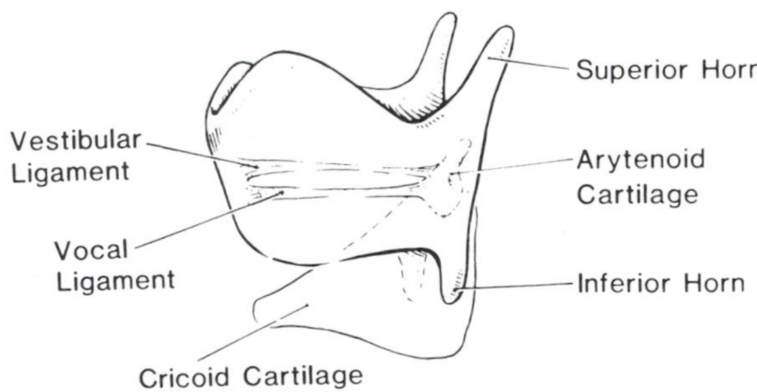

FIGURE 13–2. Demonstrates the relationship of thyroid, cricoid, and arytenoid cartilages. (Reproduced with permission from Smith C, Ramsey RG. Xeroradiography of the lateral neck. Radio Graphics 1982;2:306–328.)

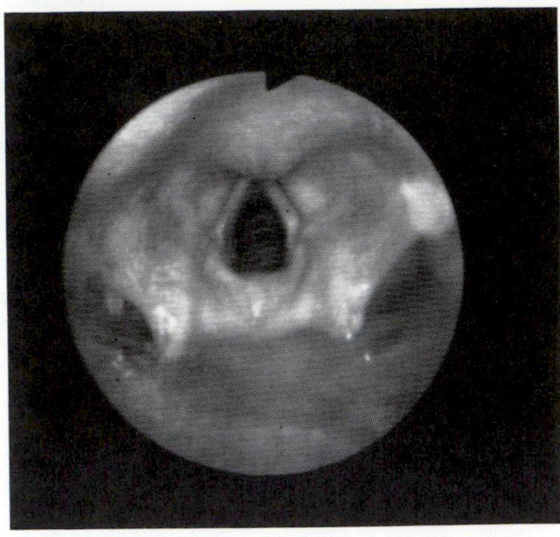

FIGURE 13–3. Endoscopic view of the larynx. Black triangle at 12 o'clock indicates the tubercle of epiglottis, below which true and false vocal cords with laryngeal ventricle appear. Pyriform sinuses represented by deepest part of hypopharynx lateral to aryepiglottic folds bilaterally.

The superior thyroid notch is the most distinctive landmark on the anterior surface of the neck, though it may be subtle in women and children. Identified as the depression between the thyroid and cricoid cartilages, the cricothyroid ligament is used for translaryngeal injection of local anesthetic, transtracheal ventilation, retrograde intubation, and cricothyrotomy (Fig. 13–4). Palpable landmarks for superior laryngeal nerve blocks are the lateral horns of the hyoid bone, found at the level of the third cervical vertebra.

Growing from 4 cm long in infancy to 10 to 14

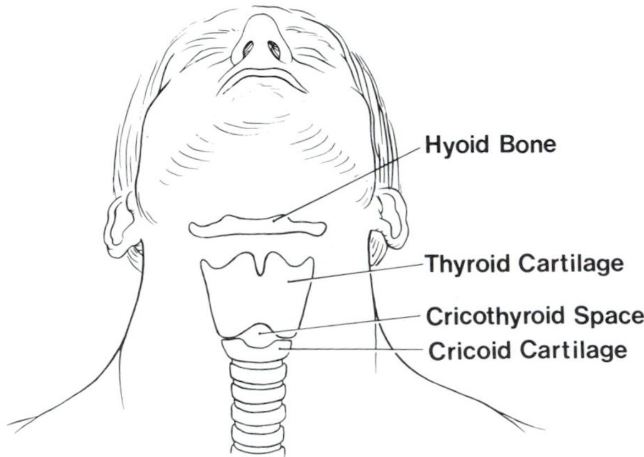

FIGURE 13–4. Front view of neck. Demonstrates the cricothyroid membrane and relation of hyoid bone to the thyroid cartilage. (Reproduced with permission from Smith C, Ramsey RG. Xeroradiography of the lateral neck. Radio Graphics 1982; 2:306–328.)

cm in the adult, the trachea extends from the lower border of the cricoid cartilage to the carina, where it divides into the right and left mainstem bronchi. A prominent aortic arch, congenital vascular anomalies, an anterior mediastinal mass, or enlarged mediastinal lymph nodes can compress and obstruct the trachea, even interfering with intubation.

In the adult, the right mainstem bronchus is 1.8 cm long and leaves the trachea at an angle of 25 to 30 degrees. The left mainstem bronchus, 5.0 cm in length, leaves the trachea at a sharper angle, about 45 degrees. In infants, the angles formed by the two main bronchi are more nearly equal than in the adult.

ASSESSMENT OF THE AIRWAY

Because airway problems are easiest to manage when they are anticipated, airway evaluation is a major part of preoperative assessment. Difficult airway management may be caused by extremes of common anatomy, specific pathologic states, or technical problems (Table 13–1). These factors may prevent a snug fit between mask and face, interfere with positioning of the head and neck, limit the opening of the mouth, narrow the airway, or fix and distort the involved tissues. Information obtained from the history may be suggestive (Table 13–2), but it is a thorough examination of the airway that enables the anesthesiologist to identify most problems (Table 13–3).

To assess airway anatomy, the anesthesiologist examines the sitting patient from the front as well as the side. The patient looks forward, opens the mouth, protrudes the tongue, closes the mouth, and then extends the head. The mouth opening (interincisal gap) and the distance from the mandibular mentum to the superior thyroid notch during neck extension are measured. The hyoid bone, superior thyroid notch, and cricothyroid ligament are each palpated, and the size, firmness, and mobility of any abnormal masses are evaluated. Listening to the patient reveals the ventilatory pattern as well as any abnormal sounds: nasal speech, hoarseness, coughing, wheezing or stridor.

Radiologic studies may be needed when examination reveals trauma, tumors, or deviation of the airway. Whereas lateal cervical spine films can confirm or exclude vertebral damage, computed tomography or magnetic resonance imaging reveals the degree of tracheal compression and upper airway abnormalities.

TABLE 13–1. Some Causes of Difficult Intubation or Difficult Mask Ventilation

1. Anatomic Features
    - Short, muscular neck
    - Protruding maxillary incisors
    - Long, high, arched palate with narrow mouth
    - Limited mobility of the neck
    - Receding mandible
    - Small mouth opening (interincisal gap less than 40 mm in adult)
2. Other Pathologic States
    - Hereditary angioedema
    - Arthritis and ankylosis
    - Cervical spine immobility
    - Temporomandibular joint disease
    - Laryngeal abnormalities
    - Congenital anomalies
        - Klippel-Feil syndrome
        - Pierre Robin syndrome
        - Treacher-Collins syndrome
    - Endocrinopathies
        - Obesity
        - Acromegaly
        - Hypothyroidism
        - Goiter
    - Infections
        - Ludwig's angina
        - Retropharyngeal abscess
        - Epiglottitis
    - Myopathies
    - Scarring
    - Trauma, swelling, hematoma
    - Tumors and cysts
3. Technical and Mechanical Factors
    - Body cast
    - Halo traction and cervical collar
    - Foreign bodies in the airway
    - Poor technique, inexperience, or haste
    - Leaks around a face mask
        - Edentulous
        - Flat bridge of nose
        - Large face and head
        - Whiskers
        - Nasogastric tubes

Quantitative estimates of airway obstruction can be obtained with flow-volume spirometry. Recognizable patterns appear in the case of extrathoracic, intrathoracic, dynamic, fixed, or combined airway obstruction.

When doubt remains about the ability to intubate, direct inspection of the airway is indicated. Fiberoptic or rigid laryngoscopy under topical anesthesia and sedation may precede awake/sedated intubation or conventional induction of anes-

TABLE 13–2. Clues from the History, Suggesting Difficult Intubation or Difficult Mask Ventilation

Finding	Result
Loud snorer	Soft tissue airway obstruction
Gastroesophageal reflux	Risk of aspiration
Undigested food in mouth	Pharyngeal pouch (Zenker's diverticulum) (poses aspiration risk)
Dry cough	Tracheobronchial compression
Easy bleeding	Epistaxis
Radiation to the neck	Fibrosis and immobility
Cigarette smoking	Salivation, coughing, and laryngospasm
Recent temporal craniotomy	Temporalis muscle scarring (limits mouth opening)
Longstanding diabetes mellitus	Stiff joints (limit positioning)

thesia, depending on the results of the examination.

HYPOVENTILATION, APNEA, AND PREOXYGENATION

Hypoventilation, one result of airway obstruction, produces hypercapnia and sometimes hypoxemia. During apnea, Pa_{CO_2} increases abruptly 6 to 8 mm Hg in the first minute, and 2 to 3 mm Hg each minute thereafter. Although hypoventilation while breathing room air leads to hypoxemia when the alveolar ventilation decreases to about 1.5 L per minute, supplemental oxygen is an effective remedy. At an F_{IO_2} of 50 per cent, normal patients can maintain oxyhemoglobin saturation above 95 per cent at an alveolar ventilation of 0.5 L per minute. At 100 per cent F_{IO_2}, the oxyhemoglobin saturation may remain near 100 per cent even during apnea, as long as an open airway provides communication between the oxygen source and the alveoli. This apneic oxygenation technique is especially useful during operations involving the airway.

Denitrogenation, often misnamed "preoxygenation," increases the margin of safety in the event of prolonged apnea. The typical adult consumes 250 ml per minute of oxygen and has a functional residual capacity (FRC) of 2500 ml. When the inspired oxygen concentration is 21 per cent, the FRC contains less than 500 ml of oxygen, enough to meet the patient's metabolic requirements for less than than two minutes. After denitrogenation by breathing 100 per cent oxygen, the FRC con-

TABLE 13–3. Physical Findings That Suggest Difficult Intubation or Difficult Mask Ventilation

Finding	Result
Obesity	Soft tissue upper airway obstruction; poor view of larynx; regurgitation risk; diminished thoracic compliance
Pregnancy	Obesity; large breasts impair laryngoscope insertion; swollen mucosae bleed easily
Ascites	Regurgitation risk; poor thoracic compliance
Mouth opens less than 40 mm	Glottis obscured by teeth, tongue, or epiglottis
Head extension produces angle at hyoid less than 160 degrees	Difficult to align mouth and pharynx for glottic exposure
Distance from thyroid notch less than 6 cm; receding chin	Difficult to displace tongue to visualize glottis
Short, thick, muscular neck	Soft tissue upper airway obstruction; difficult to mobilize neck and tongue
"Maxillary gap" caused by missing incisors with other right maxillary teeth present	Laryngoscope fits into gap, while adjacent teeth, lip, or gums obscure view of glottis and passage of tracheal tube
Edentulous, with atrophic mandible	Small face and furrowed cheeks impair mask fit; tongue and soft palate block exhalation
Whiskers, flat nasal bridge, large face	Difficult to seal mask
Prominent or protruding incisors	Teeth block view of glottis
Advanced caries, loose teeth, caps, bridges	Can be damaged or aspirated
Nasogastric tube	Difficult to seal mask
Stridor; retractions	Risk of insurmountable airway obstruction
Hoarseness	Chance of vocal cord malfunction or airway masses
"Underwater" voice	Vallecular or epiglottic cysts
Poorly visualized soft palate and fauces in upright patients with mouth fully open	Difficult to mask ventilate and to expose glottis
Immobile tumors displacing trachea; large goiter	Difficult to expose glottis; airway obstruction or tracheal collapse
Tracheostomy scar	Possible subglottic stenosis

TABLE 13–4. Steps for Effective Denitrogenation/ Preoxygenation

1. Pop-off valve open to avoid high airway pressure
2. Vaporizers off
3. Oxygen at 8 to 10 L/min
4. Leak-free face mask fit to prevent entrainment of room air. Recognize good fit when rebreathing bag fills.
5. Four vital capacity breaths, or quiet breathing for 2 to 3 minutes

tains oxygen equal to the patient's metabolic needs for eight to ten minutes (Table 13–4).

In a denitrogenated patient whose FRC contains 90 to 95 per cent oxygen and who has a sudden complete airway obstruction, the Pa_{CO_2} increases to 70 to 80 mm Hg in the eight to ten minutes it takes for profound hypoxemia to evolve. By itself, such hypercarbia is unlikely to cause morbidity as serious as the attendant hypoxemia. Infants, pregnant patients, and the obese fare less well during apnea because of their greater oxygen consumptions and smaller functional residual capacities. Nevertheless, all patients benefit from denitrogenation before anesthesia and airway manipulation.

AIRWAY MANAGEMENT WITHOUT INTUBATION

The steps in airway management by mask include assessing the adequacy of ventilation, positioning the patient to facilitate ventilation, achieving a leak-free mask seal, providing manual positive pressure mask ventilation when needed, and employing artificial airways or muscle relaxants to improve airway patency.

Assessing Adequacy of Ventilation

In the absence of arterial blood gas analysis, the anesthesiologist assesses the adequacy of ventilation by integrating many observations, especially chest wall motion (Table 13–5). Other signs of hypoventilation may be deceptive. During mask ventilation, small tidal volumes and apparatus dead space combine to impede the access of alveolar gas to a capnometer; the maximum P_{CO_2} may deceptively underestimate the alveolar P_{CO_2} during spontaneous ventilation with a face mask (Table 13–5).

Although hypoxemia is a late sign of hypoventilation, a finding of hypoxemia in an anesthetized patient prompts an immediate assessment of ventilation. Cyanosis is an unreliable sign, as it requires 5 gm per dl of deoxygenated hemoglobin to be apparent. This implies a hemoglobin oxygen saturation of 50 per cent in a patient having a hemoglobin concentration of 10 to 15 gm per dl. The cardiorespiratory signs of hypoxemia (tachycardia, hypertension, and tachypnea) may have other causes and are often blunted by anesthetics, narcotics, or other drugs such as beta-adrenergic blockers. If one misses the early signs of hypoventilation, pulse oximetry eventually warns of hemoglobin desaturation, regardless of its cause.

Positioning to Facilitate Ventilation

Upper airway obstruction is usually caused by the base of the tongue sliding posteriorly as the genioglossus and geniohyoid muscles relax during anesthesia. The sniffing position, provided by rest-

TABLE 13–5. Signs that Suggest Adequate or Inadequate Ventilation When the Trachea Has Not Been Intubated

Suggests Adequate Ventilation	Suggests Inadequate Ventilation
Normal breath sounds	Stridor, phonation, snoring
Subcostal region rhythmically rising and falling	Subcostal region motionless or rising with inspiration, but not falling
Reservoir bag refilling during exhalation at fresh gas flows under 2 L/m	Reservoir bag not filling
Spirometer registers appropriate tidal volume with each attempted breath	Paradoxical chest movement without producing a measurable tidal volume
Correct sequence of respiration: Upper chest expands before or along with subcostal protrusion	Pathologic respiratory movements: Chest retracts while abdomen rises; tracheal tug; nasal flaring; supraclavicular and intercostal retractions
Normal vital signs and oxygen saturation	Tachycardia, bradycardia, hypotension, dysrhythmia, hypertension, tachypnea, bradypnea, oxygen desaturation
Plateau-shaped capnogram with normal end-tidal CO_2	Capnogram without a plateau; increased end-tidal CO_2
Pulse oximeter reads 100%	Pulse oximeter reads less than 100%

ing the adult occiput on a firm 8 to 10 cm pillow (the large occiputs of small children eliminate the need for head support) and extending the cervico-occipital joint, opens the airway. Displacing the mandible anteriorly further expands the airway by moving the base of the tongue. Pushing the mandible anteriorly and upward toward the maxilla may impede ventilation, especially in the edentulous patient. This maneuver forces the tongue against the hard palate, while the soft palate and posterior pharyngeal wall form a one-way flap valve. Positive pressure mask ventilation pushes gas into the lungs via the nasopharynx, but exhalation is checked. This soft tissue airway obstruction can be corrected by inserting an oral airway.

When airway patency cannot be achieved with the chin in the midline, turning the patient's head to one side may prove effective. Roentgenographic and fiberoptic examinations have shown that the epiglottis itself rarely may produce obstruction unrelieved by maneuvers of the head and jaw or placement of artificial airways. Such patients require prompt tracheal intubation.

Once the airway obstruction is recognized, there are three reasons why efforts to relive it must begin immediately. First, even after denitrogenation, hypoxemia will follow in a matter of minutes. Second, attempts to inhale against a closed glottis increase the gastroesophageal pressure gradient and predispose to regurgitation. Third, brief periods of increased negative airway pressure, caused by inhaling against an obstructed airway, can result in pulmonary edema, even in healthy patients.

To decrease upper abdominal pressure, improve thoracic compliance, and maintain the FRC, the head-up position is advantageous for patients who are pregnant or obese or who suffer from ascites.

Achieving a Good Mask Fit

Without a tight seal between mask and face, positive pressure ventilation is difficult, anesthetic gases may pollute the environment, and room air may dilute the inspired gases. To achieve a good fit, several steps are needed. The cushion on the mask is filled with air (Fig. 13–5). The superior angle of the mask is fitted to the depth of the bridge of the nose, while the inferior margin of the mask is applied to the chin. One's middle and ring fingers pull the mandible anteriorly, and the thumb and index finger, placed one above and one below the connector, lightly press the mask to the face. Excessive submandibular pressure may completely obstruct the airway.

Maintaining a mask fit—even for hours—is possible if one holds the mask correctly and the patient's anatomy is favorable. Mask straps are helpful, but they present hazards, including pressure damage to facial structures and retention of secretions or vomitus under the mask.

Clear masks reveal any secretions, vomitus or cyanosis of the lips and the fogging that accompanies ventilation. The large, soft cushions on disposable masks fit patients with flat noses. In small children, a molded, cushion-free mask (Rendell-Baker Soucek) minimizes dead space; thumb and forefinger are used as in the conventional mask grip, but only the third finger is needed to lift the chin and soft tissues into the mask.

In edentulous patients with furrowed cheeks, a mask seal may be achieved by inserting an oral airway to separate the mandible from the maxilla, filling out the cheeks with gauze sponges or pulling the lower lip onto the inferior rim of the mask. Leaving snug dentures in place fills out the cheeks, but this risks loss or damage to the dentures.

In challenging patients, an airway and mask seal may be established only by using the two-handed jaw thrust. Both thumbs and possibly the anesthetist's chin press on the mask while all fingers apply anterior traction to the angles and the rami of the mandible. An assistant manages ventilation and the remainder of anesthetic care.

Positive Pressure Ventilation

Positive airway pressure applied by mask in excess of 20 cm H_2O (15 mm Hg) may force air into the esophagus. Gentle, shallow breaths minimize this likelihood and are better tolerated by lightly anesthetized patients than are abrupt, large breaths. A stethoscope in the suprasternal notch helps to confirm gas movement.

Positive pressure ventilation is best begun gradually as anesthesia is induced and deepened. The ideal progression is from spontaneous ventilation with the mask on the face, to assisted ventilation, to controlled ventilation. Assisted breaths must be in phase with the patient's spontaneous breathing. The advantage of this gentle progression is that steps can be retraced if ventilatory problems

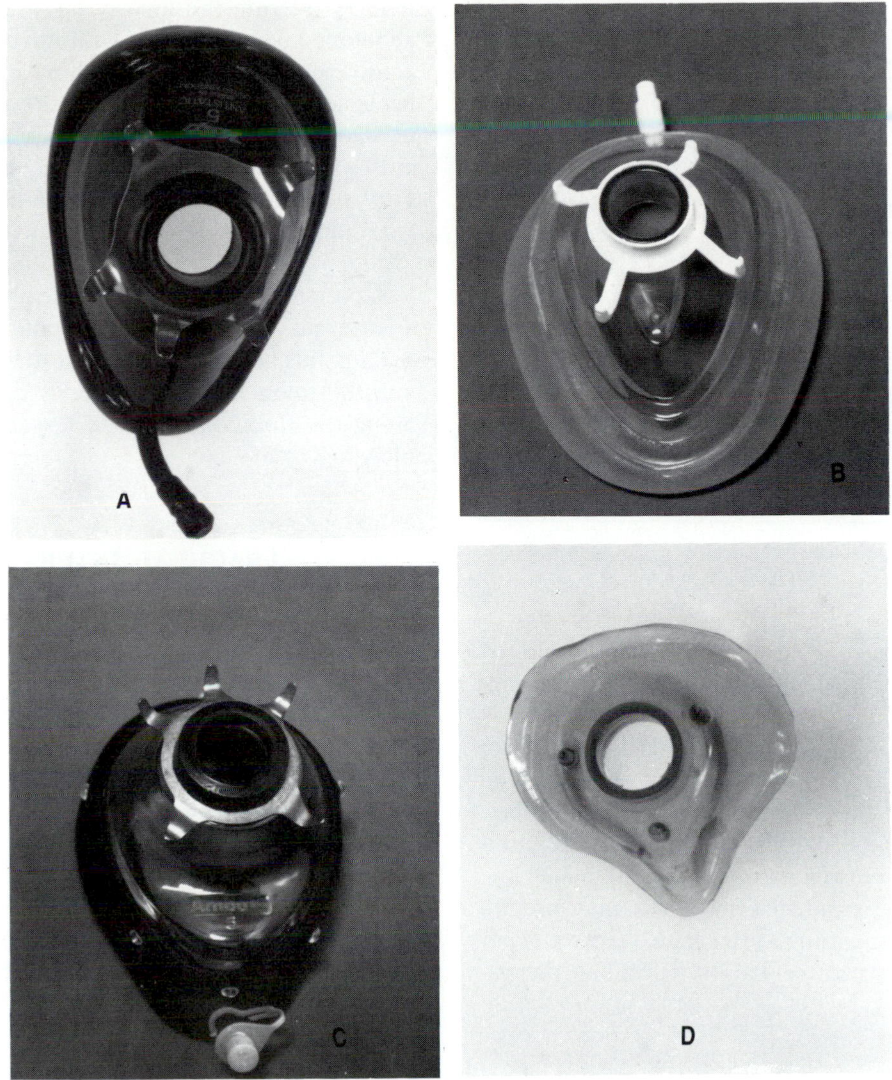

FIGURE 13–5. Selection of face masks: A, deformable, padded mask; B, universal disposable mask; C, Ambu transparent mask; D, Rendell-Baker Soucek pediatric mask.

occur. Drugs that produce apnea must not be given unless one is confident of one's ability to ventilate the patient.

Muscle Relaxants

Muscle relaxants confer both risks and benefits in managing the airway. They eliminate responses that complicate airway control, such as coughing, laryngospasm, and rigidity of airway and chest wall muscles. Administration of 5 to 20 mg of intravenous succinylcholine relaxes the muscles of the upper airway and permits ventilation during laryngospasm. Yet, in patients with airway tumors, obesity, edema, inflammation, or extrinsic compression of the airway by mediastinal masses, airway patency can be lost irretrievably when muscle tone is abolished. The anesthesiologist must choose from a spectrum of options in managing the patient suspected of being difficult to ventilate by mask (Table 13–6).

Artificial Airways

Artificial airways (Fig. 13–6), intended to separate the obstructing tongue and soft palate from

TABLE 13–6. Strategies To Manage the Patient Suspected of Being Difficult To Ventilate by Mask

"Awake" intubation, most useful when intubation is likely to be difficult
Slow, progressive induction of anesthesia
- Preoxygenation and denitrogenation, always
- Inhalation induction, *or*
- Small dose of ultra-short hypnotic, followed by inhalation agent, maintaining spontaneous ventilation, *or*
- Use of ultra–short-acting relaxants for brief attempt at intubation, intending if intubation fails to allow the patient to awaken before hypoxemia occurs

Transcricothyroid jet ventilation to assist intubation or to conduct total intravenous anesthesia: useful in emergencies when, unexpectedly, ventilation by mask and intubation are both impossible
Tracheostomy under local anesthesia: useful in the patient in whom efforts to intubate or ventilate by mask may produce abrupt loss of the airway

the posterior pharyngeal wall, must be employed cautiously to minimize trauma, coughing, gagging, and laryngospasm.

An oropharyngeal airway is inserted with the aid of a tongue blade when obstruction occurs and the muscles attached to the mandible are felt to relax, suggesting that the patient will tolerate the stimulus. If the patient reacts to the tongue blade, the artificial airway is not inserted, as it may precipitate vomiting, coughing, or laryngospasm. Deeper anesthesia or muscle relaxants will allow the patient to tolerate the airway later. If the patient is spontaneously breathing and adequately oxygenated, efforts to assist breathing may be stopped because they may compound the airway irritability. Continuous positive airway pressure of 5 to 15 cm H_2O applied to the airway by closing the pop-off valve is often enough to open the upper airway when anesthetic depth is insufficient to allow an artificial airway.

A patient who cannot tolerate an oropharyngeal airway may tolerate a nasopharyngeal airway, making this airway aid the first to be used by some anesthesiologists. Lubrication and gentle insertion along the floor of the nose lessen the chance of bleeding.

TRACHEAL INTUBATION

Although general anesthesia by mask is safe and effective for many patients, the requirements of the operation, the anesthesia plan, or the patient's medical condition may require intubation (Table 13–7). Over the years, the percentage of anesthetized patients subjected to intubation has increased steadily. This trend largely reflects a growing appreciation of the frequency with which anesthetized patients suffer unrecognized hypoventilation, hypoxia, and aspiration. Nevertheless, most clinicians can provide examples to contradict the listed indications for intubation. For example, it

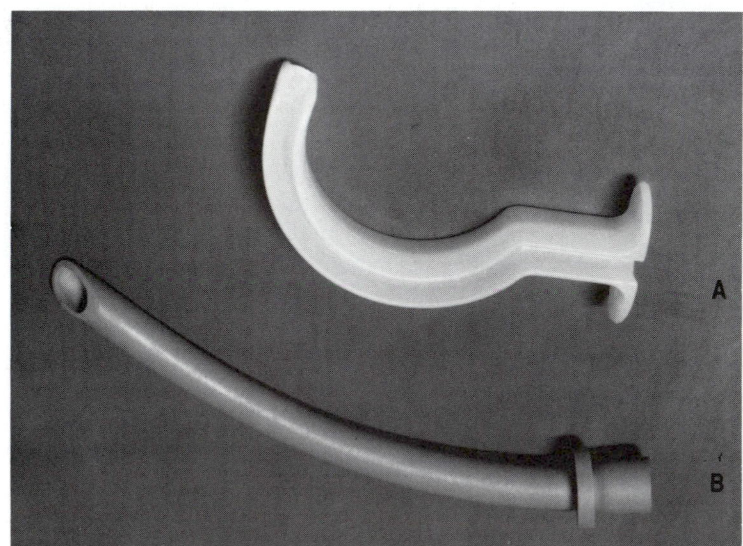

FIGURE 13–6. *Artificial airways: A, oropharyngeal; B, nasopharyngeal.*

TABLE 13–7. Indications of Tracheal Intubation of Patients Undergoing Operations

To prevent hypoventilation or to assure an increased inspired oxygen concentration when patients are affected by
- Anesthetics
- Muscle relaxants
- Coexisting cardiac or pulmonary disease
- Positions or operations that limit diaphragmatic motion

To free the operator's hands for other tasks

To guarantee airway patency with
- Airway operations
- Prolonged anesthesia
- Unfavorable airway anatomy
- Surgical positions that obstruct the airway or make access to it difficult

To protect against aspiration of gastric contents with
- The patient with a full stomach
- Obstetrical anesthesia
- Prolonged anesthesia
- Intraabdominal operations
- Positions that predispose to regurgitation

To ensure oxygenation in patients at risk of fluid overload from massive transfusion or at risk of pulmonary emboli during operations.

may be warranted to offer general anesthesia without intubation for a brief elective abdominal procedure to a professional singer who fears regional anesthesia but for whom the consequences of vocal cord damage would be devastating.

Equipment

LARYNGOSCOPES

The anesthesia laryngoscope consists of a handle and a blade. The handle contains batteries for a light; interchangeable blades attach to the handle (Fig. 13–7). Laryngoscope blades with a fiberoptic light guide provide brighter, more reliable illumination than do traditional blades with the bulb near the tip.

Although many varieties and sizes of laryngoscope blades exist, successful intubation in the majority of adult patients can be accomplished by using just two of them. Among the curved blades, a Macintosh No. 3 fits most adults; among the straight blades, a No. 2 or No. 3 Miller usually suffices. Single-use plastic laryngscopes are available when needed for patients with contagious diseases. Otherwise, it is usual simply to soak laryngoscope blades in a germicidal solution between uses.

TRACHEAL TUBES

Most endotracheal tubes are disposable and are made of clear, inert polyvinyl chloride that molds to the contour of the airway after softening at body temperature. Their lengths are marked in centimeters and their internal diameters in millimeters. Cuffs are used in adults and larger children; when inflated, the cuff produces an airtight seal with the

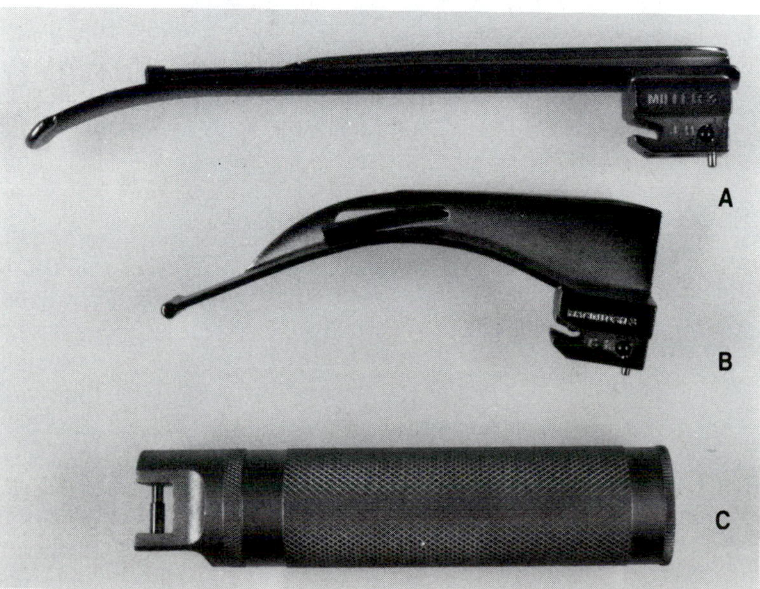

FIGURE 13–7. Laryngoscope set. A, the Miller straight blade; B, Macintosh curved blade; C, laryngoscope handle.

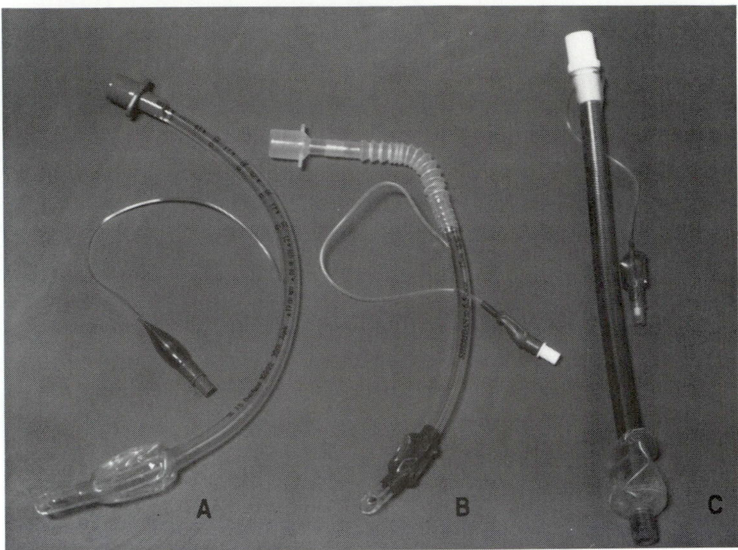

FIGURE 13–8. Tracheal tubes: A, cuffed oral/nasal tracheal tube; B, cuffed oral tracheal tube with flexible connector; C, armored (anode) cuffed tube with imbedded wire to prevent kinking.

trachea, guarding against aspiration and facilitating positive pressure ventilation. Filled so as to permit a small leak at maximum positive airway pressure (''mini-leak technique''), low-pressure large-volume cuffs are intended to avoid mucosal ischemia resulting from pressure on the tracheal wall. Types of tracheal tubes (Figs. 13–8 and 13–9) include (1) standard single-lumen tubes, available in varying sizes with a Magill or Murphy tip (the latter with an opening opposite the bevel to minimize the chance of occlusion); (2) armored (or anode) tubes, wire-reinforced to prevent compression; (3) performed tubes for nasal, oral, or tracheostomy insertion, designed to avoid kinking and displacement.

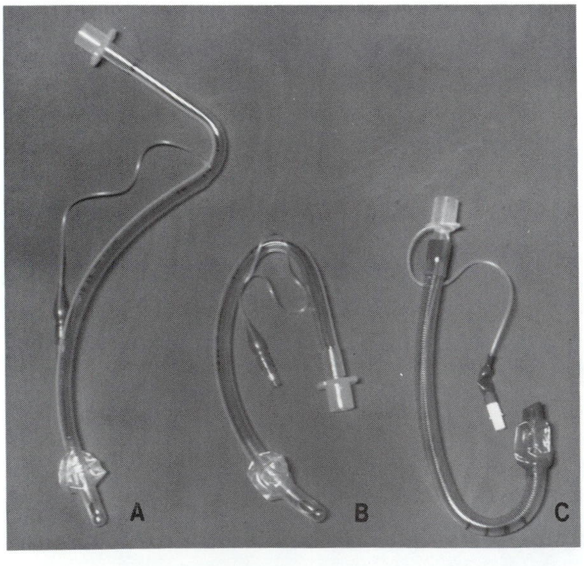

FIGURE 13–9. Preformed tracheal tubes: A, RAE (right angle) cuffed nasal tracheal tube; B, RAE (right angle) cuffed oral tracheal tube; C, armored (anode) cuffed tracheostomy tube shaped to prevent bronchial intubation.

For normal women, a tube 7.0 or 7.5 mm in diameter commonly is chosen; for men, 8.0 mm is chosen. Tracheal tubes trimmed for oral insertion can be slightly longer than needed, keeping in mind that proper depth in adults is usually 21 cm for woman and 23 cm for men, measured at the central incisors. A final step in preparing the tube is to inflate the cuff to test for leaks.

INTUBATING FORCEPS AND STYLETS

Magill intubating forceps are inserted in the mouth along with a laryngoscope to guide an endotracheal tube passed through the nose into the glottis.

An intubating stylet alters the curve of a tracheal tube, aiding its entry into a difficult-to-reach glottis. The stylet is bent 5 cm from its tip to produce a ''hockey stick'' shape. Before using the tube and stylet, the stylet must be tested to prove that it can be withdrawn from the tube. Because the stylet makes the endotracheal tube stiffer, one must be even more careful than usual to avoid trauma when using one. Unsheathed stylets can break, leaving the distal segment in the trachea; newer plastic sheathed stylets are safer. Some are meant to protrude beyond the tip of the tube, so as to enter a narrow or unseen glottis and provide a guide for the tube, but this maneuver is reserved for skilled clinicians.

Techniques of Tracheal Intubation

Intubation is attempted only after careful preparation. Except in emergencies, adequate preparation includes all the customary equipment and supplies for general anesthesia. The patient must be sedated or anesthetized (as tolerated) and adequate ventilation established by mask. Denitrogenation and monitoring with pulse oximetry guard against hypoxia.

Rigid Laryngoscopic Intubation

Tracheal intubation in a patient undergoing general anesthesia is usually performed with a rigid laryngoscope, the endotracheal tube passing through the mouth into the glottis under direct vision.

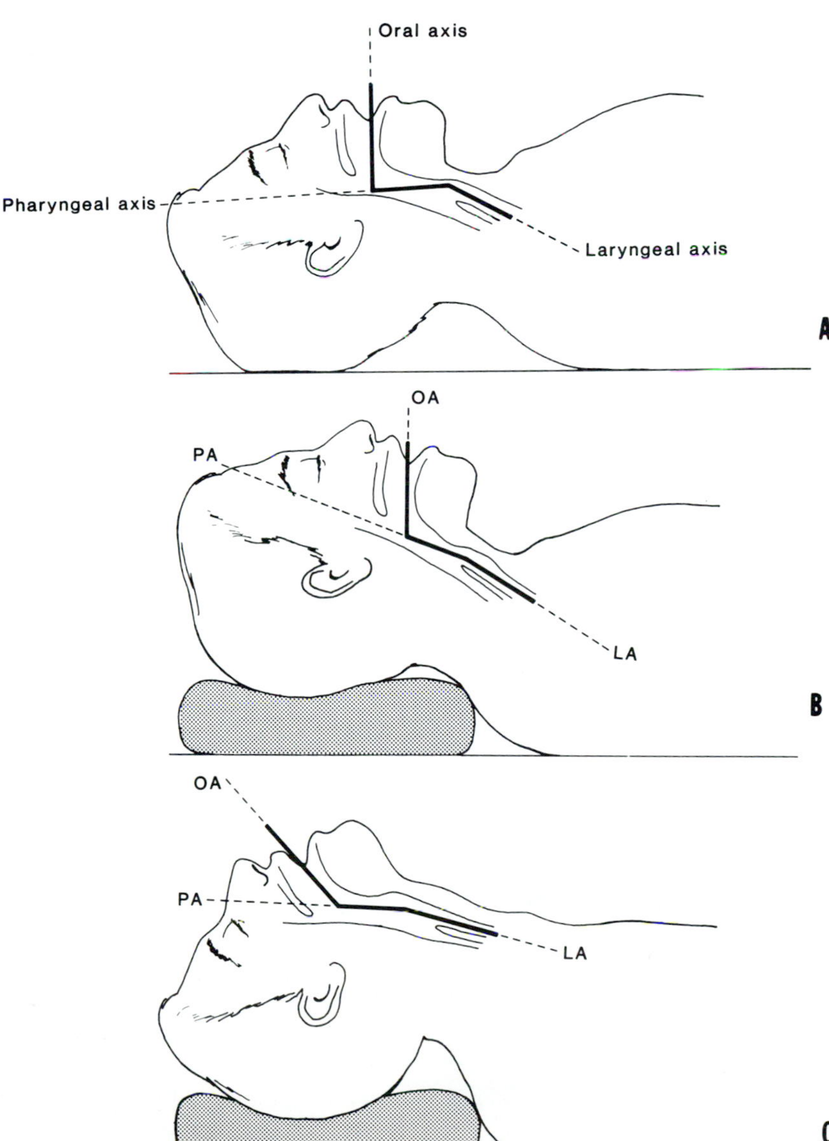

FIGURE 13–10. Intubating position during rigid laryngoscopy; A, Supine patient without head rest; B, Head elevation and neck flexes bring the pharyngeal and laryngeal axes into line. Head rest 8–10 (3–4) inches cm high is usually optimal; C, Extension of head at occipitocervical joint aligns the oral axis with the other two.

1. The operator works best if not forced to bend and if far enough from the glottis to preserve binocular vision. The operating table is adjusted to provide these condition.

2. The sniffing position (Fig. 13–10), 8 to 10 cm occipital elevation and cervico-occipital extension, aligns the axes of the mouth, pharynx, and larynx.

3. The operator's right hand opens the patient's mouth, pushing the lips away from the teeth to prevent bruising.

4. Held in the left hand, the laryngoscope with a curved blade is introduced at the right side of the mouth and advanced so as to displace the tongue to the left, until the right tonsillar fossa is located. The epiglottis is identified medially, at the base of the tongue. The tip of the blade is advanced into the vallecula (Fig. 13–11B). Intubation with a straight blade requires identical maneuvers, except that after locating the epiglottis, the blade tip is slipped beneath the epiglottis.

5. While keeping the wrist rigid to avoid using the upper teeth as a fulcrum for the blade of the laryngoscope, forward and upward traction on the laryngoscope handle attached to a curved blade stretches the hyoepiglottic ligament, folding the epiglottis upward to reveal the glottis. The straight blade lifts the epiglottis directly.

6. The tracheal tube is introduced from the right so as not to obstruct the view, and inserted through the rima glottidis and into the trachea until the cuff passes 1 to 2 cm beyond the vocal cords.

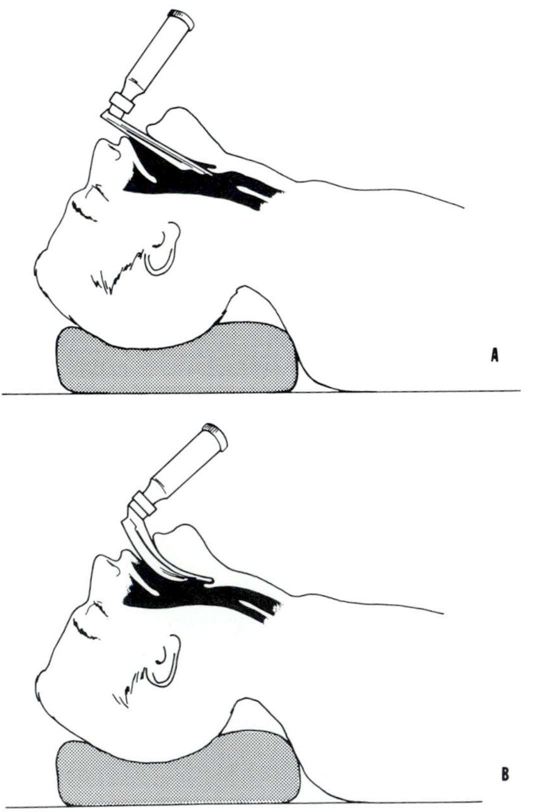

FIGURE 13–11. Demonstrates the different placements of straight (A) and curved (B) blades in relation to the epiglottis during laryngoscopy.

Although either straight or curved blades may be used in most patients, airway anatomy sometimes makes one a better choice over the other. The Macintosh curved blade retracts a large tongue well and often makes more room for passage of the tracheal tube between the teeth than do most straight blades. The curved blade also avoids contact with the sensitive laryngeal surface of the epiglottis, which makes it appropriate for awake intubation. Because it also demonstrates clearly the relation of the epiglottis to other anatomic features, the curved blade is often chosen for learning intubation.

In patients with prominent teeth and small mouth openings, exposure of the glottis may be better with a straight blade. The straight Miller blade, with its small cross section, is especially useful when the mouth is small or jaw mobility is limited.

When the corniculate and cuneiform prominences are visible, but not the glottis, intubation is possible if a stylet is used to direct the tube anteriorly. An assistant can push the thyroid cartilage in a posterior and superior direction.

With either blade, the common causes of failure include neglecting proper head position, intubating without full muscle relaxation, failing to open the mouth wide enough, off-midline placement of the blade, neglecting to locate the epiglottis, allowing the tongue to obscure the visual field, or advancing the tip of the blade too far.

Nasotracheal Intubation

Nasotracheal intubation is used when the mouth cannot be opened sufficiently, for some oral and maxillofacial operations, and in emergency situations outside the operating room (Table 13–8). It is avoided in the patient with nasal obstruction, coagulopathy, retropharyngeal abscess, or fracture of the base of the skull. The technique is ap-

TABLE 13–8. Advantages and Disadvantages of Nasotracheal Intubation

Advantages	Disadvantages
Tube better secured	Smaller-size tube, fiberoptic bronchoscopy difficult
Awake patient more comfortable	Long, narrow tubes: removing secretions difficult
Patient cannot bite tube	Higher incidence of bacteremia
Oral feeding possible	Nosebleed
	Nasal bacteria carried into traceha and lung
	Sinusitis

plicable to patients who are awake, sedated, or under general anesthesia. It is made easier by using a slightly smaller tube than usual and topical application to the nasal passage of a mixture of 3 per cent lidocaine with 0.25 per cent phenylephrine to anesthetize the mucous membranes and induce vasoconstriction.

For blind nasotracheal intubation, the patient's head is placed in an exaggerated sniffing position. One directs the lubricated tube directly posteriorly along the floor of the nose—never upward toward the cribriform plate. Advancement is slow and gentle, withdrawing and twisting the tube when resistance is met. Haste, large rigid tubes, an upward direction, or abrupt force cause bleeding.

The operator listens for breath sounds at end of the tube, while advancing the tube with one hand and palpating over the anterior neck with the other. Clues to position include intensity of breath sounds, lateral bulging produced by the tip of the tube in the pyriform sinuses, resistance to passage if the tube enters the valleculae, and disappearance of breath sounds with passage into the esophagus. Twisting the tube sweeps its tip from side to side; flexing and extending the head on the neck usually moves the tip anteroposteriorly. Entry into the trachea produces coughing, aphonia, and a typical capnograph trace. Especially in anesthetized patients, laryngoscopy and intubating forceps may be needed to place the nasotracheal tube.

Light Wand Intubation

Light wands are flexible, battery-powered devices with lighted tips. Bent into a "hockey stick" shape and placed inside the tracheal tube, the light wand is passed in the midline over the tongue, which has been pulled forward. With the room darkened, tracheal entry is signalled by a vertical beam of light appearing in the midline of the neck. Light appears above the thyroid cartilage if the tip of the tube enters the valleculae, and laterally on entry into a pyriform sinus. The transmitted light dims markedly if the tube passes into the esophagus. Although its use requires considerable skill, the light wand permits intubation in the presence of unstable neck fractures or congenital deformities.

Tracheal Intubation in the Conscious Patient

"Awake" intubation, performed blindly through the nose, under direct vision through the mouth, or with a fiberscope via either route, is indicated in several situations (Table 13–9). Prior explanation and effective sedation ensures the patient's cooperation while minimizing recall. Topical anesthesia of the upper airway eases the procedure and can be achieved by translaryngeal injection, nebulization, pledgets, superior laryngeal nerve block, or spraying under direct vision with a laryngoscope. The application of topical anesthetics and sedation obtund airway protective mechanisms, and their use must be minimized in patients at risk for aspiration of gastric contents.

Fiberoptic Laryngoscopy

The skillful fiberoptic laryngoscopist may use this instrument for routine as well as challenging intubations such as cervical spine fractures and dislocations. A variety of other applications have been described (Table 13–10).

TABLE 13–9. Indications for Awake Intubation

1. Patients at risk for aspiration who are not candidates for rapid-sequence intubation
2. When the airway is likely to be difficult to maintain without intubation
3. To assess neurologic functions after intubation (unstable neck)
4. To allow patients to position themselves after intubation
5. A patient who is unlikely to need or tolerate anesthetics.

TABLE 13–10. Other Applications of the Fiberoptic Laryngoscope

1. Evaluate upper airway obstruction or pathology
2. Evaluate vocal cord motion
3. Assess laryngotracheal injury after burns or prolonged intubation
4. Correctly position endotracheal or endobronchial tubes
5. Change from orotracheal to nasotracheal tube while maintaining a path into the trachea

Technique of Fiberoptic Tracheal Intubation

Oral and nasal fiberscopic intubation are easier in the conscious than in the unconscious patient; the tongue and epiglottis are less likely to obscure the vocal cords, and the patient can assist by phonating or protruding the tongue. Hasty maneuvers are unnecessary when the patient is adequately oxygenated. Viewed through the fiberscope, the distance to the vocal cords is exaggerated, and the true cords may not be seen until the false cords have been passed. Small amounts of secretions and blood, contact with tissues, or fogging of the lens may obscure the view completely.

Oral Approach

After the application of topical anesthetic to the tongue and oropharynx, a special oropharyngeal airway is inserted to prevent biting on the fiberscope, to keep it in the midline, and to displace the tongue. The operator then aspirates secretions from the pharynx, inserts a lubricated tracheal tube within the airway, and passes the fiberscope through the tube and the oropharynx to view the vocal cords. Spraying 2 ml of 4 per cent lidocaine via the fiberoptic laryngoscope facilitates passage of the fiberscope into the trachea, at which time the tube is advanced over the fiberscope into the trachea. For the less facile operator, translaryngeal injection of 4 per cent lidocaine prior to laryngoscopy minimizes coughing and laryngeal spasm.

Fiberoptic intubation in the anesthetized patient requires an assistant at the patient's side to hand the fiberscope to the operator and to apply jaw thrust. The intubation is interrupted to ventilate the patient as needed (Table 13–11).

Nasal Approach

Fiberoptic nasotracheal intubation in the awake patient is often easier than the orotracheal approach, because the nasopharynx is better aligned with the glottis. After applying a topical vasoconstrictor and local anesthetic to the larger nasal passage, the operator carefully advances the lubricated tracheal tube through it, into the oropharynx. After the pharynx has been cleared of secretions by a suction catheter passed through the endotracheal tube, the fiberscope is passed through the tube to view the glottis. Laryngeal anesthesia and intubation proceed as described for the oral approach.

Intubation in Patients at Increased Risk for Aspiration

Induction of anesthesia in patients who do not have empty stomachs or those with poorly functioning gastroesophageal sphincters may result in regurgitation and pulmonary aspiration. Histamine-2 blockers, metoclopramide, and possibly nasogastric suction reduce risks but may leave the patient with stomach contents of sufficient volume (>30 ml) or acidity (pH <2.5) to constitute a significant risk for classic acid aspiration syndrome. In these patients, intubation often precedes the induction of anesthesia.

Alternatively, anesthesia may begin with a "rapid sequence" of intravenous hypnotic, 1.5 mg per kg of succinylcholine, and intubation, while an assistant presses the cricoid ring against the cervical vertebrae (Sellick's maneuver). Intubation must proceed without delay to prevent aspiration.

TABLE 13–11. Practical Suggestions for Fiberoptic Intubation

1. Practice the techniques on a model and in elective cases before applying them in a difficult situation
2. When possible, administer an antisialagogue; secretions obscure the view
3. Before approaching the patient, focus on a fine test pattern by adjusting the diopter ring on the eyepiece
4. To prevent fogging, warm the tip of the fiberscope for a few minutes by immersion in tepid water
5. Avoid smearing the objective lens when applying lubricant
6. If the tip of the endotrocheal tube will not advance past the epiglottis and aryepiglottic folds, withdraw the tube, twist it by 90 degrees and advance it again

The assistant maintains cricoid pressure during cuff inflation and confirmation of tube position. If intubation is delayed, gentle ventilation at airway pressures of less than 30 cm H_2O while maintaining cricoid pressure minimizes the chance of gastric distension and regurgitation.

Coexisting diseases in patients at risk of aspiration challenge the anesthesiologist's ingenuity and skills in airway management. Table 13–12 lists some of the commonly occurring situations and some of the possible solutions for each.

TABLE 13–12. Intubation and Airway Management When Complicating Conditions Coexist with Increased Risk of Aspiration

Complicating Condition	Drugs or Techniques To Consider
Asthma	Ketamine and rapid sequence
	Beta-2 adrenergic agonists, theophylline, lidocaine, opioids, and rapid-sequence intubation
Difficult airway or intubation	Awake intubation
Succinylcholine contraindicated	Use nondepolarizer in large doses, possibly after a priming dose
	"Awake" intubation
Ischemic heart disease	Opioid, lidocaine, beta-adrenergic antagonist, nitroglycerin, hypnotic drug, and rapid sequence
	Consider slow induction of anesthesia to protect heart and accept risk of aspiration
Open eye injury	Defasiculating dose of nondepolarizer, followed by usual rapid sequence
	Large dose of nondepolarizer, with or without "prime" as substitute for succinylcholine in rapid-sequence induction.
Pharyngeal pouch	Awake intubation is first choice
Shock or moribund	Muscle relaxant alone, with or without small doses of ketamine or scopolamine
	Awake intubation
Small bowel obstruction or vomiting feces	Awake intubation first choice
Upper GI bleeding	Awake intubation first choice

THE DIFFICULT INTUBATION

Among experienced anesthesiologists, 0.5 to 2 per cent of rigid laryngoscopic intubations prove difficult. Anticipated difficult intubations are usually easier to manage than those that come as a surprise, because the forewarned anesthesiologist can apply a broad range of techniques to resolve the situation.

Predicting the Difficult Intubation

Patients in whom intubation proves difficult can be classified into four categories: those with no warning signs; those with obvious findings of a specific pathologic condition on the history or physical; those with extremes of normal anatomy giving only subtle hints of trouble; and those whose intubations are rendered unnecessarily difficult by faulty technique or inexperience.

The first group reflects such rare phenomena as masseter spasm, asymptomatic masses on the base of the tongue and epiglottis, tracheal stenosis, and partial tracheobronchial obstruction or compression. Because any patient may belong to this group, careful anesthesiologists employ denitrogenation with all patients before beginning anesthesia, and they perfect their skills at mask ventilation as well as a wide variety of techniques for tracheal intubation.

Patients presenting obvious signs or symptoms of difficult intubation (Tables 13–2 and 13–3) prompt the skilled anesthesiologist to choose an appropriate technique from among those described previously.

It is those patients with only subtle findings that suggest difficult intubation whom the anesthesiologist must strive to identify, even at the expense of an increased false-positive rate. Difficult rigid laryngoscopic intubation in the absence of obvious airway pathology occurs when the base of the tongue cannot be displaced anterior to the plane that passes perpendicular to the sagittal plane through the tips of the maxillary incisors (or alveolar ridge) and the glottis. In such a case, no more than the epiglottis and possibly the corniculate and cuneiform prominences are visible, and the patient is said to have a "high anterior larynx," a term that is probably anatomically incorrect. The preanesthetic diagnosis of difficult intubation is often subtle, and some patients whose intubations prove difficult go unrecognized (Tables 13–1, 13–2, and 13–3).

Management of the difficult intubation depends on the etiology of the problem, the patient's condition, the available equipment, familiarity of the operator with various techniques, and whether the difficulty was anticipated. Above all, ventilation and oxygenation must be maintained. If mask ventilation or first attempts at intubation cannot achieve this end, then the anesthesiologist must accomplish intubation, transcricothyroid ventilation, cricothyrotomy, or tracheostomy before hypoxia harms the patient (these latter surgical techniques are rarely required by skilled anesthesiologists). Although alternate techniques or other laryngoscopists may be employed, one must also limit repeated attempts at laryngoscopy and blind nasal intubation to avoid hemorrhage and edema.

If ventilation is satisfactory, the experienced anesthesiologist may attempt fiberoptic, light-wand-guided, or nasal intubation, remembering that a return to spontaneous ventilation facilitates fiberoptic exposure of the larynx. The pharynx is first cleared by suction and an antisialogogue administered. In one series, fiberoptic intubation was successful in 98.8 per cent of 338 difficult intubations; it failed most often in cases of distorted anatomy requiring awake tracheostomy or when blood, secretions, or equipment problems prevented an adequate view.

Difficulty in advancing a tracheal tube after it has passed between the vocal cords may indicate subglottic or tracheal stenosis. Causes of tracheal stenosis include previous prolonged intubation, congenital stenosis, and tumors invading the tracheal lumen. Extrinsic compression of the trachea may come from a large aortic arch, a substernal thyroid or an anterior mediastinal mass.

Percutaneous Transtracheal Ventilation

When both mask ventilation and tracheal intubation are impossible, ventilation via a 14- or 12-gauge venous catheter passed through the cricothyroid membrane into the trachea may be lifesaving. The technique has also been used by some as a prophylactic measure during anticipated difficult intubation. Effective oxygenation demands an intermittent flow of high-pressure oxygen (up to 50 psi). Depressing the flush valve of the anesthesia machine provides the needed pressure, but appropriate hoses and fittings are required. To prevent barotrauma, gases must escape—normally through the larynx.

Cricothyrotomy and Tracheostomy

Tracheostomy is complex and is best performed by an experienced surgeon. Even with a surgeon available, cricothyrotomy is the preferred approach if hypoxia is life-threatening. The cricothyroid ligament is palpated on the hyperextended neck. Transverse incisions through the skin, the scant subcutaneous tissue, and the ligament allow insertion of a narrow tracheal tube or a specially designed airway.

CARE AFTER TRACHEAL INTUBATION

Maintenance

After the endotracheal tube has been passed into the trachea, the cuff is inflated and the position of the tube verified. For orotracheal tubes, the typical depths given previously (21 cm for women, 23 cm for men) are almost always correct. Other tests of tube position are applied as well, and the results documented in the record. Observing chest movement and listening over the epigastrium and both sides of the chest assure that the trachea—and not the esophagus or a bronchus—has been intubated. The endotracheal tube cuff may be palpated in the sternal notch. Intubation also is confirmed by detecting appropriate levels of CO_2 in the exhaled gas over several successive breaths (5 per cent or 40 mm Hg). Carbon dioxide can enter the esophagus during mask ventilation, but its exhaled concentration rapidly decreases during ventilation of the esophagus. When in doubt, one must consider removing the tracheal tube and ventilating the lungs with a face mask. After the depth of insertion of the endotracheal tube has been adjusted, the marking on the tube opposite the upper central incisors (or alveolar ridge) is recorded in the record.

An oropharyngeal airway or soft block between the teeth prevents the patient biting the tube. Taping the tube to the skin over the maxilla secures it in ordinary circumstances. When the tube may be dislodged by movement of the head or when the face will be out of the anesthesiologist's reach, the tube may be secured by placing tape completely around the head, or by coating the tube and skin with tincture of benzoin. Nasotracheal tubes must be taped securely while avoiding pressure on the nares. The position of the tube is verified again each time the patient's position changes.

Removing Endotracheal Tubes

After verifying that criteria for safe removal of the endotracheal tube have been met (Table 3–13), the anesthesiologist removes the tape securing the endotracheal tube. With the patient's lungs fully inflated with oxygen and 10 to 20 cm H_2O positive pressure in the breathing system, the cuff is deflated just before removing the tube. This ensures that the patient will exhale, tending to move the epiglottis away from the glottis and forcing any fluid above the glottis into the mouth. In the first moments after removal of the tube, the patient is watched closely to determine that the airway is open, to assure adequate ventilation and oxygenation, and to detect promptly vomiting or laryngospasm. Supplemental oxygen is also applied.

TABLE 13–13. Checklist for Removing Endotracheal Tubes at the End of Anesthesia and Operation

1. There is no medical indication for continued intubation, such as impending respiratory failure or circulatory instability.
2. Equipment and drugs are ready to clear airway by suction, ventilation by mask, or intubation, if needed.
3. Adequate spontaneous ventilation has returned.
4. Reversal of muscle relaxants has been accomplished.
5. Desired level of consciousness has been achieved: Patient is deeply anesthetized or nearly awake.
   - Deep:
     - Obtunds airway reactivity and prevents coughing that might jeopardize results of some operations.
   - Awake:
     - Reduces risks of aspirating gastroesophageal contents or of airway obstruction.
6. Clear the pharynx with a soft suction catheter.
7. Administer high-flow oxygen for denitrogenation.
8. Deflate endotracheal tube cuff.
9. Apply positive pressure to breathing system and gently remove endotracheal tube.
10. Insert suction catheter into pharynx after extubation only if needed.
11. Apply face mask with high-flow O_2.
12. Assess airway, ventilation, and vital signs.

TABLE 13–14. Complications of Tracheal Intubation

- During intubation
  - Trauma to lips, teeth, upper airway, trachea, and esophagus
  - Cardiovascular
    - Hypertension and tachycardia
    - Arrhythmias
    - Reflex bradycardia or asystole
    - Cardiac ischemia
  - Respiratory
    - Laryngospasm
    - Bronchospasm
    - Aspiration
    - Coughing, chest wall spasm
  - Central nervous system
    - Increased intracranial pressure
    - Spinal cord injury with unstable neck
  - Unrecognized improper positioning
    - Esophageal intubation
    - Endobronchial intubation
    - Cuff between vocal cords
- While tracheal tube is in place
  - Obstruction, kinking, secretions, compressions, or biting
  - Endobronchial intubation or extubation
  - Barotrauma
  - Cuff leak
  - Disconnection from breathing circuit
- Immediately following extubation
  - Laryngospasm
  - Aspiration
  - Acute laryngotracheal edema
  - Trauma during extubation
- Late complications
  - Tracheal stenosis
  - Vocal cord polyps
  - Nosocomial infection

COMPLICATIONS

During management of the airways of anesthetized patients, trauma such as bruised lips, chipped, loosened, or dislodged teeth, and epistaxis are common (Table 13–14). More serious complications include perforation of the hypopharynx, esophagus, or trachea, which may result in mediastinitis and pneumothorax. Immediate recognition and appropriate therapeutic intervention are essential to forestall severe morbidity or death.

A major complication of intubation is airway obstruction after removal of the endotracheal tube. Causes include soft tissue upper airway obstruction, laryngospasm, bronchospasm, tracheobronchial obstruction, chest wall rigidity, and machine problems (as in attempting to use the reservoir bag with the selector valve set for the mechanical ventilator). Assessment and treatment are carried out the same as during the induction of anesthesia, including intubation if needed.

Uncontrolled autonomic responses (usually tachycardia and hypertension) result from laryngoscopy and intubation in lightly anesthetized patients, at the beginning or at the end of procedures. In susceptible patients, stroke or myocardial ischemia may result. Depending on the patient's overall condition, these responses may be blocked with deep anesthesia, short-acting adrenergic blocking drugs, or relatively large doses of opioids. Topical anesthesia of the larynx and trachea and the intravenous administration of lidocaine (1 mg per kg) are also helpful, but are usually ineffective when used alone.

Spinal cord injury has resulted from attempts at intubation in patients with unstable neck fractures or severe rheumatoid arthritis. Neurosurgeons and orthopedic surgeons can render valuable assistance during intubation or extubation by helping to prevent movement of the neck. Likewise, during intubation or extubation in patients with compromised airways, it is wise to have the surgeon present.

Sore throat is the most frequent complication of tracheal intubation, but this can follow anesthesia by mask also. Nasogastric tubes compound the problem. If sore throat is associated with persistent hoarseness, the patient must be examined to exclude vocal cord paralysis or injury. Preanesthetic teaching and sympathetic postanesthetic evaluation help patients keep this bothersome condition in perspective. Warm fluids and throat lozenges will minimize symptoms of sore throat until the expected resolution in 1 to 2 days.

REFERENCES

Birmingham PK, Cheney FW, Ward RJ. Esophageal intubation: A review of detection techniques. Anesth Analg 1986;65:886–891.

Caplan RA, Posner KL, Ward RJ, Cheney FW. Adverse respiratory events in anesthesia: A closed claim analysis. Anesthesiology 1990;72:828–833.

Finucane BT, Santora AH. Principles of airway management. Philadelphia: FA Davis, 1988.

Latto IP, Rosen M. Difficulties in tracheal intubation. Philadelphia: Bailliere Tindall, 1985.

McIntyre JWR. The difficult tracheal intubation. Can J Anaesth 1987;34:204–213.

Ovassapian A. Fiberoptic airway endoscopy in anesthesia and critical care. New York: Raven Press, 1990.

CHAPTER FOURTEEN

Conduct of General Anesthesia

Skilled anesthesiologists are recognized by other anesthesiologists, patients, and surgeons for providing "good anesthesia." This term has different meanings to different observers, but it includes making the patient comfortable, avoiding complications and near misses, managing the anesthetic so that it harmonizes with the surgical procedure, reacting calmly and decisively in emergencies, using resources efficiently, working quickly but not in haste, performing technical procedures skillfully, and maintaining pleasant, professional relationships with co-workers. Because some who have been in practice for years may not meet all these standards, and because ease and familiarity are such important components of skilled practice, trainees may feel that they cannot achieve this goal for many years. This is far from the truth; in fact, residents can begin to form the habits of good anesthesia practice starting with the first anesthetic they administer.

Because this volume seeks to relate the scientific foundations of anesthesia to the principles of safe practice, much of it already concerns the conduct of anesthesia. But much remains unwritten in anesthesiology textbooks. The folklore, routines, and advice for the management of anesthesia handed down orally from instructor to resident are important to good practice. Those elements of quality practice that do not derive directly from scientific disciplines such as physiology, pharmacology, or anatomy are the subject of this chapter.

Planning Anesthesia

A good anesthetic begins with a good plan. Indeed, in discussions with colleagues and in the oral examination of the American Board of Anesthesiology (ABA), an anesthesiologist's medical judgment is tested by the quality of the anesthesia plan, the degree to which it is based on scientific principles, its adaptability to changing circumstances, and the clarity with which the anesthesiologist can explain it. There is no rigid format for planning anesthesia. Rather, each plan is adapted to the case at hand.

Goals

The fundamental goals of anesthetic management are unchanging: safety, comfort, and convenience (in that order), first for the patient, and second for those caring for the patient. Rarely can one satisfy all these perfectly; compromise is the rule. Depending on the case, the specific goals that dominate planning may include teaching, research, or minimizing malpractice exposure, but the patient's interests remain paramount. As an example consider the following patient:

> A 64-year-old woman is to undergo revision of a total hip arthroplasty because of increasing pain due to loosening of a prosthesis that was originally placed for treatment of a fracture-dislocation. Problems for management include: (1) obesity, at 5′4″ tall and 180 pounds, weight distributed in hips and thighs; (2) mild hypertension, of five years' standing, BP 150/95, no ECG changes, no history of stroke, angina, or MI, BUN/Cr normal; (3) she refuses blood products, Hb 12.4 gm per dl; (4) she says she is quite anxious and warns she may refuse to get on the operating room table at the last minute. She takes no medication, has no allergies, and her dentition and airway anatomy are normal. A prior general anesthetic with enflurane was uneventful and she has refused regional anesthesia of any kind.

The major safety-related goal in this case is prevention of postoperative anemia; as many as several liters of blood might be lost in a revision of a total hip arthroplasty, and the patient refuses blood. A related goal is to prevent extremes in blood pressure and heart rate, which might produce myocardial ischemia in this untreated hypertensive patient with anemia. The third goal of this case, relief of her anxiety, fortunately does not conflict with the approaches needed to achieve the other goals. In fact, relief of anxiety may help reduce tachycardia and hypertension in the preoperative period. If obesity had compromised her airway, this patient might not be offered preoperative sedation because of the fear of airway obstruction.

Kinds of Plans for Anesthesia

In a recent monograph, Muravchick has presented a set of formal algorithms for choosing elements of a anesthetic plan. Flow diagrams of logical thought processes form excellent bases for teaching and provide the ultimate justification for a plan, but anesthesiologists often use other styles of planning, based on experience and suited to the particular case at hand. Some of these patterns of thought include:

1. Formal algorithms, which have the advantage of being thorough, are a great benefit for the trainee, but have the disadvantage of slowness for those who are more experienced.

2. A list of problems and a method for managing each often provides a valuable summary, and can serve to point out conflicting goals and approaches.

3. Planning forward involves imagining the course of the anesthetic and the problems that might arise in sequence. One proceeds in order from preoperative evaluation to premedication, monitoring, induction, airway management, maintenance of anesthesia, management of surgical stress, emergence, and postoperative care. This approach serves well as a checklist, but it relies on experience and is not oriented to physiologic problems.

4. Planning backward requires that the anesthesiologist imagine the state to be achieved for the patient at the end of the case and work back in time to plan the needed steps to achieve that state. As does forward planning, this relies on experience, but it may alert one to conflicts and inconsistencies in elements of the plan. This style of planning is most valuable when the major goal is to achieve a specific postoperative state. For example, if a patient must awaken promptly at the end of an anesthetic to allow evaluation of the results of neurosurgery, then everything in the anesthesia plan must take this goal into account and backward planning is appropriate.

5. To focus the plan on a major issue is useful when there is too much or too little in a case to encourage a complex plan. For example, one might plan in an elderly patient with a recent MI and renal failure undergoing abdominal aortic aneurysmectomy to avoid myocardial ischemia, even at the risk of compromising renal perfusion. Such singular plans cannot be complete of themselves, but can help organize thinking in a confusing case.

6. Planning by routine is an appropriate choice when patients and cases are similar; it is likely that laparoscopy in a healthy patient can be accomplished successfully using an anesthetic that has worked well in healthy patients previously. The benefit of following a routine is the chance to refine the technique based on prior experience. The danger is that by following routines, one may overlook the needs of the unusual patient.

The patterns of thinking listed nearer the top of this list are more academic, more time consuming, more useful for beginners, more defensible in court, and less likely to lead one astray in novel situations. Skilled anesthesiologists use all of these methods at one time or another, depending on what seems to suit the case at hand. Often, it is appropriate to use several methods for planning a single case.

For example, the description given previously of the patient for revision of a total hip arthroplasty already includes a problem list; the list of goals provides a therapeutic objective for each problem. Adding the planned therapy to each completes a problem-oriented description of an anesthesia plan and includes the following:

1. *Obesity*. Cimetidine and metoclopramide, as prophylaxis for aspiration of gastric contents, but no rapid sequence intubation because of hypertension; general anesthesia and intubation to assure adequate ventilation, oxygen.
2. *Hypertension*. Intubate with deep anesthesia plus intravenous lidocaine to blunt hypertension during intubation; fluids after induction of anesthesia to correct hypovolemia; monitor V_5 of the electrocardiogram (ECG) for ischemia; warming blankets to prevent hypothermia, postoperative vasoconstriction.
3. *Refuses blood*. Deliberate hypotension (isoflurane, nitroprusside, esmolol) to minimize losses; central venous pressure (CVP), arterial, and Foley catheters to monitor fluid balance and BP; limit hypotension to 90/50 because of Hx of hypertension; blood salvage permitted by patient; saline and hetastarch for fluid therapy.
4. *Anxiety*. Oral midazolam 2 hours before operating room; intravenous midazolam in holding area, before entering operating room; avoid regional anesthesia because patient wants guarantee of amnesia.

Although this plan was formulated as a list of problems and solutions, it was backward planning that reminded the anesthesiologist of the need for special attention to warming the patient. The choice of general anesthesia was based not only on the patient's need for amnesia, but on the need to assure ventilation and oxygenation in a potentially prolonged procedure in an obese subject. Isoflurane is a popular choice for induced hypotension because hypotension with this agent is characterized by decreased peripheral vascular resistance and sustained cardiac output.

Characteristics of a Good Plan

Good anesthesia plans share certain characteristics. First, they take into account interpatient variability. For example, one might anticipate that this patient's blood pressure will decrease to a satisfactory degree with a nitroprusside infusion of 1 μg per kg per minute, but this is not the planned starting dose, which might be one fourth or less of the anticipated dose, so that the patient will not become excessively hypotensive if she should prove sensitive to the drug. Alternatively, this patient might require 20 μg per kg per minute of nitroprusside, a rate that may risk cyanide toxicity. Adding the beta adrenergic blocker would reduce this excess requirement. Thus, good anesthesia plans anticipate extreme responses, not just average responses. Just as a pilot is required to plan for an alternate destination and to carry enough fuel to reach it, so must the anesthesia plan always incorporate an alternate approach.

Second, good anesthesia plans do not assign the same importance to various goals. For example, our anxious patient for hip revision might be more comfortable if she were made unconscious by large doses of midazolam before leaving her room. Because the goal of preventing airway obstruction is more important than the goal of relieving anxiety, she will not receive the final doses of midazolam until she reaches the holding area outside the operating room, where the anesthesiologist can observe the effect of the drug and monitor oxygen saturation. Also, even if a plan is likely to have a good outcome, the possibility of rare but a severe complications may make the plan unwise. An example in our patient might be the decision to use a central venous pressure catheter. In all likelihood, her blood volume can be managed without such monitoring, but the consequences of inadequate volume replacement or overhydration in this woman are potentially severe (because of anticipated anemia and suspected heart disease), making it unacceptable to many anesthesiologists to proceed without a CVP or Swan-Ganz catheter.

Third, a plan for anesthesia recognizes that the various elements interact, even in a simple anesthetic plan. In our patient, the decision to use H_2 blockers preoperatively was a response to the decision not to use a rapid sequence intubation, which in turn resulted from the fear of hypotension or myocardial ischemia in this patient. It is usually necessary to make reasonable compromises in the management of one problem in order to allow successful management of another. Beginners in anesthesia sometimes error when they mix elements of two unrelated plans without considering the interactions. As an example, a patient might simultaneously be given large doses of muscle relaxant, high levels of epidural anesthesia with 0.75 per cent bupivacaine, and increased concentrations of isoflurane in an effort to relax abdominal muscles. Hypotension, prolonged emergence, and postoperative weakness might result, but the relaxation would likely be no better than that produced by any one of these treatments alone.

Fourth, a good anesthesia plan is practical; it does no good to frame a plan that cannot be accomplished with the people and equipment at hand. For example, this patient's blood could be conserved by reinfusing blood lost during the operation; without the necessary equipment, this part of the plan would be impractical.

Preparing for Anesthesia

After a good plan, a good anesthetic requires adequate preparation. For our patient, adequate preparation includes all of the routine measures listed in the checklist given in Chapter 5, as well as the following special steps:

1. Verifying that the equipment and technicians are available for intraoperative recovery of shed blood.
2. Preparing the nitroprusside and esmolol infusions, calculating appropriate pump settings for various dose rates, and posting a table of doses with the pumps.
3. Having ready the monitors, transducers, and insertion kits for the arterial and central venous cannulae.

Whereas minor problems may become major ones if the anesthesiologist is not ready to deal with them, there is waste and delay in overpreparation. Thus, neither a nitroglycerine infusion nor trimethaphan is prepared ahead of time for the patient, despite the possibility that signs of myocardial ischemia might prompt the use of the one, and hypoxemia from nitropruside the other (although these drugs are available in unopened vials if needed). On the other hand, rare but life-threatening complications may require advance preparations even though they are rarely needed; an example is the immediate availability in the operating suite of a defibrillator for this patient.

Bringing The Patient Into The Room

Before bringing the patient into the operating room, the anesthesiologist verifies the patient's identity, the planned operation, and the site of the operation, if necessary. With tact, this patient is asked to give her name; in conversation, it can be established that she expects a second operation on her right hip. At this time, another review of the chart reveals any overnight events, new laboratory data, or consultants' reports. Also, the patient can be questioned as to the time of the last meal and any medications received.

Depending on staffing and available space, the intravenous catheter and ECG pads or other monitoring can be placed (and some regional anesthetics performed) before bringing the patient into the operating room. This can improve operating room efficiency if it can be accomplished during the preceding operation, or while the operating room is being cleaned. This is an appropriate time to administer any needed intravenous sedatives or narcotics; the anxious woman for hip revision receives midazolam intravenously in 2 mg increments to a total of 6 mg.

All of the preparations are completed before the patient enters the room, thereby keeping to a minimum the time during which the awake anxious person must lie on the operating table. This also allows the anesthesiologist to focus attention on the patient rather than technical preparations.

Once the patient is in the room, the remaining monitoring equipment is attached as quickly and deftly as possible. Not all of the monitoring devices that will be used intraoperatively need be attached or inserted before inducing anesthesia. Invasive monitors not needed for induction are often inserted after anesthesia has begun. In the case of our patient for hip surgery, the arterial catheter, the CVP catheter and the urinary bladder catheter can all be placed after anesthesia begins, because they are needed only to monitor the effects of blood loss and deliberate hypotension; a smooth induction is anticipated.

During this time, the patient may breathe oxygen, if denitrogenation is required. Before proceeding with induction, the immediate preoperative vital signs are recorded on the anesthesia record. Also before proceeding, the anesthesiologist evaluates these initial findings in light of the problem list for that patient. For example, this woman might be found to have a peripheral oxygen saturation of 94 per cent, not unexpected in view of the midazolam given in the holding area. Her blood pressure might be 180/105 just before induction. This is higher than her preoperative blood pressure, but not unexpected in the circumstances. Because leads V_2 and V_5, properly calibrated for voltage, appear identical to the preoperative ECG and the patient has no complaints of chest pain, anesthesia begins.

Induction of Anesthesia

The practical and scientific considerations involved in planning the induction of anesthesia are considered extensively throughout this text, including the chapters on intravenous anesthetics, opioids, muscle relaxants, the airway and spinal and epidural anesthesia, as well as the chapters on special management concerns such as pediatrics, obstetrics, and trauma. The topic recurs because it is the most crucial maneuver in managing an anesthetic. Because of the sometimes unpredictable responses to routine doses of drugs required to establish the proper depth of anesthesia, it seems appropriate to give incremental doses of anesthetics until the proper depth of anesthesia is reached, as in titrating a chemical reaction to a desired endpoint. Ordinarily, this is good advice for drug administration in anesthesia practice, but during the induction of anesthesia, to proceed too slowly can be as dangerous as to proceed too quickly. Patients in very light stages of anesthesia (Stage II) are hyperreflexic and may be harmed by catecholamine excess, uncontrolled and sometimes violent movement, vomiting, and laryngospasm.

The patient for hip repair comes to the operating room in some discomfort. Rather than induce anesthesia with the patient in bed (sometimes done for patients with fractures), the anesthesiologist administers oxygen by nasal prongs and 100 μg of fentanyl intravenously before moving the patient to the operating table with the help of five people; the anesthesiologist stands at the head, another person holds the feet, and two people on each side lift the sheet on which the patient lies.

Working With The Surgeon

Anesthetics are not conducted in isolation; the anesthetic and the operation must be coordinated for best results. Before the operation begins, the anesthesiologist must be fully informed about the operation: the anatomy, the duration, the expected blood loss, and the physiologic effects that can be expected. If these matters are not clear, consultation between anesthesiologist and surgeon before the patient comes into the operating room is in order. When surgeon and anesthesiologist share the airway, this need for cooperation is most evident, but it remains important no matter what the procedure. An anesthesiologist's lack of knowledge about the surgical procedure not only leads to a clumsy anesthetic, but also impairs the relationship between surgeon and anesthesiologist.

In the case of our patient undergoing a hip operation, even though the surgeon and the anesthesiologist have worked together before on similar cases, they confer preoperatively about measures to reduce and treat blood loss, and about postoperative care (intensive care may be needed). During the operation, it is important for the anesthesiologist to keep the surgeon advised of this patient's condition, especially the hemoglobin concentration and the patient's tolerance of anemia, so that together they can consider whether the procedure can be completed safely.

Maintenance of Anesthesia

Maintaining Vigilance

Although it is during maintenance that anesthesia appears most uneventful, there are often profound changes in the patient's condition during this phase of anesthesia. In studies of critical incidents in anesthesia, it was found that significant problems with patients went unrecognized during maintenance and were not detected until another individual replaced the dulled observer. The antidote to this problem is vigilance, the motto of the American Society of Anesthesiologists; unfortunately, vigilance is the very quality that is lost to boredom.

To overcome this effect, skilled anesthesiologists manage the maintenance of anesthesia aggressively. The first element in this approach is to make vigilance an active process. Instead of waiting for alarms to sound, one surveys at regular intervals the monitoring data (see Chapter 6), recording the results in the record, seeking to interpret any changes. A valuable approach to improve vigilance is to establish a systematic pattern of reviewing the data, beginning at the patient (operative site, chest excursion, IV site, nerve stimulator), and progressing to the airway (endotracheal tube, breathing circuit, valves, airway pressure), and then to the various monitors at or on the anesthesia machine (ECG, oxygen saturation, blood pressure, gas flows).

The intervals between observations and the attention given to each item vary according to circumstances. Selection of monitoring for a procedure not only entails choosing at the start of the case the devices to be used, but also directing one's attention to the most important data of the moment during the procedure. During this patient's hip operation, such moments might occur with intubation, when changes in heart rate, rhythm, ST segment elevation, and blood pressure might all be expected, and during placement of the cement for the femoral component of the new prosthesis, when pulmonary embolization and hypotension can be expected, and attention is directed to the pulse oximeter and the arterial pressure.

The second element in active vigilance is to approach the anesthetic as a scientific experiment, framing hypotheses to explain observed changes and taking steps to confirm them. For example, during our patient's hip operation, the amount of nitroprusside needed to maintain the mean arterial pressure at 70 mm Hg might increase from 0.5 to 3.0 μg per kg per minute over the course of 45 minutes. Several explanations are possible. If it has been an hour since the initial dose of fentanyl was given, perhaps the loss of analgesia is responsible; a positive response to a second dose of fentanyl might support this hypothesis. On the other hand, perhaps intact barostatic reflexes have responded to increase the heart rate and renin secretion. If a review of the record shows that the heart rate has increased from 68 to 107 over the same 45 minutes, and there is a positive response to esmolol, this is a likely explanation. Perhaps cyanide toxicity is resulting from nitroprusside infusion; a review of the total dose given and the arterial blood gas and pH value can help identify this possibility.

A third element of active vigilance is to change the anesthetic periodically to verify requirements and responses, even if all is going smoothly. When a system remains unchanged for a time, it can be helpful to introduce a change to verify the accuracy of the monitoring and the efficacy of the treatment. For example, if our patient undergoing a hip operation has experienced no change in her blood pressure for an hour, it may be appropriate to reduce the rate of administration of nitroprusside to verify that the present dose is needed.

Depth of Anesthesia

The concept of depth of anesthesia has been introduced elsewhere. In modern practice, the depth of anesthesia is best thought of as corresponding to the degree of depression of reflex responses to surgical stimuli. At light depths of anesthesia, patients develop tachycardia and hypertension in response to surgical stimuli, and may even move; at deeper levels of anesthesia, responses are less vigorous. Cardiovascular responses are monitored as indications of depth of anesthesia, but these can be deceptive when there are reasons other than deep anesthesia to explain depressed blood pressure or when a narcotic-based anesthetic blunts hypertensive responses without rendering the patient fully unconscious.

Because stimulation varies throughout an operation, and because blood concentration of infused or inhaled anesthetics changes with time, it is wise to test periodically the depth of anesthesia by decreasing the concentration of an inhaled anesthetic or the infusion rate of an intravenous one. When a reflex response signifying light anesthesia (changes in heart rate, blood pressure, respiratory rate or depth, or even movement) appears, the amount of anesthetic can be increased, with the assurance that the patient is not anesthetized too deeply. The measurement of the concentration of anesthetic in end-tidal gas is an effective means of quantifying the dose, but is not a direct measure of the depth of anesthesia, which represents a pattern of patient responses and not a drug concentration.

In a skillfully administered anesthetic, the depth of anesthesia varies throughout the operation to meet the needs of the moment and in anticipation of the planned emergence. For our hypertensive patient undergoing a hip operation with general anesthesia and deliberate hypotension, anesthesia begins with the intravenous sedation (6 mg midazolam) administered outside the operating room, and the fentanyl (100 μg) given just before moving her to the operating table. These render the patient indifferent and somnolent, but still able to respond to commands. These drugs also decrease the doses of other anesthetics needed, and will depress respiration during the procedure; the planned use of controlled ventilation means that respiratory depression will not pose a threat to the patient. Because the procedure is expected to last four or five hours, postoperative somnolence and respiratory depression are not expected from these small doses of short-acting drugs given at the start of the procedure. Had this patient been an elderly, less robust woman with a fractured hip, the same drugs might have been used for the same purpose, but perhaps in markedly reduced amounts (0.5 mg midazolam, 10 to 20 μg of fentanyl).

After denitrogenation, thiopental is injected into a free-running intravenous infusion at about 100 mg per minute. (The induction could be completed with midazolam, but the anesthesiologist fears postoperative somnolence with large doses of this drug.) The slow infusion of thiopental allows the anesthesiologist to stop short of the usual dose (4 mg per kg or 300 mg for this patient) if the patient loses consciousness (because of the midazolam) or becomes hypotensive or apneic (because of her hypertension or the other intravenous drugs she has received). After 125 mg of thiopental, the patient stops breathing and fails to respond to commands to open her eyes; at this point, she is lightly anesthetized. After cautious efforts at controlled ventilation, the anesthesiologist finds that the patient's airway is patent and that she accepts controlled ventilation without coughing or breath holding. For several minutes, manual ventilation continues with a mixture of 50 per cent nitrous oxide, 48 per cent oxygen and 2 per cent isoflurane; the goal is to deepen anesthesia so that the patient will not respond to intubation with excessive hypertension or tachycardia, and to do so slowly, to avert abrupt and severe hypotension.

Intubation might be accomplished without the aid of a muscle relaxant, but experience has taught that it will be difficult to achieve deep enough anesthesia for intubation without hypotension in a patient such as this. Instead of succinylcholine, curare is chosen for the intubation because it is the relaxant to be used for the remainder of the procedure. (For a prolonged operation, curare or pancuronium are better choices than the shorter-acting relaxants; for deliberate hypotension, curare is a better choice than pancuronium because of the tachycardia induced by the latter.) To prevent histamine release and hypotension, the curare is given in divided doses (0.1 to 0.2 mg per kg each) a minute or two apart. After the response to the nerve stimulator has decreased to post-tetanic facilitation (PTF) only, and six minutes of isoflurane administration have decreased the blood pressure to 90/50, the depth of anesthesia is sufficient to permit intubation (intravenous lidocaine may be administered to blunt the hypertension associated with laryngoscopy).

After intubation, the arterial catheter, CVP catheter, extra intravenous cannula and urinary bladder catheters are placed. Anesthesia of adequate depth to deal with these mild stimuli may not require isoflurane, which is reduced in concentration or turned off to prevent hypotension. Amnesia and analgesia are provided by the combination of nitrous oxide, midazolam, fentanyl, and thiopental. When the cannulae have been inserted, the same light depth of anesthesia probably will be sufficient for turning the patient to the lateral position and for the surgical preparations.

Just before the incision, the alveolar isoflurane concentration is again increased in anticipation of the patient's response to this painful stimulus. If the patient has shown no tendencies to hypotension so far, alveolar concentrations of as much as 1.5 times minimum alveolar concentration (MAC) may be required; more likely, lesser concentrations will suffice. During the majority of the procedure, the fresh gases added to the breathing circuit consist of 0.5 L per minute of nitrous oxide, 0.5 L per minute of oxygen, and enough isoflurane to maintain an end-tidal concentration of about 0.8 per cent. Less isoflurane is not used because when it is decreased, the patient's blood pressure increases, requiring that more nitroprusside be given. Just before the surgeon closes the wound, the nitroprusside is discontinued and the inspired concentration of isoflurane decreased to allow the blood pressure to return to preoperative values. This helps the surgeon to assure adequate hemostasis.

About 15 minutes before the anticipated time of applying the dressing, the fresh gas flows are increased to a total of 6 L per minute and the isoflurane vaporizer turned off. Beginning the emergence from anesthesia this early may require that the isoflurane vaporizer be turned on again later, but it also helps ensure against delayed awakening at the end of the procedure. Curare administration has been discontinued and the response to the train-of-four impulses from the nerve stimulator has increased to three or four twitches. No muscle relaxation is needed for this portion of the procedure, but dislocation of the hip is possible if the patient moves violently, so the surgeon is warned to control the leg as the patient awakens. Well before the end of the operation, as the blood concentrations of curare and isoflurane decrease, the patient is allowed to regain spontaneous or assisted ventilation. To control the anticipated pain on awakening, morphine is given intravenously in doses of 1 to 5 mg, guided by the respiratory rate.

This patient's anesthesia might be managed in many ways; a supplemental regional anesthetic might have been quite helpful if the patient had permitted it. However, no matter what drugs or overall plan are chosen, management of the depth of anesthesia will resemble the pattern described here. During most of the procedure, even during maintenance, the depth of anesthesia and the rates of administration of the drugs producing anesthesia are changed to meet circumstances. The management of emergence, removal of the endotracheal tube, and transport to the recovery room are described in Chapter 35.

Transferring the Patient's Care to Another During the Anesthetic

Ideally, it might seem that the patient's best interests are served when the same individual attends to the anesthetic throughout the operation. In practice it is often desirable to have another person take over the anesthetic during a lunch break or at the end of the day. There is no doubt that fatigue impairs performance, and the new person often sees problems and solutions overlooked by a tired predecessor. To make this transfer of care safe, a systematic review is needed, including at least:

1. A summary of the preoperative evaluation of the patient.
2. The anesthetic plan.
3. The course of the overall anesthetic and any changes which have been made in the plan, including any unresolved problems.
4. The current state of the operation and its anticipated course.
5. Every item being monitored, including the findings and their interpretation.
6. A note in the anesthesia record documenting the transfer of care.

Error, Chaos, and Emergencies

The testimony of experienced anesthesiologists, case presentations at departmental conferences, analysis of closed malpractice claims, Cooper's studies of critical incidents in anesthesia, and experience in high-technology industries all provide insight into accidents and near misses. Several facts are clear:

1. Error is unremitting. Something is always going wrong, but usually nothing comes of it. These background errors do not propagate themselves, either because they are of little consequence in the first place (0.5 mg of atropine is given instead of 0.3 mg), or because the problem is noticed and corrected (the endotracheal tube becomes disconnected and is immediately reattached). These problems crop up continually during even the most routine cases.
2. Healthy patients undergoing usual operations may withstand many such errors without harm, but sick patients are more vulnerable.
3. Catastrophes tend to occur when errors summate. For example, if the endotracheal tube becomes disconnected from the breathing circuit, while at the same time the airway pressure alarm fails and the anesthesiologist is distracted by a phone call from the blood bank, hypoxia may occur. If the pulse oximeter also fails, the patient might suffer a cardiac arrest.
4. Most problems are due to human error, not mechanical malfunctions or patient aberrations.
5. Complex, highly interlinked processes are more vulnerable to disruption than are less complex ones. When the plan calls for a rapid succession of linked treatments, then a minor occurrence has serious consequences. For example, unexpected infiltration of an intravenous infusion, of

no consequence in a healthy young patient undergoing arthroscopy of the knee, might have led to disaster in our patient undergoing hip reconstruction; loss of intravenous access might have meant loss of nitroprusside effect and inability to give fluids, with hypertension, hemorrhage and inability to replace lost blood. One of the reasons for using a second peripheral intravenous cannula as well as a CVP catheter was to prevent this sort of occurrence.

These insights suggest several remedies to reduce the harm patients suffer from accidents.

Protect the Patient First, Diagnose the Problem Second. If a problem is simple (ventilator disconnected), correct it (reattach the hose); if the origin of the problem is not obvious immediately (mysterious ventilator malfunction), do not focus on the problem, but focus instead on preventing harm to the patient (institute manual ventilation). Later, it is important to find an explanation for what happened. No maloccurence and no abnormal finding can be left unexplained, lest a small problem grow into a large one. For example, if our patient's arterial pressure decreases suddenly to 50/30, the first step is to discontinue the anesthetics and the nitroprusside, not to seek causes; later, investigation might show that a bolus of nitroprusside had been inadvertently flushed into the patient.

Take More Precautions for Sick Patients. Since the consequences of misadventure are graver for them, sick patients require more precautions. For example, if our patient for the hip operation had been healthier and had been willing to accept blood if needed, then invasive monitoring might not have been needed.

Keep Errors From Summating. When several things go wrong at once, take definitive steps to break the chain of events and assure the patient's safety. For example, if one undertook a rapid sequence induction in our patient and misjudged the dose of thiopental, she might become hypotensive. If at the same time, a novice anesthesiologist could not see the glottis, the right course of action would be to have an experienced person intubate the trachea immediately, to assure adequate oxygenation and interrupt a chain of events leading to cardiac arrest.

Since prompt action often prevents maloccurrences from summating, anesthesiologists mentally rehearse their responses to some common problems. It is a good idea to plan rational responses to each of these;

1. Abrupt decrease in peripheral oxygen saturation.
2. Abrupt onset of hypotension.
3. Loss of breath sounds.
4. Increased airway pressures.
5. Wheezing.
6. Cardiac arrest.
7. High fever, increased CO_2 production.
8. Bradycardia.
9. Tachyarrhythmias.

Minimize Chances for Error. Attention to detail, checklists, mechanical alarms, redundancy (e.g., using stethoscope, capnograph, and pulse oximeter), retrospective analysis of critical incidents, and other compulsive steps are natural responses to the problem of error. In addition to improved equipment and checklists, those giving anesthesia must cultivate imagination and innovation, if for no other reason than to ward off boredom and inattention.

Avoid Complex Plans. If at all possible, avoid tightly linked management schemes; good plans for anesthesia management offer easy alternatives for unexpected contingencies. Rapid sequence intubation was not chosen for the induction of anesthesia for our woman undergoing hip surgery because this plan is unnecessarily complex and its steps are tightly linked; the plan is therefore vulnerable to disruption (wrong thiopental dose, failed intubation), but offers her no appreciable benefits in compensation for the increased risk. The plan chosen offered more alternatives: the chance to limit the dose of thiopental or the dose of isoflurane, and the chance to abort the induction if airway difficulties arose.

Complex Cases

Anesthesia for some operations and for some patients cannot be managed by simple means. Many cardiac procedures, large-scale abdominal procedures, liver transplants, some trauma or other emergency cases, some operations on the great vessels, and any patient whose condition deteriorates rapidly or who is near death may require more care than a single anesthesiologist can give. Some anesthesiologists who perform well while alone do poorly when teamwork is required. A useful analogy is that the analysis of cockpit tapes recorded in the minutes before airplane crashes have shown that capable pilots have made mistakes that might have been averted if they had used more effectively the help available to them from copilots, flight engineers, and air traffic controllers. Experience with complex cases has shown how an anesthesia team can function most effectively.

First, the effort must be organized; an uncontrolled group of well-intentioned assistants will not be effective. Some of the job descriptions to be filled are:

1. *Head of table*. Stands at the head of the operating table, administers drugs, watches the patient and makes adjustments to the anesthesia machine and ventilator.
2. *Record keeper*. Keeps an accurate contemporaneous record.
3. *Thinker*. Stays aloof from manual tasks and minute-to-minute worries and considers the overall care of the patient.
4. *Worker(s)*. Prepares IV drips, hangs blood, places intravenous cannulae, all at the direction of the anesthesiologist in charge.
5. *Aide*. Runs errands.
6. *Pump technician(s)*. Even if cardiopulmonary bypass is not needed, rapid infusion of blood often is required in this type of case. A pump and technicians to run it are a vital part of the team.
7. *Anesthesiologist in charge*. This is usually the attending anesthesiologist of record, who might be the one at the head of the table, the "thinker," or the record keeper. Though in charge of the anesthetic, this person must accept help from others.

Each of these jobs must be assigned clearly to someone. In most instances, one person will fulfill several of these functions; in truly massive cases, the anesthesia team may indeed number 4 to 6, with a correspondingly large number of surgeons and nurses.

Second, just as in the studies of behavior in the cockpits of airplanes, members of the anesthesia team must communicate effectively with each other and with the surgeons, so that their efforts are coordinated. Extraneous chatter must be suppressed, but everyone must be able to share data and ideas. Surgeons and anesthesiologists must understand each other's thinking and plans. The blood bank must receive advance notice of the blood products needed. Speaking slowly and calmly can help control the atmosphere in the room, reducing the ill effects of anger, frustration, and anxiety on the group's performance. From time to time, someone must summarize the case. "We have a healthy 22-year-old man with a gunshot wound to the upper abdomen. The aorta is clamped and the heart is full, but not contracting. There is something wrong besides hypovolemia. What?"

Despite a calm, orderly approach, a massive case sometimes becomes confusing. If the situation can be salvaged at all, attention to simple measures is usually effective:

1. Adequate ventilation with oxygen.
2. Support of the circulation with fluids, pressors, inotropes, or cardiac massage as required.
3. Correction of acidemia and hyperkalemia.
4. Consideration of possible pneumothorax or cardiac tamponade.

COSTS

Anesthesiologists feel that their primary responsibility is to the patient, and not to the hospital or third-party payer. Thus, anesthesiologists often prefer the most effective, most recent, and most expensive drugs and equipment available. The cost differences among anesthesia drugs are significant: older drugs such as halothane, enflurane, curare, pancuronium, thiopental, fentanyl, and morphine are much cheaper than patented drugs such as isoflurane, vencuronium, atracurium, propofol, alfentanil, and sufentanil. The more modern drugs offer important advantages, but in most clinical settings, the older and less expensive drugs will yield satisfactory results.

Money can be saved in the conduct of anesthesia without compromising results by reserving the more expensive drugs for those situations in which their special advantages justify their use. As an example, the woman who underwent the hip operation received the cheaper muscle relaxant curare, whereas another patient, with renal failure, electrolyte abnormalities, and receiving gentamicin, might require atracurium. It is also important to remember that the cost of drugs does not represent the entire cost of care. If the use of an inexpensive drug prolongs the patient's stay in the recovery room, the total cost may be greater than if a more rapidly metabolized drug had been used.

Anesthesia Record

A properly conducted anesthetic includes a good record, a necessary tool for keeping track of what has been done and the patient's responses. Good records improve the conduct of anesthesia in the same way that accurate laboratory notebooks improve experiments: they focus attention and oblige one to confront data objectively. An adequate record meets these criteria:

1. Every space or box is completed, legibly.
2. All significant findings and therapies are recorded with no gaps in monitoring.
3. Any anesthesiologist can reconstruct the case from the record.
4. The record gives the rationale for various actions. For example, the record not only records that the endotracheal tube was removed, but also that the patient responded to command, supported his head for five seconds, and breathed freely through an open airway when the tube was removed.

The Conduct of the Anesthesiologist

Some anesthesiologists who give technically excellent care do not inspire confidence in patients, surgeons, or co-workers. Sometimes, this is because of behavior that is not obviously related to competent anesthesia. There has already been advice given on the need for sympathetic relations with patients and collegial communication with surgeons; these are major aspects of behavior that can inspire confidence. Others are less obvious.

Dealing with the awake patient in the operating room requires a different approach than is used during the preoperative visit. The patient is at a marked disadvantage: unclothed, supine, drugged, frightened, and helpless when everyone else in the room is dressed, upright, alert, at ease, and in control of events. The anesthesiologist must speak gently and reassuringly, informing the patient ahead of time of each step in preparing for induction of anesthesia, projecting at least an air of calm, if not of confidence, and avoiding frightening exclamations (such as "oops").

A neat and orderly approach to the work also improves one's professional standing. A long list of advice could follow this general injunction without enlarging on the basic concept: neatness counts. Speed and efficiency are also valuable attributes for an anesthesiologist, given the increasing economic pressures for more efficient use of operating room time. While a calm, orderly approach must not be sacrificed, and shortcuts that risk patient safety are not appropriate, much can often be done to work quickly. Important ways of improving speed safely include:

1. Varying speed according to the task (opening a spinal anesthesia kit quickly, but mixing the drugs and placing the needle with deliberation).
2. Performing tasks in parallel, not in series (asking the patient to breath oxygen while waiting for the automated blood pressure cuff to produce the first reading).
3. Anticipating coming steps (drawing up the neostigmine and atropine before the end of the anesthetic).
4. Keeping surgeons informed of the progress of the anesthetic so that they can keep pace (encouraging the surgeon to begin the skin preparation after induction but before intubation, if this seems safe).

In all, the efficient and safe conduct of anesthesia is a complex undertaking. The person who does it well must strive to perfect the practices described here, as well as the ordinary technical and intellectual skills of anesthesia.

References

Cooper J, Long CD, Newbower RS, Philip JH. Critical incidents associated with intraoperative exchanges of anesthesia personnel. Anesthesiology 1982;56:456.

Muravchick S. The anesthetic plan: From physiologic principles to clinical strategies. St. Louis: Mosby Year Book, 1991.

Perrow C. Normal accidents. New York: Basic Books, 1984.

CHAPTER FIFTEEN

Managing Fluids, Electrolytes and Blood Loss

Fluids and Electrolytes

Before, during, and after major operations, surgical patients may suffer life-threatening blood and fluid losses, along with derangements of acid-base physiology, electrolyte balance, and hemostasis. Impaired function of heart, lungs, liver, and kidney makes these problems more urgent and difficult to treat. Even for minor operations in healthy patients, an intravenous infusion is part of good management, if only for emergency administration of drugs. Knowledge of the relevant physiology and skill at placing intravenous cannulae takes second place in the anesthesiologist's armamentarium only to the skills of airway management.

The Body Fluid Compartments

Anesthesiologists are primarily concerned with monitoring the patient's intravascular volume, assessing it by such routine measurements as blood pressure, pulse, urine output, central venous pressure, and pulmonary capillary wedge pressure. Interpreting these observations depends on an understanding of the relation between total body water and its major subcompartments, intracellular (ICF) and extracellular (ECF) volumes, and the subdivisions of the latter into the intravascular (IVC) and interstitial (ISS) compartments. (Fig. 15–1)

Total body water is usually expressed as a fraction of total body weight. Approximately 60 per cent of the adult lean body mass consists of water; the variable amount of additional fat, with its lesser water content, accounts for interpatient variability and the systematic differences among men, women, and children (Table 15–1).

Physiologic mechanisms maintain the balance between the capacity of the intravascular space and the intravascular fluid volume. In acute blood loss, homeostatic mechanisms include mobilization of extravascular protein via the lymphatics, and vasoconstriction, primarily in the venous system. In addition, hormonal responses mediated via the central nervous system (CNS) cause release of antidiuretic hormone (ADH), which increases

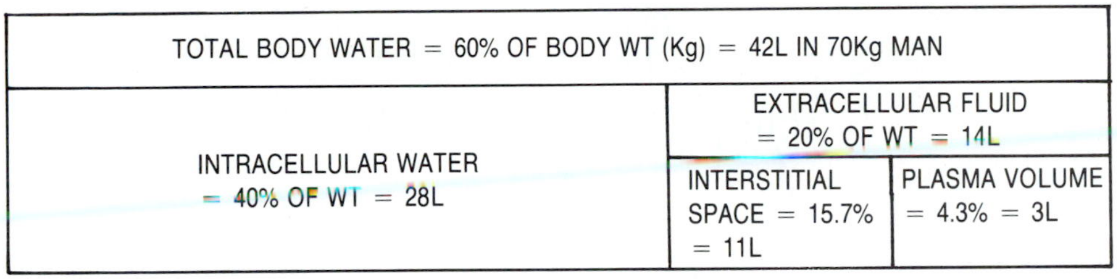

<table>
<tr><td colspan="3">TOTAL BODY WATER = 60% OF BODY WT (Kg) = 42L IN 70Kg MAN</td></tr>
<tr><td rowspan="2">INTRACELLULAR WATER
= 40% OF WT = 28L</td><td colspan="2">EXTRACELLULAR FLUID
= 20% OF WT = 14L</td></tr>
<tr><td>INTERSTITIAL
SPACE = 15.7%
= 11L</td><td>PLASMA VOLUME
= 4.3% = 3L</td></tr>
</table>

FIGURE 15–1. *Distribution of total body water for a normal 70 kg man with 60 per cent water (range can be 40 to 68 per cent).*

renal tubular water reabsorption as well as sodium reabsorption mediated by the renin-angiotensin-aldosterone mechanism. Conversely, in cases of fluid overload, stretch of atrial cardiac muscle fibers releases atrial natriuretic factor, producing vasodilation. (Fig. 15–2)

The major ECF cations are sodium, calcium, and magnesium; the ICF cations are potassium and magnesium (Table 15–2). Because of large total stores, major losses in total body potassium occur before a significant decrease in serum potassium is detectable. Similarly, changes in serum calcium and magnesium produce neurologic and cardiac signs before osmotic effects are observed. The clinical problems produced by common extracellular cation abnormalities, and their treatment, are summarized in Table 15–3.

The major ECF anions are chloride and bicarbonate, frequently referred to as exchangeable anions. When renal reabsorption of one anion is increased, renal excretion of the other is enhanced. For example, patients with chronic obstructive lung disease and carbon dioxide retention may have bicarbonate values between 35 and 40 mEq per L and chloride values between 85 and 95 mEq per L. The major ICF anions include phosphates, organic acids, and the negatively charged intracellular proteins. Because proteins cannot move freely between compartments, these solutes play a major role in the distribution of water.

Normally, the sum of plasma sodium and potassium concentrations (mEq per L) does not exceed the sum of chloride and bicarbonate concentrations by more than 15 mEq per L. Should a larger difference exist, increased amounts of other unmeasured anions, such as lactate, ketones, or anions from an exogenous source, such as salicylate or ethylene glycol, are suspected. This anion gap is a reflection of the differences in unmeasured cations and anions:

$$\text{anion gap} = [NA^+] + [K^+] - [HCO_3^-] - [Cl^-]; \text{ normally } <15 \text{ mEq/L}.$$

TABLE 15–1. Average Fluid Volumes

Measurement	Absolute Value		Relative Value (% Body Weight)	
	Men	*Women*	*Men*	*Women*
Weight (kg)	70	60	100	100
Hematocrit whole blood (%)	42	30	—	—
Plasma volume (ml)	3150	2700	4.5	4.5
Red blood cell volume (ml)	2100	1500	3.0	2.5
Blood volume (ml)	5250	4200	7.5	7.0
Extracellular water (L)	16.4	14.2	23.4	23.7
Total body water (L)	42	30	60	50

TABLE 15–2. Representative Values of the Major Solutes in the Respective Fluid Compartment (mEq/L)

Solute	Fluid Compartment		
	Plasma	*Interstitial Fluid*	*Intracellular Fluid*
Na^+	142	142	10
K^+	4	4	140
Ca^{++}	5	5	<1
Mg^{++}	3	3	58
Cl^-	103	106	4
HCO_3^-	27	27	10
(HPO_4^-, $H_2PO_4^-$)	4	4	75
$SO_4^=$	1	1	2
Organic acid$^-$	7	7	25
Proteins$^-$	17	2	66

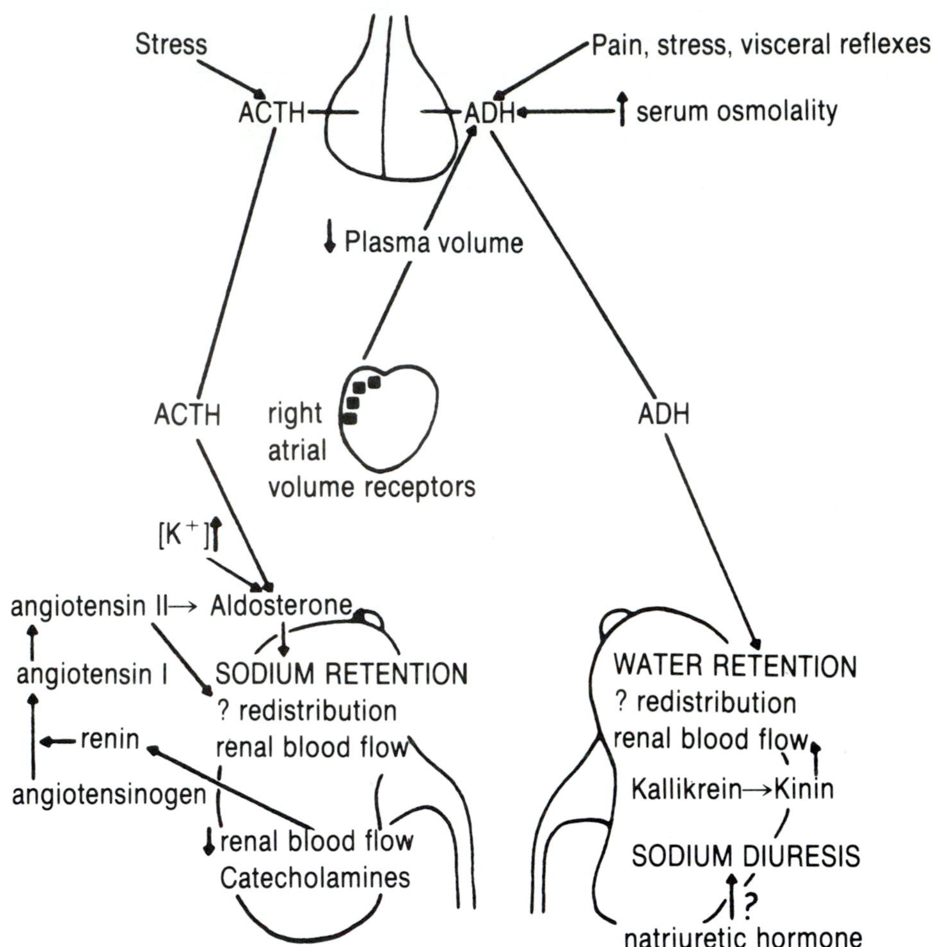

FIGURE 15–2. Schematic overview of hormonal and CNS interaction in the control of fluid and electrolyte balance. ACTH is secreted from the anterior pituitary and ADH from the posterior pituitary gland. (Reproduced with permission from Twigley AJ, Hillman KA. The end of the crystalloid era? Anaesthesia 1983;40:800–871.)

Intravenous Fluid Therapy

Most patients are denied food and water for 8 to 12 hours before elective operations; this practice can result in considerable solute and water loss. Insensible losses from the lungs and skin range from 800 to 1000 ml daily in the normal adult. An obligatory 500 ml of urinary water is required for excretion of waste products, while average urine volume is 1.0 ml per kg of body weight per hour, or approximately 1700 ml daily in a 70 kg adult. The water-conserving capability of the kidney provides a generous margin of safety and is the major means of adjustment when body water must be conserved. Although renal mechanisms limit losses in the fluid-restricted adult, infants are less able to deal with unreplaced losses, because the immature kidney concentrates urine poorly and the increased ratio of body surface area to volume increases relative insensible loss.

Unless gastric emptying is abnormally delayed, feedings of clear liquids up to a few hours before operation do little to increase the volume in the stomach or the risk of pulmonary aspiration. For adults scheduled for afternoon operations, an early morning clear-liquid breakfast seems safe and appropriate. However, if delayed gastric emptying is a concern, an intravenous infusion is safer. Infants and young children in whom prolonged fasting may result in severe dehydration are fed clear fluids two

Table 15–3. Extracellular Cation Abnormalities and Their Treatment

	↑ K^+	↓ K^+	↓ Ca^{++}	↓ Mg^{++}
Major clinical problems	Cardiac arrhythmias: ultimately sinus arrest	Cardiac arrhythmias: Ultimately ventricular fibrillation	Inotropic cardiac failure	Hyperreflexia and tetany
		Muscle weakness or loss of reflexes	Hyperreflexia and tetany	Psychiatric symptoms Neuromuscular weakness Increased arrhythmias with digitalis, inability to defibrillate ventricular fibrillation
Most common causes	Renal failure	Diuretic therapy; steroid therapy	Alkalosis	Alcoholism
	Acidosis	Treatment of acidosis; nasogastric suction	Hypoparathyroidism	Diuretic therapy
	Iatrogenic	Alkalosis Dehydration	Massive transfusion (rare)	Chronic renal disease GI losses
Laboratory values*	>5 mEq/L	<3.0 mEq/L	<4.5 mEq/L >9 mg/100 ml	<1.5 mEq/L <1.8 mg/100 ml
ECG changes	Peaked T waves	ST segment depression	Prolonged Q-T interval	Prolonged Q-T interval, Nonspecific St-T wave changes
	Loss of P wave Loss of peaked T wave	T wave inversion U wave (may be a positive or negative wave)		
	Bradycardia Spread of QRS			
Acute therapy in 70-kg adult (life-threatening situations only)	100 mEq $NaHCO_3$, IV over 2 min 50 gm glucose, 20 U regular insulin IV	K^+IV at 1 mEq/min	CaCl 250 mg IV every 5 min until symptoms reverse; if calcium gluconate is used, multiply dose by 3	$MgSO_4$ 5 gm/hr IM or IV (may aggravate preexistent hypocalcemia)

* These are threshold values; the severe forms of the syndromes appear only at more abnormal values.

or three hours prior to elective operation in most pediatric centers.

In view of the preoperative fluid deficit, the administration of one third to one half of the estimated 24-hour fluid requirement parenterally during the course of a major operation in the adult is logical. Thus, an average 70 kg adult would receive approximately 1000 ml during a brief operation, even without operative blood or fluid loss. To minimize the hazard of excess free water, at least one third of the fluid can be a solute-containing solution such as saline or lactated Ringer's solution. As most of these patients have had no caloric intake over the preceding 10 to 12 hours, adding 25 to 30 gm of dextrose is also logical. In healthy patients undergoing minor operations, compensatory mechanisms make acceptable any reasonable fluid regimen that avoids extremes.

Patients presenting with a history of vomiting, diarrhea, prolonged gastric suction, or intestinal fistulae may have sustained massive fluid losses from the gastrointestinal tract. In addition, those with peritonitis or bowel obstruction may sequester large volumes of protein-rich fluid in the abdominal cavity or lumen of the gut. In the diabetic patient with hyperglycemia and acetonuria, and in some types of renal failure, impressive fluid deficits occur as a result of renal salt and water losses. Extensive burns result in major losses of water, salt, and protein into the involved areas. Among febrile patients or in hot climates, insensible losses are increased by sweating and through the respiratory tract. Finally, chronically ill, elderly, anorectic, and psychotic patients frequently fail to maintain adequate fluid intake and oral nourishment.

Chronically ill, malnourished patients suffer a "depletion syndrome" consisting of major losses of essential substrates, amino acids, glycogen, fat, and caloric reserves. There is a significant decrease in intracellular water, a slight increase in the interstitial volume, and a decrease in the intravascular or plasma volume. These patients have deficiencies in total body potassium, phosphate, sodium and serum proteins, and a tendency toward a decreased serum osmolarity. Frequently, such patients appear stable until subjected to anesthesia and operation. Under these circumstances cardiovascular function rapidly deteriorates and may fail to respond promptly to standard fluid resuscitation.

Useful signs in evaluating a patient with these problems include the state of consciousness and the cardiovascular response to changes in posture (orthostatic hypotension). A fully conscious patient who can sit upright for at lest a minute without any significant increase in pulse rate or decrease in mean arterial pressure is unlikely to have more than a 10 per cent deficit in ECF. At the other extreme, an obtunded patient with peritonitis, who demonstrates hypotension and tachycardia while lying supine, is obviously deficient in extracellular fluid. In the operating room, a final test of intravascular volume may be made, the "tilt test", in which the operation table is tilted to place the patient head-up for one minute. An increase in pulse rate of more that 10 beats per minute or a decrease in blood pressure of more than 10 mm Hg indicates hypovolemia.

Failure to restore intravascular volume before proceeding may produce catastrophe when the sympathoplegia, vasodilation, and decreased cardiac output that accompany anesthesia are added to preexisting hypovolemia. Restoration of intravascular volume toward normal before operation is essential to preserve adequate cardiovascular, cerebral, and renal function.

In the hypotensive, dehydrated patient with adequate cardiovascular reserves, the ECF can be replenished rapidly with isotonic saline or lactated Ringer's solution. It may be necessary to give 1 L of crystalloid solution every 15 minutes, up to 3 to 4 L. In the patient with limited cardiovascular reserves, careful replacement with incremental fluid challenges of 200 ml of crystalloid over a period of ten minutes, with observation for sequential changes in CVP or pulmonary artery wedge pressures (PAWP) is performed. Fluids are continued at this rate until vital signs improve and urine output reaches 0.75 to 1.0 ml per kg per hour or CVP or PAWP increases excessively with each fluid bolus.

If signs of intravascular fluid overload appear before cardiovascular stability or adequate urine output, the rate of fluid administration is reduced. Under these circumstances it is likely that the primary fault is inadequate myocardial function and a positive inotropic drug, such as dopamine, must be considered. A diuretic may help eliminate excess water. Under these circumstances, monitoring of left and right ventricular function using a pulmonary artery catheter is helpful in judging the effects of therapy. Stability is best achieved before anesthesia, because of the cardiovascular action of the anesthetic. If the patient has not been resuscitated before operation, only the lightest general anesthesia or local anesthesia is possible.

Some physicians prefer colloid solutions over crystalloid solutions for treatment of dehydrated patients with peritonitis, bowel obstruction, or severe burns, because of the large internal losses of protein-rich fluid. Provided that sufficient amounts are administered, crystalloid alone is almost always effective in restoring circulatory stability. However, large amounts of crystalloid may be required, carrying risks discussed later. Thus, there is a rationale for the use of colloid solutions in volume replacement.

Similarly, some physicians prefer balanced salt solutions, which more nearly mimic the chemical composition of ECF, to simple isotonic saline. The composition of the commonly available parenteral fluid solutions is given in Table 15–4. There is little proven advantage or disadvantage in using more expensive and complex salt solutions. Acid-base evaluation is essential in patients receiving major fluid therapy regardless of the solution chosen, because hemostasis is best achieved only near pH 7.40.

It is unwise to administer potassium routinely to dehydrated patients without first measuring the serum potassium, as they may suffer either hypokalemia or hyperkalemia. Available balanced salt solutions supply insufficient potassium to cor-

TABLE 15–4. **Comparison of Extracellular Fluid and Various Replacement Solutions**

Solution	Na^+ (mEq/L)	K^+ (mEq/L)	Cl^- (mEq/L)	Total Base (mEq/L)	pH	Ca++ (mEq/L)	Mg++ (mEq/L)	Calories per Liter
Extracellular fluid	138	5	108	27	7.4	5	3	12
5% Dextrose/water	0	0	0	0	4.5	0	0	200
Normal Saline	154	0	154	0	6.0	0	0	0
Lactated Ringer's	130	4	109	28	6.5	3	0	9
Normosol	140	5	98	50	7.4	0	3	24
5% Albumin	145	0			7.4	0	0	—
Hetastarch	154	0	154	0	5.5	0	0	—

rect hypokalemia, which requires 40 mEq of potassium per L in replacement solutions. Potassium is not given more rapidly than 1 mEq per minute per 70 kg to avoid impairing cardiac conduction. Should the dose exceed 1.5 mEq per minute per 70 kg, the ECG is monitored continuously and serum potassium measured every two hours.

Medical treatment may cause salt and water excess or deficiency. Patients treated with salt restriction and diuretics for hypertension or congestive heart failure frequently suffer volume depletion that becomes evident only after induction of anesthesia. If both arterial hypotension and a decrease in venous filling pressure follow induction, intravenous fluids are indicated. The added intravascular volume necessary to maintain cardiovascular stability during anesthesia may not be tolerated once the vasodilating effects of anesthetic agents are eliminated. When this occurs, fluid restriction, diuresis, and ventilatory support may be required immediately after operation.

Hazards of Excess Fluid and Electrolyte Administration

As a substitute for blood transfusion, to treat shock, and to protect the kidneys by maintaining diuresis during major operations, anesthesiologists administer parenteral fluids in excess of probable losses. This therapy is associated with several potential hazards (Table 15–5).

WATER INTOXICATION

Release of ADH occurs in response to stress, general anesthesia, opioids, pain, blood loss, and positive pressure ventilation so that postoperative patients may have increased ADH levels despite normal or decreased ECF tonicity. This inappropriate ADH secretion, combined with administration of excess free water, can result in dilutional hyponatremia and expansion of intracellular volume, including neuronal swelling. Cerebral symptoms range from mild lethargy and disorientation to delirium, coma, and convulsions. The condition may be worsened by opioids given in an effort to treat delirium.

Symptoms of water intoxication usually begin on the first to third postoperative day; if convulsions occur, the fatality rate is high. The syndrome is more common in patients over 60 years of age and is rarely seen in adults with normal renal function if they receive on any one day less than 2 L of free water, including water absorbed during transurethral resection of the prostate. Although serum sodium levels at the onset of symptoms are usually less than 130 mEq, the rapidity of the change is more relevant than the sodium concentration. Urine osmolarity is inappropriately increased (>500 mOsm per L), while serum osmolarity is decreased (<240 mOsm per L).

Treatment includes restricting fluids to less than 1 L of isotonic saline per day, with no free water intake. Serum osmolarity can be increased more quickly by the use of diuretics or by the administration of hypertonic saline. In the absence of serious symptoms, fluid restriction alone is effective. Symptoms may persist for several days despite return of serum sodium levels to normal. Because of the hazard of water intoxication, sodium-free water should be limited to that needed to replace losses, including those caused by overnight fluid restriction.

TABLE 15-5. **Effect of Administering Too Little or Too Much Water and Certain Solutes***

Substance	Amount Administered	
	Too Little	*Too Much*
Water	Hyperosmolar hyponatremia Concentrated, sparse urine Thirst Oliguria Fever Circulatory failure	Hypoosmolar hyponatremia Very dilute urine Polyuria Intracranial hypertension Headache, confusion, nausea, and vomiting Weakness Muscle twitching and cramps Convulsions Coma
Sodium	Extracellular fluid volume decreased Hemoconcentration Lost tissue elasticity Hypotension Circulatory failure Uremia	Extracellular fluid volume increased Edema formation and congestive heart failure Tendency to potassium deficiency
Phosphorus	Hypophosphatemia Other effects	Hyperphosphatemia Hypocalcemia
Carbohydrate	Ketosis Protoplasmic catabolism augmented Tendency to greater water and electrolyte losses	Hyperglycemia Glycosuria Hepatic failure

* Reproduced in part with permission from Talbot NB, et al. N Engl J Med 1955; 252:856.

EXCESS SALT ADMINISTRATION

Just as ADH secretion may be increased postoperatively despite decreased extracellular tonicity, adrenocorticoid production may increase in spite of increased ECF volume. As with ADH, increases in circulating glucocorticoids and aldosterone are in part related to stress. In part, these increases are provoked by response to a functional decrease in ECF due to loss of fluid to sites from which it cannot be mobilized rapidly (third space losses). Such functional decreases in ECF follow major operations or trauma, and the concomitant tendency toward renal salt conservation can be overcome by a copious saline loading. In contrast, postoperative renal free water conservation is not overcome with administration of additional free water.

Nevertheless, administration of large amounts of sodium is not without hazard. Previously healthy individuals given relatively large doses of isotonic salt solution (3000 ml or more) for the treatment of shock can develop pulmonary edema. Lesser volumes may cause deterioration in pulmonary gas exchange even in the absence of overt edema. Pulmonary symptoms may not occur until several days postoperatively when healing allows sequestered third space fluid to be mobilized. Although most patients tolerate excess saline better than excess free water, indiscriminate use of salt solutions without demonstrable indication is inappropriate.

INDICATIONS FOR CRYSTALLOID SOLUTION OTHER THAN AS REPLACEMENT THERAPY

Several situations justify the use of crystalloid solutions in amounts modestly exceeding probable fluid loss. In relatively healthy patients, blood losses of less than 15 to 20 per cent of the blood volume can be replaced with crystalloid given in amounts three to four times the volume of shed blood. Salt-containing solutions are substituted for much of the blood formerly used to prime heart-lung machines, decreasing the hemolysis seen during cardiopulmonary bypass and conserving limited blood supplies.

Salt-containing solutions may also be used for rapid expansion of the intravascular volume prior to spinal or epidural anesthesia, decreasing the se-

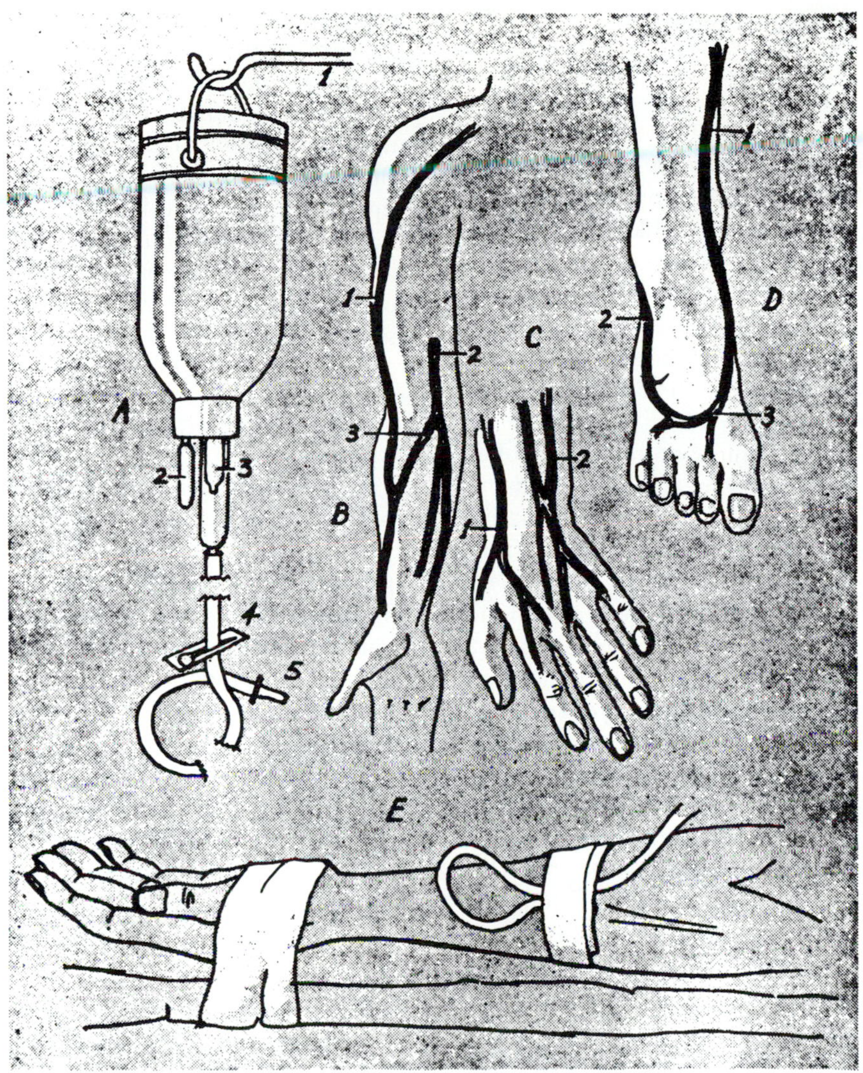

FIGURE 15–3. Important elements in intravenous catheter placement. A, Components of intravenous apparatus: *1*, hook on pole of adjustable height; *2*, air inlet; *3*, drip chamber; *4*, pinch clamp for controlling flow of fluid; *5*, adapter for insertion into needle or catheter. *B*, Veins of arm: *1*, cephalic; *2*, basilic; *3*, antecubital. *C*, Veins of dorsum of hand: *1*, cephalic; *2*, basilic. *D*, Veins of dorsum of foot: *1*, great saphenous; *2*, small saphenous; *3*, dorsal venous arch. *E*, Fixation of intravenous needle and tubing to arm.

verity of hypotension and the need for vasopressors after neural blockade. Finally, fluid administration beyond replacement of measured loss is commonly used to protect the kidneys. An intraoperative diuresis of 50 ml per hour or more decreases the risk of postoperative renal failure, especially in adults with major trauma or those undergoing resection of an aortic aneurysm. Usually, crystalloid solutions are used to increase urine output. Because excessive fluids can lead to pulmonary edema, mannitol or furosemide may be preferable to large volumes of fluid when the initial response to crystalloid solutions is inadequate. Exact figures on the limits of fluid administration above measured losses are not available. Limits are determined by what is known about each patient's renal, pulmonary, and cardiac function, by the results of cardiovascular and pulmonary function monitoring, and plans for postoperative mechanical ventilation.

Intravenous Technique

Plastic intravenous catheters inserted over a needle are used routinely for almost all procedures, no matter how minor. They are much less likely to become dislodged than are metal needles. The major disadvantages are sepsis and thrombophlebitis, which become more likely the longer the catheter is left in place. Catheters are changed or discontinued if possible within 72 hours of insertion. A 20-gauge catheter is the smallest that is used routinely in adults undergoing anesthesia, but larger catheters are indicated when blood replacement is required.

Skin preparation for venipuncture with alcohol or iodine solution provides mechanical cleansing and a bactericidal action. Gloves worn during intravenous cannulation protect the operator from unnecessary exposure to the patient's blood. A small skin wheal is first raised with local anesthetic through a 27-gauge needle to minimize pain of the large catheter. The veins on the dorsum of the hand are often excellent from the standpoint of size, visibility, and minimal chance of inadvertent arterial cannulation, but it is sometimes difficult to maintain immobilization in the immediate postoperative period. Veins of the mid-forearm are more suitable for immobilization over long periods (Fig. 15–3).

A wide tourniquet applied without pinching the skin or pulling on hair provides adequate venous engorgement. The vein is fixed distally by stretching the skin. The needle, bevel up, is inserted through the skin and advanced at a shallow angle directly at the vein. When penetration occurs the catheter is pushed over the needle into the vein, using a slight rotatory movement. The appearance of blood in the catheter indicates successful puncture. The tourniquet is released before the infusion is started.

If a vein is torn, the operator first removes the tourniquet, and then the needle, applying pressure to the site and elevating the arm to decrease the size of the hematoma. Following successful cannulation, the catheter is connected to the intravenous tubing. To prevent accidental disconnection, adhesive tape is used to reinforce the connection if the preferred locking connection is not used. After insertion, and at frequent intervals, the system is checked for infiltration. A clear dressing facilitates checking the infusion site. Tape is never applied completely around the limb, for it may interfere with venous return and produce limb ischemia.

Anxious patients with constricted veins occasionally may benefit from delaying venipuncture until after the inhalation induction of anesthesia. This is certainly more pleasant for the patient than repeated unsuccessful attempts at venipuncture, but it carries risks. If vasoconstriction is due to hypovolemia or the patient has a full stomach or a difficult airway, intravenous access is mandatory before induction.

Managing Blood Loss

Well over 50 per cent of the blood collected in the United States is administered to surgical patients in the perioperative period, much of it intraoperatively. Administration of blood products is a common task in the practice of anesthesia, one which requires careful consideration of risks and vigilance to prevent error. Modern practice is to limit transfused blood to the minimum required for safe care.

Allowable Blood Loss

In the past, many anesthesiologists insisted that patients have hemoglobin levels of 10 gm per dl or greater before the beginning of anesthesia. The rigid adherence to any prescribed value is illogical, in that no one value can be applied to all patients or settings. However, safe lower limits are now thought to be in the range of 7.0 to 8.0 gm per dl, depending on the patient and the surgical procedure. Two groups of patients, Jehovah's Witnesses and those with end-stage renal failure, have demonstrated clearly that hemoglobin values of 5 gm per dl or less can be tolerated when necessary.

It is a common practice in otherwise healthy patients to replace blood loss with either crystalloid (at a rate of 3:1) or colloid solution (rate of 1:1) until transfusion is required. An approximation of the allowable loss is given by:

$$\text{allowable loss} = \text{EBV} \times (\text{Hb}_{\text{initial}} - \text{Hb}_{\text{target}})/\text{Hb}_{\text{initial}}$$

where

$\text{Hb}_{\text{initial}}$ is the hemoglobin at the start of blood loss:

Hb_{target} is the target hemoglobin level; and
EBV is the estimated blood volume

For example, in a patient with an EBV of 4500 ml and a hemoglobin of 15.0 gm per dl, the target hemoglobin of 9.0 gm per dl would be achieved by replacing the first 1800 ml of blood loss with colloid or crystalloid solutions (4500 ml × [15 − 9]/15 = 1800 ml). This estimate errs on the conservative side in that each subsequent ml of blood lost is further diluted by the crystalloid or colloid that is administered to maintain normal blood volume.

Blood Component Therapy Versus Whole Blood

Over 80 per cent of blood collected in the United States is fractionated. Each donor unit provides specific components for several patients, thus promoting goal-directed specific therapy in lieu of whole-blood administration, and permitting the available blood supply to serve a larger population. However, the resulting scarcity of whole blood has complicated the treatment of massive hemorrhage, because whole blood must be approximated by component therapy, exposing these patients to a greater number of donor units and slowing the process of transfusion.

Autologous Blood Transfusion

Autologous transfusion has several advantages. Not only does this practice save bank blood, but compatibility and disease transmission are not issues, unless errors result in giving the wrong blood. There are several variants of autologous blood transfusion.

Preoperative collection and storage of blood at weekly intervals before elective cases involving blood loss can produce a store of 4 units of autologous blood. In some patients with rare blood types this may be the only way to provide compatible blood; freezing can provide even more units. To avoid anemia, these patients must receive iron treatment; erythropoietin also increases the volume of blood that can be collected. To ensure against clerical errors, at least ABO and Rh matching of patients and their analogous units is required.

Acute isovolemic hemodilution is a form of autologous transfusion unique to the operating room and to the practice of anesthesia. At the start of the operation, some portion of the allowable loss is drawn off through the arterial line or a large bore central IV, while intravenous fluids are infused simultaneously. The remaining blood lost during operation has a lesser hemoglobin content. Reinfusion of the stored blood near the end of the operation increases the hemoglobin and provides fresh platelets stored for only a few hours.

Intraoperative scavenging of blood shed during operation is especially valuable in trauma patients and other emergency cases where there is no time to cross-match homologous units. Available commercial devices use various anticoagulants and provide either washed red blood cells (RBCs) or all the blood collected. Bacteria or tumor cells in the shed blood rule out intraoperative blood scavening with open bowel or malignancy.

Postoperative salvage of blood collected from chest tubes and other wound drains also decreases use of homologous blood.

External hemoconcentration refers to the practice of centrifuging and washing the blood remaining in a heart-lung machine after cardiopulmonary bypass to remove the heparinized plasma, and reinfusing the RBCs to increase the hemoglobin level.

Designated Donors

Fear of acquired immune deficiency syndrome (AIDS) has led patients to name the donors who provide blood for their operation. The blood bank community has resisted, contending that any given population of relatives, neighbors, or co-workers will provide blood no safer than does the nation's volunteer blood donor population. Indeed, in a study of 12,000 donors, the incidence of serologic markers of infection was identical to that in the donor pool at large. Despite these arguments, in the face of considerable public pressure and even legislation, most blood banks have developed a system to designate donors when requested.

The Safety of the Blood Supply

INFECTION

Although bacterial and parasitic infections such as malaria can be transmitted via transfusion, the commonly occurring transmissible infections are viral in origin. Commercial blood collected from paid donors imposes an increased risk of hepatitis and is rarely used today. All units collected are tested for markers of hepatitis A, B, and C human immunodeficiency virus (HIV). Unfortunately, blood collected from an infected donor during the incubation period before development of antibodies may transmit the disease. AIDS is transmitted with an estimated incidence of between 1:40,000 and 1:1,000,000. Lawsuits have been brought following such infections; some authorities recommend specific written informed consent prior to elective blood transfusion or elective procedures where transfusion is likely.

COMPATIBILITY

The first step in ensuring against incompatible transfusions is to identify carefully the intended recipient and then collect a blood sample that is clearly marked with the name, hospital number, and date of collection. The final step, when the unit of blood is administered to the patient, requires equally careful patient identification and matching of patient name and hospital number to that on the unit to be transfused. These procedures prevent the most common cause of fatal transfusion reactions, the administration of ABO-incompatible blood.

Type and crossmatch is a procedure in which a patient's serum and a potential donor's cells are incubated together (major crossmatch) for 30 minutes with Coombs' reagent to detect gamma G immunoglobulin (IgG)–antibody coating of the red cell surface. Agglutination is a sign that the patient's antibodies react to donor antigens and are therefore incompatible. The mixing of the patient's cells and the donor's serum (minor crossmatch) is no longer performed routinely.

Type-and-screen, used when a need for blood is unlikely, is performed by incubating the patient's serum with RBCs with known antigens to detect recipient antibodies. Units of compatible blood are then made available in case a need for blood occurs intraoperatively. Units of blood are not reserved for the exclusive use of one patient when the likelihood of their being needed is small, reducing the overall inventory in the blood bank. In some centers, type-and-screen is the only compatibility testing done if the antibody screen is negative. A full crossmatch offers little additional safety over simple testing for ABO-Rh compatibility when the antibody screen is negative.

Immunologic Consequences

Renal transplant recipients are less likely to reject a donor kidney if they have previously been transfused. Transfusion clearly affects the immune system, to the benefit of these patients. Conversely, transfusion has been correlated with early recurrence and poor prognosis in several forms of malignancy, as well as increased risk of bacterial infection. The logical suggestion that the need for blood is correlated with more advanced disease has been refuted by other detailed studies. This effect is more marked following whole blood transfusion than after RBCs, and has been attributed to an unidentified component of stored plasma or associated cellular debris.

Emergency Transfusion

When an emergency precludes even an antibody screen, O-negative blood ("universal donor") can be administered without any testing. If time permits, uncrossmatched ABO-Rh type-specific blood is superior. The use of O-negative RBCs instead of whole blood decreases the administered volume of plasma containing anti-A and anti-B antibodies that would hemolyze recipient A, B, or AB cells. Prior to administration of type-specific blood to patients who have received O-negative blood as an emergency measure, the levels of anti-A and anti-B must be demonstrated to have decreased to levels less than those that may produce hemolytic transfusion reactions.

Blood Substitutes

The use of electrolyte or colloid solutions to replace initial blood loss is the first step in blood substitution. Plasma protein fraction (PPF), 5 per cent albumin, dextran, and starch solutions are colloidal solutions commonly used. Plasma protein fraction and 5 per cent albumin have the same on-

TABLE 15–6. **Signs and Symptoms of Transfusion Reactions**

Type of Reaction	Awake Patient	Anesthetized Patient
Acute hemolytic	Pain at infusion site, anxiety, chest pain, dyspnea, chills, headache, flank pain	Fever, hemoglobinemia, hemoglobinuria, shock, DIC
Febrile	Chills, faintness	Fever, shock (rare)
Hypervolemic	Dyspnea, headaches, palpitations	Pulmonary edema, hypertension, arrhythmias
Allergic	Pruritus, hoarseness, faintness, urticaria	Urticaria, stridor, hypotension
Delayed hemolytic	Fever, malaise, decreasing hematocrit, increased indirect bilirubin, increased urine urobilinogen	Not applicable

Abbreviation: DIC, disseminated intravascular coagulation.

cotic pressure as plasma, whereas dextran and starch have a slightly greater oncotic effect. None of these products provide coagulation factors or transport oxygen efficiently, but they may be stored at room temperature, transmit no diseases, and require no compatibility testing.

Potential acellular carriers of oxygen, often referred to as "artificial blood," include stroma-free hemoglobin, perfluorocarbon compounds, and (potentially) recombinant hemoglobin.

Stroma-free hemoglobin, from which all red cell membranes have been removed, delivers oxygen to tissues at ambient barometric pressure and also supports oncotic pressure; the preparation is not antigenic, and compatibility testing is not required prior to infusion. However, the hemoglobin is excreted by the kidneys within hours and colors plasma and urine red, potentially masking pathologic conditions associated with hemoglobinemia or hemoglobinuria. Experimental recombinant hemoglobin is a promising alternative because it is retained in the intravascular compartment for considerably longer intervals (at least in animals) and the molecule can be altered to influence its oxygen dissociation characteristics.

Perfluorocarbon compounds currently available do not carry sufficient oxygen to justify their clinical use. They are rapidly exhaled by the lungs, must be stored frozen, and may cause pulmonary insufficiency and complement activation. They do not provide oncotic or coagulation properties.

Recombinant erythropoietin has been used to stimulate red cell production in anemic patients with end-stage renal failure. The hormone is now approved for use in such patients; its use in surgical patients may further decrease the demand for homologous blood.

Treatment of Hemolytic Transfusion Reaction

The various transfusion reactions are listed in Table 15–6. Acute hemolytic reactions are usually the result of incompatible RBC transfusion (most often clerical error), incompatible fluids infused with RBCs, and gram-negative sepsis from contaminated blood. Unexplained bleeding at an operative site is an important clinical sign of acute disseminated intravascular coagulopathy (DIC) secondary to a hemolytic transfusion reaction. Table 15–7 outlines the treatment of a hemolytic transfusion reaction.

Delayed hemolytic reactions derive from incompatibility involving non-ABO antigens and require only monitoring of the hematocrit level, renal function, and coagulation profile. Febrile and allergic reactions are elicited by antibodies to white blood cells (WBC), platelets, and plasma proteins, including gamma A immunoglobulin (IgA). Treatment consists of antipyretics, antihistamines, vasopressors if needed, and use of washed RBCs in

TABLE 15–7 **Management of a Suspected Hemolytic Transfusion Reaction**

1. Discontinue the blood transfusion, but do not remove the intravenous catheter.
2. Maintain intravenous catheter flow with normal saline.
3. Notify the blood bank.
4. Send a newly collected and labeled blood specimen to the blood bank.
5. Send the blood unit and administration set to the blood bank.
6. Recheck any other units set up for this patient.
7. Send a urine specimen to the laboratory for hemoglobin analysis.

TABLE 15–8. **Tests of Hemostasis**

Test	Comment
Primary (Screening) Tests of Hemostasis Used to Confirm the Presence of a Disorder of Hemostasis	
1. Activated coagulation time (ACT)	Can be done in OR; observe for clot retraction and lysis
2. Fibrinogen level	Depressed in DIC
3. Prothrombin time (PT)	Prolonged in liver disease, vitamin K deficiency, coumarin anticoagulation, DIC
4. Partial thromboplastin time (aPTT)	Prolonged in Factors V, VIII deficiency (massive transfusion), the hemophilias, or the presence of heparin
5. Platelet count	Decreased in thrombocytopenia and DIC
Secondary Tests of Hemostasis Used to Identify the Cause of a Disorder of Hemostasis	
1. Bleeding time	Widely accepted clinical test of platelet function
2. Platelet aggregation	A more refined test of platelet function using various agents to determine the responsiveness of the platelets
3. Protamine titration	Definitive test used to confirm heparin effect
4. Individual factor levels	Used to diagnose and follow therapy with hemophilia
5. Fibrin split products	Confirmatory test for DIC

future transfusion. Hypervolemia, caused by excessive or too-rapid transfusion, is treated with phlebotomy, diuretics, tourniquets, intravenous morphine, and cardiopulmonary support.

Diagnosis of Hemostatic Disorders

The best means of detecting a hemorrhagic diathesis preoperatively is to review the history, especially the hemostatic response to prior operations or dental extractions. In the absence of a positive history or physical findings such as petechiae or ecchymosis, routine screening tests usually are not indicated, because they yield few true-positive results and the false-positive tests produce further dilemmas.

When such findings are present, when large blood losses are anticipated, or when bleeding during operation appears excessive, the tests outlined in Table 15–8 permit a specific diagnosis and rational therapy. Repeating the tests after treatment ensures that the abnormality has been corrected.

TABLE 15–9. **Blood Products for Hemostatic Disorders**

Hemostatic Factor	Minimal Level Needed for Surgical Hemostasis (% Normal)	In Vivo Half Life	Therapeutic Agent
I	50–100	3–6 days	Cryoprecipitate
II	20–40	3–4 days	Plasma
V	5–20	12 hours	Fresh plasma Fresh frozen plasma
VII	10–20	4–6 hours	Plasma
VIII	30	10–18 hours	Cryoprecipitate Antihemophilic factor
von Willebrand's	30		Desmopressin Plasma
IX	20–25	18–24 hours	Plasma Prothrombin complex concentrate
X	10–20	2–4 days	Plasma
XI	20–30	2–3 days	Plasma
XII	0		Plasma
XIII	1–3	5+ days	Plasma
Platelets	50,000–100,000	variable	Platelet concentrates

Management of Hemostatic Disorders

Table 15–9 lists the blood products available to treat specific hemostatic deficiencies. The first step in treatment is meticulous surgical hemostasis.

1. *Fresh Frozen Plasma (FFP)* is the acellular portion of blood that has been separated and frozen within six hours of collection. Fresh frozen plasma differs from single donor plasma (which has not been frozen) in that it contains adequate levels of Factor V and VIII, which decay with storage at room temperature. Fresh frozen plasma also replaces Factors II (prothrombin), V, VII, IX, X, and XI, to reverse the effects of warfarin, and to provide antithrombin III. In massive blood transfusion, especially when red cells are used in lieu of whole blood, FFP is also required. To replace clotting factors, 15 to 20 ml of plasma per kg body weight are required to provide a 25 per cent increase, which suffices for all factors except Factor VIII. Attempts to raise levels of clotting factors more than 25 per cent by infusion usually result in fluid overload, a problem which may be overcome by exchange transfusion.

2. *Platelet concentrates* are indicated for the treatment of bleeding due to thrombocytopenia or abnormal platelet function, but are relatively ineffective in idiopathic autoimmune thrombocytopenic purpura (ITP), septicemia, and hypersplenism. One unit of platelets usually provides an increase of 5000 to 10,000 in the platelet counts of adults not actively consuming platelets. The usual adult dose is 6 to 8 units. In patients who have received multiple platelet transfusions, platelet alloimmunization requires HLA-matched platelets. In Rh-negative girls and women with childbearing potential, ABO-Rh compatible platelets are transfused to prevent Rh immunization.

3. *Cryoprecipitate* is the residual when FFP is thawed at 4° C, and is rich in Factor VIII/von Willebrand factor and fibrinogen. One unit of plasma will generally yield 100 units of Factor VIII and 300 mg of fibrinogen. Ten such bags provide a 25 per cent increment in the Factor VIII level of the 70 kg individual and increase the fibrinogen by 100 mg per dl.

4. *Antihemophilic factor (AHF) concentrates* used to treat Factor VIII-deficient hemophiliacs are prepared by plasma fractionation and lyophilized for storage. The large pool of donors from which the product is derived considerably increases the risk of disease transmission, especially hepatitis or AIDS.

5. *Prothrombin complex concentrate (PCC)* is available to treat the deficiencies of Factors II (prothrombin), VII, IX, and X. Theoretically, this product can be used for neutralization of coumarin, but since it is a pooled product that carries a great risk of disease transmission, PCC is reserved almost exclusively for patients with severe Factor IX deficiency.

6. *Desmopressin (DDAVP)* is a vasopressin analogue that acts by releasing Factor VIII/von Willebrand factor from endothelial cells; it raises levels of that factor in patients with von Willebrand's disease. It has also been used in a large variety of patients ranging from those undergoing cardiac surgery to patients with uremia in order to improve hemostasis, presumably by improving platelet function.

References

Consensus Conference: Perioperative red blood cell transfusion. JAMA 1988;260:2700–2703.

Moore FD, Shires GT. Moderation. Editorial. Ann Surg 1967;166:300–301.

Myhre BA, Bove JR, Schmidt PJ. Wrong blood—a needless cause of surgical deaths. Anesth Analg 1981;60:777–778.

Randall HT. Fluid, electrolyte and acid-base balance. Surg Clin North Am 1976;56:1019–1058.

Toy PTCY, Strauss RG, Sterling LG, et al. Predeposit autologous blood for elective surgery, a national multicenter study. N Engl J Med 1987;316:517–520.

Twigley AJ, Hillman KA. The end of the crystalloid era? Anaesthesia 1985;40:800–871.

CHAPTER SIXTEEN

Positioning the Surgical Patient

The patient's position during an operation is chosen to provide the optimum exposure of the anatomical target. Unfortunately, a single position is unlikely to be ideal for surgeon, patient, and anesthesiologist. The absence of pain under anesthesia allows positions that patients would not tolerate when awake; most surgical positions have potentially deleterious cardiovascular and respiratory effects, as well as complications such as backache, alopecia, or peripheral nerve injury. The anesthesiologist and the surgeon must work together to position the patient in a way that will do the least harm, yet allow the operation to proceed.

Safe positioning of patients requires a knowledge of the advantages and disadvantages of various surgical positions, and an understanding of the physiological consequences of each. Positioning problems anticipated during the preanesthetic visit, as well as measures undertaken in the operating room (OR), must be documented on the record. A sufficient number of trained people must help with positioning to minimize risk to patient and OR personnel. Lastly, all necessary positioning equipment must be present at the start of the procedure.

Patients are positioned just after the induction of anesthesia, before surgical stimulation begins. These postural changes often produce hypotension owing to vasodilation and peripheral pooling of blood, while compensatory reflexes are obtunded by anesthesia. Deficits in circulating volume, preexisting illnesses, and rapid changes in posture make hypotension more severe. Frequent determination of blood pressure allows the anesthesiologist to detect any changes and to judge whether the new posture is acceptable. If hypotension occurs, further changes in posture are postponed until the blood pressure is corrected by fluid infusions, decreasing concentrations of anesthetic drugs, or vasopressors. When these measures fail, the position must be adjusted to one that the patient tolerates.

At the end of operation, when patients are again moved, intravascular volume deficits or electrolyte abnormalities acquired during operation may again produce hypotension, especially when venous return is compromised by return to the supine position from the Trendelenburg or lithotomy positions. Conversely, lightly anesthetized patients may become hypertensive from airway stimulation or pain with movement, requiring appropriate treatment with anesthetics, opioids, or vasodilators.

The Supine Position

People spend the majority of their lives upright; changes in cardiopulmonary dynamics occur within minutes of assuming the supine position. External forces acting on the lung change; in the supine position, the abdominal contents limit diaphragmatic movement and force it cephalad, reducing functional residual capacity (FRC) by 20 per cent. An additional 20 per cent loss of FRC occurs after induction of anesthesia, probably because of changes in diaphragmatic and abdominal muscle tone.

This decreased lung volume produces small airway closure. In the anesthetized, supine patient, the FRC is markedly less than in the sitting position, whereas the closing volume (the lung volume at which airway closure begins in dependent regions of lung) remains the same. Therefore, closing volume may exceed FRC in the supine position, producing closure that occurs during tidal breathing (Fig. 16–1). Airway closure leads to gas trapping, and hypoxemia results from venous admixture. This is particularly likely in elderly patients because closing volume increases with age. These adverse effects on lung volume are partially offset by positive pressure ventilation.

Gravitational effects on pulmonary arterial pressure, described in Chapter 22, are minimized in the supine position, so that pulmonary blood flow is more homogenous than in the erect state. The distribution of ventilation (see Chapter 22) is also affected by position. Pleural pressure is more uniform in the supine position, so variation in ventilation/perfusion ratios is less than when the patient is erect. In the erect position, the base to apex ratio is 1.5:1 for ventilation and 3:1 for perfusion. In the supine position, the base to apex ratio is 0.9:1 for ventilation and 1.3:1 for perfusion.

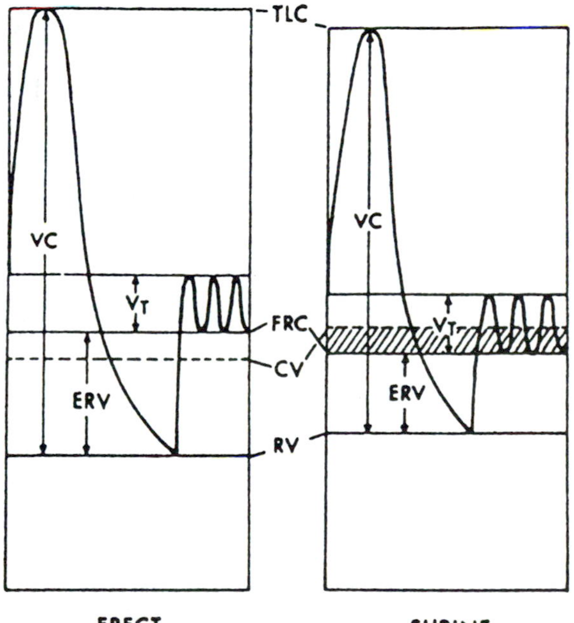

FIGURE 16–1. Spirometric tracing imposed on lung volumes in erect and supine positions. The ordinate represents lung volume and the abscissa, time. In the supine position, the closing volume is greater than functional residual capacity so that tidal volume and closing volume overlap. Abbreviations: TLC, total lung capacity; VC, vital capacity; VT, tidal volume; ERV, expiratory reserve volume; RV, residual volume; FRC, functional residual capacity; CV, closing volume. (Reproduced with permission from Martin JT. Positioning in anesthesia and surgery. 2nd ed. Philadelphia: WB Saunders Co., 1987.)

Circulatory effects of the supine position are unremarkable except when the patient suffers obesity, or has an abdominal mass, ascites, or a gravid uterus. These conditions compress the inferior vena cava and impede venous return in the supine position, decreasing cardiac output and causing hypotension. Rolling the patient with an abdominal mass into a 10-degree left lateral tilt using the operating room table or a pelvic wedge shifts the abdominal weight from the vena cava, relieving the obstruction.

In the supine position, when the head is poorly padded or in the presence of hypotension, pressure on the occipital scalp, can cause pain, swelling, and alopecia, which may last for months or be permanent. Skin biopsies in these cases show obliterative vasculitis. Appropriate padding and frequent turning of the head (every 30 minutes) can prevent this complication. This condition is to be differentiated from the generalized hair loss that rarely follows anesthesia and operation, for which the etiology is unknown.

The lithotomy position (Fig. 16–2) is a variation of the supine position; the patient is supine with the legs flexed at the knee and elevated so the perineum and rectum are accessible to the surgeon. The principal hazard of the lithotomy position is peripheral nerve injury (see Peripheral Nerve Injury). Circulatory and respiratory effects are similar to the supine position. Vital capacity and FRC are further decreased from restriction of diaphragmatic movement if the patient's knees are flexed onto the abdomen or if the patient is placed head-down. Circulatory effects are minimal unless a mass or abdominal obesity obstructs the inferior vena cava. Hypotension can occur when the patient's legs are lowered at the conclusion of surgery as the venous capacitance vessels of the lower extremities refill with blood. This relative hypovolemia is accentuated by untreated surgical blood loss or cardiac disease.

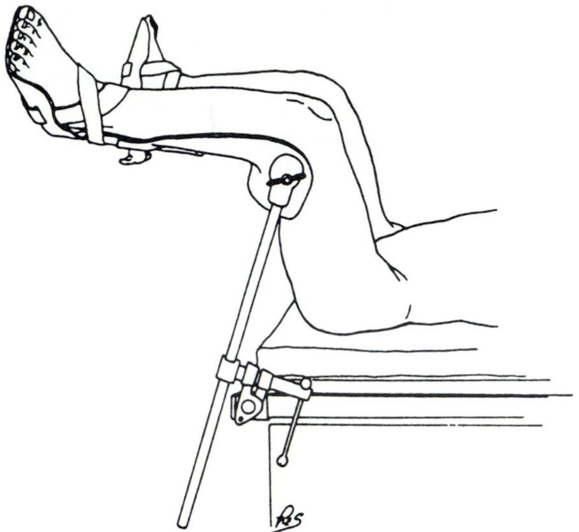

FIGURE 16–2. *Proper lithotomy position: minimal external rotation of legs, thighs minimally flexed toward abdomen, symmetric position of legs. Protective padding not shown. (Reproduced with permission from Martin JT. Positioning in anesthesia and surgery. 2nd ed. Philadelphia: WB Saunders Co, 1987.)*

PRONE POSITION

The prone position (Fig. 16–3) is used for operations on the rectum, spine, or the dorsum of the body. Respiratory effects of this position may be severe if the patient is not appropriately positioned, as compression of the abdominal viscera against the operating table causes several ill effects. Inspiratory movement of the diaphragm is restricted by abdominal contents so the patient must raise his thoracic weight to expand the chest, increasing the work of breathing. During positive pressure ventilation, increased airway pressures are required and there can be excessive movement of the patient's back in the surgical field. Compression of the inferior vena cava decreases cardiac output and increases central venous pressures (Fig. 16–4). Venous return from the extremities is diverted into pathways offering less resistance, such as the venous plexus of the vertebral column (Batson's plexus). During spinal operations, this may be a source of increased intraoperative bleeding.

A wide variety of devices and frames are used to redistribute body weight to the shoulders and hips, so that the abdomen hangs free and can de-

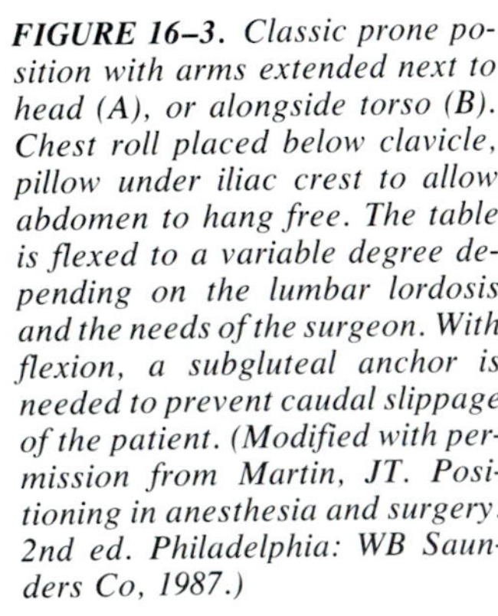

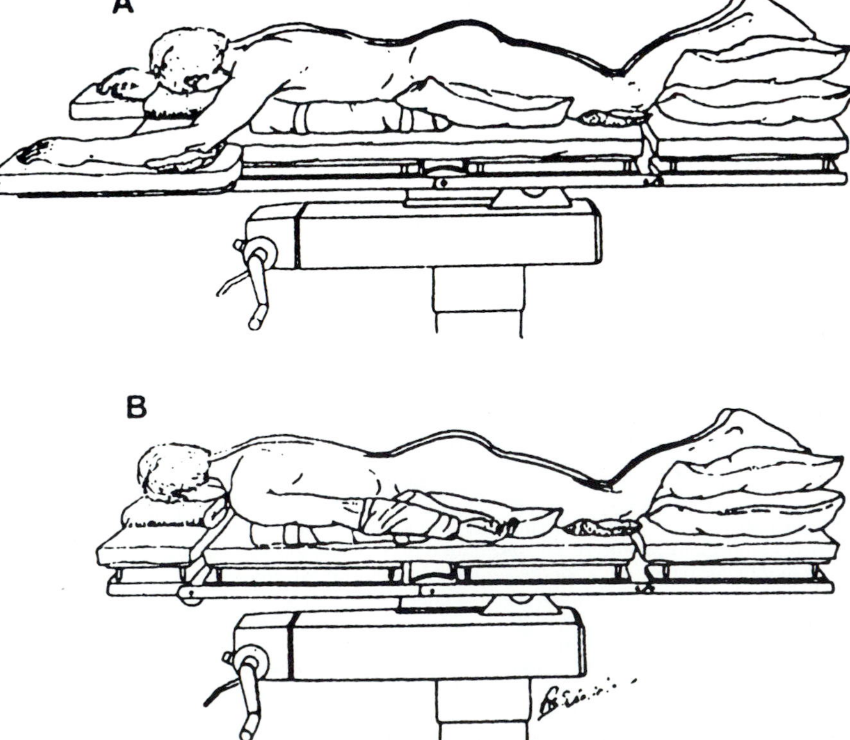

FIGURE 16–3. *Classic prone position with arms extended next to head (A), or alongside torso (B). Chest roll placed below clavicle, pillow under iliac crest to allow abdomen to hang free. The table is flexed to a variable degree depending on the lumbar lordosis and the needs of the surgeon. With flexion, a subgluteal anchor is needed to prevent caudal slippage of the patient. (Modified with permission from Martin, JT. Positioning in anesthesia and surgery. 2nd ed. Philadelphia: WB Saunders Co, 1987.)*

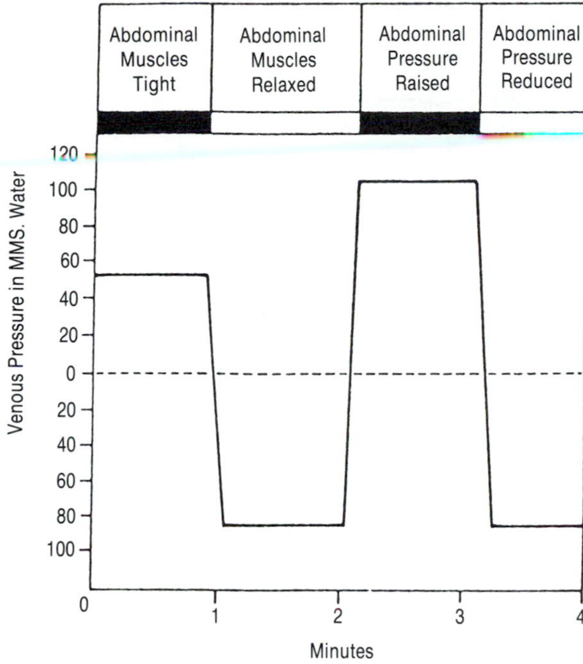

FIGURE 16–4. Venous pressure changes in the prone, supported position. When abdominal muscles are tight, or abdominal pressure is raised, there is an increase in central venous pressure. (Reproduced with permission from Pearce DJ. The role of posture in laminectomy. Proc Roy Soc Med 1957; 50:109.)

scend with expansion of the chest. These include rolls placed longitudinally from clavicle to pelvis along the lateral edges of the torso, or kneeling arrangements using the patient's buttocks and thighs as supports for the pelvis (Fig. 16–5). All these devices require adequate padding of pressure points, free abdominal and chest expansion, and no greater than 90-degree abduction of the arms.

With proper positioning, the weight of the freed abdomen draws the diaphragm downward, so the FRC is greater in these prone positions than in either the supine or the lateral positions. Pulmonary blood flow is as homogeneous as in the supine position. Studies of pulmonary shunting show no change when anesthetized patients are turned from supine to prone.

Other circulatory effects depend on the positioning device in use. If the legs are horizontal, there is no pressure gradient between the legs and the torso. When the patient is kneeling, significant venous pooling is likely in the dependent legs, which suggests the use of elastic stockings.

Positioning the patient's head is a challenge in the prone position (Fig. 16–6). Rotation of the head and neck may produce ischemia by occluding the carotid or vertebral arteries; an 80-degree rotation of the head may completely obstruct the contralateral vertebral artery. Patients with intact vascular anatomy compensate by increased flow through the opposite vertebral artery or the circle of Willis, but those with vessels partially obstructed by atherosclerosis may suffer ischemia, thrombosis, or an embolic stroke. When cerebral arterial disease or arthritis is suspected, the patient's head must not be turned from the sagittal plane. This is usually accomplished by using a Mayfield headrest, the horseshoe shaped pad that supports the periphery of the face without pressing on the eyes.

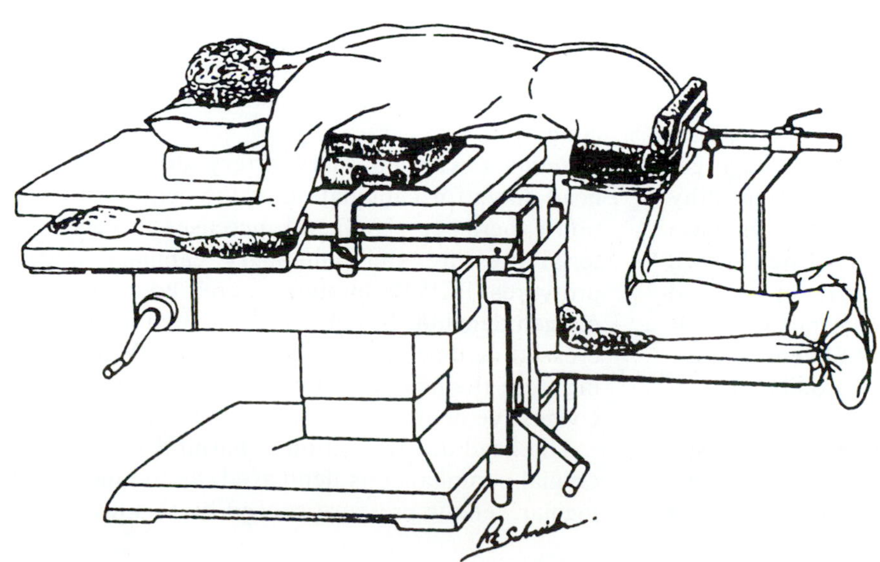

FIGURE 16–5. The Andrews frame, which supports the chest and buttocks, with the knees padded. The knees are never flexed more than 90 degrees on the thighs. (Reproduced with permission from Martin JT. Positioning in anesthesia and surgery. 2nd ed. Philadelphia: WB Saunders Co, 1987.)

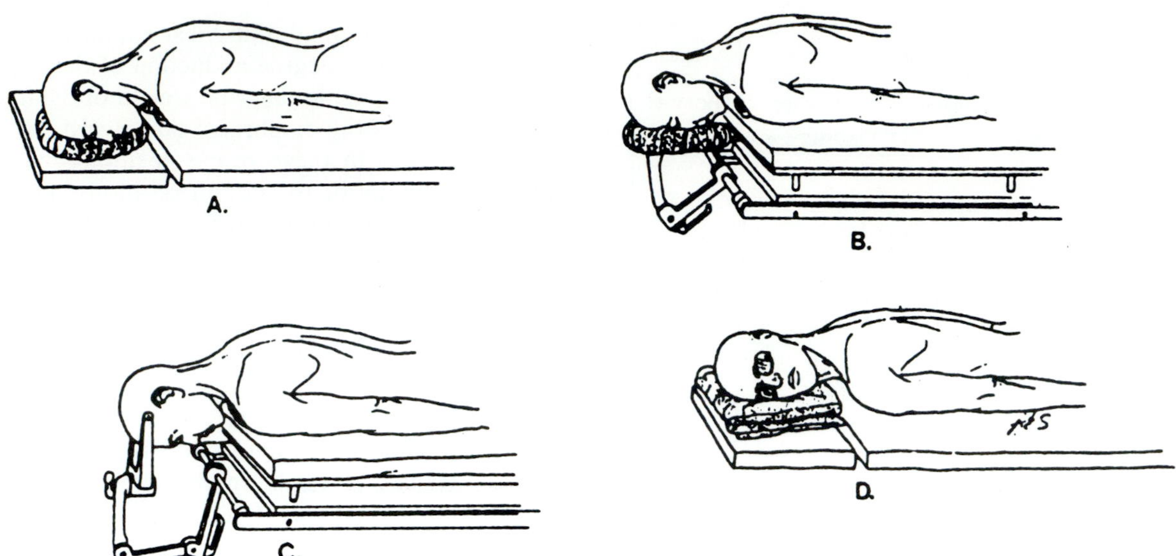

FIGURE 16–6. Methods of avoiding excessive turning of the head in the prone position. (A), (B), and (C) are acceptable. Extreme rotation of the neck (D) may be dangerous in patients with cervical spine disease or cerebrovascular disease. The eyes themselves must be free from pressure, since pressure on the globe may reduce flow in the retinal vessels enough to produce permanent retinal blindness. (Reproduced with permission from Martin JT. Positioning in anesthesia and surgery. 2nd ed. Philadelphia: WB Saunders Co, 1987.)

THE HEAD-DOWN (TRENDELENBURG) POSITION

This position results in a cephalad shift of large and small bowel and improves exposure of pelvic organs. The classic Trendelenburg position's steep 30 to 40-degree tilt necessitated some means of preventing patients from sliding off the table. Historically, wrist cuffs or shoulder braces were used, but both can stretch or compress the brachial plexus. At present, the tilt is usually limited to 10 to 15 degrees, which does not require patient restraints.

The head-down position causes decreased arterial pressure in the legs, and relative engorgement of the vessels of the mediastinum. In healthy patients, baroreceptor reflexes keep this increase small; volunteers placed 15 degrees head-down show only a 2 per cent central increase in blood volume and no significant hemodynamic changes. Although cardiac output and central venous pressure are increased transiently, vasodilation and bradycardia soon follow.

Although the head-down position is widely used to treat hypotension and shock, studies of patients with acute cardiac disease, hypotension, sepsis, or shock do not show a consistent beneficial effect. In hypotensive patients in shock (placed head-down), there was either no effect or a decrease in mean arterial pressure; left heart filling pressures (PCWP) and cardiac output did not change. Animal data suggest that all forms of shock are made worse by the Trendelenburg position. When hypovolemia is present, the Trendelenburg position does not improve blood pressure but may improve cardiac output slightly. Many clinicians elevate the patient's legs while keeping the body level to increase venous return without triggering harmful baroreceptor changes or risking cerebral venous congestion.

Patients with coronary artery disease placed head-down for cannulation of the central circulation experience significant increases in mean arterial pressure and pulmonary capillary wedge pressures (PCWP), implying increased myocardial oxygen demand. In patients with significantly decreased cardiac reserve, increased PCWP resulting from the head-down position can cause acute congestive heart failure or myocardial ischemia.

The head-down position is harmful when intracranial compliance is decreased, as the increased jugular venous pressure caused by this maneuver increases intracranial pressure. Increased cerebral venous pressures may also decrease cerebral perfusion pressure, which is the difference between mean arterial pressure and either central venous pressure or intracranial pressure, whichever is greater.

In the head-down position, abdominal contents compress the lung bases so that, compared to the supine position, FRC and pulmonary compliance are decreased and the work of breathing is increased. Left atrial pressure increases in relation to alveolar pressure, making pulmonary edema, congestion, and atelectasis more likely. This tendency to develop atelectasis and hypoxemia is greatest in obese or elderly patients, or when surgical retractors are placed in the upper abdomen.

Endotracheal tube position must be verified after any change in the patient's position, but particularly after patients are placed head-down. Gravity displaces the lungs and carina cephalad, causing the tip of the endotracheal tube to lie more distally in the trachea. Even a tube that is appropriately anchored at the mouth can enter the right mainstem bronchus.

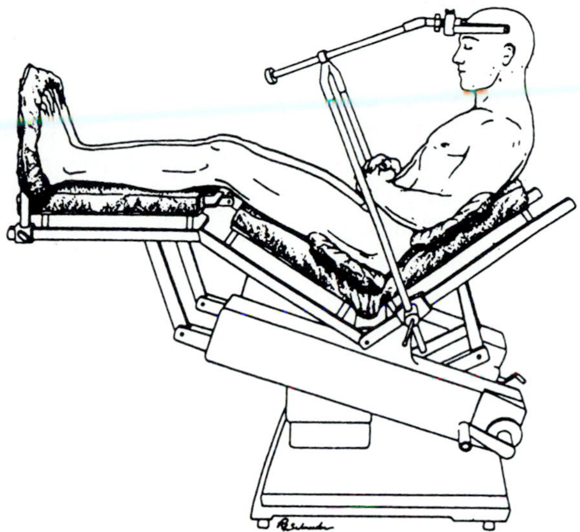

FIGURE 16–7. *Neurosurgical sitting position. The legs are slightly flexed and raised to the level of the heart. The feet are padded to maintain a dorsiflexed position. The sciatic nerve is protected by gluteal padding. The frame of the head holder is clamped to the back section of the table so that the patients head can be lowered in case of air embolization. (Modified with permission from Martin JT. Positioning in anesthesia and surgery. 2nd ed. Philadelphia: WB Saunders Co, 1987.)*

THE STTING POSITION

The sitting position (Fig. 16–7) is used during posterior fossa craniotomy and surgery on the cervical spine, face, neck, and shoulders to facilitate exposure and enhance venous drainage. The full sitting position is uncommon; patients are usually semireclining with the head flexed and legs elevated.

In the anesthetized patient, hemodynamic changes are not usually significant at head-up angles less than 60 degrees, although cardiovascular changes progress for an hour after the position is established. Gravity impedes venous drainage from the legs, shifting blood from the upper body to the lower extremities; atrial filling decreases, decreasing cardiac output by 20 to 40 per cent. In healthy unanesthetized subjects, these changes are opposed by increases in sympathetic tone, tachycardia, and increases in systemic vascular resistance. With these protective reflexes obtunded by anesthesia, postural hypotension can be sudden and severe, especially in elderly or hypertensive patients, or in the presence of dehydration or cardiac disease. Mean arterial pressure may be measured at the level of the circle of Willis instead of the right atrium to assess the cerebral perfusion.

Respiratory effects of the sitting position are often advantageous. Compared to the supine position, inspiratory movement of the diaphragm is less impeded by abdominal viscera. The work of breathing is decreased for spontaneous ventilation, and inflating pressures are decreased during positive pressure ventilation. The functional residual capacity increases, and age-related increases in closing capacity are minimized.

The risk of air embolism via open veins above the heart increases with height above the right atrium. Unappreciated or "silent" air embolism occurs frequently in head-elevated positions. Usually, the volume of air is small and detectable only by sophisticated means. Larger volumes of air are potentially lethal because they create compressible foam in the right heart, making ventricular contractions inefficient. Small bubbles also obstruct the peripheral pulmonary vasculature. Air embolism is recognized by changes in the tones produced by a Doppler probe directed at the heart from the second right interspace, decreases in expired carbon dioxide, increases in expired nitrogen, arrhythmias, hypotension, or a characteristic ''mill-wheel'' murmur.

Air embolism can be particularly dangerous in the 20 to 35 per cent of the population having a probe patent foramen ovale. In these patients, the foramen ovale is closed only when pressures in the left atrium are greater than the right. This is usually the case, but these pressures can be reversed in the sitting position. Air in the right side of the heart may then pass through the foramen ovale and enter the coronary or cerebral circulations, causing ischemia and permanent injury. The treatment of air embolism is discussed in Chapter 30.

THE LATERAL DECUBITUS POSITION

The lateral position (Fig. 16–8) is used for thoracotomy, or renal or orthopedic surgery. It is designated right or left, denoting the dependent side; for example, in the right lateral decubitus position the patient lies on the right side.

Blood pressure values in the lateral position depend on the position of the blood pressure cuff or aterial pressure transducer in relation to the heart. Because the distance between the arms of an adult patient may be as great as 40 cm, blood pressures measured in the two arms may be as different as 32 mm Hg. When measuring arterial pressure directly, this effect is avoided by opening the transducer system to air at the level of the heart while zeroing the amplifier.

Respiratory effects of the lateral position are significant. The weight of the chest and restriction of the movement of the dependent ribs, combined with the pressure of the abdominal viscera, force the dependent diaphragm cephalad, decreasing the vital capacity and the FRC of the dependent lung. However, in awake patients breathing spontaneously in this position, the cephalad displacement of the dome of the dependent diaphragm makes its contractions more efficient, providing the dependent lung with more ventilation. Because the dependent lung also receives the majority of the pulmonary blood flow, ventilation/perfusion relationships remain normal in awake patients in the lateral position.

In contrast, under anesthesia, the majority of the tidal volume is distributed to the nondependent lung, because the dependent lung's decreased FRC makes it less compliant, and positive pressure ventilation eliminates any mechanical advantage the dependent diaphragm enjoys during spontaneous ventilation. After the pleura or chest wall are opened, the upper lung becomes even more compliant and receives an even larger fraction of the tidal volume. Decreased cardiac output and compromised hypoxic pulmonary vasoconstriction under anesthesia only serve to reduce further the blood flow to the upper lung (see Chapter 22).

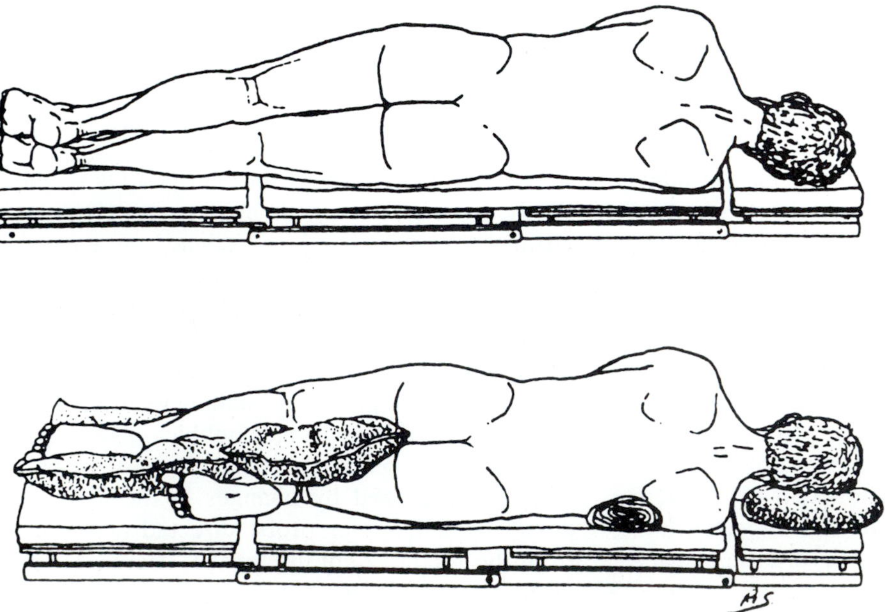

FIGURE 16–8. The right lateral decubitus position. Upper figure shows inadequate padding and improper head position. In the lower figure, there is padding over bony prominences, chest roll to protect neurovascular bundle in axilla, and proper alignment of the cervical spine. The lower leg is flexed to stabilize the patient. (Reproduced with permission from Martin JT. Positioning in anesthesia and surgery. 2nd ed. Philadelphia: WB Saunders Co, 1987.)

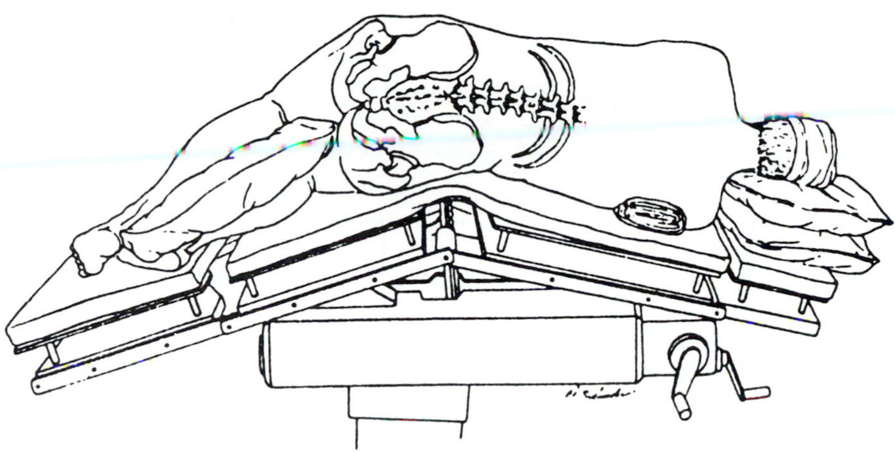

FIGURE 16–9. Flexed lateral decubitus position. The point of flexion lies beneath the dependent iliac crest to minimize interference with the dependent lung and diaphragm. (Modified with permission from Martin, JT. Positioning in anesthesia and surgery. 2nd ed. Philadelphia: WB Saunders Co, 1987.)

Thus, in the anesthetized, ventilated patient, the majority of the blood flow goes to the dependent lung and the majority of the ventilation goes to the nondependent lung. This mismatch can produce severe arterial hypoxemia.

In the lateral position, the upper arm is positioned on an elevated board, suspended from a metal frame (an "ether screen"), or supported on pillows. A small pad (axillary roll) is placed under the chest just below the axilla to support the upper part of the rib cage, to avoid compression of the axillary neurovascular bundle, and to remove pressure from the head of the humerus. The axillary roll may itself cause compression of the contents of the axilla if placed too cephalad.

A modified form of the lateral position is used for renal surgery (Fig. 16–9). The upper leg is straight and the lower leg flexed at the hip and knee. The iliac crest is positioned at the midpoint of the operating table, over a retractable fulcrum called the kidney rest. With the table flexed and the kidney rest elevated, the costal margin is separated from the iliac crest, improving surgical exposure of the kidney.

This position impairs inflation of the dependent lung, predisposing it to atelectasis. Pooling of blood occurs in the two dependent parts of the body. If abdominal flexion partially obstructs the inferior vena cava, further pooling of blood in the lower extremities occurs. These pulmonary and circulatory effects are minimized by avoiding extreme flexion, controlling ventilation, and positioning the subject properly over the kidney rest, with the fulcrum at the iliac crest. If the flexion point is placed improperly at the flank or costal margin, ventilation of the dependent lung or venous return is further compromised.

Nonneural Injury

Low back pain is frequent after either spinal or general anesthesia, occurring in as many as 37 per cent of patients. It is unrelated to the type of anesthesia but is correlated with the duration of surgery and patient positioning: the lithotomy, supine, and prone positions produce the greatest incidence. Anesthesia and neuromuscular blockers relax paraspinal muscles so that the lordosis of the lumbar spine is flattened and tension is applied to the interlumbar and lumbosacral ligaments. Postoperatively, patients complain of back pain, sometimes with radiation in the sciatic nerve distribution, lasting from a few days to several months. To avoid this injury, the hips and knees are flexed slightly in the supine position with padding under the lumbar spine (Fig. 16–10). This also increases venous return from the extremities and decreases anterior abdominal wall tension. While placing patients in the lithotomy position, the legs are raised and lowered simultaneously to avoid twisting the back.

Prolonged pressure on skin can result in ischemia and even ulceration. Skin over bony prominences where pressure will be exerted (heels, medial malleoli, sacrum, or supraorbital ridge) is vulnerable to ischemic damage and must be carefully padded.

Pressure on the eye may occur in the prone or lateral positions and may cause thrombosis of the retinal artery or retinal ischemia when pressure

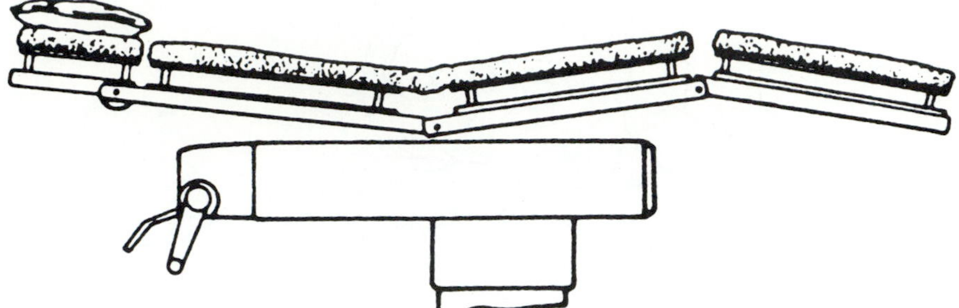

FIGURE 16–10. The lawn chair position with flexion of the hips, minimal knee flexion, and trunk section level. (Modified with permission from Martin JT. Positioning in anesthesia and surgery. 2nd ed. Philadelphia: WB Saunders Co, 1987.)

transmitted through the eye is sufficient to occlude the retinal artery. Intraoperative hypotension or a history of glaucoma make this complication more likely. Irreversible blindness results from these insults; the anesthesiologist must guarantee that the patient's eyes are free from pressure. The ear may also be injured if it is pinched or folded, particularly in the lateral position or when a mask strap is used.

Whenever parts of the operating table are moved, the patient may be injured. When the foot of the surgical table is returned to the horizontal position after a procedure in the lithotomy position, the patient's fingers may be crushed between the two sections of the operating table. When the surgical table is raised, overhanging equipment, such as a Mayo stand, may injure the patient.

PERIPHERAL NERVE INJURY

Peripheral nerve injuries occur during anesthesia because the patient may assume unphysiologic positions and does not feel the discomfort they produce. Injury occurs as a result of direct trauma from surgery or nerve blocks, compression by surgical retractors or against hard operating room table surfaces, pressure from tourniquets, or from stretching of nerves around bony prominences (e.g., the head of the humerus displaces the brachial plexus when the arm is abducted). The most common mechanisms of nerve damage are ischemia from direct compression, or rupture of small capillaries caused by stretching.

Nerve damage is the second most common complication related to anesthesia resulting in a malpractice suit, as reported from the American Society of Anesthesiologists (ASA) Closed Claims Study, although the mechanism of damage was not apparent in the majority of cases. Ulnar and brachial plexus injuries usually occurred during general anesthesia; lumbosacral neuropathies mostly occurred during regional anesthesia (Fig. 16–11). Nerve damage is a significant risk; the incidence reported in several studies lies between 0.1 and 13 per cent.

Other factors contributing to nerve injury include congenital anomalies (such as anomalous derivation of the brachial plexus), diabetes, hematoma formation secondary to blood dyscrasia or anticoagulant therapy, hypothermia, and use of a tourniquet. The differential diagnosis of postoperative nerve damage includes preexisting damage, misplaced needles (percutaneous angiograms through the axillary artery) or surgical manipulation (femoral nerve injury from self-retaining retractors).

When a patient suffers a nerve palsy after surgery, a neurologic examination is recorded and a neurologist consulted so that nerve conduction studies can be obtained and the patient can receive follow-up care. An accurate recording in the preanesthesia note of any neurological deficiencies that may exist is clearly essential in postoperative management.

Peripheral nerve injuries occur in three classifications. (1) *Transient ischemic nerve block* is temporary paralysis that follows compression of a nerve, as from a blood pressure cuff. This is commonly described by patients as the extremity "going to sleep," usually lasts 20 minutes or less, and is not associated with structural damage. (2) *Neuropraxia* also constitutes temporary paralysis or sensory loss, although recovery takes four to six weeks or longer. Pathologically, nerve fibers become demyelinated near the periphery of the nerve trunk, but continuity of the nerve trunk and the endoneurial sheath is preserved. Remyelinization parallels clinical recovery. (3) After severe stretch injury or cutting of a nerve, complete dis-

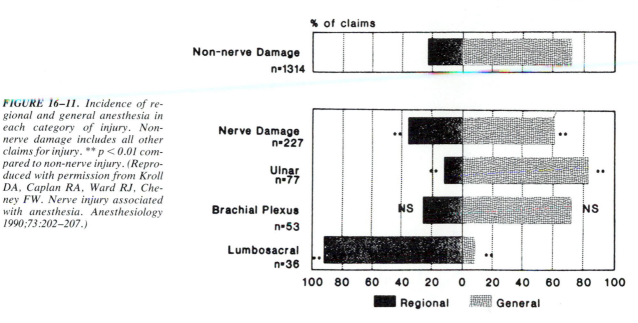

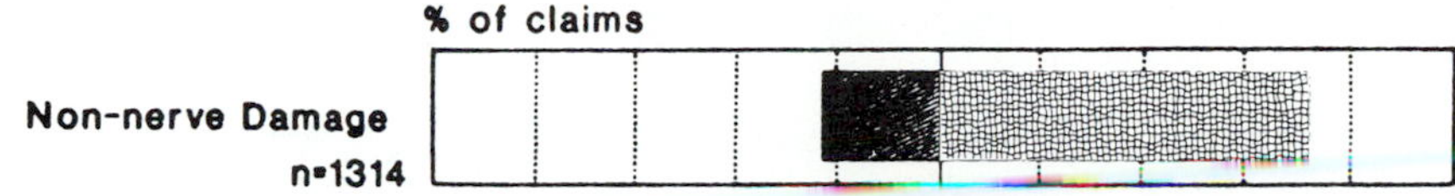

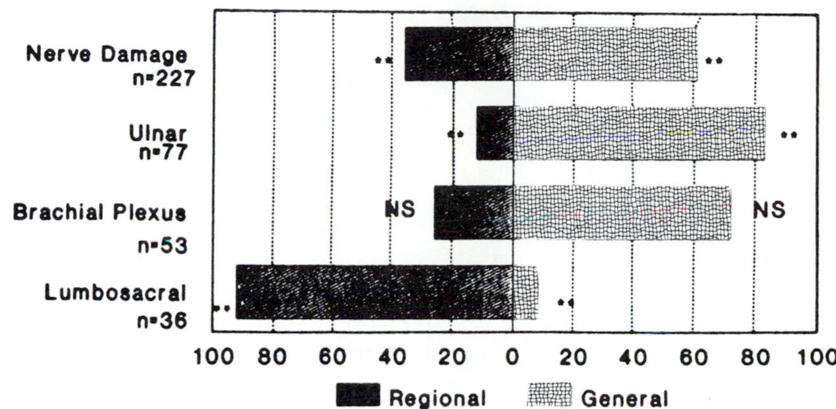

*FIGURE 16–11. Incidence of regional and general anesthesia in each category of injury. Non-nerve damage includes all other claims for injury. ** $p < 0.01$ compared to non-nerve injury. (Reproduced with permission from Kroll DA, Caplan RA, Ward RJ, Cheney FW. Nerve injury associated with anesthesia. Anesthesiology 1990;73:202–207.)*

ruption of the axons within an intact sheath or of the entire nerve trunk occurs (*axotmesis or neurotmesis*). Wallerian degeneration of the peripheral nerve distal to the site of injury takes place and complete recovery is much less likely than in injuries that do not affect axonal continuity.

The ulnar nerve is the most commonly injured peripheral nerve; damage occurs when the nerve is compressed against the posterior aspect of the medial epicondyle of the humerus. This can happen when the patient's elbow slips off the operating table mattress, encountering the edge of the table. The ulnar nerve can also be compressed in the cubital tunnel when the elbow is fully flexed as the arm is secured across the abdomen or chest. On an armboard, the hand is best supinated rather than pronated; this maneuver rolls the ulnar nerve into a more protected position. In 20 per cent of individuals, the ulnar nerve has a more medial course than is described in anatomy texts, passing behind the tip of the epicondyle rather than in the more protected groove.

Results from the ASA Closed Claims Study shed some new light on postoperative ulnar nerve injury. Ulnar injury accounted for 34 per cent of the claims, but the mechanism of damage was apparent in only 6 per cent. For 18 per cent of cases, the file contained the specific information that the arm was padded over the ulnar nerve. Symptoms of ulnar nerve injury also occurred late, suggesting that injury occurred during the postoperative rather than intraoperative period. Patients with postanesthetic ulnar nerve lesions frequently have abnormalities of nerve conduction testing in both the affected and the unaffected arms, perhaps owing to a chronic neural disorder exacerbated by positioning, the blood pressure cuff, or the intravenous line. Patients who experience ulnar paresthesia or dysesthesia preoperatively must be warned that a surgical procedure may aggravate this condition. Although more women than men appear in the Closed Claims database as a whole, in several studies three times as many men as women suffered ulnar nerve damage, suggesting an anatomic predisposition among men.

After the ulnar nerve, the second most common neurologic injury is to the brachial plexus, which is susceptible because of its long course between two firm points of fixation, the vertebral fascia above and the axillary fascia below. In addition, the clavicle and the humerus serve as fulcrums to further stretch the nerves. Stretching of the brachial plexus occurs when the neck is extended, the head is turned to the side opposite, or the arm is abducted to greater than 90 degrees (Fig. 16–12).

Patients with stretch injuries to the brachial plexus may complain of mild shoulder pain in the supraclavicular area, but usually there is a nearly painless motor deficit. Any combination of roots can be affected; the upper roots are involved more frequently than the lower.

The radial nerve may be injured as it passes lat-

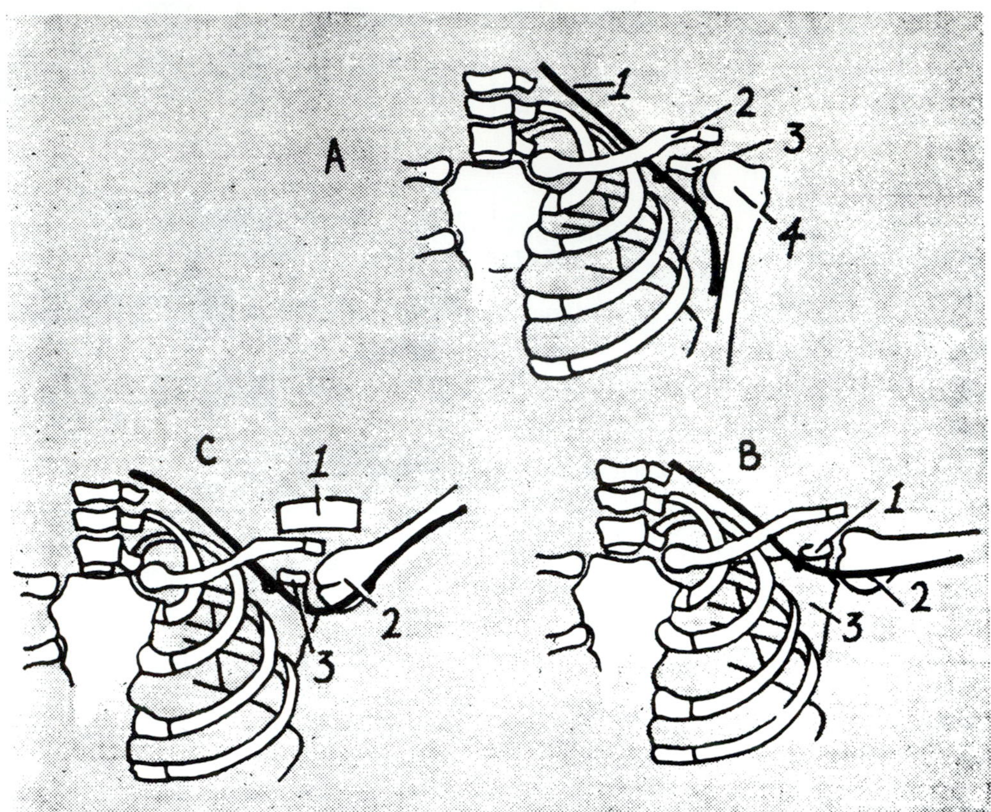

FIGURE 16–12. Brachial plexus in relation to surrounding structures. A, Arm at side: (1) brachial plexus; (2) clavicle; (3) coracoid process; (4) head of humerus. B, Arm at right angle. C, Arm hyperextended by shoulder brace, which depresses scapula, stretching brachial plexus beneath coracoid process and around humeral head. (Reproduced with permission from Dripps RD, Eckenhoff JE, Vandam LD. Introduction to anesthesia: the principles of safe practice. 7th ed. Philadelphia: WB Saunders Co, 1988.)

erally around the humerus by pressure against operating table hardware. Injury is followed by wrist drop, weakness of abduction of the thumb, and inability to extend the metacarpophalangeal joints.

The median nerve in the antecubital fossa is close to the medial cubital and basilic veins. It may be injured by intravenous needles or the extravasation of drugs such as sodium pentothal. Median nerve injury causes decreased sensation on the palmar surface of the first three and one half fingers, inability to oppose the thumb and little finger, and weakness of thumb abduction.

The common peroneal nerve is the most frequently injured nerve in the lower extremity. Injuries usually occur when patients are in the lithotomy position; the nerve is compressed between the head of the fibula and the stirrup that suspends the leg. Proper padding of the head of the fibula avoids this complication. Nerve damage causes foot drop and loss of extension of the toes. Injury can also occur in a thin patient in the lateral position after prolonged pressure against a poorly padded operating room table.

Prolonged pressure on the popliteal fossa can also produce a compartment syndrome. Although this syndrome can develop without any intraoperative findings, frequent examination of the lower extremities for diminished distal pulses, edema, or color changes is required during any procedure requiring more than four hours in the lithotomy position. If there is a question of inadequate circulation, the legs must be returned to the horizontal position. This syndrome arises because of direct local muscle pressure, which produces ischemia, loss of capillary integrity, and massive edema within the compartment, eventually leading to a tissue necrosis.

The femoral nerve can be injured by excessive angulation of the thigh on the abdomen in the lithotomy position or by the blade of a self-retaining retractor during a laparotomy. This injury results in loss of hip flexion and extension of the knee; sensation is diminished over the anterior thigh and anteromedial calf.

If the ankles are plantar flexed during anesthesia in the sitting or prone positions, the anterior tibial nerve in the ankle is vulnerable to stretch injury. Plantar flexion increases the distance the nerve travels over the anterior ankle joint. To prevent this injury, a foot support or ankle roll maintains a dorsiflexed position.

The sciatic nerve can be injured in patients in the lithotomy position if the thighs and legs are externally rotated or if the knees are not flexed. Both maneuvers increase the distance between the sciatic noch and the neck of the fibula, stretching the nerve. Patients in the sitting position must have their knees slightly flexed for the same reason. Sciatic nerve damage causes weakness of all the muscles below the knee and numbness of the lateral calf and entire foot except the inner arch.

Airway equipment and the anesthesiologist's hand may also cause nerve injury on the face. Excessive pressure from the mask or head strap results in paralysis of the buccal branch of the facial nerve with loss of function of the orbicularis oris muscle. If forward pressure on the ascending ramus of the mandible is required to maintain a patent airway, the facial nerve may be compressed, resulting in loss of muscle tone on the affected side of the face. The supraorbital nerve can be compressed medial to the eyebrow by a metal endotracheal tube connector, producing eye pain, photophobia, and forehead numbness.

Although complications from positioning have been described since the early days of anesthesia, they still constitute a large portion of anesthetic complications. Most positioning injuries are preventable by padding bony prominences, moving patients slowly and gently, avoiding positions that strain ligaments or nerves, and proper attention to the physiologic effects of positioning.

References

Britt BA, Gordon RA. Peripheral nerve injuries associated with anesthesia. Can Anaesth Soc J 1964;11:514–536.

Coonan TJ, Hope CE. Cardiorespiratory effects of changes of body position. Can Anaesth Soc J 1983;30:424–437.

Dawson DM, Krarup C. Perioperative nerve lesions. Arch Neurol 1989;46:1355–1360.

Kroll DA, Caplan RA, Posner K, Ward RJ, Cheney FW. Nerve injury associated with anesthesia. Anesthesiology 1990;73:202–207.

Lincoln JR, Sawyer HP. Complications related to body positions during surgery. Anesthesiology 1961;22:800–809.

Martin JT. *Positioning in anesthesia and surgery*. 2nd ed. Philadelphia: WB Saunders Co, 1987.

Wilcox S, Vandam LD. Alas, poor Trendelenburg and his position—a critique of its uses and effectiveness. Anesth Analg 1988;67:574–578.

SECTION 5

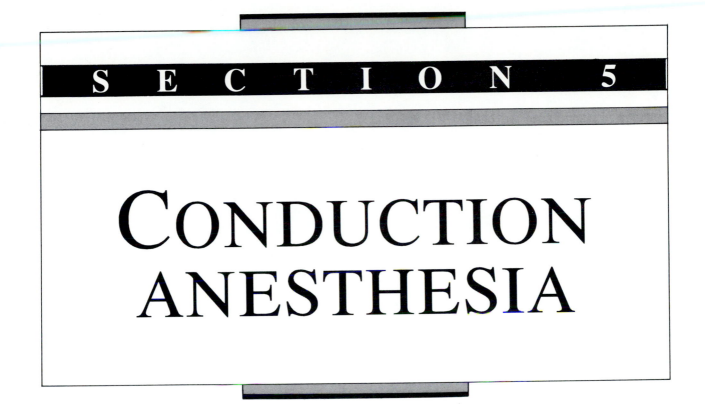

CONDUCTION ANESTHESIA

CHAPTER SEVENTEEN

Pharmacology of Local Anesthetics

Local anesthetics cause loss of sensation by inhibiting excitation at nerve endings or by blocking conduction in peripheral nerves. Regional anesthesia originated in 1884, when Koller described the topical anesthetic properties of cocaine, an alkaloid isolated from the leaves of the *Erythroxylin coca* bush. In 1905, Einhorn synthesized procaine, the first clinically useful local anesthetic. After the introduction of procaine, many ester derivatives of para-aminobenzoic acid (e.g., tetracaine and chloroprocaine) were developed. In 1943, Lofgren synthesized lidocaine, the prototype amide derivative of diethylamino acetic acid. Since then, many other amide local anesthetics, such as mepivacaine, prilocaine, bupivacaine, and etiodocaine have come into use, each with its own pharmacological profile.

Conduction of Nerve Impulse

The sequence of events that leads to the conduction of nerve impulses is as follows:

1. **Stimulus.**
2. **Increased sodium conductance.**
3. **Depolarization of nerve membrane.**
4. **Critical (threshold) level reached.**
5. **Spontaneous rapid phase of depolarization.**
6. **Action potential generation.**
7. **Propagation of action potential.**
8. **Decreased sodium conductance.**
9. **Decreased potassium conductance.**
10. **Repolarization.**
11. **Reestablishment of ionic equilibrium.**
12. **Resting state.**

Mechanism of Action of Local Anesthetics

Impulse conduction is due to changes in the electrical gradient across the nerve membrane. This results from the movement (conductance) of ions, particularly sodium and potassium, across the membrane. An adequate stimulus that reduces the resting membrane potential from approximately −90 mV to approximately −60 mV (the threshold potential level) produces a spontaneous rapid phase of depolarization (action potential). Depolarization in one segment of an unmyelinated nerve propagates to adjacent segments because of the difference in electrical potential between the depolarized and polarized areas. In this way, an action potential generated by a stimulus applied to one end of a nerve is transmitted along the entire length of the nerve fiber. In myelinated nerves the impulse jumps from one node of Ranvier to the next adjacent node (saltatory conduction). Repolarization returns the nerve membrane potential to the original resting level.

Depolarization is due to the inward passage of sodium ions from the extracellular to the intracellular space via specific sodium channels in the membrane. The flow of potassium ions from the interior to the exterior of the nerve causes repo-

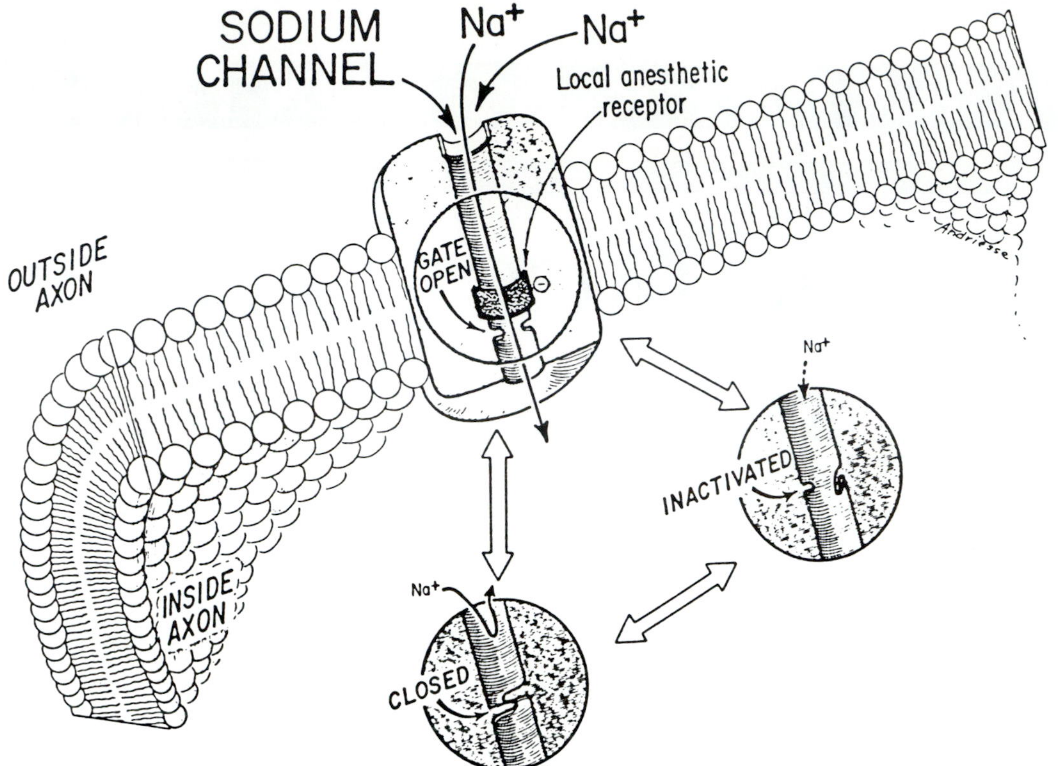

FIGURE 17–1. The sodium channel in nerve. The channel probably traverses a protein structure that spans the entire thickness of the axonal membrane. A gating mechanism located on the internal aspect of the sodium channel controls the inward transit of sodium ions. In the resting axon, the gate is closed and does not permit passage of sodium ions. During action potential development, the gate opens to allow the inward rush of sodium responsible for initial axonal depolarization. The gating mechanism may be inactivated by local anesthetics that bind to specific receptors in the sodium channel. A single receptor on the inner aspect of the channel binds all types of local anesthetics, although the route of arrival of the various types of local anesthetic molecules to the receptor may differ (From Savarese JJ, Covino BG. Basic and clinical pharmacology of local anesthetic drugs. In Miller RD, ed. Anesthesia. 2nd ed. New York: Churchill Livingstone, 1986; 994, with permission.)

CONDUCTION BLOCKADE

Local anesthetic agents produce conduction blockade in peripheral nerves by this sequence:

1. **Diffusion of the local anesthetic base across the nerve sheath and membrane into the axoplasm.**
2. **Reequilibration between the base and cation in the axoplasm.**
3. **Penetration of the cation into the sodium channel and attachment to a receptor site.**
4. **Blockade of the sodium channel.**
5. **Inhibition of sodium conductance.**
6. **Decrease in the rate and degree of the depolarization phase of the action potential.**
7. **Failure to achieve the threshold potential.**
8. **Lack of development of a propagated action potential.**
9. **Conduction blockade.**

larization. At the completion of the action potential, ionic equilibrium is reestablished by the membrane sodium-potassium pump. Local anesthetic agents prevent depolarization of the nerve membrane by blocking the flow of sodium ions, with little effect on potassium currents. For example, lidocaine completely inhibits sodium conductance but decreases potassium conductance only 50 per cent.

Sodium Channel/Local Anesthetic Receptor

The site of action of local anesthetic agents undoubtedly involves the sodium channel in the nerve membrane (Fig. 17–1). Local anesthetics such as lidocaine apparently penetrate the lipoprotein membrane matrix to the axoplasm and then enter the sodium channel where they likely interact with a specific receptor. The sodium channel exists in three states: closed, open, and inactive. At rest the channel is closed so that neither sodium ions nor drugs can enter. Stimulation of the nerve opens the channel, allowing sodium ions and local anesthetics to enter its interior. As the frequency of stimulation increases, the sodium channels remain in an open state for relatively longer periods. Therefore, at higher stimulation frequencies, the local anesthetic agent, which has diffused across the membrane into the axoplasm, has greater opportunity to penetrate the interior of the sodium channel. For example, lidocaine demonstrates frequency-dependent block, producing greater degrees of block at higher stimulating frequency.

Membrane Expansion

Other mechanisms for conduction blockade also exist. The *ionized* (cation) form of the conventional local anesthetics causes conduction block by binding to a receptor site in the sodium channel. However, benzocaine and benzyl alcohol are un-ionized compounds that possess local anesthetic activity. Conduction block with benzocaine and benzyl alcohol is reversible by high atmospheric pressures, whereas the block produced by conventional local anesthetics is only partially reversed. Also, the anesthetic potency of the un-ionized agents relates to the amount of drug taken up by the nerve membrane, which is a function of their lipid solubility. Agents such as benzocaine and benzyl alcohol appear to act much like general anesthetics, inhibiting sodium flux and blocking nerve conduction by expanding or altering the configuration of the nerve membrane, thus decreasing the diameter of the sodium channel.

Diffusion to the Receptor

Diffusion of local anesthetics to the site of action depends largely on the degree of ionization of the various agents. In solution, local anesthetic agents exist as uncharged molecules and as positively charged cations. The relative proportion of uncharged base to charged cation depends on the pKa of the specific local anesthetic and the pH of the solution, and is governed by the Henderson-Hasselbalch equation. The pKa of a given agent being fixed, the relative proportion of free base and charged cation depends on the pH of the local anesthetic solution. As the pH of the solution decreases, equilibrium shifts toward the charged cationic form and more cation is produced from free base. Conversely, as the pH increases, the equilibrium shifts toward the free base form.

$$\text{pH} = \text{pKa} + \log \frac{[\text{base}]}{[\text{cation}]}$$

The uncharged base and the charged cationic form of the local anesthetic are both important to the process of conduction blockade. Only the base diffuses readily through the nerve sheath and membrane into the axoplasm. In the axoplasm, a new equilibrium is established between base and cation and the charged cation binds to the receptor site in the sodium channel, inhibiting sodium conductance. Although the cation plays the major role in conduction blockade, the free base may contribute by causing expansion of the nerve membrane in a fashion similar to benzocaine.

DIFFERENTIAL NEURAL BLOCKADE

The goal of regional anesthesia is to block conduction of nociceptive impulses. Nerve fibers are classified according to diameter and conduction velocity. The large A fibers are subdivided into four groups (alpha, beta, gamma, and delta). The myelinated fibers have nodes and the internodal distance is directly related to the fiber diameter. The larger myelinated fibers conduct impulses more rapidly than the smaller nonmyelinated fibers (Fig. 17–2).

In vitro, smaller C fibers are more resistant to block than are the larger A fibers. In patients and intact animals, the larger, myelinated fibers seem to be the more resistant, so that dilute local anesthetics produce differential neural blockade with some sensation blocked but motor function intact. This paradox is likely due to the fact that in vivo diffusion of local anesthetic to the membrane receptor site influences the apparent sensitivity of the various fiber types. Depending on the anatomy of the nerve being blocked, it may appear that smaller fibers are more sensitive to the local anesthetic than the larger fibers. For example, if the smaller fibers are located close to the nerve surface and the larger fibers deeper in the nerve, then the smaller fibers may appear to be more sensitive than the larger ones because it takes longer for the local anesthetic to reach the deeper, larger fibers.

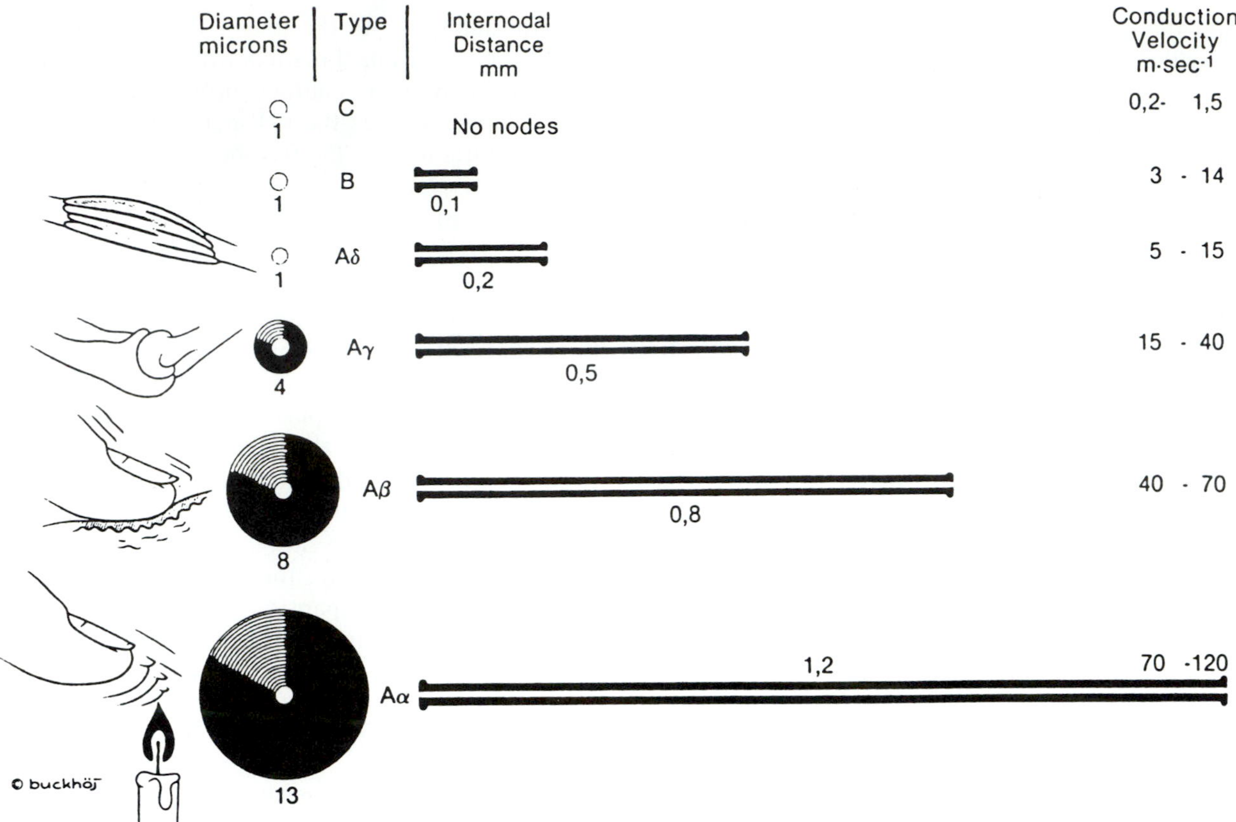

FIGURE 17–2. Description of the difference in size and conduction velocity of various types of nerve fiber. (From Covino BG, Scott DB. Handbook of epidural anesthesia and analgesia. Orlando: Grune & Stratton, 1984; 42, with permission.)

PHARMACOLOGY OF LOCAL ANESTHETICS

Esters and Amides

Local anesthetics consist of an aromatic end linked by an intermediate chain to an amide end. The clinically important local anesthetics are divided into two distinct chemical groups (Table 17–1). Amino esters are local anesthetics with an ester link between the aromatic and amine ends: procaine, chloroprocaine, and tetracaine. Amino amides are local anesthetics with an amide link between the aromatic and amine ends: lidocaine, mepivacaine, prilocaine, bupivacaine, and etidocaine.

The esters and amides differ in regard to metabolism, stability, and allergic potential (Table 17–2). The ester agents are hydrolyzed in plasma by pseudocholinesterase, whereas the amide compounds undergo enzymatic degradation in the liver. The amino esters are somewhat unstable in solution whereas amides are extremely stable. Para-aminobenzoic acid is a metabolite formed from the hydrolysis of ester type compound and this substance causes allergic reactions in a few patients. The amide drugs are not metabolized to para-aminobenzoic acid, and allergy to these agents is extremely rare.

Characteristics of Local Anesthetic

The pharmacologic characteristics of a local anesthetic are due to:

1. Lipid solubility.
2. Protein binding.
3. pKa.
4. Intrinsic vasodilator activity.

TABLE 17–1. Chemical Structure, Physical Chemical Properties, and Pharmacological Properties of Local Anesthetic Agents

	Chemical Configuration			Physicochemical Properties				Pharmacological Properties		
Agent	*Aromatic Lipophilic*	*Intermediate Chain*	*Amine Hydrophilic*	*Molecular Weight (base)*	*pK (25°C)*	*Partition Coefficient*	*Per Cent Protein Binding*	*Onset*	*Relative Potency*	*Duration*
Esters										
Procaine	H—N(H)—⟨benzene ring⟩	—$COOCH_2CH_2$—	$N(C_2H_5)(C_2H_5)$	236	8.9	0.02	6	Slow	1	Short
Tetracaine	$H_9C_4N(H)$—⟨benzene ring⟩	—$COOCH_2CH_2$—	$N(CH_3)(CH_3)$	264	8.5	4.1	76	Slow	8	Long
Chloroprocaine	H_2N—⟨benzene ring⟩, Cl	—$COOCH_2CH_2$—	$N(C_2H_5)(C_2H_5)$	271	8.7	0.14	—	Fast	1	Short
Amides										
Prilocaine	⟨benzene ring⟩, CH_3	—NHCOCH(CH_3)—	$N(H)(C_3H_7)$	220	7.9	0.9	55	Fast	2	Moderate
Lidocaine	⟨benzene ring⟩, CH_3, CH_3	—$NHCOCH_2$—	$N(C_2H_5)(C_2H_5)$	234	7.9	2.9	64	Fast	2	Moderate
Mepivacaine	⟨benzene ring⟩, CH_3, CH_3	—NHCO—	⟨piperidine ring⟩ N—CH_3	246	7.6	0.8	78	Fast	2	Moderate
Bupivacaine	⟨benzene ring⟩, CH_3, CH_3	—NHCO—	⟨piperidine ring⟩ N—C_4H_9	288	8.1	27.5	96	Moderate	8	Long
Etidocaine	⟨benzene ring⟩, CH_3, CH_3	—NHCOCH(C_2H_5)—	$N(C_2H_5)(C_3H_7)$	276	77	141	94	Fast	6	Long

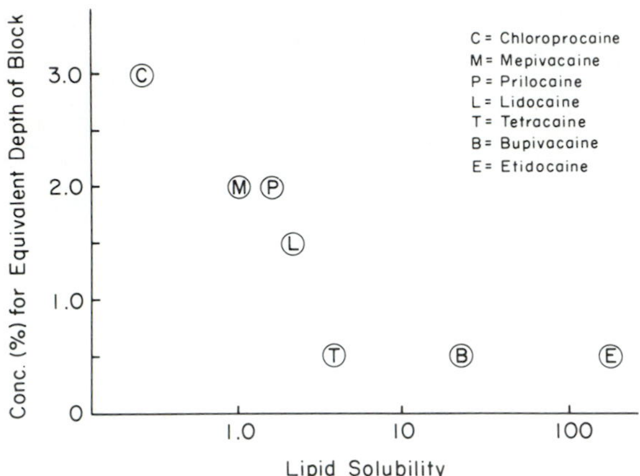

FIGURE 17–3. Relation between lipid solubility and inherent potency of local anesthetic agents. (From Covino BG. Clinical pharmacology of local anesthetic agents. In *Cousins MJ, Bridenbaugh PO, eds. Neural blockade. Philadelphia: JB Lippincott, 1988; 114, with permission.)*

LIPID SOLUBILITY

The relationship of lipid solubility to relative anesthetic potency is shown in Figure 17–3 and Table 17–1. The lipid solubility of chloroprocaine is less than one; it is one of the least potent local anesthetics. On the other hand, the partition coefficients of bupivacaine, tetracaine, and etidocaine are very great, varying from 4 to 141. These lipid-soluble agents produce conduction blockade in isolated nerves at very dilute concentrations. Their intrinsic anesthetic potency is approximately 16 times greater than that of chloroprocaine. Lidocaine, mepivacaine, and prilocaine are intermediate in lipid solubility and potency. Local anesthetic agents that are lipid soluble penetrate the nerve membrane readily and have greater intrinsic anesthetic potency.

TABLE 17–2. Metabolism, Stability, and Allergic Potential of Esters and Amides

	Metabolism	Stability in Solution	Allergic Reactions
Esters	Plasma Esterase	Unstable	Rare
Amides	Hepatic Enzymatic	Stable	Very rare

PROTEIN BINDING

Protein binding of local anesthetic agents primarily influences their duration of action (Fig. 17–4). Agents of short duration, such as procaine, bind poorly to proteins. Conversely, tetracaine, bupivacaine, and etidocaine avidly bind to proteins and display the longest duration of anesthesia.

Lidocaine, mepivacaine, and prilocaine are intermediate in protein binding and duration of anesthesia. Agents that penetrate the axolemma and attach more firmly to membrane proteins have a prolonged duration of anesthetic activity.

pKa

The pKa of a local anesthetic is the pH at which the concentration of ionized and un-ionized forms

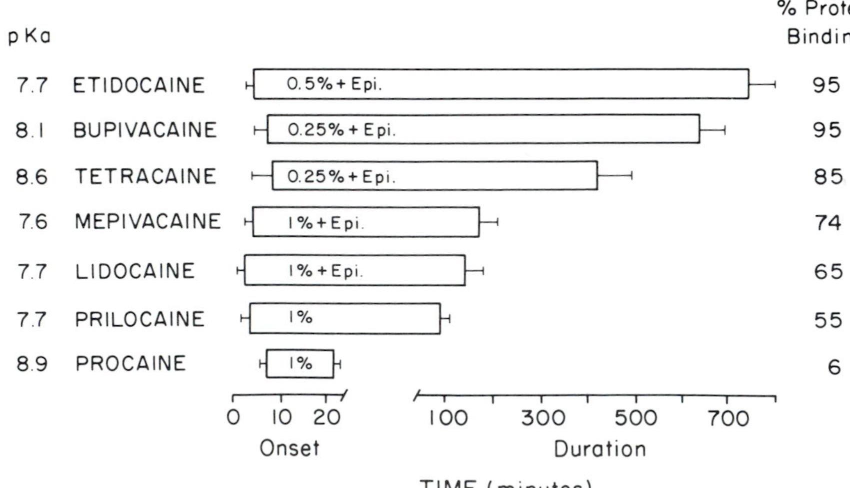

FIGURE 17–4. Relation between pKa and onset of anesthesia (left side of figure) and relation between protein binding and duration of anesthesia (right side of figure). (From Covino BG. Clinical pharmacology of local anesthetic agents. In *Cousins MJ, Bridenbaugh PO, eds. Neural blockade. Philadelphia: JB Lippincott, 1988; 115, with permission.)*

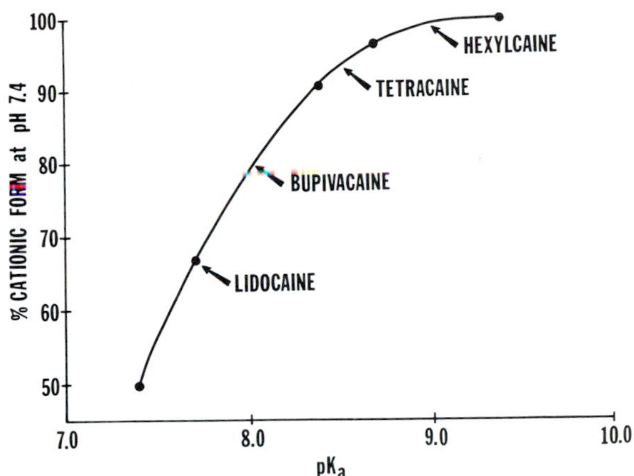

FIGURE 17–5. The fraction of local anesthetic in the protonated, cationic form of aqueous solution at physiologic pH (7.4), as a function of the pKa of the drug. (From Covino BG, Vassallo HG. Local anesthetics. Mechanism of action and clinical use. New York. Grune & Stratton, 1976; 44, with permission.)

are equal (see above). Because the uncharged base is primarily responsible for diffusion across the lipoid nerve sheath, the rapidity of onset of anesthesia depends on the amount of drug in the base form. The percentage of local anesthetic in the base form when injected into a tissue with pH is 7.4 is inversely related to the pKa of that agent (Fig. 17–5). For example, lidocaine, with pKa of 7.74, is 65 per cent ionized, at a tissue pH of 7.4, whereas tetracaine, with pKa of 8.5, is 95 per cent ionized. Both in vitro and in vivo studies confirm that local anesthetic drugs like lidocaine, whose pKa is closer to tissue pH, have a more rapid onset than agents with a greater pKa, such as tetracaine (Fig. 17–4).

INTRINSIC VASODILATOR ACTIVITY

Intrinsic vasodilator activity of the local anesthetic agents also influences potency and duration of action in vivo. After injection of a local anesthetic agent, some drug is taken up by the nerve and some is absorbed by the vascular system. The degree of vascular absorption corresponds to the blood flow through the area in which the drug is injected. Except for cocaine, local anesthetic drugs cause vasodilation. Yet the degree of vasodilation produced by the various agents differs. Although the intrinsic anesthetic potency of lidocaine is significantly greater than that of mepivacaine, in vivo it is no more potent than mepivacaine and has a shorter duration of action. The greater vasodilator activity of lidocaine results in greater vascular absorption, so that less lidocaine is available for nerve blockade.

Structure alterations (Table 17–1) within a homologous group of local anesthetic agents produce quantitative changes in physicochemical properties, such as lipid solubility and protein binding, which alter the anesthetic properties of the compounds. For example, in the ester series, the addition of a butyl group to the aromatic end of the procaine molecule produces tetracaine, an agent of increased lipid solubility and protein binding that has greater intrinsic anesthetic potency and longer duration of action. In the amide series, the addition of a butyl group to the amine end of mepivacaine transforms this agent into bupivacaine. Similarly, substitution of a propyl group for an ethyl group at the amine end of lidocaine, and the addition of an ethyl group to the alpha carbon in the intermediate chain yields etidocaine. Bupivacaine and etidocaine are more lipid soluble, more protein bound, and therefore have greater intrinsic potency and longer duration of action than mepivacaine and lidocaine.

Specific Local Anesthetic Agents

AMINO ESTERS

Cocaine. This compound, isolated from the *Erythroxylin coca* bush, was the first to be successfully used for clinical local anesthesia. Problems with systemic toxicity and addiction led to this agent's abandonment for most regional anesthetic techniques, but it remains an excellent topical anesthetic and is the only agent that produces vasoconstriction at clinically useful concentrations. Anesthesiologists and otolaryngologists still use it to anesthetize and constrict blood vessels in the nasal mucosa prior to nasotracheal intubation and during nasal operations.

Procaine. This was the first synthetic local anesthetic agent; it is of weak potency, with slow onset and short duration of action. This weak potency and the drug's rapid hydrolysis by plasma pseudocholinesterase account for its minimal systemic toxicity. Procaine is hydrolyzed to para-aminobenzoic acid, the cause of allergic reactions seen with repeated use. At present, procaine is used primarily for infiltration anesthesia, differential spinal blocks for diagnosis of pain syndromes, and occasionally for spinal anesthesia.

Chloroprocaine. This agent demonstrates rapid onset of action, short duration, and little systemic toxicity. Because of its rapid onset and lesser toxicity in mother and fetus, chloroprocaine is primarily employed for obstetrical epidural analgesia and anesthesia. Because frequent injections of chloroprocaine are required, obstetrical epidural analgesia is often begun with chloroprocaine but continued with a longer acting agent such as bupivacaine. Chloroprocaine is also of value in ambulatory patients when the duration of operation is not expected to exceed 30 to 60 minutes.

Tetracaine. Because of the slow onset of analgesia and potential for systemic toxicity when large doses are used, tetracaine is primarily used for spinal anesthesia where the onset of anesthesia is intrinsically rapid and the amount of drug required is small. It may be employed as an isobaric, hypobaric, or hyperbaric solution for spinal blockade, although the hyperbaric solution is probably employed most commonly. Tetracaine provides a rapid onset of spinal anesthesia, good sensory anesthesia, and profound motor blockade. Isobaric solutions of tetracaine produce two to three hours of spinal anesthesia, and the addition of epinephrine can extend the duration to four to six hours. Tetracaine is also an excellent topical anesthetic, and is useful for corneal and endotracheal topical anesthesia. Rapid absorption of this drug from the tracheobronchial tree has produced fatalities. Minimizing the dose prevents this complication.

AMINO AMIDE AGENTS

Lidocaine. Lidocaine was the first drug of the amino amide type to be introduced into clinical practice. Its potency, rapid onset, moderate duration of action, and topical anesthetic activity make this agent the most versatile and commonly used local anesthetic. Solutions of lidocaine are available for infiltration, peripheral nerve block, spinal and epidural anesthesia; ointment, jelly, and aerosol forms are applied topically. Intravenous lidocaine is of value as an antiarrhythmic, an antiepileptic, an analgesic, and as a supplement to general anesthesia.

Mepivacaine. This agent is similar to lidocaine and produces profound anesthesia with rapid onset and moderate duration of action. Mepivacaine is used for infiltration, peripheral nerve block, and epidural anesthesia. In some countries, where a 4 per cent hyperbaric solution is available, mepivacaine is used for spinal anesthesia. Mepivacaine is not effective as a topical anesthetic. Because its metabolism is markedly prolonged in the fetus and the newborn, it is not normally employed for obstetrical epidural anesthesia. In adults, mepivacaine is apparently less toxic than lidocaine. Because of its reduced vasodilator activity, mepivacaine produces a somewhat longer duration of anesthesia than does lidocaine.

Prilocaine. Prilocaine is also similar to lidocaine: it rapidly produces profound block of moderate duration. Prilocaine causes significantly less vasodilation than does lidocaine. Therefore, the duration of prilocaine without epinephrine is similar to that of lidocaine with epinephrine, making prilocaine particularly useful in patients in whom epinephrine is contraindicated. Because prilocaine is the least toxic of the amino amide local anesthetics, it is particularly useful for intravenous regional anesthesia, as central nervous system (CNS) toxic effects rarely occur after tourniquet release.

Methemoglobinemia may occur following the use of large doses (more than 600 mg) of prilocaine. Although prilocaine does not cause adverse effects in mother, fetus, or newborn, it is not used in obstetric anesthesia because of the potential for methemoglobinemia and cyanosis in the newborn.

Bupivacaine. Bupivacaine provides intermediate onset, long duration of action, and profound blockade. Depending on the type of block, the average duration of anesthesia with bupivacaine varies from three to ten hours, the longest duration occurring with major peripheral nerve blocks (i.e., brachial plexus block). Unlike most local anesthetics, in dilute concentrations it produces excellent sensory anesthesia with little motor blockade, a major advantage during labor, where epidural bupivacaine provides prolonged pain relief yet allows the patient to "push" during delivery. This differential blockade of sensory and motor fibers is also the basis for the widespread use of bupivacaine for postoperative epidural analgesia and to treat chronic pain states.

Etidocaine. This agent exhibits extremely rapid onset, prolonged duration of action, and profound sensory and motor blockade. It is useful for infiltration anesthesia, peripheral nerve block, and epidural anesthesia. The onset of anesthesia with etidocaine is significantly more rapid than with bupivacaine, but concentrations of etidocaine necessary for adequate sensory anesthesia produce intense motor blockade. As a result, etidocaine is primarily used for operations where muscle relaxation is necessary, and not for obstetrical epidural analgesia and postoperative pain relief.

Ropivacaine. This investigational drug is similar in structure to mepivacaine and bupivacaine. It is prepared as an isomer, whereas mepivacaine and bupivacaine are racemic mixtures. Onset is similar, but potency and duration of motor blockade are slightly less than that of bupivacaine. Ropivacaine is cleared more rapidly and the elimination half-life is shorter than that of bupivacaine. It depresses the myocardium less than does bupivacaine, but more so than lidocaine, making it a desirable alternative to bupivacaine.

CLASSIFICATION BASED ON POTENCY AND DURATION

Based on differences in anesthetic potency (lipid solubility) and duration of action (protein binding), the local anesthetic compounds can be classified into three categories:

Group I. Agents of weak anesthetic potency and short duration of action:
- Procaine
- Chloroprocaine

Group II. Agents of intermediate anesthetic potency and duration of action:
- Lidocaine
- Mepivacaine
- Prilocaine

Group III. Agents of high anesthetic potency and long duration of action:
- Tetracaine
- Bupivacaine
- Etidocaine
- Ropivacaine

PHARMACOKINETICS OF LOCAL ANESTHETIC AGENTS

The rate of absorption from the site of injection, the rate of tissue redistribution, and the rate of metabolism and excretion determine the concentration of local anesthetic in blood. Patient-related factors such as age, cardiovascular status, and hepatic function also influence physiological disposition and therefore the blood concentration of location anesthetic agents (Table 17–3).

TABLE 17–3. **Factors Affecting the Plasma Concentration of Local Anesthetics**

Absorption	Distribution	Metabolism/ Excretion
Site of injections	$t\frac{1}{2}_{\alpha}$	Ester-hydrolysis
Dose	$t\frac{1}{2}_{\beta}$	Amide-enzymatic degradation
Vasoconstrictors		$t\frac{1}{2}_{\gamma}$
Physicochemical characteristics	Patient status	Patient status

Absorption

The site of injection, dosage, addition of vasoconstrictor agent, and the characteristics of the drug control the systemic absorption of local an-

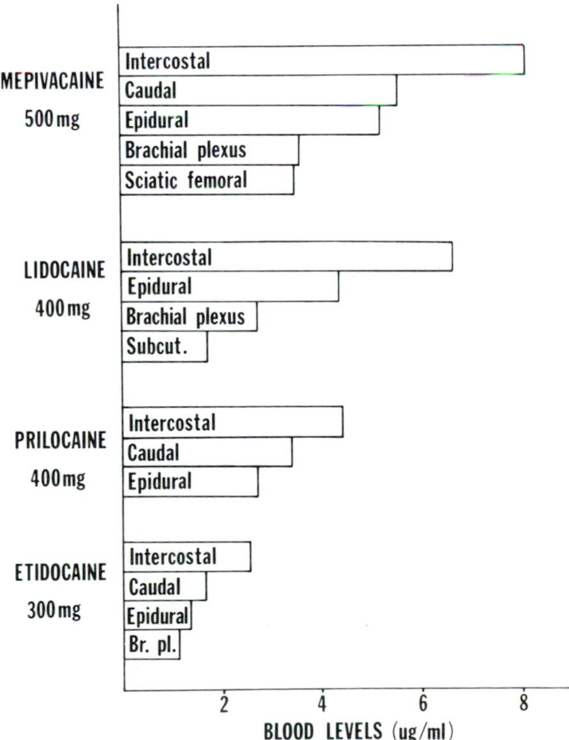

FIGURE 17–6. Comparative peak blood levels of several local anesthetic agents following administration into various anatomic sites. (From Covino BG, Vassallo HG. Local anesthetics. Mechanism of action and clinical use. New York: Grune & Stratton, 1976; 97, with permission.)

esthetic agents. The blood concentration of lidocaine is greatest after intercostal nerve blockade, followed in order of epidural, brachial plexus, and subcutaneous tissue (Fig. 17–6). The increased blood concentrations after intercostal administration may be due to the multiple injections enhancing vascular absorption. This relationship of injection site to rate of absorption implies that a dose of local anesthetic agent safe at one site may be toxic when given at another. For example, 400 mg of lidocaine given without epinephrine for intercostal nerve block results in peak venous plasma concentration of approximately 7 μg per ml, causing CNS toxicity in some patients. In contrast, 400 mg of lidocaine given for brachial plexus block yields a maximum blood concentration of only 3 μg per ml, rarely causing toxicity.

The blood concentration of local anesthetic also depends on the total dose of drug administered at a given site of administration. For most local anesthetics a linear relationship exists between the amount of drug administered and the resultant peak blood concentration. For example, the mean venous blood concentration of lidocaine increases from approximately 1.5 μg per ml to 4 μg per ml as the total dose injected into the lumbar epidural space increases from 200 to 600 mg. Depending on the site of injection, blood concentrations of 0.5 μg per ml to 2.0 μg per ml are achieved for each 100 mg of lidocaine or mepivacaine injected.

Local anesthetic solutions frequently include a vasoconstrictor agent, usually epinephrine in a concentration of 5 μg per ml. The vasoconstrictor may prolong the duration of action of some local anesthetics by decreasing the rate of absorption, which also decreases the potential for systemic toxicity. A dose of 5 μg per ml of epinephrine (1:200,000) significantly reduces the peak blood concentrations of lidocaine and mepivacaine, regardless of the site of administration. However, the peak blood concentrations of prilocaine, bupivacaine, and etidocaine following injection into the lumbar epidural space are minimally influenced by the addition of epinephrine (see below). Yet epinephrine significantly reduces the rate of vascular absorption of these agents when used for peripheral nerve blocks such as brachial plexus blockade.

The pharmacological characteristics of the specific local anesthetic drug also influence the rate and degree of vascular absorption, as described above. After epidural administration, etidocaine produces lesser peak blood concentrations than bupivacaine, yet both have similar vasodilator activity. The greater lipid solubility of etidocaine may result in sequestration by epidural fat, decreasing vascular absorption, and decreasing peak blood concentrations.

Pharmacokinetic Distribution

The distribution of local anesthetic agents can be described by a two- or three-compartment model. The rate of disappearance from blood is usually described in terms of the time required for a 50 per cent reduction in blood concentration ($t\frac{1}{2}$). The rapid disappearance ($t\frac{1}{2}_{\alpha}$) phase is due to uptake by tissues that have plentiful vascular perfusion (Fig. 17–7). The slower phase of disappearance is due to distribution to slowly equilibrating tissues ($t\frac{1}{2}_{\beta}$), and metabolism and excretion ($t\frac{1}{2}_{\gamma}$). Prilocaine redistributes more rapidly from blood to tissues than do lidocaine and mepivacaine (Table 17–4), and the $t\frac{1}{2}_{\beta/\gamma}$ disappear-

TABLE 17–4. **Pharmacokinetic Properties of Various Amide Local Anesthetics**

Agent	$t\frac{1}{2}_{\alpha}$(min)	$t\frac{1}{2}_{\beta}$ (min)	Vdss† (L)	$t\frac{1}{2}_{\gamma}$ (hrs)	$t\frac{1}{2}$‡ Cl (L/min)
Pilocaine	0.5	5.0	261	1.5	2.84
Lidocaine	1.0	9.6	91	1.6	0.95
Mepivacaine	0.7	7.2	84	1.9	0.75
Bupivacaine	2.7	28.0	72	3.5	0.47
Etidocaine	2.2	19.0	133	2.6	1.22

* $t\frac{1}{2}$ = Half-life time.
† Vdss = Volume of distribution at steady state.
‡ Cl = Clearance.

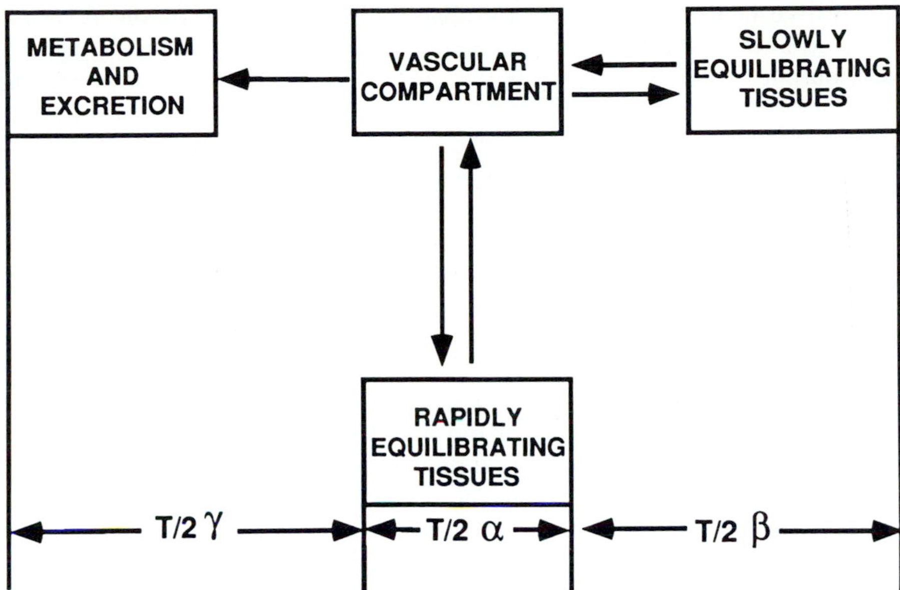

FIGURE 17–7. Pharmacokinetic phases according to a three-compartment model. (From Covino BG, Vassallo HG. Local anesthetics. Mechanism of action and clinical use. New York: Grune & Stratton, 1976; 110, with permission.)

ance phase from blood also occurs more rapidly with prilocaine, suggesting a more rapid rate of metabolism. Differences also exist between bupivacaine and etidocaine. Etidocaine shows a more rapid rate of tissue redistribution and metabolism than bupivacaine.

Local anesthetic agents distribute themselves throughout all body tissues, but the relative concentration in different tissue varies. The better perfused organs generally take up more local anesthetic than less well-perfused organs. Thus, greater concentrations occur in vascularized organs such as lung and kidney, but skeletal muscle constitutes the largest reservoir.

Metabolism and Excretion

The metabolism of local anesthetics depends on their chemical structures. The ester drugs undergo hydrolysis in plasma by pseudocholinesterase, but the rate of metabolism varies markedly between agents in the same chemical class. Chloroprocaine undergoes the most rapid hydrolysis, 4.7 μmol per ml per hour, compared to 1.1 μmol per ml per hour for procaine and 0.3 μmol per ml per hour for tetracaine. Less than 2 per cent of procaine appears unchanged in the urine; 90 per cent of the primary metabolite, para-aminobenzoic acid, appears in the urine. On the other hand, only 33 per cent of diethylaminoethanol, the other major metabolite of procaine, is excreted unchanged.

The amide local anesthetics undergo enzymatic degradation in the liver: prilocaine most rapidly, lidocaine at an intermediate rate, and mepivacaine somewhat more slowly. Hepatic clearance of etidocaine is significantly more rapid than that of bupivacaine.

The metabolism of the amide local anesthetics is more complex than that of the esters. Although many metabolites of the various amide agents are known, the complete metabolic pathways for all compounds in this class are not yet determined. The main metabolic pathway for lidocaine in humans appears to involve oxidative de-ethylation to monethylglycinexylidide, followed by subsequent hydrolysis of xylidine. The amide local anesthetics undergo renal excretion, but less than 5 per cent of drug appears unchanged in the urine.

The physiological disposition of local anesthetic depends on the patient's age and health. The half-life of lidocaine in patients 22 to 26 years is 81 minutes, compared to 139 minutes in patients 61 to 71 years. Greater blood concentrations of amide agents occur in patients with decreased liver blood flow or hepatocellular disease. For example, the half-life of lidocaine is 1.5 hours in normal volunteers, compared to 5.0 hours in patients with liver disease. Finally, the rate of lidocaine disappearance from blood is prolonged in patients with congestive heart failure. This is probably due to reduced liver blood flow owing to diminished cardiac output.

CHOOSING A LOCAL ANESTHETIC

Table 17–5 lists the majority of local anesthetics, their primary uses (injection site), onset time, and duration of action. This table provides the criteria necessary for selecting an appropriate local anesthetic.

The choice of a local anesthetic depends largely on (1) the site of injection, (2) the duration of the operation, and (3) the speed of onset required. The site of injection influences the choice of local anesthetic agent. Agents commonly used for spinal anesthesia are procaine, lidocaine, bupivacaine, or tetracaine; for epidural anesthesia, chloroprocaine, lidocaine, mepivacaine, bupivacaine, or etidocaine. Lidocaine, mepivacaine, and bupivacaine are often used for brachial plexus block, but etidocaine is not.

Local anesthetic selection is also based on the duration of anesthesia required. Consider, for example, epidural anesthesia for knee operations. Whereas chloroprocaine might be ideal for a brief arthroscopic procedure, bupivacaine or etidocaine would be more appropriate for a knee reconstruction, because of their longer durations of action. Because onset of action is an important consideration and bupivacaine is slow in onset, the epidural might be started with chloroprocaine, mepivacaine, or lidocaine, which have a rapid onset,

TABLE 17–5. Characteristics Useful for Choosing a Local Anesthetic

Agent	Uses	Onset	Duration
Cocaine	Topical		
Procaine	Infiltration Differential spinal Spinal	Slow	Short
Chloroprocaine	Brachial plexus Epidural	Fast	Short
Lidocaine	Topical Infiltration IV regional Brachial plexus Spinal Epidural	Intermediate	Intermediate
Mepivacaine	Infiltration Brachial plexus Spinal Epidural	Intermediate	Intermediate
Prilocaine	Infiltration IV regional Brachial plexus Epidural	Intermediate	Intermediate
Bupivacaine	Infiltration Brachial plexus Spinal Epidural	Slow	Long
Etidocaine	Infiltration Epidural	Fast	Long
Tetracaine	Topical Brachial plexus Spinal	Slow	Long
Ropivacaine*	Infiltration Brachial plexus ? Spinal Epidural	Intermediate–fast	Intermediate–long

* Investigational.

and then continued with bupivacaine to take advantage of its extended duration. Etidocaine combines both rapid onset and long duration.

Similar principles apply to drug selection for spinal, brachial plexus anesthesia, and other regional anesthetic techniques. However, conduction blockade is so rapid with spinal anesthesia, that speed of onset of an agent is not as important as it is with epidural or brachial plexus anesthesia.

IMPROVING ONSET OF ANESTHESIA

One of the drawbacks of regional anesthesia is the slow onset of anesthesia, owing to the time required for the local anesthetic to reach the sodium channel inside the nerve. Because diffusion into the interior of the axon depends on the un-ionized lipophilic base, the onset of anesthesia can be hastened by increasing the base concentration by carbonating the local anesthetic solution or increasing its pH.

Increasing pH with Bicarbonate

Local anesthetic solution are manufactured with a pH of 3.5 to 6.5 to enhance shelf life and solubility. The pH can be increased by adding small amounts of sodium bicarbonate just prior to injection. Large changes in pH cause major increases in the amount of free base available and a decrease in onset time. Unfortunately, the un-ionized base forms of local anesthetics tend to be insoluble, which limits the amount of sodium bicarbonate that can be added to local anesthetic precipitates. Table 17–6 provides guidelines for adding sodium bicarbonate to the various local anesthetics to shorten onset of action. Addition of sodium bicarbonate to local anesthetic solutions also increases the P_{CO_2} and this "carbonation" may also contribute to the decreased onset time (see below). Another beneficial aspect of increasing the pH of local anesthetic solutions is that less pain is felt during injection.

Local anesthetic solutions supplied with epinephrine added have a pH of 3.5 to prevent oxidation of the epinephrine; the speed of onset of anesthesia provided by these solutions is greatly improved by increasing their pH. An alternative to adjusting the pH with sodium bicarbonate is to add the epinephrine to the plain local anesthetic (pH = 6.5) just before injection.

Carbonation

Carbonation of local anesthetic *base* solutions speeds onset, enhances spread, and improves quality of conduction blockade. Unfortunately, carbonated local anesthetics are only commercially available in Canada and some European countries. There are several mechanisms by which carbonation might enhance blockade: carbon dioxide may have a direct membrane depressant effect; the increase in CO_2 inside the nerve decreases the pH causing local anesthetic cation trapping; loss of CO_2 as the vial is opened increases the pH of the solution from 6.5 to greater than 7.0, making more free base available for nerve penetration. The first two of these mechanisms are predicated on the rapid diffusion of CO_2 through the nerve membrane into the axoplasm.

TOXICITY OF LOCAL ANESTHETIC AGENTS

Local anesthetic agents produce few side effects when given in appropriate dosage at the proper anatomical site. Most toxic reactions occur after the accidental intravascular or subarachnoid injection of a large dose of local anesthetic, although an excessive dose given into the appropriate anatomical location can lead to systemic toxicity, owing to the expected vascular absorption.

Systemic Toxicity

The major systemic toxicity of local anesthetic agents involves the CNS and the cardiovascular system. CNS is more susceptible to the systemic effects of local anesthetics than is the cardiovascular system. Studies in dogs and sheep demonstrate that significantly smaller blood concentrations of local anesthetic are required to produce CNS toxicity than are required to cause circulatory collapse; most toxic reactions to local anesthetic in humans involve the CNS. Although less common, cardiovascular toxicity is more serious and more difficult to manage.

TABLE 17–6. **Suggested Alkalinization Doses and pH Achieved**

Local Anesthetic	(%)	HCO_3^-, ml/20 ml Anesthetic‡	HCO_3^-, mEq/20 ml Anesthetic	pH after HCO_3^-
2-Chloroprocaine	2	4.0	1.92	7.51
	3	4.0	1.92	7.43
Mepivacaine	1	4.0	1.92	7.26
	1.5	2.0	0.96	7.00
Etidocaine	1	0.015	0.007	5.90
	1 + epi*	0.100	0.048	5.73
	1 + epi†	0.015	0.007	5.85
	1.5 + epi*	0.100	0.048	5.76
Bupivacaine	0.25	0.10	0.048	6.97
	0.5	0.05	0.024	6.62
	0.5 + epi*	0.30	0.144	6.37
	0.5 + epi†	0.05	0.024	6.78
	0.75	0.05	0.024	6.56
	0.75 + epi*	0.30	0.144	6.32
	0.75 + epi†	0.05	0.024	6.58
Lidocaine	1	4.0	1.92	7.43
	1 + epi*	4.0	1.92	7.21
	1 + epi†	4.0	1.92	7.37
	1.5	4.0	1.92	7.31
	1.5 + epi*	4.0	1.92	7.16
	1.5 + epi†	4.0	1.92	7.35
	2	4.0	1.92	7.24
	2 + epi*	4.0	1.92	7.08
	2 + epi†	4.0	1.92	7.26

* Commercially added epinephrine 1:200,000.
† Freshly added epinephrine, 1:200,000.
‡ Data compiled for sodium bicarbonate, 4% (wt/vol), (0.48 mEq/ml).
No precipitation before 1 hour with HCO_3^- at these doses.
Adapted with permission from Peterfreund RA, Datta S, Ostheimer GW. pH Adjustment of local anesthetic solutions with sodium bicarbonate: Laboratory evaluations of alkalinization and precipitation. Reg Anesth 1989; 14:265–270.

Central Nervous System Toxicity

The signs and symptoms of local anesthetic-induced CNS toxicity are summarized in Table 17–7. Volunteers receiving intravenous infusions of local anesthetics describe feelings of lightheadedness and dizziness, often followed by visual and auditory disturbances such as difficulty in focusing and tinnitus. Other subjective CNS symptoms include disorientation and feelings of drowsiness. Objective signs of CNS toxicity include shivering, muscular twitching, and tremors involving muscles of the face and extremities; ultimately, gen-

TABLE 17–7. **Signs and Symptosm of Local Anesthetic-Induced CNS Toxicity**

Initial events
Tinitus
Lightheadedness
Confusion
Circumoral numbness
Excitation phase
Tonic-clonic convulsions
Depression phase
Unconsciousness
Generalized CNS depression
Respiratory arrest

eralized tonic-clonic convulsions occur. If an excessive dose of local anesthetic is administered systemically, the initial signs of CNS excitation are rapidly followed by generalized CNS depression. Seizure activity ceases and respiratory depression and respiratory arrest occur. Occasionally, CNS depression occurs without a preceding excitatory phase, particularly if other CNS depressant drugs are given concomitantly.

The initial CNS excitation by local anesthetics results from the selective blockade of inhibitory pathways allowing facilatory neurons to function unopposed, causing increased excitatory activity and convulsions. If the dose is further increased, inhibition of both facilatory and inhibitory pathways results in generalized CNS depression.

The intrinsic anesthetic potencies of local anesthetics correlate with their ability to cause CNS excitation. The relative CNS toxicities of bupivacaine, etidocaine, and lidocaine are approximately 4:2:1, similar to the relative potencies of these agents for producing regional anesthesia.

Cardiovascular Toxicity

Local anesthetic agents can produce profound effects on the cardiovascular system (Table 17–8), depressing both cardiac muscle and peripheral vascular smooth muscle. The primary effect of local anesthetics on isolated cardiac muscle is to decrease the maximum rate of depolarization by decreasing sodium conductance in the fast sodium channels. Bupivacaine markedly depresses the rapid phase of depolarization so that when the heart rate exceeds 10 beats per minute, bupivacaine prevents complete restoration of V_{max} between action potentials (beats). Similar effects are not observed with lidocaine, which does not provoke the arrhythmias bupivacaine does.

TABLE 17–8. Signs and Symptoms of Local Anesthetic-Induced Cardiovascular Toxicity

Initial Events
- Hypertension and tachycardia during the CNS excitation phase

Intermediate phase
- Myocardial depression
- Decreased cardiac output
- Mild–moderate hypotension

Terminal phase
- Peripheral vasodilation
- Profound hypotension
- Sinus bradycardia
- Conduction defects
- Ventricular arrhythmias
- Circulatory collapse

All local anesthetics exert a dose-dependent negative inotropic action on cardiac muscle, proportional to their ability to suppress conduction in peripheral nerves. The most potent local anesthetic agents depress cardiac contractility at the least concentrations, whereas the least potent of the local anesthetics are also least depressant to contractility.

Local anesthetic agents exert a biphasic action on smooth muscle of peripheral blood vessels. Lesser concentrations of lidocaine and bupivacaine cause vasoconstriction, whereas greater concentrations cause vasodilation.

As the blood concentrations of local anesthetic increases, cardiovascular events follow in sequence. At nontoxic blood concentrations, slight increases in blood pressure may occur owing to a small increase in cardiac output and heart rate with sympathetic stimulation, or to the vasoconstrictor action of local anesthetics at lesser concentrations. Concentrations of local anesthetics that cause CNS toxicity result indirectly in a marked increase in heart rate, blood pressure, and cardiac output because of the seizures. Further increases in the blood concentration of local anesthetic causes cardiovascular depression. Initial hypotension owing to the negative inotropic effect of the agents and decreased cardiac output is transient in most patients. However, excessive amounts of local anesthetic cause profound cardiovascular depression, due to negative inotropy, peripheral vasodilation, and depressant effects on the excitability of cardiac tissue, decreasing sinus rate and inducing arteriovenous (AV) conduction block. In addition, agents such as bupivacaine may precipitate ventricular arrhythmias as well.

PREVENTING TOXICITY DURING MAJOR REGIONAL ANESTHESIA

Monitoring

Whenever patients receive local anesthetics, systemic toxicity is possible, and appropriate pre-

cautions are indicated. The means used to monitor the systemic effects of the local anesthetic depend on the blood concentration anticipated, considering the drug, dose, and site of injection. If only a few milligrams of lidocaine are to be injected in the skin around a leg wound, and no sedation is used, monitoring may consist only of maintaining verbal contact with the patient. On the other hand, for major blocks involving large doses of drug and significant physiologic sequelae from blockade, such as brachial plexus block, or spinal or epidural anesthesia, monitoring includes verbal contact as well as all the usual monitoring appropriate for a general anesthetic in the same circumstances.

Precautions

Preparations for administering a local anesthetic include the items listed below.

Preparation for Local or Regional Anesthesia

1. **Equipment needed for cardiopulmonary resuscitation (CPR), including at least oxygen, suction, airway equipment, all standard resuscitative drugs.**
2. **Equipment and drugs to induce general anesthesia, if needed, as an alternative to a failed block.**
3. **CNS depressants for treating seizures: thiopental, midazolam, diazepam.**
4. **An intravenous infusion in place before the block is performed.**

Toxic reactions are best avoided by frequent aspiration for blood during slow intermittent injection of the local anesthetic. Aspiration may not always detect that a needle or catheter is within a blood vessel. Local anesthetic containing epinephrine (5 μg per ml) usually produces an increase in heart rate and blood pressure if the solution is injected intravascularly, unless the patient is taking beta blocker medications. However, by administering the drug slowly and intermittently (2 to 5 ml every 30 seconds) while asking the patient about symptoms related to local anesthetic-induced CNS toxicity (such as ringing in the ears, circumoral numbness, feelings of lightheadedness), one can halt the injection at the first signs of intravascular injection, before a large amount of local anesthetic is administered intravenously. Further, the slow injection allows the local anesthetic to be diluted in the blood, decreasing the peak concentration. Local anesthetic systemic toxicity is rare in the absence of intravascular injection or overdose. When CNS and cardiovascular reactions are promptly treated, the outcome of local anesthetic systemic toxicity is usually benign.

Maximum Recommended Doses of Local Anesthetics

The maximum recommended doses for local anesthetics (Table 17–9) are intended to prevent systemic toxic reactions by setting safe limits on the amount of drug to be used. However, because peak plasma-drug concentration depends so strongly on the site of injection, a single recommended dose cannot be correct for all uses of the drug. For example, injecting lidocaine, 300 mg in the intercostal region, 500 mg epidurally, 600 mg in the brachial plexus, or 1000 mg subcutaneously, each result in plasma concentrations of approximately 5 μg per ml, which usually does not cause toxic reactions. However, the maximum dose of lidocaine that is recommended by the manufacturer is 4 mg per kg (approximately 300 mg) regardless of the injection site. This maximum recommended amount is insufficient for brachial plexus and epidural anesthetic procedures, and does not take into account factors such as the site of injection.

The addition of epinephrine (5 μg per ml) reduces vascular absorption and peak plasma concentrations of lidocaine by 20 to 30 per cent after intercostal, brachial plexus, or lumbar epidural injection, and 50 per cent after subcutaneous injection. The maximum recommended dose for lidocaine with epinephrine is 7 mg per kg (approximately 500 mg). This amount is sufficient for epidural anesthesia but may be insufficient for brachial plexus blockade. Some expert anesthesiologists question the logic behind these recommended dosages and may exceed them, depending on the circumstances. For example, some experts perform brachial plexus anesthesia with 50 ml of 1.5 per cent plain mepivacaine, more than twice the recommended dose, arguing that the increased dose increases the success of the block. However, medicolegal problems arise when the maximum

Table 17–9. Manufacturers' Single Injection Maximum Recommended Doses for Local Anesthetics

Drug	Concentration (%)	mg/kg Plain/(EPI)†	mg/70 kg pt Plain/(EPI)†	ml/70kg pt Plain/(EPI)†
Chloroprocaine	3.00	11(14)	770(980)	25(33)
Lidocaine	1.00	4(7)	280(490)	28(50)
Lidocaine	1.50	4(7)	280(490)	19(33)
Lidocaine	2.00	4(7)	280(490)	14(25)
Mepivacaine	2.00	4(7)	280(490)	14(25)
Prilocaine	3.00	7(8.5)	500(600)	17(20)
Bupivacaine	0.75	2.5(3.2)	175(225)	23(30)
Etidocaine	1.00	6(8)	420(560)	42(56)
Etidocaine	1.50	—(8)*	—(560)	—(37)†

* Etidocaine, 1.5% is *not* available without epinephrine.
† The doses in parentheses apply when epinephrine 5 μg/ml is added to the solution.

recommended dose is exceeded and systemic toxicity occurs.

The expert is technically adept and less likely to misplace the local anesthetic than is the beginner. Likewise, experienced practitioners recognize signs of toxicity promptly and are prepared to treat these reactions and to defend their actions in court. Although the maximum recommended doses may be illogical and too small, they are regarded as safe and appropriate limits for the neophyte. Adding epinephrine to the local anesthetic often permits increasing the dose without exceeding the manufacturer's recommendations.

EFFECT OF CNS DEPRESSANTS

Some anesthesiologists medicate patients with a benzodiazepine prior to regional anesthesia to increase the seizure threshold and decrease the chance of systemic toxicity. This controversial practice may increase the seizure threshold to local anesthetics, but will not prevent the cardiotoxic effects of agents such as bupivacaine, should systemic toxic concentrations occur. Although there is a theoretical advantage to premedication with benzodiazepines before regional anesthesia, it does not substitute for careful technique and care in dose selection to avoid local anesthetic toxicity.

Management of CNS and CVS Toxicity

If CNS toxicity is detected during the slow injections recommended here, presumably owing to intravascular injection, treatment is simple and effective. Halting the injection of local anesthetic and administering oxygen and reassurance are usually all that is needed, because the drug is quickly redistributed and the blood concentration decreases immediately. If CNS excitability appears slowly, after the full dose of drug has been given, then the blood concentration of local anesthetic may continue to increase for some time. The later the symptoms appear, the more likely the associated blood concentration represents the peak. Patients with late and mild symptoms can be managed with oxygen and small doses of anticonvulsants such as thiopental or benzodiazepines. Patients with more severe, early, and progressive symptoms may require the same therapy as those who develop frank convulsions.

Convulsions or cardiac arrest due to local anesthetic systemic toxicity require establishment of a patent airway, adequate ventilation, and support of the circulation. If the patient cannot be ventilated adequately, 20 to 40 mg of intravenous succinylcholine may allow insertion of an oral airway and success with mask ventilation. Should mask ventilation not be possible, or if the patient has a full stomach, immediate intubation of the trachea is required. Central nervous system excitability is treated with small amounts of barbiturate (thiopental 25 to 50 mg) or benzodiazepine (midazolam 1 to 2 mg or diazepam 5 to 10 mg). Hypotension is treated with alpha and beta agonists as required. For life-threatening cardiac dysrhythmias, electrical cardioversion or bretylium (up to 20 mg per kg) may be required.

MISCELLANEOUS SYSTEMIC EFFECTS

A variety of miscellaneous systemic actions have been attributed to local anesthetic drugs, most of which relate to their membrane-stabilizing effects. For example, local anesthetics produce neuromuscular block, ganglionic block, and anticholinergic activity. There is little evidence to suggest that any of these miscellaneous effects are clinically significant under usual conditions.

Allergy

The amino ester agents such as procaine can produce allergic-type reactions. These agents are derivatives of para-aminobenzoic acid, which is allergenic. The amino amide local anesthetics are not derivatives of para-aminobenzoic acid and rarely cause allergic reactions. Solutions of the amino amide agents may contain a preservative, methylparaben, whose chemical structure is similar to para-aminobenzoic acid, and is often responsible for allergic reactions attributed to amide local anesthetics.

Occasionally, patients indicate that they are allergic to local anesthetics. Because true local anesthetic allergies are rare, these reactions usually represent systemic toxicity, the effect of added epinephrine, a psychological reaction, or a simple faint. Often, a careful history elicits the cause of the reaction. Further investigation of local anesthetic allergy consists of testing for wheal formation following intradermal injection of small amounts (0.1 ml) of dilute solutions of the local anesthetic in question. Complete testing includes injecting increasing doses of the local anesthetic and testing the preservative methylparaben.

Local Tissue Toxicity

Although the primary toxic effect of local anesthetics involves the systemic administration of excessive doses, the potential local irritant action of these agents is also of interest. Local anesthetics rarely produce localized nerve damage in the concentrations employed clinically. However, prolonged sensorimotor deficits have occurred in a few patients following the epidural or subarachnoid injection of large doses of chloroprocaine. This neural toxicity associated with the use of chloroprocaine presumably relates to the acidity and the sodium bisulfite that functions as an antioxidant in chloroprocaine solutions. Solutions of chloroprocaine without sodium bisulfite have not caused neural damage, and recently, sodium bisulfite free solutions of chloroprocaine have become commercially available.

REFERENCES

Butterworth JF, Strichartz GR. Molecular mechanisms of nerve block by local anesthetics. Anesthesiology 1990;72:711.

Covino BG. Pharmacology of local anaesthetics. Br J Anaesth 1986;58:717–731.

Covino BG. Toxicity of local anesthetics. Adv Anesth 1986;3:37–65.

Clarkson CW, Hondeghem LM. Mechanism for bupivacaine depression of cardiac conduction: Fast block of sodium channels during the action potential with slow recovery from block during diastole. Anesthesiology 1985;62:396–405.

Peterfreund RA, Datta S, Ostheimer GW. pH adjustment of local anesthetic solutions with sodium bicarbonate: Laboratory evaluations of alkalinization and precipitation. Reg Anesth 1989;14:265–270.

Tucker GT. Pharmacokinetics of local anaesthetics. Br J Anaesth 1986;58:717–731.

CHAPTER EIGHTEEN

Spinal and Epidural Anesthesia

Clinical spinal and epidural anesthesia were first reported at the turn of the 20th century. In 1899 in Germany, August Bier and an assistant injected cocaine into their subarachnoid spaces to produce spinal anesthesia; each developed a headache. In 1901, Cathelin in France administered the first caudal epidural; in 1921, Pages described the lumbar approach to the epidural space. Today, spinal and epidural administration of local anesthetics are the most common techniques in regional anesthesia, used for anesthesia for operations, labor and delivery, management of postoperative pain, and diagnosis and treatment of acute and chronic pain syndromes. Spinal or epidural anesthesia may also be combined with general anesthesia. The use of intraoperative conduction anesthesia and postoperative intraspinal analgesia may attenuate endocrine and metabolic responses to operation and thereby improve outcome.

Anatomy

The spinal canal lies within the vertebral column between the foramen magnum and the sacral hiatus, bounded anteriorly by the vertebral bodies, laterally by the pedicles, and posteriorly by the laminae. The spinal cord proper extends within the canal from the brain stem to its termination at the L2 vertebral level in the adult. It is anchored to the sacrum by the filum terminale, a band of connective tissue running parallel with the cauda equina in the lumbar cistern. The cord is invested concentrically by the three meningeal layers: the pia, arachnoid, and dura mater (outermost). Between the pia and arachnoid mater lies the subarachnoid space, which contains the spinal nerve roots and cerebrospinal fluid. It extends caudally to the termination of the dural sac at S2 (Fig. 18–1).

The epidural space is the potential space between the dura mater and the bony and ligamentous walls of the spinal canal. It contains areolar connective tissue as well as the internal vertebral plexus of veins (Batson's plexus), also called epidural veins, which drain the meninges and vertebral bodies. Another much smaller potential space between the dura and arachnoid mater, the spinal subdural space, has been identified radiologically. Unintentional injection into it may explain an occasional failure of spinal anesthesia or high spinal anesthesia after attempted epidural block. Important ligamentous structures include the supraspinous ligament, interspinous ligament, and the ligamentum flavum. These structures join and reinforce the spinous processes and laminae,

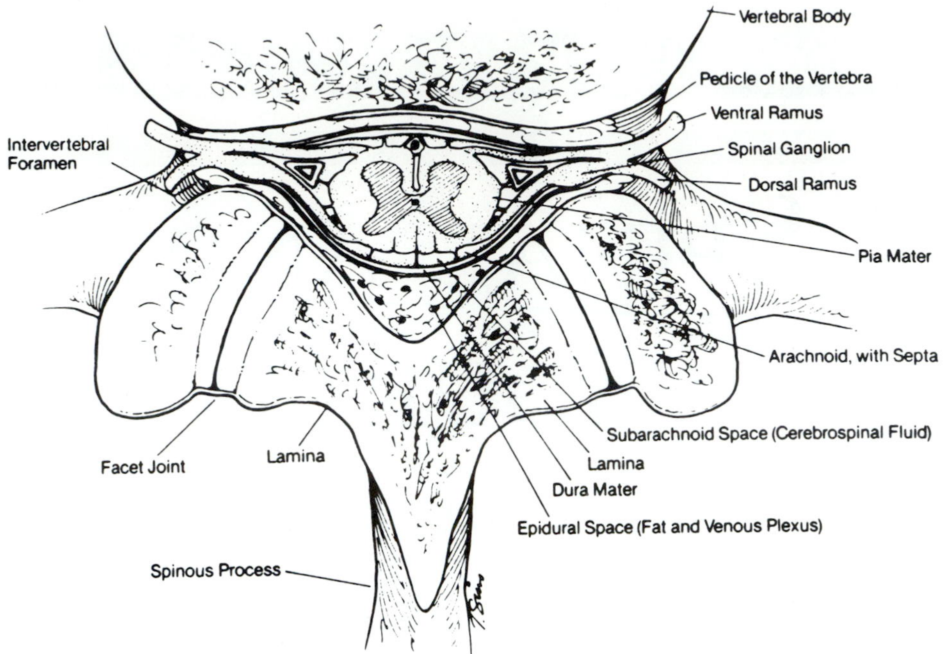

FIGURE 18–1. Transverse section through lumbar spine. (Reproduced with permission from Raj PP. Handbook of regional anesthesia. New York: Churchill Livingstone, 1985.)

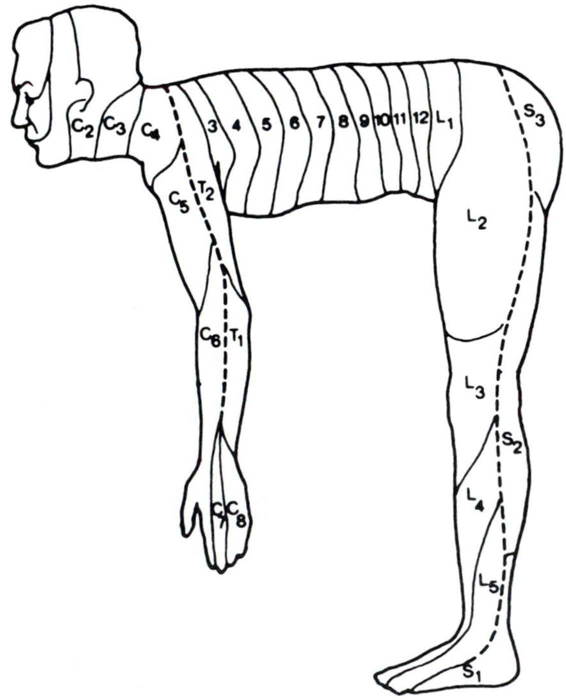

FIGURE 18–2. In the quadrupedal position, the dermatomes lie on order. (Reproduced with the permission of the publisher, Oxford University Press, from Foerster I. Brain 1933; 56:1.)

and are traversed in sequence by the needle tip as it passes toward the dura.

Paired somatic spinal nerves exit the canal through the intervertebral foramina bilaterally, each supplying a region of skin (dermatomes) and skeletal muscle (myotomes) (Fig. 18–2). Visceral nervous pathways are more complex. Sympathetic afferents return from end organs via prevertebral plexuses and the paravertebral chain ganglia, and reach the spinal cord at multiple levels. These levels may be higher than the corresponding somatic dermatomal level. For example, although the incision for operations on the testis is at a dermatomal level of T12, it is necessary to have at least a T10 level to ensure adequate visceral analgesia. Planning the extent of spinal and epidural anesthesia must take into account the innervation of the area of the incision and the innervation of the affected viscera as well (Table 18–1).

PREOPERATIVE EVALUATION

As with other sorts of anesthesia, the preoperative evaluation of a patient before spinal or epi-

Table 18–1. Spinal Levels of Preganglionic Afferent Visceral Innervation*

T1	Eye T1–2	
T2		Head T1–3
T3	Heart T1–5	Arm T1–6
T4		Lungs T2–6
T5		
T6		
T7		
T8	Upper GI T7–9	
T9		
T10	Lower GI T10–11	Gonads T10–11
T11		
T12	Lower limb T11–L2	Kidneys T12–L1
L1	Rectum, bladder, uterus T12–L2	Ureter L1–L2
L2		

* Data modified with permission from Last RF. Anatomy, regional and applied. 6th ed. Edinburgh, Churchill Livingstone, 1978.

dural anesthesia takes into account the planned operation, the patient's physical condition, the patient's feelings, and any contraindications to regional techniques.

Operations for which spinal or epidural anesthesia alone is appropriate are those on the lower abdomen, inguinal region, lower extremities, or perineum. Operations involving the upper abdomen and chest are not usually suitable for spinal or epidural anesthesia used alone, because to relieve visceral pain, very high levels of anesthesia are required (T2), despite which patients are often uncomfortable. In addition, the need for protection of the airway and for assisted ventilation make intubation of the trachea desirable during such procedures. Spinal or epidural anesthesia may be combined with light general anesthesia for these patients.

In some instances, it is the choice of surgeon and not the site of the operation that argues for or against regional anesthesia. Some surgeons enjoy working while the patient is awake and use techniques that minimize visceral pain; others find it preferable to have an unconscious patient.

An important element of the patient's condition that affects planning is a history of coagulopathy or the use of anticoagulants or antiplatelet drugs. Specific tests of coagulation are required for such patients because of the irreversible damage that can result from an epidural hematoma (see Chapter 15, Table 15–8).

The patient must be questioned about symptoms of preexisting neurological deficits. Although there is little evidence that spinal or epidural anesthesia causes or worsens neurologic diseases, it is wise to avoid these techniques when postoperative exacerbation of an existing problem is possible.

Because so many patients suffer backache after operations (see Chapter 16), some anesthesiologists do not offer spinal or epidural anesthesia to patients with histories of back pain or operations on the back, so that postoperative back pain will not be attributed to the anesthetic. In addition, it is possible that nerve roots immobilized by scar tissue are more liable to damage by the needle. It can be difficult to perform lumbar puncture or to identify the epidural space in patients with previous back operations, as well as in those with kyphoscoliosis or obesity.

During preoperative evaluation, some patients express fear of spinal or epidural anesthesia. If spinal or epidural anesthesia offer no significant advantages for such a patient, it may be best simply to direct the discussion toward general anesthesia. Otherwise, careful and sympathetic questioning may elicit a reason for the patient's fears, giving the anesthesiologist the opportunity to reassure the patient. Fear of major neurologic damage arises in part from episodes almost a half century old; injury often was due to contaminated equipment or drugs. With the use of factory-prepared kits containing dilute solutions of modern local anesthetics, free of preservatives, major neurologic injury attributable to skillfully conducted spinal or epidural anesthesia is virtually nonexistent. One review published in 1981 of 65,304 patients undergoing spinal or epidural anesthesia documented only one permanent nerve injury possible related to spinal anesthesia.

Some patients fear the needle itself, others dread being awake in the operating room, and some worry about inadequate analgesia; information about the use of local anesthetics during lumbar puncture, and the availability of sedation or general anesthesia when needed may reassure these patients. If reassurance fails, pressing a patient to accept a regional anesthetic against his wishes invites a strong reaction to the slightest maloccurance.

An absolute contraindication to regional anesthesia is the patient's refusal; relative contraindications are listed in Table 18–2. As with any other therapy, spinal or epidural anesthesia rarely may

TABLE 18–2. Contraindications to Spinal or Epidural Anesthesia*

Patient refusal (the only absolute contraindication)
Untreated coagulation defect severe enough to worsen surgical bleeding
Infection at the site of the block
Bacteremia (risks provoking meningitis)
Neurological disease, especially involving the spinal cord or roots
History of back pain or back operation
Hypovolemia

* Except for the patient's refusal, all of these are relative contraindications. Spinal or epidural anesthesia may still be the first choice in spite of these conditions, especially if appropriate treatment for the condition has been given, as in the treatment of hypovolemia.

be appropriate in the face of these contraindications, but in each case the potential benefits of regional anesthesia must outweigh the risks, and the patient must give fully informed consent.

TECHNIQUES COMMON TO SPINAL AND EPIDURAL ANESTHESIA

Operating room preparation and machine testing before spinal or epidural anesthesia are identical to those preceding general anesthesia, which may be required if the block is inadequate. A vasopressor is prepared to treat hypotension if necessary.

Upon the patient's arrival in the operating room, the usual noninvasive monitors are applied, and baseline vital signs recorded. Supplemental oxygen, usually via nasal cannulae, helps prevent hypoxemia, which may be due to sedatives or to the effects of the anesthesia itself. Sedatives or opioid analgesics are given as needed before the block; patients must remain sufficiently awake to report any parasthesias during the block.

If the block is to be performed with the patient sitting, an assistant supports the patient, who may faint because of the sedatives and narcotics or because of simple vagal syncope. Intravenous fluids or prophylactic vasopressors may be given to blunt the hypotension expected after the block, depending on circumstances. Throughout the procedure, the operator and the assistant warn the patient of each step to be taken and provide constant reassurance, as well as monitor the patient for bradycardia, hypotension, or faintness.

After positioning, there follows careful palpation of landmarks, preparation of the skin over a wide area with a bactericidal solution, and draping. Sterile gloves and meticulous aseptic technique are required. The sterilization indicator in the kit is examined and the drugs identified carefully before mixing the required solutions, to prevent administration of the wrong drug or the wrong dose.

SPINAL ANESTHESIA

Technique

Positioning for lumbar puncture is determined by patient comfort, the surgical site, and the density of the planned local anesthetic solution. Lumbar puncture may be performed with the patient in the sitting, lateral decubitus, or prone positions. Regardless of positioning, the lumbar spine should be as flexed as possible to spread the spinous processes and enlarge the interlaminar spaces. In the prone position, this may be facilitated by placement of a pillow beneath the hips to flex the sacrum on the lumbar spine.

A line perpendicular to the spine through the iliac crests passes through the L4-L5 interspace, or intersects the spinous process of L4. Because the spinal cord proper ends at L2 in adults, performing the puncture below this level avoids the risk of spinal cord injury.

A midline approach to lumbar puncture is most commonly used. The index and middle fingers of the operator's nondominant hand straddle the chosen interspace perpendicular to the spinal column. The skin over the interspace is infiltrated with local anesthetic through a fine needle (25 to 27 gauge). The spinal needle is advanced through the skin into the ligaments in the midline sagittal plane, directed slightly cephalad. As the needle tip advances through the ligamentum flavum, an increase in resistance is felt, followed by a "pop" as the needle punctures the dura, at an average depth of 4 to 6 cm (Fig. 18–3).

After the stylet is removed, free flow of clear cerebrospinal fluid (CSF) as the needle is rotated through 360 degrees confirms that the bevel of the needle has fully penetrated the dura. If the CSF is blood tinged, it should clear rapidly; otherwise, the

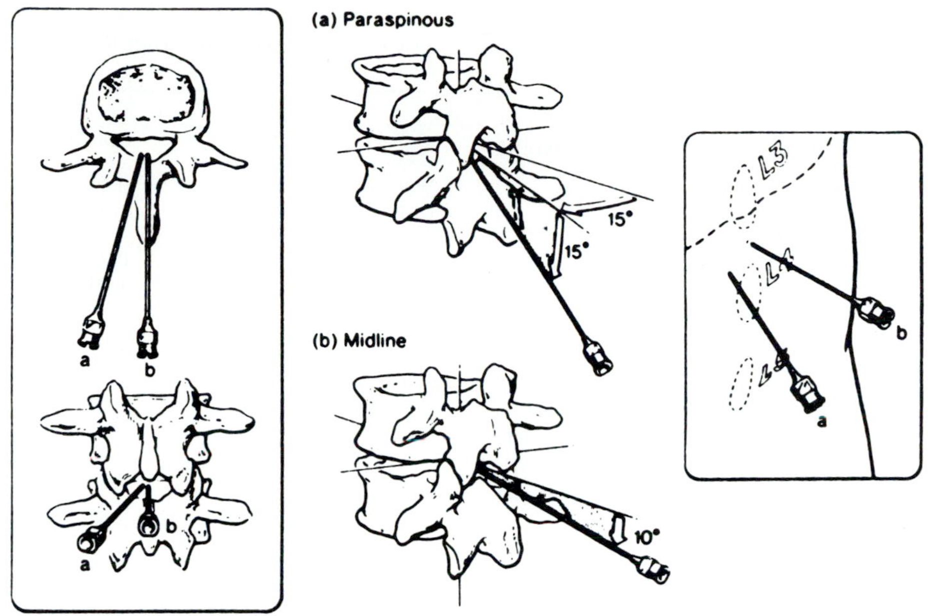

FIGURE 18–3. The midline and paramedian approaches for spinal or epidural anesthesia. (From Cousins MJ, Bridenbaugh, PO, eds. Neural Blockade. 2nd ed. Philadelphia: JB Lippincott, 1988.)

needle tip may lie in an epidural vein, and spinal anesthesia will be unsuccessful.

If the needle encounters bone instead of entering the subarachnoid space, the needle tip is withdrawn to the subcutaneous tissue and redirected (usually more cephalad), to walk off lamina or inferior spinous process into CSF. Failure of lumbar puncture is usually due to poor patient positioning, selection of a small interspace, or failure to advance in the midline.

After free flow of CSF is established, the operator anchors the needle with the nondominant hand, which rests on the patient's back with the thumb and index finger stabilizing hub position. The syringe containing the spinal anesthetic is firmly attached to the needle hub, free aspiration of CSF is confirmed, and the local anesthetic injected. Speed of injection does not appear to influence the ultimate distribution of spinal anesthesia. Confirmation of CSF back flow at the end of injection verifies delivery of the spinal anesthetic to the CSF.

When the midline approach fails, such as in elderly patients with calcified ligaments, or in patients who are difficult to position with the lumbar spine flexed, a paramedian (lateral) approach to the interlaminar space may succeed. The skin is punctured 1.5 to 2.0 cm from the midline adjacent to the spinous process below the chosen interspace and the needle advanced slightly medial and cephalad through the paraspinous muscles. Any bone the needle encounters is likely to be ipsilateral lamina, and the needle is walked off superiorly or inferiorly into CSF.

An alternative to midline or paramedian approaches is the Taylor (lumbosacral) approach, which uses the largest interspace in the vertebral column at L5 to S1. The posterior superior iliac spine is identified, and the skin entered 1.0 cm medial and 1.0 cm inferior to this point. The needle is directed medially and cephalad to enter the spinal canal in the midline at L5 to S1. If the needle contacts bony sacrum, it may be walked off into CSF.

Agents for Spinal Anesthesia

Satisfactory spinal anesthesia requires that the block extend to the dermatomes needed for the operation (described previously), last longer than the procedure, and be profound enough to block all sensory modalities (and, at times, motor function as well). In addition, spinal or epidural anesthesia that extends no farther than necessary limits side effects. Local anesthetics produce predictable results in peripheral blocks because they are delivered undiluted directly to the nerves. In subarachnoid anesthesia, local anesthetics in volumes of 1 to 10 ml are diluted, perhaps unevenly, in about 40 ml of CSF and spread from the site of injection to produce an often unpredicted extent of anesthesia.

LOCAL ANESTHETIC SOLUTIONS

As in other applications, the duration of action of local anesthetics in spinal anesthesia is greater for drugs with greater lipid solubility: tetracaine and bupivacaine are longer acting (90 to 240 minutes in usual doses); lidocaine is briefer in its effects (60 minutes). Duration also increases with increasing dose of drug and the addition of vasoconstrictors (0.2 mg of epinephrine, mixed with the local anesthetic solution).

Subarachnoid distribution of the local anesthetic and the dermatomal distribution of the resulting anesthesia are primarily influenced by the density of the injected solution relative to CSF and the position of the vertebral column during and just after injection. The density of a local anesthetic solution is a function of its concentration and the vehicle in which the drug is dissolved. The density of CSF at 37°C is 1.001 to 1.005 gm per ml. Local anesthetic solutions with densities (at 37°C) greater than 1.008 are termed hyperbaric, those with densities between 0.998 and 1.007 are considered to be isobaric, and those with densities less than 0.997 are termed hypobaric. When local anesthetics are prepared in 5 to 8 per cent dextrose, they are hyperbaric solutions; in CSF or isotonic saline they are isobaric; in dilute solution in water (less than 3 mg per ml for tetracaine or bupivacaine) they are hypobaric (Table 18–3).

TABLE 18–3. Physical Characteristics of Spinal Anesthetic Solutions at 37°C

	Density	Specific Gravity	Baricity†
Water	0.9934	1.0000	0.9931
CSF	1.0003	1.0069	1.0000
Tetracaine			
0.33% in water	0.9980	1.0046	0.9977
1.0% in water	1.0003	1.0007	1.0000
0.5% in 50% CSF	0.9998	1.0064	0.9995
0.5% in half normal saline	1.0000	1.0066	0.9997
0.5% in 5% dextrose	1.0136	1.0203	1.0133
Dibucaine			
0.066% in 0.5% saline	0.9970	1.0036	0.9976
Bupivacaine			
0.5% in water	0.9993	1.0059	0.9990
0.5% in 8% dextrose	1.0210	1.0278	1.0207
Procaine			
2.5% in water	0.9983	1.0052	0.9983
Lidocaine			
2% in water	1.0003	1.0066	1.0003
5% in 7.5% dextrose	1.0265	1.0333	1.0265

† Baricity is the ratio of the density of the local anesthetic solution to that of CSF.

Choosing appropriate doses of local anesthetic solutions of known densities, and altering the patient's position allows the anesthesiologist to influence the distribution of local anesthetic. Other factors such as age, height, needle direction, and transmission of increased abdominal pressure to the spinal column are of lesser importance than dose, density, and positioning.

In supine patients, the lumbar lordosis produces a high (anterior) point at L3-4, and the thoracic kyphosis a low (posterior) point at T5-6. Thus, if a patient is given a subarachnoid injection of a hyperbaric local anesthetic solution at L4 and placed supine immediately, the solution will distribute by gravity from the high point to the two lowest regions, the sacrum and T5-6, producing a block that extends well into the thoracic dermatomes.

Isobaric solutions tend to remain at the site of injection and produce a more localized block, usually extending only to the lower thoracic dermatomes. Isobaric solutions are appropriate for lower extremity procedures, but anesthesia of the thoracic dermatomes may be unreliable for this reason.

A "saddle block" confined to the lower lumbar and sacral dermatomes is useful for perineal procedures, and may be produced by injecting hyperbaric solutions with the patient sitting, and maintaining that position for several minutes after injection. Patients in the lateral position may receive hyperbaric solutions if the incision site is on the dependent side, and hypobaric solutions if the site is on the nondependent side. Similarly, patients in the prone position may receive hypobaric solutions if the surgical site is in the lumbosacral area, such as for hemorrhoidectomy.

These guidelines for using the density of the local anesthesia solution to control the distribution

TABLE 18–4. **Dose Ranges for Local Anesthetic in Subarachnoid Anesthesia***

Drug	Local Anesthetic Concentration (%)	Total Dose (mg)	Volume (ml)	Expected Duration Without Epinephrine (hours)	Glucose Concentration (% W/V)
Lidocaine, hyperbaric	5	25 to 100	0.5 to 2	1	7.5
Lidocaine, isobaric	2	20 to 100	1 to 5	1	0 (in water)
Tetracaine, hyperbaric	0.5	3 to 20	0.6 to 4	2	5
Tetracaine, isobaric	1 (in water)	3 to 20	0.3 to 2.0	2 to 3	0 (in water)
Tetracaine, hypobaric	<0.3	3 to 20	1 to 7	2	0 (in water)
Bupivacaine, isobaric	0.5	3 to 20	0.6 to 4	2 to 3	0 (in saline)
Bupivacaine, hyperbaric	0.75	3 to 20	0.5 to 3	2	8.5

* The doses given cover a wider range than is usually given in such tables, as explained in the text. Conventional doses lie at the midpoint of the range. The expected duration of effect is given in hours to reflect the uncertainty of such predictions.

of the anesthetic are reliable. Less reliable are rules that relate the dose to the resulting level. Hyperbaric solutions of local anesthetic, usually made up in small volumes, distribute themselves according to gravity, and not dose. In general, as compared to smaller doses, greater doses of subarachnoid local anesthetic produce more extensive anesthesia that is more profound and lasts longer. When the patient's position and the density of the local anesthetic solution strongly direct the drug to one area (as in a saddle block performed with the patient sitting for several minutes), increases in dose do not enhance the extent of the anesthetic but instead produce a more profound and longer lasting block. Because of these effects, Table 18–4 gives suggested dose ranges for spinal anesthesia, but does not correlate dose with the expected extent of anesthesia.

It is sometimes possible to predict the distribution of spinal anesthesia with single-injection techniques. If a hyperbaric drug is injected with the patient sitting, and the patient remains sitting for several minutes, the anesthesia level rarely rises above T10. If larger doses (15 to 20 mg of tetracaine or bupivacaine) in hyperbaric solution are injected with the patient in the lateral position, and the patient is turned promptly supine, high thoracic levels usually follow. If doses taken from the middle of the ranges given for hyperbaric drugs (Table 18–4) are given to patients in the lateral position, and the patient immediately turned supine, low to mid thoracic levels often result, but these intermediate levels of anesthesia cannot be guaranteed with single-injection techniques.

The effects of a given dose of drug in the subarachnoid space exhibit considerable biological variability. Using the same dose of drug for all patients and expecting the same results is as unrealistic for spinal anesthesia as for general anesthesia. Some patients cannot tolerate inadvertent high levels of spinal anesthesia, yet require regional anesthesia for best management; for these patients, a continuous subarachnoid block technique provides more predictable results.

VASOCONSTRICTORS

Vasoconstrictors such as epinephrine (0.2 to 0.3 mg), or phenylephrine (2.0 to 5.0 mg), are added to local anesthetic solutions to prolong the duration of spinal anesthesia. Vasoconstrictors in the CSF are believed to decrease spinal cord and meningeal blood flow, delaying elimination of local anesthetic. Vasodilating effects of local anesthetics may partially antagonize vasoconstrictors, but the end result is prolongation of conduction block. In addition to decreasing local blood flow, vasoconstrictors exert a direct antinociceptive effect themselves on the spinal cord, and thus may contribute to the quality of sensory anesthesia.

SUBARACHNOID OPIOIDS

Narcotic analgesics may be added to spinal anesthetic solutions to improve the quality of sensorimotor blockade, and to produce postoperative spinal analgesia. Morphine, 0.1 to 0.25 mg, produces significant postoperative analgesia; fentanyl, 5 to 25 μg, provides briefer effects; useful intraoperatively. Postoperative respiratory monitoring is necessary to detect and treat delayed respiratory depression, should this occur (see Chapters 10 and 36).

Clinical Management of Spinal Anesthesia

The minutes following local anesthetic injection into the CSF are crucial, demanding that full attention be paid to the patient. The exigent tasks are to ensure adequate distribution of spinal anesthesia, and to promptly diagnose and treat side effects, principally arterial hypotension. The patient is positioned to distribute the anesthesia as anticipated by the dose and baricity of the solution used. Sensory and motor function are assessed frequently to monitor onset and distribution of the block. Automated blood pressure cuffs are set to cycle every minute initially, and arterial hypotension is treated promptly. Supplemental oxygen is continued, and arterial oxygenation monitored via pulse oximetry.

The distribution of spinal anesthesia can be measured in several ways. The level of sympathetic block is approximated by testing somatic cold perception, which is mediated by nerve fibers of diameter and conduction velocity similar to those of sympathetic afferents. Somatosensory levels are obtained by response to pinprick. Motor function is tested by asking the patient to plantar flex the toes (S1 to S2), dorsiflex the foot (L4 to L5), raise the knees (L2 to L3), or tense the rectus muscles (T6 to T12) by lifting the head.

During spinal and epidural anesthesia, the level of sympathetic block extends higher than that of sensory block, which in turn extends higher than that of motor block. A credible explanation for this consistently observed phenomenon of "differential block" has been elusive. It is now known that myelinated, rapidly conducting, large diameter motor fibers (A-alpha) are no more resistant to conduction block than thinly myelinated, slower conducting, smaller diameter sensory and sympathetic fibers (A-delta, B, and C fibers), when exposed to local anesthetics in vitro over sufficient fiber lengths. Current hypotheses propose concentration gradients of local anesthetic and variations in exposed nerve-root lengths, to explain differential block in spinal and epidural anesthesia.

As a rule, the block from shorter acting agents such as procaine or lidocaine is fixed after about five minutes after injection, allowing only this period of time to alter patient position to influence the distribution of anesthesia. Longer acting agents such as tetracaine or bupivacaine require about ten minutes to become fixed. However, even long after these periods of time, the level of anesthesia can spread when the patient is moved, emphasizing the need for continuous monitoring and for care in repositioning patients after subarachnoid block. Vasoconstrictors may delay the onset of anesthesia, in addition to prolonging its duration.

Continuous Spinal Anesthesia

Continuous spinal anesthesia can be provided through a catheter placed into the CSF via intentional dural puncture. As compared to epidural anesthesia, this technique offers the usual advantages of spinal anesthesia: more rapid onset and more certain effect. This technique has two advantages over single-injection subarachnoid anesthesia: prolonged block may be provided for lengthy operations, and small incremental doses of local anesthetic may be given to produce precisely the desired level of anesthesia. The local anesthetic solutions and principles governing distribution of anesthesia are the same as those for singe-injection techniques, but longer acting drugs and vasoconstrictors are not required. Despite the use of larger bore epidural needles (16 to 18 gauge), the incidence of postdural puncture headache following transdural catheter placement appears to be acceptably small. This may represent an effect of the catheter producing early closure of the dural hole or the fact that anesthesiologists usually offer this technique only to older patients in whom postdural puncture headache is less common.

Complications of Spinal Anesthesia

Complications resulting from spinal anesthesia may be immediate or delayed. Immediate complications result from transient physiologic effects of neural blockade and are readily anticipated and treated; they include arterial hypotension, high spinal anesthesia with ventilatory inadequacy, and nausea. Delayed complications include postdural puncture headache, back pain, urinary retention, and neurologic injury.

ARTERIAL HYPOTENSION

Arterial hypotension results from blockade of preganglionic vasomotor efferents of the sympathetic nervous system, which traverse the subarachnoid and epidural spaces with the spinal nerve roots before diverging to the paravertebral chain ganglia as the white rami communicantes. The severity of hypotension parallels the extent of sympathetic blockade. The level of sympathetic blockade may extend as high as six dermatomes above the level of sensory blockade, accounting for hypotension occasionally seen even with lower sensory levels of spinal anesthesia.

Hypotension is caused by decreased cardiac output, resulting from decreased venous return as blood pools in the dilated venous capacitance system. Decreased arteriolar tone appears to play only a lesser role in the hypotension after subarachnoid anesthesia in healthy patients. Bradycardia after spinal anesthesia may result from blockade of the cardioaccelerator fibers at T1 to T4, and also contributes to the decrease in cardiac output.

Patients with hypovolemia, in whom the sympathetic nervous system maintains increased arteriolar and venous tone, may suffer profound hypotension and cardiac arrest with spinal anesthesia. Spinal anesthesia is unsafe in such patients and must be delayed until volume resuscitation is complete.

Frequent blood pressure determinations after beginning spinal anesthesia are required to allow early diagnosis of hypotension. Treatment is directed at maintaining adequate tissue oxygen delivery. Oxygen is administered, with monitoring via pulse oximetry. Cardiac output is supported by rapid infusion of intravenous fluids, and elevation of the legs when possible. These measures alone are adequate in the majority of cases. For refractory or profound hypotension, intravenous vasopressors (ephedrine 5 to 10 mg, or phenylephrine 50 to 100 μg) may be necessary. Atropine 0.4 mg intravenously is given for bradycardia.

HIGH SPINAL ANESTHESIA WITH VENTILATORY INADEQUACY

High levels of spinal anesthesia are associated with complete block of the preganglionic thoracolumbar (T1 to L2) outflow comprising the sympathetic nervous system. Such blocks are occasionally associated with fulminant hypotension, which transiently results in global cerebral hypoperfusion. The typical patient is hypotensive, agitated, dyspneic, and nauseated. Absence of proprioceptive input from the blocked intercostal musculature may contribute to the sensation of dyspnea, although remaining diaphragmatic function (C3 to C5 myotomes) should be sufficient to maintain adequate pulmonary ventilation. Rapid correction of the hypotension may resolve the problem; in such cases the patient may require reassurance from the anesthesiologist that ventilation is adequate. Rarely, patients require manually assisted ventilation or tracheal intubation, controlled ventilation, and light general anesthesia, in which case it can be anticipated that these patients will be sensitive to the cardiovascular depressant effects of general anesthetic agents. In choosing treatment, high spinal anesthesia with ventilatory depression is distinguished from total spinal anesthesia, which includes block of the motor innervation to the diaphragm.

In the past, prophylactic fluids and pressors were routine in managing spinal anesthesia for all patients, not just parturients and others at special risk. Lately, it has become the practice to treat the cardiovascular and respiratory sequelae of spinal anesthesia expectantly, reserving pressors and fluids that engender complications of their own until a clear need appears. However, as demonstrated recently in an analysis of closed claims involving sudden death among healthy patients undergoing spinal anesthesia, what appears to be mild hypotension and appropriate sedation can progress abruptly to cardiac arrest. This may be due to the synergistic effects of sedatives, opioids, sympathectomy, and partial respiratory paralysis. These cases emphasize the importance of vigilance and early treatment (if not prophylactic use of pressors) in managing even the usual cardiopulmonary depression of spinal anesthesia.

NAUSEA

Nausea immediately following spinal anesthesia may be the first sign of hypotension and cerebral hypoperfusion. Commonly, the patient complains of nausea before the hypotension is recognized, especially in obstetric patients. Another contributor to nausea with spinal anesthesia may be a relative excess of parasympathetic tone in the gastrointestinal tract, either related to chemical sympathectomy or surgical traction on the peritoneum. Intravenous atropine may ameliorate refractory nausea once normal blood pressure has been restored. Other antiemetics, such as droperidol or metoclopramide, may also be helpful.

URINARY RETENTION

Micturition is dependent on intact innervation of the urethral sphincter and bladder musculature. Lower extremity motor and sensory function appear to recover before bladder function, especially with the longer acting spinal agents such as tetracaine or bupivacaine. When spinal anesthesia has been accompanied by vigorous fluid administration, or is not completely resolved, bladder distention may require catheter drainage.

PAIN DURING OPERATION

Despite what appears to be successful delivery of an adequate dose of local anesthetic into the CSF (free flow of CSF from the needle before and after injection of the drug), some patients report discomfort during the surgical procedure. If pain occurs early, with skin incision, this likely represents misplaced drug; injection of radiocontrast medium between the dura and the arachnoid has been demonstrated, and such injection of local anesthetic would produce less anesthetic effect than expected from subarachnoid injection.

Later in the operation, pain usually represents recession of the spinal level. At times, patients experience pain despite a persisting level of spinal anesthesia that should be adequate to block sensation; this often involves intolerable aching at the site of a pneumatic tourniquet about the thigh ("tourniquet pain"). The classic explanation for this mysterious phenomenon is transmission of pain through sympathetic fibers entering the cord at levels above the level of the block. This seems unlikely, as tourniquet pain can be seen despite spinal anesthesia levels of T4 and higher.

The explanation may lie in incomplete assessment of the extent of spinal anesthesia. To determine that the upper level of anesthesia is apparently high enough (usually to pinprick or to cold) to block the pain involved is not the same as exploring for missed dermatomes or assessing the density of the block. One series of cases demonstrated that patients under spinal anesthesia recover the ability to sense the scratch of a finger before recovering sensitivity to pinprick; no patient experienced tourniquet pain who had not recovered the ability to sense finger scratch just proximal to the tourniquet. It seems likely that tourniquet pain, as well as other forms of pain during spinal anesthesia, represents insufficient concentrations of local anesthetic in neural tissue. Prevention of this phenomenon likely involves the use of adequate doses of local anesthetic; opioids added to the local anesthetic mixture may be of help too.

Regardless of the cause, the patient's pain requires appropriate treatment. If an epidural or subarachnoid catheter is in place, injecting additional local anesthetic solution is the best treatment. Because the pain is likely to lessen when the incision is closed or the tourniquet is deflated, postoperative oversedation is likely when large doses of sedatives and narcotics are administered intraoperatively to overcome this problem. Light general anesthesia usually is more satisfactory.

BACKACHE

Backache has been demonstrated to be no more common following spinal anesthesia than general anesthesia. It is probably caused by the ligamentous strain occurring with paraspinous muscle relaxation and positioning for operation, which accompany both regional and general anesthesia (see Chapter 16).

POSTDURAL PUNCTURE HEADACHE

Headache owing to dural puncture (spinal headache or postdural puncture headache), typically presents 24 to 48 hours following lumbar puncture. It may occur following diagnostic lumbar puncture or myelography as well as spinal anesthesia. The headache is frontal or occipital, with or without visual or auditory symptoms, worsened by sitting or standing, and relieved by lying down. Spinal headache must be distinguished from other forms of headache, such as tension headache, migraine headache, and cluster headache. A true spinal headache must have a postural component. Symptoms are provoked by traction on intracranial contents, including the cranial nerves, which is caused by fluid leakage across the dural rent in the lumbar cistern.

The incidence of spinal headache is greater in younger patients and women, especially during pregnancy. Any measure that results in a smaller

Table 18–5. Measures to Reduce the Incidence and Severity of Postdural Puncture Headache

- Small spinal needle: 25 to 27 gauge preferred
- Aperture in end of needle facing laterally, so that the bevel parts the longitudinal fibers of the dura, rather than transecting them
- Oblique puncture, as in paramedian approach
- Round-tipped, unbeveled needles
- Patient selection: avoiding especially the young, female, and pregnant patient.

hole in the dura or the transection of fewer dural fibers reduces the rate of CSF leak and consequently the severity and likelihood of headache (Table 18–5).

Treatment usually begins with conservative measures such as intravenous or oral hydration to encourage CSF production, abdominal binders to increase lumbar spinal canal pressures, and analgesics, and is usually effective. Keeping patients supine after spinal anesthesia does not prevent headache, but merely delays its presentation.

If headache persists despite this therapy, caffeine administered orally or intravenously (500 mg caffeine sodium benzoate in 1000 ml intravenous saline) appears to be effective in as many as 70 per cent of patients. Caffeine is a cerebral vasoconstrictor, and may work by attenuating reflex cerebral vasodilation in response to low intracranial CSF pressure.

The definitive treatment for spinal headache is an epidural blood patch. An epidural needle is placed in the epidural space at or near the level of the previous dural puncture. Ten to twenty ml of fresh, aseptically drawn autologous blood is injected slowly until the headache resolves or the patient complains of lumbar fullness or radicular pain. Blood patching is reported effective in greater than 95 per cent of cases. With one repetition in refractory cases, the success rate approaches 100 per cent. The risks include transitory backache, an inadvertent second dural puncture, and the other risks of dural puncture. Usually, this treatment is employed only after other measures have failed, but it has been applied prophylactically after inadvertent dural puncture with attempted epidural anesthesia in patients at increased risk for spinal headache.

NEUROLOGIC INJURY

Neurologic deficits after spinal anesthesia are rare. These may take the form of sensory, motor, or combined deficits. Reviews of large series of patients cite an incidence of less than 1 in 10,000, a figure similar to the incidence of major morbidity and mortality reported from general anesthesia. The majority of these are sensory deficits, and resolve spontaneously within six months. Identifiable causes include infectious meningitis, chemical arachnoiditis, spinal cord ischemia, and needle trauma. Infectious and chemical causes have been virtually eliminated since their peak incidence in the 1940s by the introduction of sterile spinal anesthesia kits containing purified, preservative-free local anesthetics in dilute concentrations. Spinal cord ischemia may be caused by systemic hypotension, surgical traction, epidural hematoma formation, or a combination of these factors. Needle trauma as a cause of neurologic deficit is difficult to document, but is rare. Nonetheless, it is prudent to reposition the needle tip when the patient reports a paresthesia, as this may indicate that the needle tip lies in a nerve.

Some neurologic diseases such as multiple sclerosis may worsen after operation and anesthesia. Although a direct cause-and-effect relationship has not been established, for medicolegal reasons regional anesthesia is often avoided in patients with chronic neurologic disease, unless it is specifically indicated and the patient gives informed consent.

When a neurologic deficit presents following spinal or epidural anesthesia and operation, rapid diagnosis and treatment are essential. Neurologic consultation and spinal cord imaging via computerized tomography or magnetic resonance are obtained immediately to rule out epidural hematoma, for which an emergency operation may be indicated.

Epidural Anesthesia

Epidural anesthesia resembles subarachnoid anesthesia, but results from injection of local anesthetic into the spinal epidural space. The site of neural blockade is believed to be the spinal nerve roots where they emerge through thinnings in their dural cuffs. Local anesthetics given into the epidural space also enter the CSF by diffusion through the dura and by transport via arachnoid granulations; this may contribute to the resulting analgesia as well.

Technique

LUMBAR EPIDURAL ANESTHESIA

Epidural anesthesia is most readily performed in the lumbar region. Here the spinous processes are least angulated, the interlaminar spaces largest, and the distance between the ligamentum flavum and dura greatest, as compared to the thoracic or cervical regions. Disposable, sterile epidural anesthesia kits are widely available. The patient is positioned as for spinal anesthesia and the skin prepared. Maintaining sterile technique, an intradermal local anesthetic wheal is raised over the chosen interspace, after which a 1.5-inch needle is used to infiltrate local anesthetic in the subcutaneous tissue and to determine a suitable angle of insertion for the epidural needle.

The needle for epidural anesthesia differs from that for spinal anesthesia in that it is usually larger (18 gauge), to permit passage of a catheter, and designed with a side-facing orifice and a blunt tip, to reduce the chance of perforating the dura. A stylet or obturator occludes the orifice while the needle passes through the skin, to prevent cutting a plug of skin. The needle is inserted through the skin wheal and passed in the midline sagittal plane slightly cephalad until the spinal ligaments are engaged.

The stylet is then removed, and an air- or liquid-filled syringe with a freely moveable plunger is attached to the needle. The dorsum of the nondominant hand is braced on the patient's back, while the thumb and index or middle finger grasp the needle shaft or hub.

The nondominant hand controls the advance of the epidural needle in 1 to 2-mm increments, while the thumb of the dominant hand intermittently depresses the plunger of the syringe. As long as the tip of the needle is buried in the ligaments, the fluid in the syringe cannot escape. As the needle tip penetrates the ligamentum flavum, it becomes easier to advance the needle, and the plunger of the syringe is easily depressed as the air or liquid enters the epidural space (''loss of resistance''). An alternative method of identifying the epidural space is to substitute a drop of sterile fluid in the needle hub for the syringe, and observe the drawing-in of this ''hanging drop'' by the negative pressure in the epidural space, which results from tenting of the dura by the needle tip or transmission of subatmospheric intrathoracic pressure.

As with spinal anesthesia, when the midline approach is unsuccessful, the paramedian or Taylor approaches may be used as alternatives.

For brief procedures, a single dose of appropriate local anesthetic solution may be injected and the needle removed. An epidural catheter allows maintenance of anesthesia for procedures of long or uncertain duration, as well as allowing for postoperative spinal analgesia with local anesthetics, narcotics, or other agents (see Chapter 36).

Plastic epidural catheters, with or without stylets and usually with depth markings, are passed 2 to 4 cm into the epidural space. The epidural needle is then removed over the catheter. Catheters must never be withdrawn through the needle, as they may shear off and remain in the epidural space. Catheters are usually secured with tape, and syringe adapters with bacterial filters attached to the proximal end. Upon removal of the catheter, the entry site is dressed and a note made recording that the tip of the catheter was removed intact.

THORACIC EPIDURAL ANESTHESIA

For upper abdominal or thoracic procedures, thoracic epidural anesthesia offers more direct access for the local anesthetic to the nerve roots to be anesthetized. Principles and procedures are the same as for lumbar epidural anesthesia. Midline or paramedian approaches may be used.

The greater angulation of the spinous processes requires steeper angles of needle insertion in this region than in the lumbar spine (hub of the needle depressed 45 degrees instead of 10 to 15 degrees in the lumbar spine). Because of the ready transmission of negative pressure to the thoracic epidural space from the chest cavity, the hanging drop method is frequently employed.

The advantage of the thoracic epidural technique over the lumbar epidural route is that it produces more localized effects, sparing the lower extremities and permitting lesser total drug doses. Because the distance from the ligamentum flavum to the dura and spinal cord is less in the thoracic region, thoracic epidural anesthesia is a demanding technique reserved for those who have mastered the lumbar technique.

Agents for Epidural Anesthesia

The choice of local anesthetic agent for epidural anesthesia is primarily determined by the duration of the surgical procedure and the desired intensity of motor blockade (see Chapter 17, Table 17–5). For epidural anesthesia, a popular short-acting local anesthetic is chloroprocaine; lidocaine and mepivacaine are intermediate in their actions; bupivacaine and etidocaine are long acting. Increasing the concentration of a given agent produces a shorter latency, greater intensity of motor blockade, and a longer duration of action. Bupivacaine is remarkable among the agents in producing a less intense motor blockade for any degree of sensory blockade, which makes it useful for analgesia during labor.

EPINEPHRINE

Addition of epinephrine to epidural local anesthetics in a concentration of 5 μg per ml (1:200,000 W/V) intensifies the sensorimotor block and increases by 50 per cent the duration of the block produced by the short- and intermediate-acting anesthetics. Epinephrine produces little prolongation of the actions of long-acting drugs such as bupivacaine and etidocaine. The use of epinephrine also results in decreased systemic blood concentrations of all local anesthetics following epidural administration.

Small amounts of epinephrine absorbed from the epidural space produce predominantly beta-adrenergic effects, decreasing systemic vascular resistance and increasing heart rate. The addition of epinephrine to local anesthetic solutions exacerbates the hypotension accompanying epidural anesthesia.

TEST DOSES

Much greater volumes of local anesthetic solution are required in the epidural space than in the subarachnoid space. Because of these large doses, before each epidural injection special precautions are required to be sure that the drug will not be injected inadvertently into the CSF or into an epidural vein. Before each injection, one draws back the plunger of the syringe. If no blood or CSF returns from the epidural needle or catheter, a small dose of local anesthetic solution is administered, chosen to produce safe but observable effects if given into the CSF or a vein.

This test dose consists of 3 ml of local anesthetic of a concentration appropriate for epidural anesthesia, containing 15 μg of epinephrine (1:200,000 W/V). Subarachnoid injection is recognized by the prompt onset of motor paralysis and sensory block, consistent with spinal anesthesia. Following administration of 15 μg of epinephrine, an increase in heart rate of 20 beats per minute or greater occurring within two minutes and lasting 35 seconds is sensitive and specific for intravenous injection. In the presence of beta-adrenergic blockade, the alpha-adrenergic effects of epinephrine are manifest, producing an increase of 15 mm Hg or greater in systolic blood pressure, with no change or even a reflex slowing of heart rate.

ANESTHETIC DOSES

Appropriate volumes of local anesthetic solution for lumbar epidural anesthesia range from 15 to 25 ml. Studies in young volunteers indicate a mean requirement of 1.6 ml per spinal segment anesthetized. Doses in the smaller thoracic epidural space are approximately one half this. Older patients require lesser volumes of local anesthetic solution to achieve a given distribution of epidural anesthesia. This is probably due to infiltration of connective tissue in the epidural space in later years with decreased leakage of drug around dural cuffs.

In contrast to spinal anesthesia, studies in humans usually fail to demonstrate a significant effect of posture on the subsequent distribution of epidural anesthesia. Instead, the dermatomal distribution of epidural anesthesia tends to be centered about the tip of the needle or catheter. Cephalad spread occurs more readily than caudad spread following lumbar epidural injection.

SUCCESSIVE DOSES OF LOCAL ANESTHETIC

The need for additional doses of epidural local anesthetic is determined by clinical observation. When anesthesia has regressed by two dermatomes, the addition of one third to one half the initial dose of local anesthetic maintains adequate anesthesia. Interpatient variability requires individualized dosing regimens. The ability to adjust the duration and distribution of continuous catheter epidural anesthesia is advantageous in some cases.

TACHYPHYLAXIS

Tachyphylaxis during epidural anesthesia denotes decreasing dermatomal spread and duration of epidural block following repeated administration of a given dose of local anesthetic. The basis for this apparent acute tolerance is unclear. Possible explanations include a decreased effect of local anesthetic at the cellular level, increased drug elimination from the epidural space over time, or altered distribution of drug within the epidural space itself. The phenomenon may be overcome by increasing drug delivery to the epidural space, bearing in mind the limitations imposed by systemic local anesthetic toxicity.

OPIOIDS

Opioids may be added to local anesthetic mixtures used in the epidural space, just as they are used in spinal anesthesia, with the same benefits, but in appropriately greater doses (see Chapters 10 and 36).

Clinical Management of Epidural Anesthesia

Immediate management of epidural anesthesia is similar to that of spinal anesthesia, except that anesthesia develops more slowly, allowing the onset of hypotension to be detected more readily and treatment to be begun before profound hypotension ensues. As position has little effect on the spread of drugs in the epidural space, assessment of the level of anesthesia is not made as frequently and the patient's position is not changed to alter the distribution of anesthesia. Monitoring of heart rate, blood pressure, oxygenation, and the level of anesthesia are similar, as is treatment with fluids, vasopressors, oxygen, and sedatives.

COMPLICATIONS

The immediate and delayed complications of epidural anesthesia are similar to those of spinal anesthesia with the added risks of local anesthetic toxicity and unwanted dural puncture.

Systemic Local Anesthetic Toxicity. The large doses of local anesthetic used in epidural anesthetics impose the risk of immediate and delayed systemic local anesthetic toxicity. Immediate local anesthetic toxicity results from direct intravascular administration. Delayed local anesthetic toxicity follows systemic uptake of large amounts of local anesthetic. In either case, the syndrome usually presents as CNS toxicity with or without cardiovascular changes (see Chapter 17).

This risk is reduced by the use of test doses to detect intravascular injection, and epinephrine to reduce uptake of the local anesthetic from the epidural space. In addition, longer operations are best managed with longer acting agents such as bupivacaine, so that frequent reinjection and summation of successive peaks of blood-drug concentration does not occur. The addition of opioids to the local anesthesia mixture allows the use of smaller doses of local anesthetic as well.

Headache and Inadvertent Dural Puncture. The risk of headache following inadvertent dural puncture during epidural anesthesia is great, because of the large diameter of epidural needles. In such an event, four courses are possible. (1) A subarachnoid catheter can be passed and the anesthetic managed as a continuous spinal anesthetic; (2) a single dose of local anesthetic in appropriate dose can be administered to produce spinal anesthesia; (3) the needle can be removed and epidural analgesia attempted at another interspace; or (4) the needle can be withdrawn to the epidural space and an epidural catheter passed at the same site. The choice will depend on a number of factors, including at least the patient's age, the duration of the operation, and the severity of illness. If an epidural catheter is successfully placed following dural puncture, a prophylactic epidural blood patch may be considered.

CAUDAL ANESTHESIA

Because of delayed and sometimes unsatisfactory caudad spread of local anesthetics from the lumbar epidural space, epidural anesthesia for procedures involving the lower lumbar or sacral dermatomes (ankle or anorectal procedures) may be accomplished via the caudal route. The needle passes through the sacral hiatus to reach the caudal portion of the epidural space.

Anatomy

The sacrum is formed by the fusion of the five sacral vertebrae (Fig. 18–4). This triangular bone

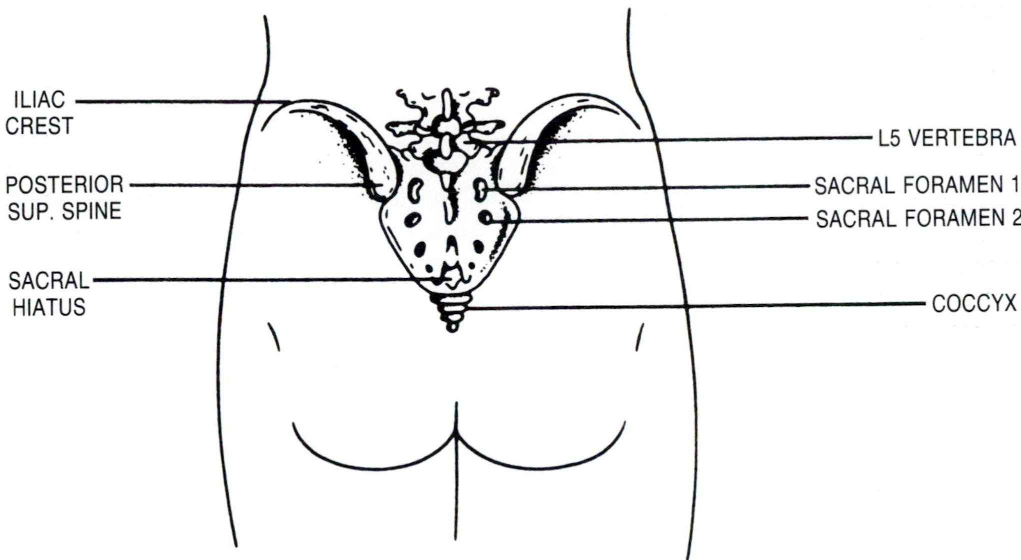

FIGURE 18–4. *View of the sacrum, showing the sacral hiatus.*

articulates with the lumbar spine superiorly, the iliac bones laterally, and the coccyx inferiorly. The sacral (caudal) canal is the inferior continuation of the spinal canal and terminates at the sacral hiatus, which is bounded bilaterally by the bony prominences of the sacral cornua. The hiatus results from lack of fusion with, or absence of, the fourth and fifth sacral vertebrae. It is covered by the sacrococcygeal ligament, which is formed from the supraspinous ligament, interspinous ligament, and ligamentum flavum.

Technique

Caudal anesthesia is usually performed with the patient prone and the heels turned outward to relax and separate the buttocks and expose the hiatus. After sterile skin preparation and draping, the sacral cornua are identified and the skin and underlying ligaments between them infiltrated with local anesthetic. An epidural (or other) needle is inserted at a 45-degree angle to the sacrum between the two cornua. After passing through the sacrococcygeal membrane with a loss of resistance, the needle tip will contact the ventral plate of the sacral canal. The needle is then withdrawn a few millimeters from the periosteum, the hub depressed 5 to 15 degrees, and the needle tip advanced 2 cm into the canal.

If the needle tip is correctly positioned within the osseous sacral canal below the dural sac, CSF cannot be aspirated and a few milliliters of air can be injected without a sensation of crepitus over the needle tip.

The anesthetic is conducted as for lumbar epidural, although approximately twice the volume (3 ml per spinal segment) of drug is required because of the large size of the sacral canal and the free leakage of solution through the sacral foramina.

Applications

Caudal anesthesia has declined in popularity for adults because of a failure rate of 10 to 15 per cent, which is related to anatomic irregularities of the sacrum. The technique is more useful in pediatric patients, in whom the landmarks are easier to identify, and in whom anesthetic spread is more consistent (see Chapter 25).

THE CHOICE OF SPINAL OR EPIDURAL ANESTHESIA

Almost always, if major conduction anesthesia is appropriate, either spinal or epidural anesthesia can be made to work. However, there are differences in the techniques that favor one over the other for some applications.

Epidural anesthesia is often chosen over spinal anesthesia to avoid headache, especially in patients at increased risk for headache (parturients). Although a successful epidural anesthetic by definition avoids dural puncture and postdural puncture headache, even in experienced hands the risk of dural puncture during epidural anesthesia is not zero (perhaps 1 per cent). After such a puncture, the risk of headache is greater than after a spinal anesthetic with a small needle. If regional anesthesia is required and even a small risk of headache is unacceptable, lumbar plexus block or specific nerve blocks of the lower extremity are preferred (see Chapter 19).

When very rapid onset of anesthesia is required, subarachnoid block is faster than epidural. Also, because it is sometimes impossible to thread a catheter into the epidural space and the distribution of epidural anesthesia is sometimes incomplete, spinal anesthesia may be the better choice when a failed or incomplete regional anesthetic must be avoided. Because spread of local anesthetic caudad from the lumbar epidural space is sometimes poor, spinal or caudal epidural anesthesia may be preferred to lumbar epidural anesthesia when anesthesia of sacral roots is required.

Because of the rapid spread of local anesthetic in the CSF and the immediate onset of hypotension after subarachnoid block, epidural anesthesia is sometimes chosen when sudden changes in blood pressure are anticipated. The advantage enjoyed by epidural anesthesia in this regard is slight, and choosing epidural anesthesia does not replace correction of hypovolemia, careful monitoring, and timely treatment of changes in blood pressure.

If the total dose of local anesthetic must be kept to a minimum, as has been recommended in the management of anesthesia for women in the first trimester of pregnancy, spinal anesthesia can be provided with much smaller doses of local anesthesia than can epidural. There is no direct evidence to support this recommendation, however.

Lastly, some patients accept epidural anesthesia who refuse spinal anesthesia. Provided the patient has a real understanding of the nature of epidural anesthesia and the risk of inadvertent dural puncture, the patient's prejudice may be a reason to choose epidural anesthesia.

REFERENCES

Bromage PR. Epidural analgesia. Philadelphia: WB Saunders, 1978.

Cousins MJ, Bridenbaugh PO, eds. Neural blockage. 2nd ed. Philadelphia: JB Lippincott, 1988.

Greene NM. The physiology of spinal anesthesia. 3rd ed. Baltimore: Williams & Wilkins, 1983.

Raj PP. Handbook of regional anesthesia. New York: Churchill Livingstone, 1985.

CHAPTER NINETEEN

Nerve Blocks

Peripheral nerve blocks are used by themselves to produce surgical anesthesia, as supplements to general anesthesia, and to provide postoperative analgesia. Selected blocks are used for diagnosis and treatment of chronic pain syndromes (see Chapter 32). Although only specialists seek to master the many nerve blocks that have been described, all anesthesiologists benefit from understanding the technical fundamentals of a basic group of nerve blocks for adult patients, as described in this chapter. (Pediatric applications are discussed in Chapter 25.)

Fundamentals Common to All Nerve Blocks

The considerations in choosing a nerve block to replace or supplement general anesthesia are similar to those described for spinal or epidural anesthesia. In contrast to spinal or epidural anesthesia, the physiologic changes that result from peripheral neural blockade are usually negligible, and the areas of the head, neck, and upper extremity may be blocked safely; these factors make peripheral nerve blocks more widely applicable than spinal or epidural anesthesia. It is sometimes more difficult and time consuming to locate peripheral nerves than the subarachnoid or epidural spaces, perhaps accounting for the lack of popularity of peripheral nerve blocks.

Patient Preparation

Preoperative evaluation before peripheral nerve block is similar to that preceding general anesthesia, as an alternative plan for airway control and safe general anesthesia is always required. In addition, the physical examination includes examination of the site of the planned block and a search for preexisting neurological defects. Specific laboratory tests of the coagulation system are indicated only when suggested by the history and physical examination.

Relative contraindications to regional anesthesia include local or systemic infection, and coagulopathy. As with spinal anesthesia, there is little reason to fear that a peripheral nerve block will worsen nerve damage already present. Nevertheless, some anesthesiologists withhold regional anesthesia from patients with neurological disease. In many cases, one can anticipate differentiating (rare) nerve damage due to the block from damage owing to operation or medical disease; for example, there can be no confusion between damage to the median nerve due to axillary block and that owing to exploration at the wrist. In cases such as this, regional anesthesia can be performed with no fear of diagnostic confusion postoperatively.

The only absolute contraindication to nerve block anesthesia is the patient's refusal, but often this can be averted by appropriate reassurance. Patients are told that sedation can be provided during the procedure, that they will not actually observe the operation, and that general anesthesia will be available if needed. As described in Chapter 4, premedication often consists of intravenous sedation administered in the operating suite. Full disclosure to the patient of potential risks and benefits is documented in the preanesthetic note.

Equipment

Proper performance of regional anesthesia requires appropriate needles, syringes, and other ancillary equipment. Sterile, disposable nerve block trays or their individual components are widely available.

NEEDLES

Needles for nerve blocks are small in diameter (22 gauge or smaller) and long enough to reach the intended target. Short bevel needles, such as the 45-degree block needles or the 23-degree "B bevel" needles, are superior to the long-bevel needles used for intramuscular injections (17-degree "A bevel"), because they more readily transmit changes in resistance as the needle passes through tissue (Fig. 19–1). Also, their shorter cutting edges may do less damage to nerves. A security bead on the needle shaft prevents retraction of a distal needle segment below the skin if the shaft breaks at the hub. Needles for use with nerve stimulators include an attachment for the electrode, and are usually insulated along the shaft.

SYRINGES

Syringes with finger rings allow single-handed loading and frequent aspiration during injection of local anesthetic solution, while the opposite hand stabilizes the needle. Standard syringes may require an assistant to aspirate and inject, as well as the use of flexible extension tubing to prevent needle-tip movement during the process.

Locating the Nerve to be Blocked

Successful nerve blocks depend on placing the needle tip near the target nerve and keeping it there throughout the injection of the local anesthetic, while avoiding vital structures near the nerve, such as blood vessels. Thorough knowledge of relevant anatomy is essential. There are several methods used to locate the nerve to be blocked.

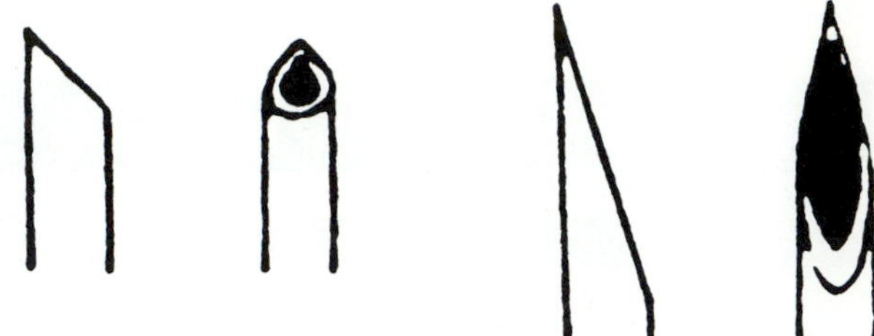

FIGURE 19–1. *On the right is shown the long "A bevel" needle tip, the long edge of which seems to do more nerve damage than the shorter edge of the 45-degree bevel of the block needle on the left. (Modified with permission from Selander D, Dhuner KG, Lundborg G. Peripheral nerve injury due to injection needles used for regional anesthesia. Acta Anesthesiol Scand 1977, 21:186.)*

INFILTRATION

Simple infiltration of local anesthetic solution around bony, vascular, or fascial landmarks can produce a successful block when the precise location of the nerve is uncertain. Only the small fraction of local anesthetic contacting the nerve produces the anesthesia, while the remainder serves to maintain the block. It is especially important to use large volumes of local anesthetic solution with this technique.

PARESTHESIAS

Contact between the needle tip and nerve produces a paresthesia, often described by patients as "electricity" or "hitting the funny bone." Although a paresthesia in the distribution of the nerve sought is good evidence that the needle is in the right place, in some blocks the occurrence of paresthesias is associated with an increase in the (rare) incidence of neuropraxia, which may result from trauma during localization and injection. If paresthesia persists, or recurs when the injection is begun, the needle is moved slightly, on the presumption that it is located in the nerve. Some patients do not distinguish paresthesias from other sensations, and others, especially when oversedated, may not report them at all.

NERVE STIMULATORS

Stimulation with weak electrical currents passed through the needle serves to locate peripheral nerves that include motor fibers. Nerve stimulators used for monitoring of neuromuscular blockade are usable if they can provide 0.1 to 3.0 ma, with a display of the current.

An electrical field at the tip of a stimulating needle induces depolarization of myelinated motor efferents as the needle tip approaches a peripheral nerve. The density of such fields decreases markedly with distance from the needle tip; the current required to produce a response decreases as the needle tip nears the nerve. When the current required to elicit a response is 1.0 ma or less, the tip of the needle is close enough to the nerve to assure success of the nerve block.

Advantages of the technique include an objective endpoint that allows more liberal use of sedatives, and the ability to systematically guide the needle tip closer to the nerve by observing changes in electrical current requirements. In addition, the technique may be used for patients who are intoxicated, anesthetized, or unable to communicate effectively. Properly conducted nerve stimulation is painless for the conscious patient, because the depolarization threshold for myelinated motor efferents is less than for unmyelinated sensory afferents. It has been suggested that the probability of neural injury is lessened with this technique, since the needle tip can be directed close to the nerve, but need not touch it.

Conduct of Anesthesia

Some operating suites include holding areas where nerve blocks may be performed to save operating room time and to facilitate teaching. These areas are equipped at a minimum with electrocardiogram (ECG) and blood pressure monitoring, pulse oximeters, intravenous supplies, oxygen, drugs for treating local anesthesia toxicity, and drugs and equipment for airway control and cardiopulmonary resuscitation. Otherwise, blocks may be performed in the operating room itself.

PREMEDICATION

All patients benefit from reassurance and support during nerve blocks. In addition, some patients benefit from sedation and analgesia; midazolam and fentanyl are appropriate medications. Small intravenous doses given repeatedly to produce the desired effect are safest. For some blocks, patient cooperation is needed; for others, where paresthesias are not expected, profound sedation is feasible. During the block, an assistant can support the patient in the required position, as well as provide additional reassurance.

NEEDLE PLACEMENT

The skin is prepared with an antiseptic solution, sterile drapes are applied, and the operator wears sterile gloves. An intradermal wheal of local anesthetic without epinephrine (with added epinephrine these injections are more painful), placed through a 25- or 27-gauge needle, anesthetizes the skin where the block needle is to be placed. The appropriate needle is then advanced toward the neural target. The thumb and index finger of the dominant hand hold the needle, while the wrist rests on an adjacent surface to steady the hand.

When the desired endpoint is reached (paresthesia, motor response to electrical stimulation, or other landmarks), the needle is halted. Success now depends on holding the needle tip near the nerve during the injection. Potential pitfalls include patient movement, failure to hold the needle firmly in place, or recoil of the needle with injection.

CHOICE OF LOCAL ANESTHETIC SOLUTION

As with spinal and epidural anesthesia, the choice of local anesthetic solution depends on the expected duration of the operation and the degree of motor block needed. Chapter 17 contains information on the available local anesthetics; the section on the maximum doses is especially important in managing peripheral nerve blocks, because the use of larger volumes usually produces more certain neural blockade. For some blocks, increasing the pH of the local anesthetic solution (usually with sodium bicarbonate) speeds the onset of the block.

Because of possible direct neurotoxicity and because of limited total volumes possible, the greatest available concentrations of local anesthetics (0.75 per cent bupivacaine, 2.0 per cent lidocaine) are little used for peripheral neural blockade. Moderate concentrations, such as 1 to 1.5 per cent lidocaine or 0.25 to 0.50 per cent bupivacaine, are used more commonly for nerve blocks. Dilute solutions, such as 0.5 per cent lidocaine and 0.125 per cent bupivacaine, are used for infiltration when large volumes are required.

As in the epidural space, epinephrine (5 μg per ml) slows vascular absorption of the local anesthetic, decreasing the blood concentration and prolonging the block. The expected duration of blockade depends on the perfusion of the space into which the drug is injected, and varies depending on the specific block. For lidocaine, peripheral nerve blocks last for 60 to 90 minutes; adding epinephrine may extend these times by 50 per cent. For bupivacaine, blocks may last more than three hours; with epinephrine, blocks may extend for more than 12 hours. Epinephrine is not used for digital blocks or other blocks in which distal circulation may be compromised.

It is not always wise to choose the longest acting local anesthetic mixture. First, the numb part may be at risk of injury postoperatively (e.g., from a tight cast). Second, prompt neurovascular evaluation may be important after some operations; residual neural blockade may interfere. Third, the onset of anesthesia is often delayed with such long-acting local anesthetics; this can delay the start of the operation unnecessarily.

LOCAL ANESTHETIC INJECTION

For many blocks, the total dose of local anesthetic far exceeds the dose that can be given safely as an intravenous bolus. Nevertheless, appropriate precautions during the injection can prevent severe toxicity. For infiltration blocks, the use of dilute solutions of local anesthetic and moving the needle about the target area ensures that only a small amount of local anesthetic will be injected if a blood vessel is entered inadvertently.

For blocks in which the needle is held in one place, one draws back on the plunger of the syringe (aspiration) before beginning the injection. If blood returns, the needle is moved slightly. Absence of blood on aspiration does not entirely rule out the possibility of intravascular injection. The local anesthetic solution is injected in increments of 5 to 10 ml, with pauses between doses so that early symptoms of intravascular injection can be detected and the injection halted.

These signs and symptoms include tinnitus, circumoral numbness, a metallic taste, tremors, garrulousness or a vague sensation patients sometimes express as "I feel funny." The ECG and blood pressure monitors are observed for signs of cardiovascular toxicity (arrhythmia, hypotension) or epinephrine effect (tachycardia, hypertension). If mild toxic symptoms appear, the block can be completed after appropriate treatment and repositioning of the needle.

TESTING THE BLOCK

Anesthesia is heralded by decreased sensitivity to cold, loss of pinprick sensation and, with concentrated local anesthetic solutions, motor block. Sufficient time is needed for local anesthetic diffusion through connective tissue barriers to reach neural axons. Repetitive, premature testing of an unblocked area can provoke anxiety for the patient and must be avoided. Proprioception is often impossible to block and patients must be reassured if they feel movement during the skin preparation and draping. At the time of incision, the surgeon tests the incision site (gentle probing with the scalpel or clamp) to determine the adequacy of the block. Expeditious induction of general anesthesia is required if the block is inadequate; if general anesthesia is hazardous, the block can be repeated or supplemented with other blocks (e.g., adding a block of the ulnar nerve at the elbow if brachial plexus block leaves the little finger with sensation).

INTRAOPERATIVE MANAGEMENT

Patients with adequate blocks may be sedated; supplemental oxygen is often appropriate. Monitoring during regional anesthesia is identical to that for any patient undergoing general anesthesia. It focuses on delayed local anesthetic toxicity from excessive tissue absorption (usually 40 to 60 minutes), ventilation and oxygenation, and the consequences of surgical stress such as tourniquet pain or blood loss.

CERVICAL PLEXUS BLOCK

Indications and Anatomy

Cervical plexus block is indicated for procedures about the neck and supraclavicular fossa between the mandible and clavicle, such as lymph node biopsy or carotid endarterectomy. Sensory and motor fibers of the cervical plexus arise from the anterior primary rami of the first four cervical nerves, with the first cervical nerve being motor only. The fibers exit in the sulcus of their corresponding transverse processes and diverge. Deeper motor branches supply the strap muscles of the neck, while the sensory branches gather at the posterior midpoint of the sternocleidomastoid

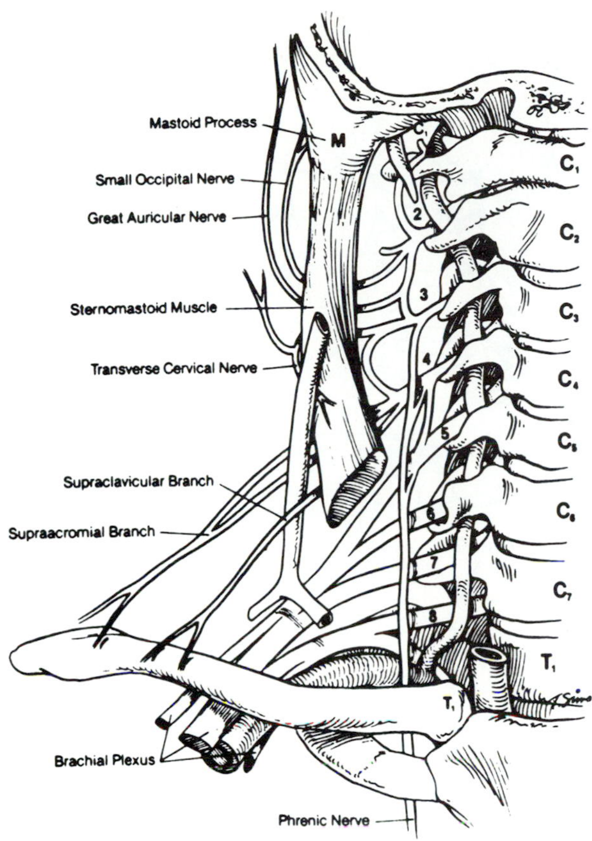

FIGURE 19–2. The anatomy of the cervical plexus and its branches. (From Raj PP with permission. Handbook of regional anesthesia. New York: Churchill Livingstone, 1985.)

muscle as the superficial cervical plexus, and ramify from there (Fig. 19–2).

Technique and Complications

DEEP CERVICAL PLEXUS BLOCK

For procedures requiring both sensory and motor block, the nerve roots of C2 to C4 are infiltrated as they pass in the sulcus of their corresponding transverse processes. The patient's head is turned to the opposite side to displace the sternocleidomastoid muscle and carotid sheath anteriorly. A line is drawn from the mastoid process of the temporal bone to the anterior tubercle of the sixth cervical vertebra (Chassaignac's tubercle), which lies at the level of the cricoid cartilage. The transverse process of C2 lies one finger's breadth below the mastoid process. The transverse processes of C3 and C4 lie deeper, 1.5 cm inferior to C2 and from each other.

Skin wheals are raised over the transverse processes of C2 to C4. A 22-gauge 1.5-inch needle is introduced perpendicular to the skin and slightly caudad until it touches the transverse process. Paresthesias may occur but are not required for success of the block. Five ml of local anesthetic are injected with the needle point in each sulcus, after careful aspiration.

Complications of the deep cervical plexus block include vertebral artery injection, since the artery runs in foramina immediately posterior to the transverse processes of the cervical vertebrae. Directing the needle caudad decreases the possibility of arterial injection. Other complications include epidural, subarachnoid, phrenic nerve, or laryngeal nerve block resulting from spread of local anesthetic solution to these adjacent neural structures.

SUPERFICIAL CERVICAL PLEXUS BLOCK

For superficial procedures, the sensory branches of the cervical plexus may be infiltrated at the posterior midpoint of the sternocleidomastoid muscle. Ten to twenty ml of local anesthetic are infiltrated in a complete circle centered on this point, both subcutaneously and beneath the fascia, to reach all the nerve fibers.

Brachial Plexus Block

Indications and Anatomy

Brachial plexus block is indicated for procedures involving the upper extremity from the shoulder to the hand. The plexus supplies all motor, sensory, and autonomic innervation to the arm. It originates from the anterior primary rami of C5-T1 and extends from the transverse processes to the apex of the axilla. The five roots of the plexus lie in the space between the anterior and middle scalene muscles and form the superior, middle, and inferior trunks as they pass over the first rib in the supraclavicular fossa. Each of these three trunks bifurcates into anterior and posterior divisions as the plexus passes under the midpoint of the clavicle. The six divisions rejoin to form the anterior, lateral, and posterior cords just proximal

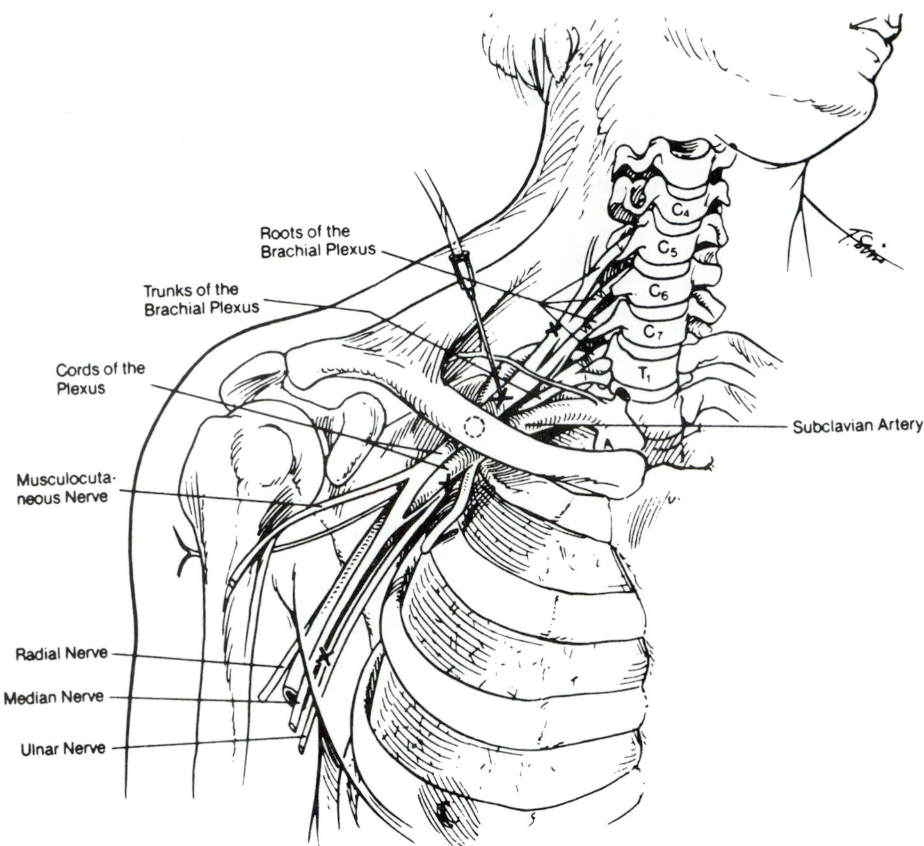

FIGURE 19–3. The course of the brachial plexus from its roots in the neck to the terminal nerves in the axilla. The needle is in the position for the supraclavicular block; the X above is at the site of the interscalene approach; the most distal X denotes the site of the axillary approach. (From Raj PP with permission. Handbook of regional anesthesia. New York: Churchill Livingstone, 1985.)

to the axilla. In the axilla itself, the four distal nerves of the brachial plexus (the musculocutaneous, median, radial, and ulnar nerves) encircle the axillary artery as they pass distally to the arm (Fig. 19–3).

Throughout its course the brachial plexus is accompanied by an artery (the subclavian proximally, becomes the axillary distally), which provides an important landmark. These structures are enveloped throughout their course by a connective tissue sheath that originates from the prevertebral fascia proximally, and extends to the axilla distally, known as the neurovascular sheath. Local anesthetic solutions are confined within this space, spreading proximally and distally from the point of injection to anesthetize the elements of the plexus.

Three approaches to the plexus are commonly used: interscalene, supraclavicular, axillary. As each approach produces a somewhat different distribution of anesthesia, the choice of technique depends on the surgical procedure and the desired pattern of anesthesia.

Techniques and Complications

INTERSCALENE BLOCK

The interscalene approach is indicated for procedures involving the cephalad roots of the brachial plexus. This includes those about the anterior shoulder, lateral elbow, and forearm. Because of the relatively lengthy cephalad-caudad dimension of the plexus in this location, the nerve roots of C8 and T1 are frequently spared, which makes this approach less reliable for procedures on the ulnar aspect of the hand and forearm.

The patient's head is turned to the opposite side, with a roll placed between the shoulders to bring

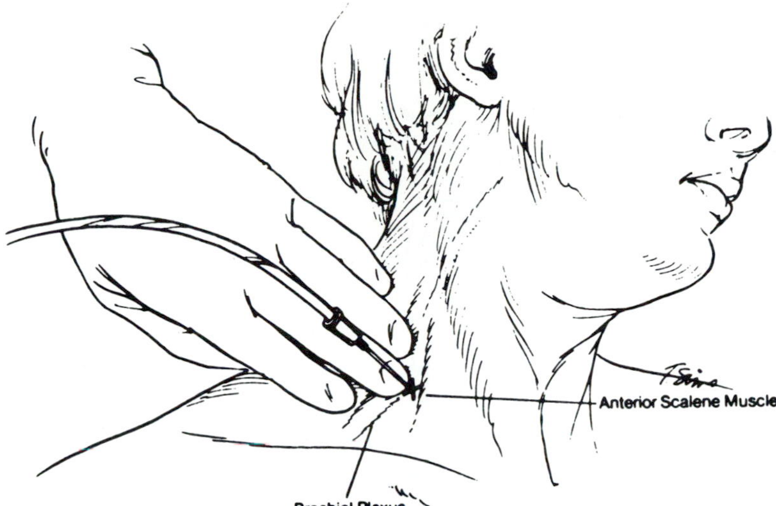

FIGURE 19–4. In the interscalene approach to the brachial plexus, the needle is directed caudad between the anterior and middle scalene muscles at the level of C6, as shown. (From Raj PP with permission. Handbook of regional anesthesia. New York: Churchill Livingstone, 1985.)

the strap muscles of the neck into relief, and the ipsilateral hand placed on the thigh to depress the clavicle. At the level of the cricoid cartilage (C6), the posterior border of the clavicular head of the sternocleidomastoid muscle is identified. A palpating finger is rolled posteriorly over the belly of the anterior scalene muscle to sense the groove between the anterior and middle scalene muscles. This can be confirmed by asking the patient to sniff, which causes preferential contraction of the scalene muscles.

The needle is directed perpendicular to the plane of the skin, in a direction caudad, mesiad, and dorsad (Fig. 19–4). The needle contacts the cephalad roots of the plexus within the neurovascular sheath as they emerge from the neck between the anterior and middle scalene muscles. Proper position of the needle may be signaled by paresthesias extending into the arm or by responses to a nerve stimulator.

Thirty to forty ml of local anesthetic is injected in divided doses, with frequent aspiration. With the injection of larger volumes, the local anesthetic spreads cephalad in the interscalene groove to the nerve roots of C2, C3, and C4 to produce anesthesia of the cervical plexus as well.

Complications of the interscalene approach include Horner's syndrome and unilateral phrenic and laryngeal nerve block (hoarseness), which are common and usually well tolerated. The complications of epidural, subarachnoid, or intravascular injection (carotid or vertebral arteries) are rare, but may require airway control and appropriate resuscitative maneuvers.

SUPRACLAVICULAR BLOCK

The roots of the brachial plexus merge to form the superior, middle, and inferior trunks as they pass over the first rib in the supraclavicular fossa. At this point the subclavian artery lies immediately anterior and inferior to the plexus within the neurovascular sheath, providing a vascular landmark. The supraclavicular approach is appropriate for procedures involving the entire upper extremity, with the exception of the ulnar aspect of the hand (inferior trunk), which is frequently spared (Fig. 19–5).

Patient positioning is the same as for interscalene block. The midpoint of the clavicle is identified, and the subclavian pulsation behind it palpated. Deeper palpation will reveal the shelf of the first rib, over which the subclavian artery and the brachial plexus travel as they pass laterally. The needle is introduced immediately posterior to the subclavian artery and directed caudally. The superior trunk of the plexus is most commonly encountered as it courses within the neurovascular sheath. If the first rib is encountered, the needle is withdrawn and "walked" anteriorly along it into the plexus.

Needle position is confirmed by paresthesias or by response to a nerve stimulator. Alternatively, the subclavian artery may be punctured and the needle withdrawn a few millimeters outside the vessel (but still within the sheath). With either method, 30 to 40 ml of local anesthetic is injected after aspiration.

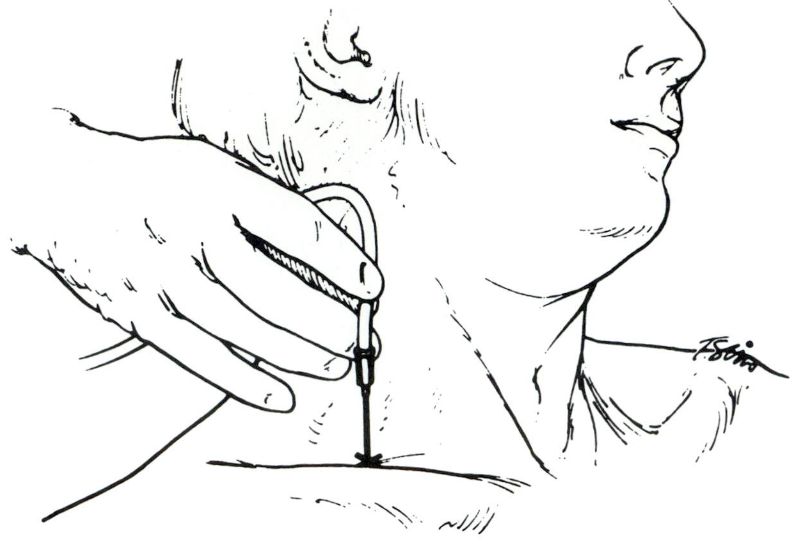

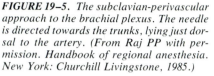

FIGURE 19–5. The subclavian-perivascular approach to the brachial plexus. The needle is directed towards the trunks, lying just dorsal to the artery. (From Raj PP with permission. Handbook of regional anesthesia. New York: Churchill Livingstone, 1985.)

Complications of the supraclavicular approach are similar to those of the interscalene approach, but include pneumothorax as well. Pneumothorax may be avoided by accurately identifying the first rib, and advancing the needle directly toward it and not in a medial direction toward the cupola of the lung.

AXILLARY BLOCK

In the axilla, the distal nerves of the brachial plexus (musculocutaneous, median, radial, and ulnar) are arranged circumferentially about the axillary artery. In contrast to the others, the musculocutaneous nerve lies outside the neurovascular sheath in the belly of the coracobrachialis muscle. The axillary approach is indicated for any procedure distal to the elbow, especially for hand operations (Fig. 19–6).

The arm is externally rotated and the shoulder abducted to 90 degrees or greater, as in a salute. The axillary artery is identified lateral to the pectoralis major and fixed between the index and middle fingers of the nondominant hand. The needle is inserted in a cephalad direction by the dominant hand at an angle of 45 degrees in the long axis of the artery. In the transarterial approach the artery is punctured directly and the needle tip advanced just beyond the wall of the artery to lie within the neurovascular sheath. Twenty ml of local anesthetic is injected deep to the artery, while firm pressure on the distal axillary artery promotes cephalad spread of the local anesthetic. The needle is then withdrawn to a position just outside the superficial wall of the artery, and another 20 ml of local anesthetic solution is injected superficial to the artery.

If paresthesias are to be sought, or if a nerve stimulator is used, the needle is directed immediately tangential to the artery to contact nerves within the sheath. At this point, the entire dose of local anesthetic may be injected. Some advocate multiple, smaller injections into the sheath to ensure local anesthetic spread beyond septae that separate the nerves. However, the functional significance of these anatomic septae is controversial. Single-injection axillary block undoubtedly can block all of the terminal nerves, indicating that the septae may not always prevent spread of local anesthetic; equally undoubtedly, single-injection techniques sometimes result in delayed onset of block in nerves other than the one closest to the needle tip.

Following local anesthetic injection, the shoulder is adducted and the axilla massaged to promote flow toward the musculocutaneous nerve, which provides sensory innervation to the lateral aspect of the forearm and the proximal thenar eminence. If this maneuver fails to block the musculocutaneous nerve, it may be blocked separately. Some anesthesiologists routinely include separate musculocutaneous nerve block when performing axillary block.

Complications of the axillary approach include a small hematoma when the artery is punctured,

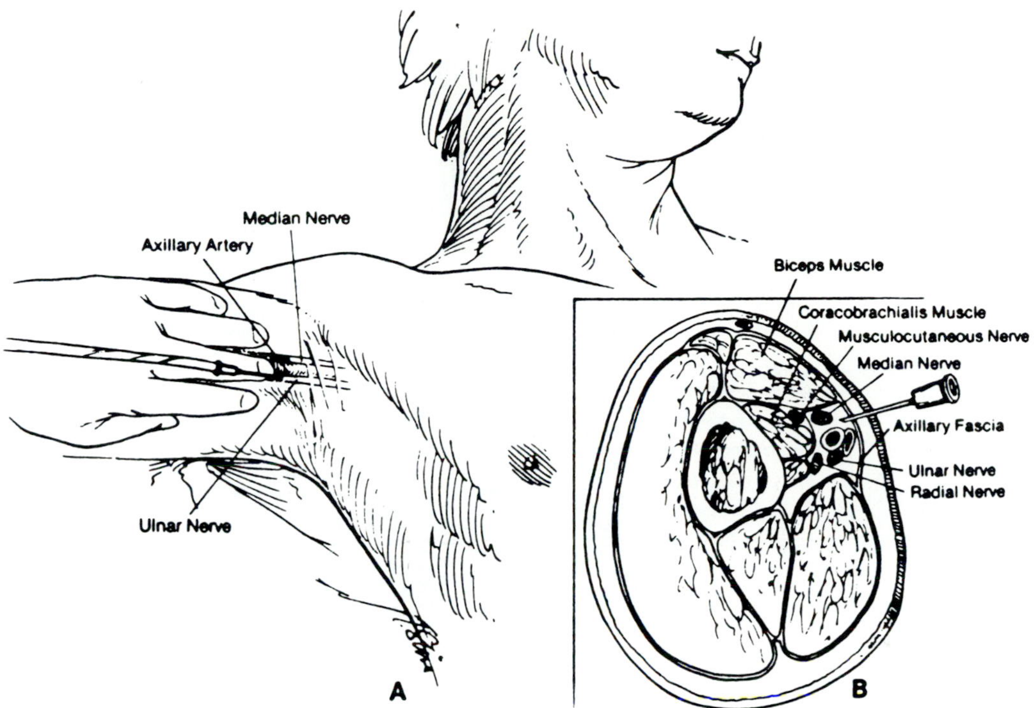

FIGURE 19–6. The surface anatomy of the axillary approach to the brachial plexus and a cross-section of the proximal right arm, viewed from distal toward proximal. Note the position of the musculocutaneous nerve in the coracobrachialis. (From Raj PP with permission. Handbook of regional anesthesia. New York: Churchill Livingstone, 1985.)

and intravascular injection, which can be detected by frequent aspiration and administration of small increments of local anesthetic while observing the patient.

MUSCULOCUTANEOUS NERVE BLOCK

The musculocutaneous nerve supplies motor fibers to the biceps and sensory innervation to the skin of the lateral forearm. It exits the neurovascular sheath above the axilla, and proximal spread of local anesthetic from the axilla may be inadequate to reach it.

In the axilla, the nerve lies within the belly of the coracobrachialis muscle, which originates from the coracoid process of the anterior scapula and inserts onto the proximal humerus. The bulk of the muscle is palpable in the axilla immediately adjacent and cephalad to the neurovascular bundle. The nerve is blocked by wide infiltration into the belly of the coracobrachialis.

Intercostobrachial Nerve Block

Any of these approaches to the brachial plexus leave unanesthetized the medial aspect of the upper arm, which is served by the intercostobrachial nerve. This nerve is not part of the brachial plexus, but derives from T1 and T2. Block of this nerve is important when a pneumatic tourniquet is to be used or when operations extend to the medial upper arm. The nerve passes through the axilla parallel to the neurovascular bundle, but superficial to the fascia. It is often blocked inadvertently during axillary block; infiltration with 5 to 10 ml of local anesthetic solution superficial to the fascia just over the axillar artery suffices to block the nerve.

Distal Nerve Blocks of the Arm

Separate blocks of the median, ulnar, and radial nerves at the wrist produce anesthesia in the hand (Fig. 19–7). Accordingly, they are indicated only for procedures about the hand or to supplement

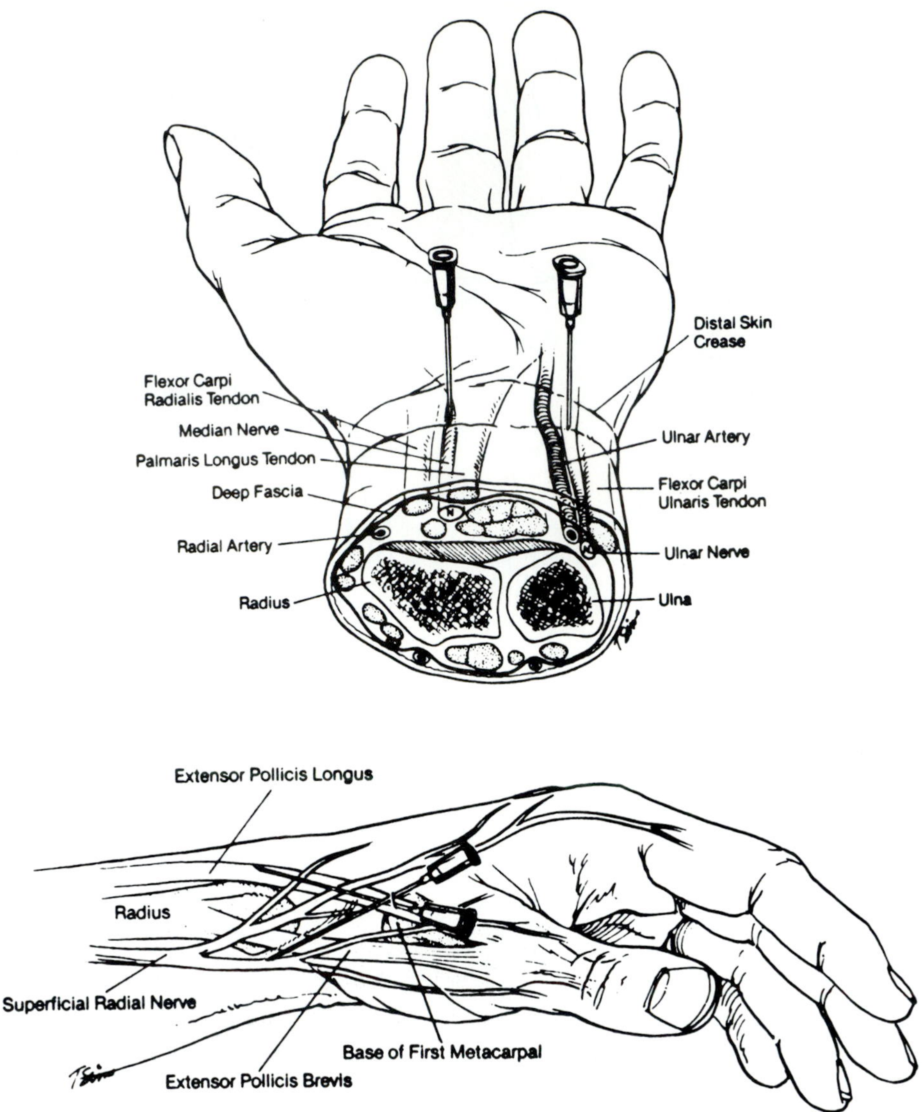

FIGURE 19–7. Cross-section and ulnar views of wrist showing blocks of median, ulnar, and radial nerves at the wrist. (From Raj PP with permission. Handbook of regional anesthesia. New York: Churchill Livingstone, 1985.)

an unsatisfactory brachial plexus block. Block at the elbow is technically more difficult than at the wrist, except for the ulnar nerve, which is palpable at the elbow and is easily blocked with 5 to 10 ml of local anesthetic solution.

MEDIAN NERVE BLOCK

The median nerve lies deep to the flexor retinaculum between the palmaris longus and flexor carpi radialis tendons. The patient flexes the wrist against counter-pressure with the fingers in extension. A ⅝-inch 25-gauge needle is inserted perpendicularly between the tendons to pierce the retinaculum. Three to five ml of local anesthetic are injected when a paresthesia is produced. If no paresthesia is produced, 5 to 8 ml are injected fanwise between the tendons.

ULNAR NERVE BLOCK

The ulnar nerve lies between the ulnar artery and the flexor carpi ulnaris tendon, which lies medial to the artery. The needle is directed between these two structures at the wrist crease. After aspiration, 3 to 5 ml of local anesthetic are infiltrated in a fan.

RADIAL NERVE BLOCK

At the wrist, the radial nerve diverges from the artery laterally and dorsally and pierces deep fascia. Three ml of local anesthetic are deposited lateral to the radial artery after negative aspiration. An intradermal and subcutaneous wheal is then extended laterally and dorsally over the wrist to reach those branches that have diverged near the anatomical snuff box to supply the dorsum of the hand.

BLOCKS OF THE THORACIC AND ABDOMINAL WALLS

Intercostal Nerve Block

INDICATIONS AND ANATOMY

Intercostal nerve blocks are most commonly used for relief of the pain caused by rib fractures or intercostal or subcostal incisions, such as for thoracotomy or cholecystostomy. Multiple bilateral intercostal blocks, in conjunction with celiac plexus block (described in Chapter 32), give anesthesia for intra-abdominal surgical procedures.

The 12 paired intercostal nerves are formed by the anterior primary rami of T1 to T12. They course circumferentially in the inferior groove of each rib, supplying skin and musculature of the chest and anterior abdominal wall (Fig. 19–8). The nerve and accompanying artery and vein are enclosed by the ribs above and below and by the external and internal intercostal musculature; this constitutes a space into which local anesthetics may be injected.

TECHNIQUE AND COMPLICATIONS

Intercostal nerve block is best performed with the patient in the prone or lateral position, with the shoulder abducted to rotate the scapula superiorly and laterally. Lateral to the posterior midline the angle of the rib is easily palpable, and lat-

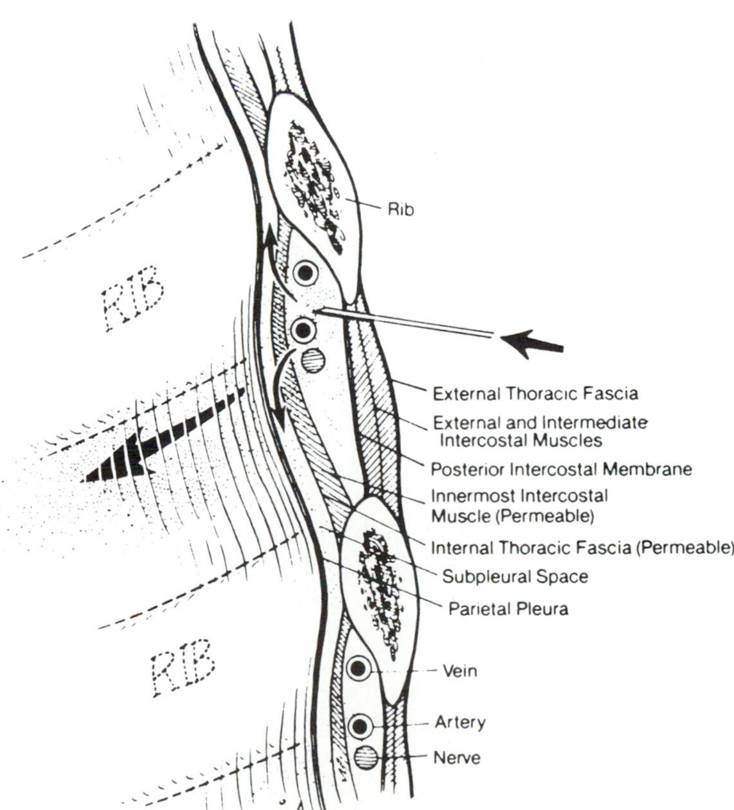

FIGURE 19–8. Views of the tissue planes defining the space around the neurovascular bundle for the intercostal nerve block. (From Raj PP with permission. Handbook of regional anesthesia. New York: Churchill Livingstone, 1985.)

eral cutaneous branches have not yet left the intercostal space. Skin wheals are raised in the intercostal spaces and pulled cephalad with the nondominant hand so they rest over the rib corresponding to the nerve to be blocked. A 22-gauge 1.5-inch needle mounted on a three ring control syringe is inserted at a slight cephalad angle to reach the periosteum of the rib, and then walked off the inferior margin to an additional depth of 3 to 5 mm. A loss of resistance may be appreciated as the needle tip penetrates the intercostal space. Paresthesias may be elicited, but are not necessary.

The syringe barrel is stabilized with the nondominant hand and 5 ml of local anesthetic injected after aspiration for blood. Intersegmental neural communication at the spinal cord necessitates that at least one nerve above and below the intended site be blocked as well.

Complications of intercostal nerve block include intravascular injection and pneumothorax owing to laceration of lung parenchyma by the needle tip. Both are rare when this procedure is performed by experienced personnel and may be avoided by maintaining strict control of the needle. Local anesthetic is taken up rapidly from this site, so that the resulting blood concentration of local anesthetic is great if many intercostal nerves are blocked. Epinephrine is added routinely to local anesthetic mixtures used for this block.

Block of the Inguinal Region

INDICATIONS AND ANATOMY

Inguinal field block is most commonly indicated for herniorrhaphy. The technique is especially useful for outpatients, debilitated patients, or as an adjunct to general anesthesia to reduce anesthetic requirements and provide postoperative pain relief.

Innervation of the inguinal region is supplied by the ventral rami of T11 to L2. The peripheral nerves of interest include the subcostals (T11 to T12), ilioinguinal (T12 to L1), iliohypogastric (T12 to L1), genitofemoral (L1 to L2), and subcutaneous ramifications of other local nerves. Autonomic fibers from the lower thoracic segments descend with and supply the spermatic cord and its contents.

TECHNIQUE AND COMPLICATIONS

The large volumes of local anesthetic solution required for the block require that dilute concentrations (1 per cent lidocaine or 0.25 per cent bupivacaine) be used to limit the total dose of local anesthetic.

Block of the iliohypogastric and ilioinguinal nerves is essential. As they descend and pierce the muscles of the anterior abdominal wall, they are blocked 2.5 cm medial to the anterior superior iliac spine. A 22-gauge 1.5-inch needle is advanced through a skin wheal and directed laterally and inferiorly to touch the inside shelf of the iliac bone. Ten ml of local anesthetic are deposited as the needle is moved in and out in a fan to infiltrate the external oblique, internal oblique, and transversalis muscles. With experience, distinct "pops" may be felt as the needle tip pierces all three layers of muscular fascia. When the depth of the muscles is sounded, the needle is directed medially through the same puncture and 5 ml infiltrated in similar fashion to complete the block, bearing in mind that the peritoneal cavity becomes progressively more superficial toward the midline.

The subcostal nerves T11 and T12, as well as stray fibers from T10, are blocked with a 3.5-inch 22-gauge needle introduced through the same point. Solution is distributed from just lateral to the anterior superior iliac spine to the umbilicus intradermally, subcutaneously, and intramuscularly. Thorough infiltration compensates for the variable penetration of these nerves as they descend toward the midline.

A subcutaneous wheal is then raised from the umbilicus to the pubic tubercle, and from the anterior superior iliac spine inferiorly 4 cm, and then medially back to the pubic tubercle. Genitofemoral nerve block is accomplished by directing a 22-gauge 1.5-inch needle superior to the lateral pubic tubercle and infiltrating 5 ml of local anesthetic.

During the procedure, the surgeon injects the incision line, as well as the spermatic cord, to prevent visceral pain. The keys to success with this block include limiting its use to smaller reducible hernias, meticulous infiltration of the various layers of the abdominal wall, and gentle technique by the surgeon to avoid pain from peritoneal traction.

Nerve Blocks of the Lower Extremity

Indications and Anatomy

Virtually any surgical procedure on the lower extremity can be accomplished with a proper combination of peripheral nerve blocks. In contrast to the upper extremity, where the nerves of the brachial plexus course together, multiple blocks are required to block the lower extremity because both the lumbar and sacral plexuses are involved.

The lumbar plexus and its terminal branches, the obturator, femoral, and lateral femoral cutaneous nerves, originate from the anterior primary rami of L1 to L4, form within the belly of the psoas muscle, and ramify widely to supply the anterior compartment of the thigh (Fig. 19–9). The obturator nerve originates from L1 to L4 and exits the pelvis through the obturator foramen to supply the adductors of the thigh. The femoral nerve is also derived from L1 to L4 and enters the thigh deep to the inguinal ligament, just lateral to the femoral artery. It provides motor innervation to the thigh extensors and sensory innervation to the skin of the anterior thigh. The continuation of the femoral nerve as the saphenous nerve provides sensory innervation to the anteromedial aspect of the leg below the knee. The lateral femoral cutaneous nerve enters the thigh medial to the anterior superior iliac spine and eventually pierces the fascia lata to supply the skin of the lateral thigh.

The sacral plexus forms from the anterior rami of L4 to S3, and lies on the anterior surface of the sacrum in a relatively inaccessible location. Its collateral branches supply the pelvis and buttocks locally, while the remaining branches give rise to the sciatic nerve. The sciatic nerve supplies the posterior thigh compartment, and through its terminal branches, the posterior tibial nerve and common peroneal nerves, the posterior and lateral compartments of the lower leg, as well as the ankle and foot.

Technique and Complications

LUMBAR PLEXUS BLOCK

All three terminal nerves of the lumbar plexus (femoral, lateral femoral cutaneous, and obturator) may be blocked with a single injection in the psoas compartment within the belly of the psoas muscle. The patient assumes the lateral position, as for spinal or lumbar epidural anesthesia. A line connecting the iliac crests perpendicular to the spine is drawn. A second line runs parallel to the spinal column and passes through the posterior superior iliac spine. At the intersection of these two lines, 4 to 5 cm from the midline and superior to the iliac crest, a 5- or 6-inch needle is inserted perpendicular to the skin in all planes. At a depth of 5 to 8 cm a paresthesia to the lower extremity or a thigh motor response to electrical nerve stimulation will be obtained.

Twenty to thirty ml of local anesthetic is injected; complete anesthesia of the lumbar plexus reliably results. If the procedure requires a sacral

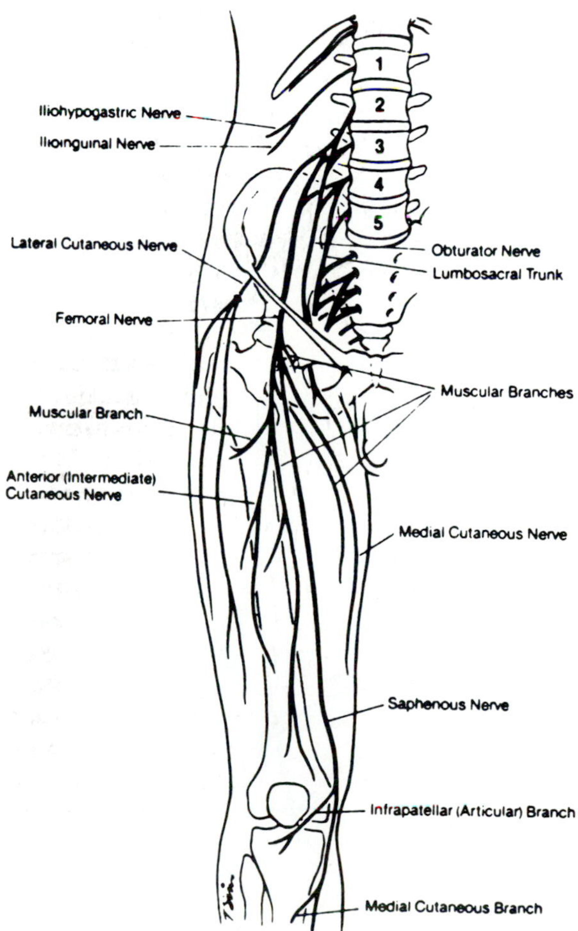

FIGURE 19–9. The formation of the lumbar plexus and its branches. (From Raj PP with permission. Handbook of regional anesthesia. New York: Churchill Livingstone, 1985.)

plexus or sciatic nerve block, this must be done separately, as local anesthetic does not spread reliably to these structures from the psoas compartment, even when given in large volumes.

FEMORAL NERVE BLOCK

The femoral nerve lies immediately lateral to the femoral artery as both structures enter the leg deep to the inguinal ligament. Infiltration, paresthesia, and nerve stimulation techniques have all been described. Ten ml of local anesthetic are injected after careful aspiration for blood. Injection of larger volumes with cephalad needle direction, which encourages proximal spread along the fascial sheath of the femoral nerve, produces anesthesia of the lateral femoral cutaneous nerve as well. It was originally thought that the obturator nerve was also blocked, but subsequent studies failed to confirm this. Apparently, the divergence of the obturator nerve from the lumbar plexus is too proximal to allow blockade from an inguinal perivascular approach.

LATERAL FEMORAL CUTANEOUS NERVE BLOCK

The lateral femoral cutaneous nerve is blocked deep to the fascia lata 2 cm medial and 2 cm inferior to the anterior superior iliac spine. A pop is felt as the needle tip pierces the fascia and 8 ml of local anesthetic are injected in a fan medially and laterally to cross the long axis of the nerve. Another 2 ml is injected superficial to the fascia to contact any superficial branches.

OBTURATOR NERVE BLOCK

Obturator nerve block is seldom used for surgical anesthesia. The obturator nerve is predominantly a motor nerve, with a variable but minimal sensory distribution on the medial side of the thigh. Gaining access to the obturator foramen is difficult and uncomfortable for the patient. If block of the obturator nerve is desired, usually in combination with femoral and lateral femoral cutaneous nerve

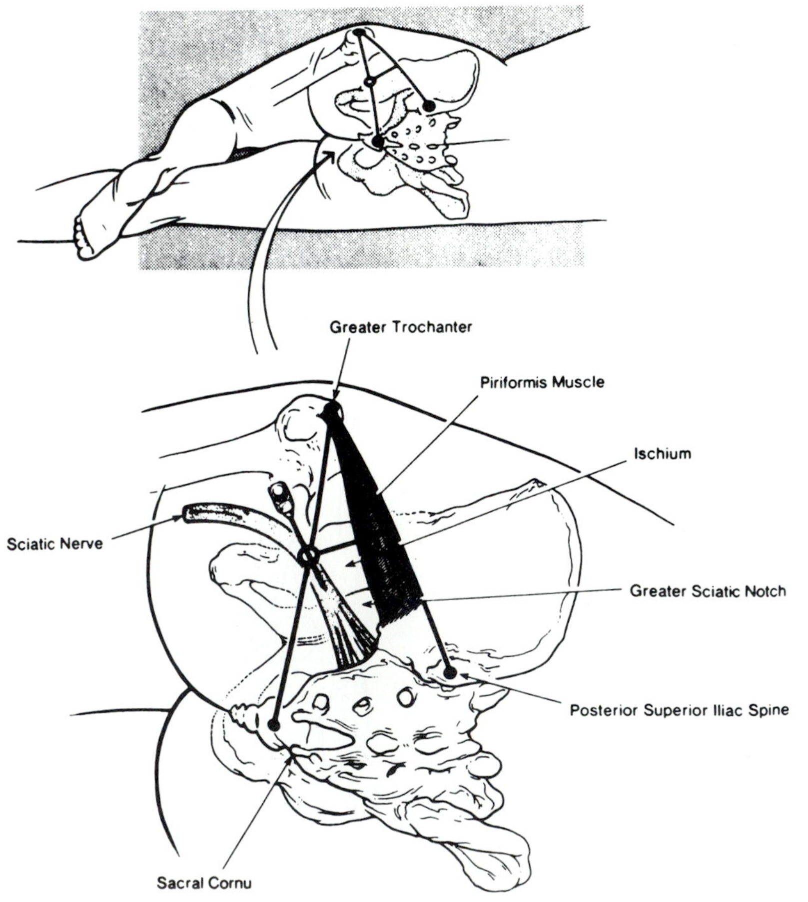

FIGURE 19–10. *The classic site for the posterior approach to the sciatic nerve is found by drawing a line between the greater trochanter and posterior superior iliac spine. From the midpoint of that line, a line extending perpendicularly downward for 5 cm should intersect a line drawn between the greater trochanter and the distal sacrum. At this point, a needle is inserted perpendicularly in all planes to reach the sciatic nerve. (From Raj PP with permission. Handbook of regional anesthesia. New York: Churchill Livingstone, 1985.)*

blocks, it may be produced reliably with a posterior lumbar plexus block.

SCIATIC NERVE BLOCK

Sciatic nerve block is usually combined with other nerve blocks to provide complete anesthesia of the lower extremity. It is also necessary for orthopedic procedures employing a thigh tourniquet to prevent tourniquet pain. A number of anterior and lateral approaches have been described, but the posterior approach of Labat is used most often (Fig. 19–10).

The patient assumes the lateral Sims' position, lying on the side opposite the one to be blocked with the bottom leg extended and the top leg flexed at the knee and hip. A line is drawn on the top leg between the greater trochanter of the femur and the posterior superior iliac spine. From the midpoint of this line, a second line is extended perpendicularly downward for 5 cm, to the point of needle insertion. Ten to twenty ml of local anesthetic is injected after elicitation of a lower leg paresthesia or motor response to nerve stimulation.

ANKLE BLOCK

Infiltration block at the ankle is indicated for procedures distal to the malleoli. The terminal branch of the femoral nerve, the saphenous nerve, and the four terminal branches of the sciatic nerve, the posterior tibial, deep and superficial peroneal, and the sural nerve, are readily accessible in the subcutaneous tissue as they cross the ankle joint (Fig. 19–11).

The patient is positioned prone or supine with the ankle to be blocked elevated. Epinephrine is not added to the local anesthetic mixture, to avoid arterial vasoconstriction and possible ischemia. The posterior tibial nerve is infiltrated behind the medial malleolus as it passes posterior to the pulsation of the posterior tibial artery. The sural nerve is blocked superficially by infiltration from the lateral malleolus to the achilles tendon. The deep per-

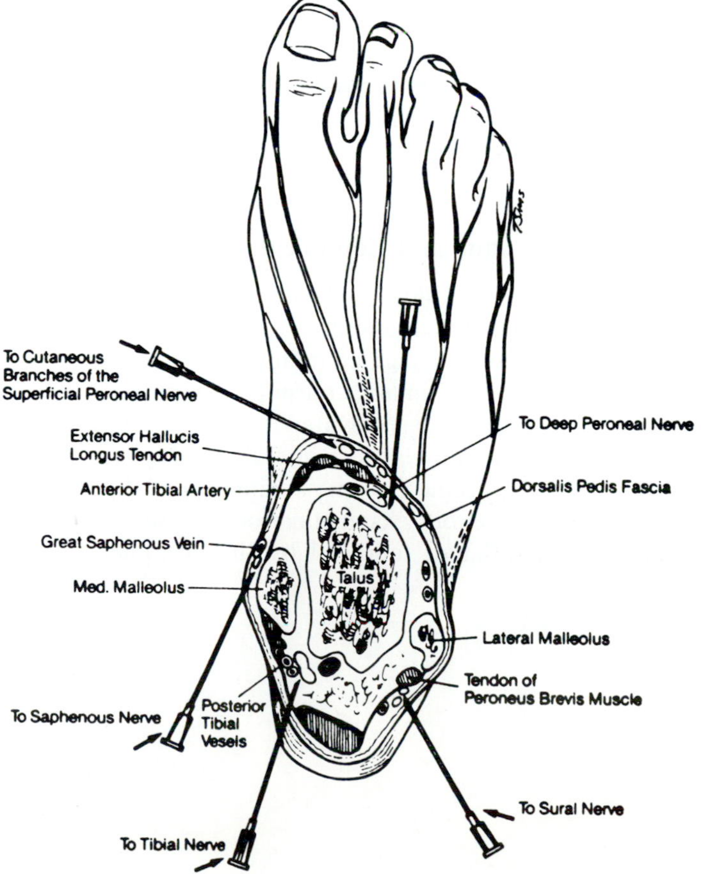

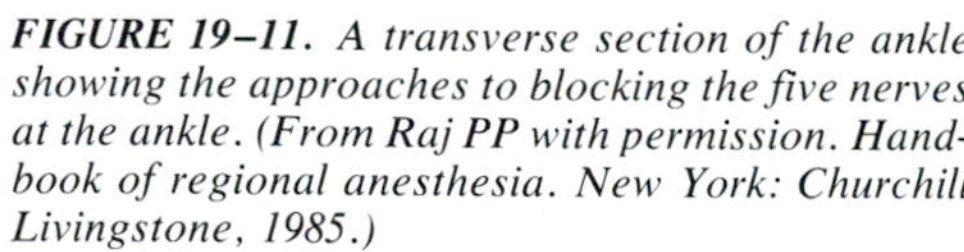

FIGURE 19–11. A transverse section of the ankle showing the approaches to blocking the five nerves at the ankle. (From Raj PP with permission. Handbook of regional anesthesia. New York: Churchill Livingstone, 1985.)

oneal nerve is blocked as it lies deep to the extensor retinaculum between the tendons of the extensor hallicus longus and tibialis anterior muscles. Superficial infiltration from this point to the medial and lateral malleoli blocks the saphenous and superficial peroneal nerves, respectively.

INTRAVENOUS REGIONAL ANESTHESIA

Indications and Anatomy

Intravenous regional anesthesia entails intravenous injection of large volumes of dilute local anesthetic while the circulation to the extremity is isolated by a tourniquet. The apparent mechanism of action is diffusion of local anesthetic across blood vessels to local nerves. The technique is indicated for brief procedures, especially about the forearm or hand, such as ganglion cyst removal. The duration of anesthesia is limited not by the duration of the effect of the local anesthetic, but by the patient's tolerance of the tourniquet, usually 40 to 60 minutes. Lidocaine 0.5 per cent is used most commonly. Chloroprocaine has been associated with thrombophlebitis. Bupivacaine is avoided because of its lesser therapeutic index for cardiovascular toxicity.

Technique and Complications

An intravenous cannula is placed distally in the limb to be anesthetized, and it is attached via extension tubing to a syringe containing local anesthetic. A double pneumatic tourniquet is placed proximally and the limb is elevated to drain venous blood. If possible, an elastic Esmarch bandage is wrapped tightly around the limb beginning distally to complete the venous exsanguination. The distal tourniquet is inflated, followed by the proximal tourniquet, both to 300 mm Hg. The distal tourniquet is then released. At this point, the extremity has a mottled, cadaveric appearance.

Lidocaine 0.5 per cent without epinephrine, 3 mg per kg (approximately 40 ml in a 70 kg patient), is then injected slowly from the reservoir syringe. Onset of anesthesia is virtually immediate. Usually, tourniquet pain develops after 40 minutes. Additional time may be gained by inflating the distal tourniquet and then deflating the proximal tourniquet. This will extend the duration of anesthesia to approximately 60 minutes.

At the conclusion of the procedure, the tourniquet is deflated. As circulation returns to the limb, the local anesthetic is washed into the systemic circulation and sensation returns within minutes. Deflation of the tourniquet must be delayed a minimum of 30 minutes after injection to allow fixation of the local anesthetic to tissues; premature deflation of the tourniquet results in toxic blood concentrations of local anesthetic. Peak blood concentrations can also be minimized by releasing the local anesthetic from the limb in small aliquots, by deflating the tourniquet intermittently for no more than ten seconds at a time.

Toxic reactions are rare, but do occur. They usually take the form of transient cardiovascular changes, such as bradycardia. The most feared complication is premature accidental tourniquet release leading to fulminant local anesthetic toxicity. For this reason, a separate intravenous cannula in another extremity and the immediate availability of resuscitation equipment are required.

REFERENCES

Cousins MJ, Bridenbaugh PO, eds. Neural blockade. 2nd ed. Philadelphia: JB Lippincott, 1988.

Raj PP. Handbook of regional anesthesia. New York: Churchill Livingstone, 1985.

Winnie A. Plexus anesthesia. Vol I. Perivascular techniques of brachial plexus block. Philadelphia: WB Saunders Co, 1984.

SECTION 6

PATIENTS WITH SPECIAL REQUIREMENTS

CHAPTER TWENTY

CARDIOPULMONARY RESUSCITATION

Modern cardiopulmonary resuscitation (CPR) employs temporary measures to deliver oxygen to the heart and brain while specific therapies are administered to restore the native circulation and ventilation. Cardiopulmonary resuscitation is an essential skill for everyone who administers anesthetics or other sedative or analgesic medications that depress consciousness, ventilation, or circulation.

CARDIOPULMONARY RESUSCITATION: RESTORATION OF OXYGEN DELIVERY

Deficiency of oxygen delivery is fundamental to all cardiopulmonary arrests, regardless of the initial cause. If an oxygen deficiency of sufficient magnitude occurs in the central nervous system, heart, or both, then ventilation, cardiac output, and oxygen transport to the body will cease. This sequence becomes a progressive spiral leading to death. The solution is rapid restoration of oxygen delivery to the brain and heart.

Basic life support (BLS) consists of temporarily providing oxygen delivery to the lungs with airway opening and rescue breathing, and providing oxygen transport from the lungs to the body tissues with cardiac compression (Table 20–1). Advanced cardiac life support (ACLS) adds specific treatments that restore natural cardiopulmonary function so the patient's ventilation and circulation maintain oxygen delivery to the body. In the final phase of resuscitation, postresuscitation life support, the primary cause of the arrest is defined and treatment provided to achieve long-term recovery.

Basic life support with manual airway opening, mouth-to-mouth exhaled air ventilation, and closed chest compression has been taught to the public and medical personnel alike as a first step in the treatment of cardiopulmonary arrest. However, BLS produces arterial oxygenation and cardiac output that are far less than physiologic, which do not permit successful resuscitation unless ACLS therapy follows rapidly (Figure 20–1).

Cardiopulmonary resuscitation outside the hospital may be limited by lack of trained medical personnel, support equipment to enhance temporary oxygen delivery, and delayed arrival of ACLS-capable providers. In the hospital, CPR administered by anesthesiologists and other trained medical personnel does not suffer these limitations. Specifically, the anesthesiologist's definition of BLS includes securing the airway by intubation, the use of 100 per cent oxygen, and the immediate use of drug therapy. Further, ACLS treatment specific to the cause of the arrest can be administered promptly to restore ventilatory and circulatory function without delay. Once ACLS begins, BLS continues until restoration of natural ventilation and circulation occurs or the resuscitation is stopped.

TABLE 20–1. **Component Parts of CPR**

BLS: Temporary Oxygen Delivery
Airway opening
Manual maneuvers
Pharyngeal airways
Tracheal intubation
Esophageal obturator airway
Cricothyrotomy
Artificial ventilation
Mouth-to-mouth
Mouth-to-mask
Manually powered ventilators
Oxygen-powered ventilators
Transtracheal jet ventilation
Artificial circulation
Closed chest compression
Cardiac back board
Epinephrine
Open chest cardiac massage
Cardiopulmonary bypass
ACLS: Restoration of Native Oxygen Delivery
Electrical therapy
Cardioversion
Cardiac pacing
Precordial thump
Vascular access
Peripheral/central venous
Endotracheal
Intraosseous
Pharmacologic therapy
Chronotropes
Antiarrhythmics
Inotropes
Vasopressors
Volume expanders/blood
Narcotic antagonists
Invasive procedures
Pericardiocentesis
Chest tube insertion
Aortic clamping
PRLS: Definition of the Primary Cause of arrest and Treatment of the Consequences of Cardiopulmonary Arrest
Continuous monitoring
Diagnostic evaluation
General intensive care
Definitive treatment of the cause of arrest

Abbreviations: BLS, basic life support; ACLS, advanced cardiac life support; PRLS, postresuscitation life support.

RESPIRATORY RESUSCITATION

Respiratory insufficiency and arrest lead to carbon dioxide retention and hypoxemia. Although extreme hypercarbia exerts arrhythmogenic and negative inotropic actions, hypoxemia is the disorder primarily responsible for the morbidity and mortality of respiratory arrest. Patient outcome from respiratory arrest depends on the duration of cerebral hypoxia and whether secondary cardiac arrest has occurred. Recovery is swift and complete if gas exchange is restored within three to four minutes of unconsciousness and prior to cardiac arrest. Outcome after secondary cardiac arrest is extremely poor in children as well as adults.

Whereas an effort is made to identify the specific cause of the respiratory difficulty in order to provide specific therapy, (e.g., narcotic antagonist or bronchodilator), several nonspecific steps apply universally:

1. Permit the conscious patient with respiratory difficulty to assume whatever body position is most comfortable. This will likely be a forward-leaning sitting position.
2. Administer 100 per cent oxygen. If apnea then occurs in a subject dependent upon hypoxic ventilatory drive (a rare occurrence), provide artificial ventilation until the F_{IO_2} is adjusted.
3. Increase the patient's minute ventilation if possible. Encourage deep breathing, or increase the tidal volume or ventilatory rate during artificial ventilation. Do not hesitate to perform tracheal intubation and begin positive-pressure ventilation in patients with impending respiratory arrest.
4. Monitor vital signs, electrocardiogram (ECG), and oxygen saturation, and establish an infusion line for subsequent intravenous drug therapy.

OPENING THE AIRWAY IN OBTUNDED AND UNCONSCIOUS PATIENTS

Airway obstruction occurs with loss of consciousness, because of relaxation of the muscles supporting the mandible, tongue, and epiglottis. The base of the tongue and epiglottis fall posteriorly into the airway, impeding gas flow into the trachea (Fig. 20–2). This can occur regardless of whether the subject is in the prone, lateral, or supine position.

Manual Airway Opening

The fundamental maneuver to open the airway is anterior displacement of the mandible to lift the

BLS Summary Performance Sheet

Cardiopulmonary Resuscitation (CPR)

	Objectives	Actions		
		Adult (over 8 yrs.)	**Child** (1 to 8 yrs.)	**Infant** (under 1 yr.)
A. Airway	1. Assessment: Determine unresponsiveness.	Tap or gently shake shoulder.		
		Say, "Are you okay?"		Observe
	2. Get help.	Call out "Help!"		
	3. Position the victim.	Turn on back as a unit, supporting head and neck if necessary. (4–10 seconds)		
	4. Open the airway.	Head-tilt/chin-lift		
B. Breathing	5. Assessment: Determine breathlessness.	Maintain open airway. Place ear over mouth, observing chest. Look, listen, feel for breathing. (3–5 seconds)		
	6. Give 2 rescue breaths.	Maintain open airway.		
		Seal mouth to mouth		mouth to nose/mouth
		Give 2 rescue breaths, 1 to 1½ seconds each. Observe chest rise. Allow lung deflation between breaths.		
	7. Option for obstructed airway	a. Reposition victim's head. Try again to give rescue breaths.		
		b. Activate the EMS system.		
		c. Give 6–10 subdiaphragmatic abdominal thrusts (the Heimlich maneuver).		Give 4 back blows. Give 4 chest thrusts.
		d. Tongue–jaw lift and finger sweep	Tongue–jaw lift, but finger sweep only if you see a foreign object.	
		If unsuccessful, repeat a, c, and d until successful.		
C. Circulation	8. Assessment: Determine pulselessness.	Feel for carotid pulse with one hand; maintain head-tilt with the other. (5–10 seconds)		Feel for brachial pulse; keep head-tilt.
	9. Activate EMS system.	If someone responded to call for help, send them to activate the EMS system.		
	Begin chest compressions: 10. Landmark check	Run middle finger along bottom edge of rib cage to notch at center (tip of sternum).		Imagine a line drawn between the nipples.
	11. Hand position	Place index finger next to finger on notch:		Place 2–3 fingers on sternum, 1 finger's width below line. Depress ½–1 in.
		Two hands next to index finger. Depress 1½–2 in.	Heel of one hand next to index finger. Depress 1–1½ in.	
	12. Compression rate	80–100 per minute		At least 100 per minute
CPR Cycles	13. Compressions to breaths.	2 breaths to every 15 compressions.	1 breath to every 5 compressions.	
	14. Number of cycles.	4 (52–73 seconds)	10 (60–87 seconds)	10 (45 seconds or less)
	15. Reassessment.	Feel for carotid pulse. (5 seconds)		Feel for brachial pulse.
		If no pulse, resume CPR, starting with 2 breaths.	If no pulse, resume CPR, starting with 1 breath.	
Option for entrance of 2nd rescuer: "I know CPR. Can I help?"	1st rescuer ends CPR.	End cycle with 2 rescue breaths.	End cycle with 1 rescue breath.	
	2nd rescuer checks pulse (5 seconds).	Feel for carotid pulse.		Feel for brachial pulse.
	If no pulse, 2nd rescuer begins CPR.	Begin one-rescuer CPR, starting with 2 breaths.	Begin one-rescuer CPR, starting with 1 breath.	
	1st rescuer monitors 2nd rescuer.	Watch for chest rise and fall during rescue breathing; check pulse during chest compressions.		
Option for pulse return	If no breathing, give rescue breaths.	1 breath every 5 seconds	1 breath every 4 seconds	1 breath every 3 seconds

FIGURE 20–1. American Heart Association (AHA) basic life support sequences for adults, children and infants. Trained rescuers incorporate use of supportive airway opening, ventilating and circulating equipment, as well as oxygen and epinephrine as soon as available. CPR, cardiopulmonary resuscitation; EMS, emergency medical system. (Reproduced with permission from the Instructors Manual for Basic Life Support. Dallas, American Heart Association, 1987, p. 181.)

epiglottis and base of the tongue from the airway. This is accomplished by the chin lift or jaw thrust maneuver (Fig. 20–3).

Pharyngeal Airways

When airway obstruction persists despite maximal mandibular displacement, an oropharyngeal or nasopharyngeal airway is indicated. These augment the elevation of the epiglottis and base of the tongue from the posterior pharyngeal wall. The oropharyngeal airway is more effective but may induce vomiting in responsive patients. Improper insertion or use of an undersized oral airway can exacerbate airway obstruction by pushing the

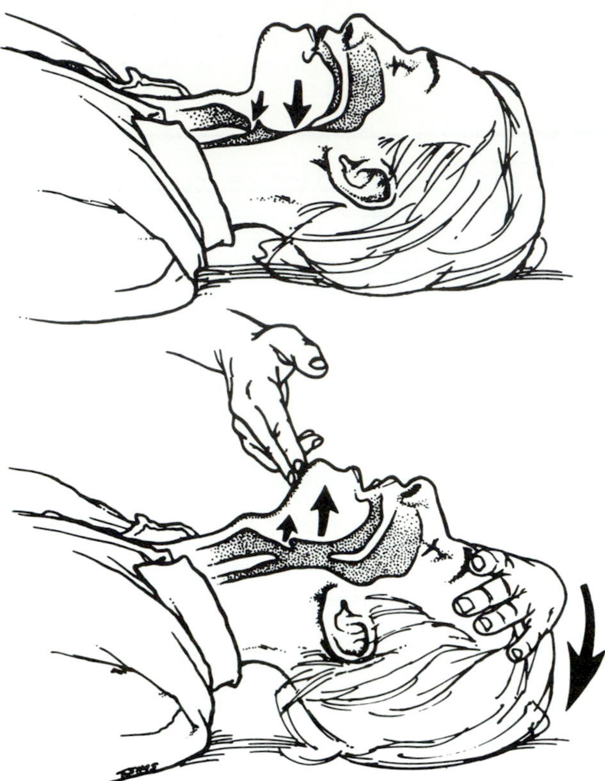

FIGURE 20–2. *Airway obstruction and the chin-lift airway opening maneuver. The fingers of one hand, grasping the mentum or ramus of the mandible, lift the jaw anteriorly. This elevates the epiglottis and lifts the base of the tongue from the posterior pharyngeal wall. Care must be taken not to compress the soft tissue under the chin thereby obstructing the airway. The rescuer's other hand is used to extend the victim's head or operate manually powered ventilating devices. If the patient has dentures, they are to be left in place to help maintain a normal facial contour, facilitating adequate lip or mask seal for ventilation. (Reproduced with permission from the Instructors Manual for Basic Life Support. Dallas, American Heart Association, 1987, p. 36.)*

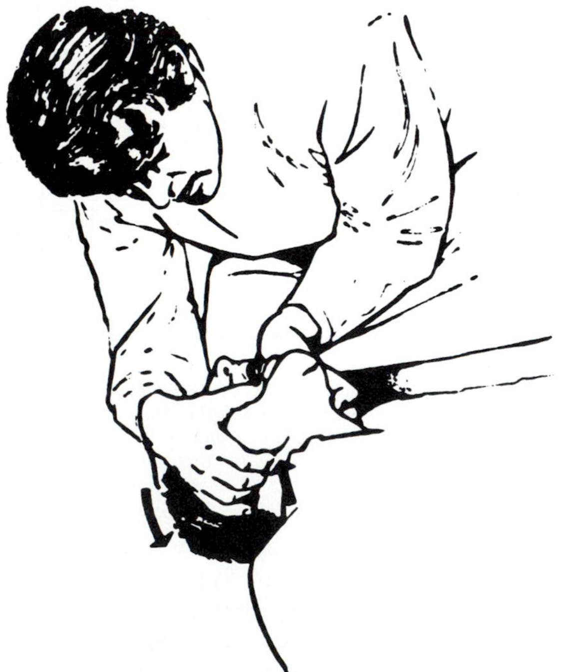

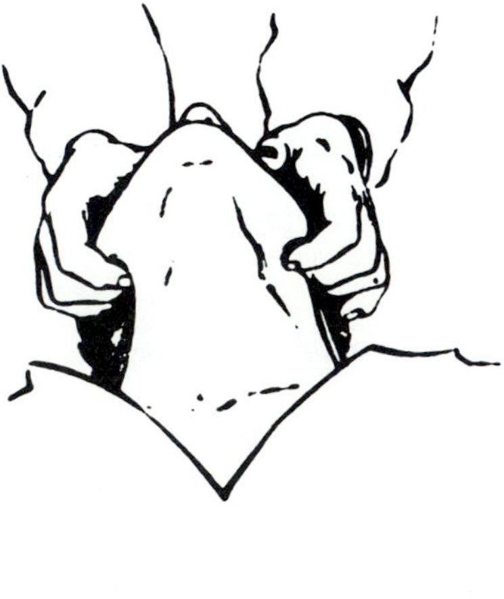

FIGURE 20–3. *Two-handed jaw thrust maneuver. The mandible is pulled forward by the fingers of both hands behind the angles of the jaw. The jaw thrust without cervical extension will often provide a patent airway in patients with suspected cervical spine injuries. (Reproduced with permission from Safar P, Bircher NG. Cardiopulmonary cerebral resuscitation. 3rd ed. London: W.B. Saunders, 1988.)*

tongue back into the posterior pharynx. Mandibular displacement must be maintained during use of pharyngeal airways.

Tracheal Intubation

When a patient's altered consciousness is not quickly reversible, measures are taken to prevent gastric inflation during artificial ventilation and protect the airway from aspiration of regurgitated gastric contents. Tracheal intubation accomplishes these goals and provides an alternative drug delivery route during resuscitation.

Attempts at tracheal intubation must not delay oxygenation of the patient; ventilation by bag and mask with manual airway opening or insertion of a pharyngeal airway precedes attempts at tracheal intubation. The technique of tracheal intubation is described in Chapter 13.

Esophageal Obturator Airway

The esophageal obturator airway (EOA) is sometimes employed by those who are not skilled at endotracheal intubation; anesthesiologists must be familiar with problems related to its use and removal in order to avoid complications (Fig. 20–4). Although the technique of EOA insertion is easily learned because laryngoscopy and glottic visualization are not required, adequate ventilation with the device is not achieved by many rescuers.

The anesthesiologist is most likely to encounter the EOA in place in an patient transported to a medical facility. It is replaced with a tracheal airway to ensure effective ventilation. After preoxygenation and ventilation using the EOA, the mask is detached from the obturator, which remains in place at the left side of the mouth during tracheal intubation, to prevent regurgitation.

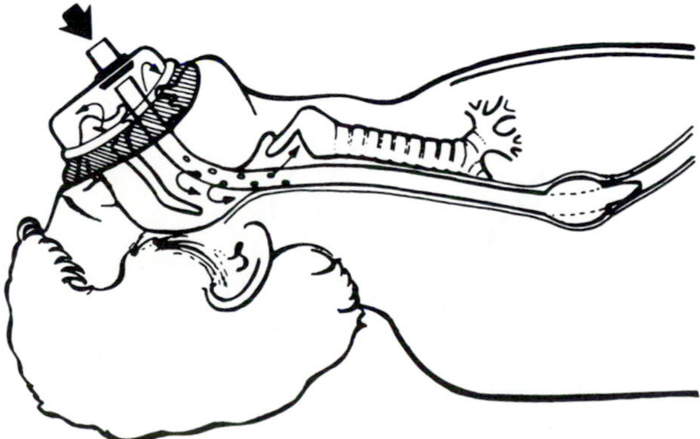

FIGURE 20–4. Structure of the esophageal obturator airway (EOA). (Reproduced with permission from Safar P, Bircher NG. Cardiopulmonary cerebral resuscitation. 3rd ed. London: W.B. Saunders, 1988.)

TABLE 20–2. Artificial Ventilation Rates

Patient Age Group	Ventilation Rate (breaths/min)
Adult (>8 yrs)	12–16
Child (1–8 yrs)	16–20
Infant (<1 yr)	20–24

Tidal volumes of 10–15 ml/kg produce observable chest expansion.

ARTIFICIAL VENTILATION

With the airway open, ventilation and oxygenation must begin immediately (Table 20–2). Without special equipment, mouth-to-mouth ventilation provides the quickest means of delivering adequate tidal volumes. Fear of infection has lead to the use of mouth-to-mask ventilating devices that include filters and non-rebreathing valves to protect rescuer and patient from direct contact and exhaled droplets.

Exhaled air ventilation techniques provide an F_{IO_2} of 0.15 to 0.18, limiting alveolar oxygen tension to less than 80 mm Hg. Decreased cardiac output and increased intrapulmonary shunting during CPR further impair arterial oxygenation. These patients require ventilation with 100 per cent oxygen as soon as possible.

Manually Powered Ventilators

Self-inflating resuscitators or portable anesthesia ventilating circuits administer oxygen and effective ventilation via mask, EOA, or endotracheal tube. The F_{IO_2} delivered by a simple self-inflating resuscitation bag (Fig. 20–5) is limited to 0.4 to 0.6 (oxygen inflow 10 to 15 L per minute) because the self-inflating bag refills itself at a rate exceeding the oxygen inflow, thereby entraining room air. Oxygen reservoirs that can be attached to these permit inspired oxygen concentrations near 0.9 to 1.0 (oxygen inflow 10 to 15 L per minute).

Portable anesthesia ventilating systems adminster an F_{IO_2} of 1.0 when supplied by an oxygen source, but oxygen inflow rates must be properly set to minimize rebreathing of exhaled gas and over- or underinflation of the breathing bag.

Gastric inflation occurs during mouth-to-mouth, mouth-to-mask, and bag-to-mask ventilation when inflation pressure exceeds esophageal opening pressure (approximately 15 to 20 cm H_2O). Distention of the stomach is minimized by using slow inspiratory flow rates (administering each breath over a 1.0- to 1.5-second inspiratory time), avoiding unnecessary positive pressure, limiting tidal volumes, and correcting airway obstruction. As soon as tracheal intubation is accomplished, more vigorous efforts at ventilation may be used, and the stomach may be decompressed by a gastric tube.

Oxygen-Powered Ventilators

Manually triggered, oxygen-powered ventilators deliver 100 per cent oxygen and prevent rebreathing. These ventilation devices administer oxygen at inspiratory flow rates greater than 100 L per minute at an airway pressure not exceeding 50 cm H_2O for as long as the control button or lever is depressed. Chest excursion is observed during inflation to avoid overinflation. These ventilation devices are used with an EOA or endotracheal airway rather than a mask, to avoid gastric distention.

Monitoring Artificial Ventilation

The efficacy of ventilation and arterial oxygenation is assessed throughout resuscitation using observation (chest excursion, cyanosis) or quantitative measures (pulse oximetry, capnography), if available, just as it is during anesthesia; any difficulties are corrected immediately (see Chapters 6 and 13).

TREATMENT OF AIRWAY OBSTRUCTION CAUSED BY FOREIGN BODY

The management of airway obstruction after foreign body aspiration depends on the degree of obstruction and adequacy of gas exchange. Partial airway obstruction with adequate gas exchange is recognized when the conscious choking victim can speak and generate an effective cough despite some respiratory distress. A rescuer does not interfere with the subject's efforts to expel the for-

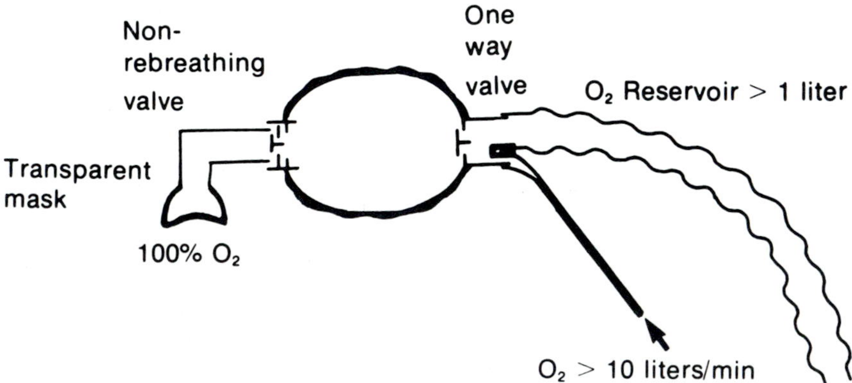

FIGURE 20–5. Manually powered self-inflating resuscitator (bag-valve device). Bag-valve devices consist of a hand-powered, self-inflating bag with inflow and nonrebreathing valves. On bag compression the intake valve closes, stopping oxygen and air inflow, and the nonrebreathing valve opens, delivering the bag's gas mixture to the patient. During exhalation, the recoil of the bag draws in oxygen and air via the opened intake valve. The nonrebreathing valve directs the patient's exhaled gases to the atmosphere preventing reentry into the bag. (Reproduced with permission from Safar P, Bircher NG. Cardiopulmonary cerebral resuscitation. 3rd ed. London: W.B. Saunders, 1988.)

eign object as long as adequate oxygenation continues. Artificial cough techniques produce less expulsive pressure and flow than natural coughs and may move the object to a more critical position in the airway, converting a partial obstruction to a more severe obstruction.

Partial obstruction with ineffective air exchange or complete airway obstruction are characterized by inability to speak and a weak or absent cough. In the unwitnessed arrest, foreign body airway obstruction is suspected if the rescuer cannot ventilate the lungs despite several attempts to open the airway. Treatment must begin immediately.

Artificial Cough Techniques

Heimlich's abdominal thrust and its variation, the chest thrust, are manual artificial cough techniques administered for the treatment of foreign body airway obstruction in adults and children over one year of age (Fig. 20–6). Back blows, an

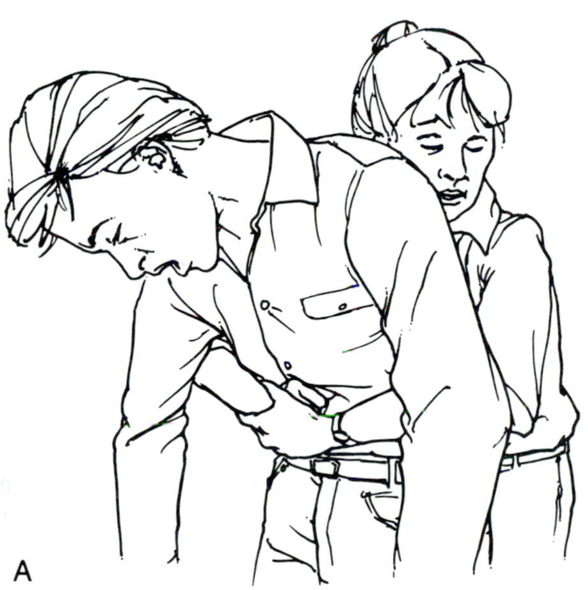

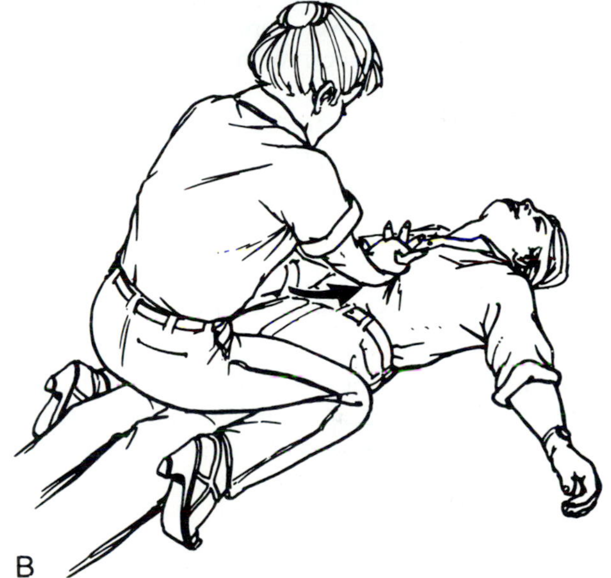

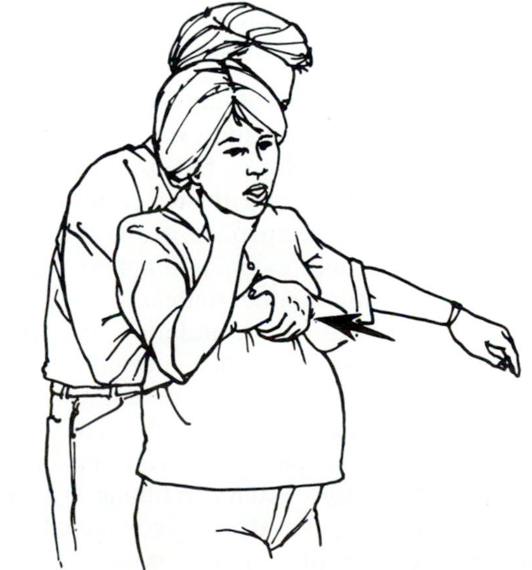

FIGURE 20–6. *Manual thrust artificial cough techniques. AB: Abdominal thrust (Heimlich maneuver), applied from the front or the back. Aspiration of a foreign body occurs during inspiration; air remaining in the lungs is forced outward to move the foreign body from its position in the airway. C: Chest thrust. In infants, obese victims, and pregnant women, chest thrusts are more effective and cause fewer complications than do abdominal thrusts. (Reproduced with permission from the Instructors Manual for Basic Life Support. Dallas, American Heart Association, 1987, pp. 56–58.)*

older artificial cough technique, are not advocated for use in adults and children.

Series of chest thrusts and back blows, in combination, are recommended for children less than one year of age with foreign body obstruction. When back blows are administered to an infant whose head and torso are supported by the opposite hand or thigh of the rescuer, intrathoracic pressure rises as a result of both the direct blow and compression of the thorax in a manner analogous to the chest thrust.

As the conscious choking victim becomes asphyxiated and unconscious, glottic muscles relax and maneuvers that were previously ineffective may dislodge the object. With relaxation it may also become possible to ventilate around the obstruction and to remove the obstructing object with a finger sweep of the posterior pharynx administered in conjunction with a tongue-jaw lift maneuver.

Direct Laryngoscopy

Direct laryngoscopy and removal of the obstructing body may be used by rescuers skilled in these techniques (e.g., anesthesiologists). Once the subject is unconscious, direct visualization can be accomplished with a laryngoscope and the object grasped with a long forceps or clamp. Blind grasping attempts in the posterior pharynx using forceps or clamps are to be avoided.

Cricothyrotomy and Transtracheal Ventilation

Percutaneous cricothyrotomy and tracheal intubation may permit ventilation when the obstruction is at or above the glottis, but this is tried only after simpler measures are unsuccessful. Subsequent tracheostomy, controlled orotracheal intubation, or endoscopic examination may be performed while ventilation continues.

Transtracheal catheter ventilation (TCV) requires an oxygen source and a specialized ventilation system through a large-bore intravenous cannula inserted into the airway through the cricothyroid membrane. The cannula is connected by a length of intravenous extension tubing to a hand-operated release valve that is connected to a source that delivers 100 per cent oxygen at 50 psi. The source may be a wall oxygen outlet, an oxygen tank with a pressure-reducing valve, or an anesthetic machine. Transtracheal catheter ventilation may also be accomplished with simplified equipment, using an ordinary wall oxygen flowmeter set at the maximum flush position (approximately 30 L per minute) and a piece of standard oxygen tubing with a side hole cut near its distal end. This end is connected via a stopcock or other connector to the transtracheal cannula. Lung inflation occurs when the side hole in the tubing is occluded by the rescuer's thumb and exhalation occurs passively when the thumb is removed.

If effective ventilation and oxygenation are to be achieved, insertion of a transtracheal cannula of adequate size and use of an appropriate ventilating device are mandatory. A 12-, 14-, or 16-gauge intravenous catheter can be used in adults and children in conjunction with jet ventilation systems. Transtracheal ventilation with bag-valve devices or anesthesia ventilating systems require a 3.0-mm inside diameter or larger cannula.

Once cricothyrotomy is performed and the catheter is connected to the ventilating device, a jet of oxygen introduced into the trachea produces lung inflation despite a retrograde air leak. Alternatively, a small endotracheal tube may be passed through the cricothyroidotomy into the tracheal lumen and conventional ventilation begun. Because exhalation during TCV occurs passively through the upper airway, complete obstruction at or above the glottis prevents exhalation and may produce dangerous airway pressures. In this situation the transtracheal cannula permits apneic oxygenation by insufflation of oxygen to meet basal metabolic requirements. Although marked hypercarbia develops, arterial oxygenation is maintained while an adequate airway is established.

CARDIOPULMONARY RESUSCITATION

The most effective therapeutic approach to cardiopulmonary arrest is immediate application of definitive treatment that restores the patient's native cardiac output and ventilation. Basic life-support measures must not delay the start of specific therapy when it is immediately available.

ARTIFICIAL CIRCULATION

Closed Chest Compression

Artificial circulation by closed chest compression accompanied by ventilation and oxygenation is indicated throughout the period of resuscitation until native circulation has been restored. Closed chest compression is not indicated for patients with palpable central pulses and systolic blood pressures greater than 50 mm Hg, even though peripheral pulses may be undetectable due to peripheral vasoconstriction. These patients are best treated with specific measures which augment circulation, such as fluids and drugs.

External chest compression can produce systolic blood pressure of 100 mm Hg and greater, but diastolic pressures range from 10 to 40 mm Hg. As a result of the decreased aortic diastolic pressures, myocardial perfusion during closed chest compression seldom exceeds 5 to 10 per cent of normal levels. Carotid artery blood flow is generally less than one third of normal. Although these blood flows temporarily sustain cerebral viability, prompt restoration of native circulation and coronary perfusion is critical for survival.

Efforts to discover more effective external chest compression techniques have lead to the understanding that two mechanisms are responsible for blood flow during CPR: compression of the heart between the sternum and spine (cardiac pump) and phasic increases in arterial perfusion pressure produced by compression of the thorax (thoracic pump). Blood flow produced by direct cardiac compression is directly related to compression rate, and thoracic pump blood flow is directly related to the magnitude and duration of intrathoracic pressure produced by sternal depression.

Survival after cardiopulmonary resuscitation is related to compression rate. Optimal blood flow and coronary perfusion during closed chest CPR are observed as compression rates of 100 to 120 per minute (Fig. 20–7). Rapid compression rates improve blood flow and aortic diastolic blood pressure as a result of rate-dependent effects on cardiac output (cardiac pump) and increases in the systolic:diastolic duration ratio (thoracic pump).

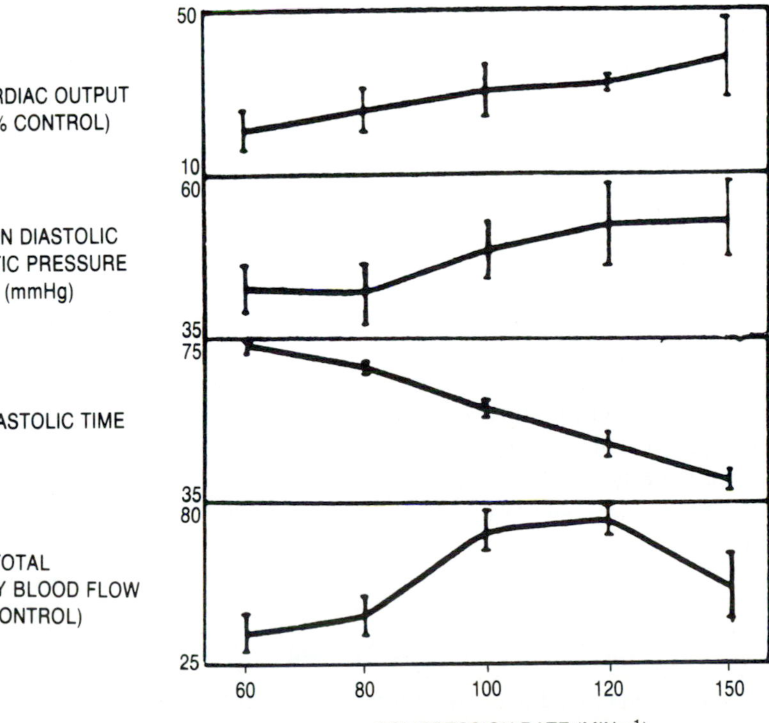

FIGURE 20–7. Influence of compression rate on hemodynamics during manually performed closed chest compression in dogs. (Modified with permission from Wolfe JA, Maier GW, Newton JR, et al. Physiologic determinants of coronary blood flow during external cardiac massage. J Thorac Cardiovasc Surg 1988; 95:523–532.)

Slightly slower compression rates, 80 to 100 per minute, have been recommended for adults and children because faster rates may not be maintained for a sufficient period by solo rescuers. Adequate depth of sternal displacement is essential to achieve complete cardiac compression (cardiac pump) and produce a substantial increase in intrathoracic pressure (thoracic pump).

Numerous alternative techniques of CPR have been proposed, but none have been shown to produce results superior to conventional chest compression. Artificial circulation is enhanced when intravenous epinephrine and the supportive equipment described below are employed to increase the cardiac output and perfusion pressure produced by closed chest compression.

TABLE 20–3. Indications for Thoracotomy and Direct Cardiac Compression

Operating room
Thorax or upper abdomen already open
Conditions prohibit effective artificial circulation by closed chest compression
Severe anatomic thoracic cage abnormalities
Flail chest
Cardiac tamponade
Tension pneumothorax
Major mediastinal shift, (after pneumonectomy, massive pleural effusion)
Cause of arrest is best treated by thoracotomy, pericardiotomy
Cardiac tamponade
Tension pneumothorax
Penetrating chest injury

Supportive Equipment and Epinephrine

The patient undergoing external chest compression must lie on a firm surface. A cardiac back board, operating table, floor, or food tray may be used.

Mechanical chest compressors reduce fatigue resulting from manual chest compression and permit longer periods of CPR. However, they provide no hemodynamic advantage over manual CPR.

Epinephrine improves cerebral and coronary blood flow during artificial circulation as a result of alpha-adrenergic-mediated vasoconstriction, which limits blood flow to peripheral tissues and increases aortic blood pressure and coronary blood flow. The enhanced myocardial oxygen delivery may result in spontaneous cardiac contraction or increased response to electrical defibrillation.

Improvements in perfusion pressure and myocardial blood flow during CPR are directly related to epinephrine dose. Although the recommended drug dose is 10 to 15 μg per kg, larger doses (45 μg per kg or greater) may further improve perfusion.

Open Chest Cardiac Massage

Although closed chest compression has replaced direct cardiac massage during CPR, direct compression of the heart generates superior cardiac output and coronary perfusion. Coronary perfusion and survival from arrest in animals are improved when open cardiac massage is instituted in place of closed chest compression within 15 minutes of cardiac arrest. There are indications for open chest cardiac massage in a hospital setting, when trained rescuers are present (Table 20–3).

Monitoring Artificial Circulation

An index of cardiac output produced during CPR would be a useful guide to chest compression rate and depth, epinephrine dose, or need for alternative artificial circulation techniques. Palpation of a central pulse during chest compressions has served this purpose, but it provides little information about blood flow and oxygen delivery.

Exhaled end-tibial carbon dioxide tension is an index of cardiac output and may predict outcome from resuscitation. When cardiac output is depressed and ventilation is constant, end-tidal CO_2 tension reflects the rate of CO_2 delivery to the lungs and is directly related to cardiac output. In humans undergoing closed chest compression, greater exhaled end-tidal CO_2 values are observed in eventual survivors than in those who do not survive. End-tidal CO_2 tensions less than 10 to 15 mm Hg obtained after tracheal intubation during closed chest compression imply a poor prognosis for survival.

Emergent Cardiopulmonary Bypass

The institution of cardiopulmonary bypass (femoral-femoral) in place of conventional artificial circulation techniques can improve resuscitation and survival when begun immediately upon cardiac arrest. This can be used when the necessary equipment and expert personnel are immediately available for hospitalized patients known to be at risk for cardiac arrest. It is also useful for the rewarming and resuscitation of victims of cardiac arrest due to accidental hypothermia.

SPECIFIC THERAPY OF CARDIAC ARREST DUE TO TACHYDYSRHYTHMIAS

Ventricular tachycardia (VT) and ventricular fibrillation (VF) are the most common cardiac dysrhythmias causing cardiopulmonary arrest. Ventricular tachycardia is a life-threatening rhythm disturbance that results in hypotension and shock. It is an electrically unstable rhythm and may degenerate to VF. Ventricular fibrillation is a lethal dysrhythmia; cardiac output is absent. Hypotension and shock may also be caused by very rapid supraventricular tachycardia (SVT). Electrical cardioversion is the most rapidly effective therapy for these rhythm disturbances and is a mainstay of advanced cardiac life support.

Synchronized and Unsynchronized Cardioversion

Electrical cardioversion, rather than pharmacologic therapy, is indicated for the treatment of tachydysrhythmias when the pulse is absent or when there is stupor or unconsciousness, severe arterial hypotension, pulmonary edema, or angina pectoris.

In instances of cardiac arrest occurring without established electrocardiogram (ECG) monitoring, the heart rate and rhythm can most rapidly be determined using defibrillator chest paddles that incorporate ECG electrodes, so that definitive therapy can be administered immediately.

Cardioversion delivers an electrical current that depolarizes a critical mass of myocardium and permits a more stable pacemaker, such as the atrioventricular or sinus node, to assume control. The amount of current passing through the heart and depolarized myocardial mass depends directly on the energy delivered from the paddles and inversely on the transthoracic resistance to current flow (Table 20–4).

TABLE 20–4. Factors That Increase Current Flow During Electrical Cardioversion

1. Paddles of large surface area that permit complete electrode contact with chest surface
2. Conductive gel, paste, or pads. Saline-soaked gauze sponges are an acceptable alternative; alcohol swabs are not.
3. Correct paddle position: The heart must lie between the paddles. In the standard paddle position, one paddle is placed on the upper right thorax below the clavicle, and the other is lateral to the apex of the heart on the lower left chest at the mid-axillary line.
4. Firm pressure on paddles
5. Exhalation of air from lungs
6. Repetitive shocks

The energy dose selected for cardioversion during cardiac arrest is based the need for rapid resolution of the rhythm disturbance. Unnecessarily large doses, however, produce myocardial injury often manifested as transient conduction blocks following cardioversion. Thus, cardioversion starts with the least energy dose that is expected to be effective for the patient's hemodynamic condition and cardiac rhythm (Table 20–5). If this dose is ineffective, the energy level is increased for each succeeding shock. A series of rapidly repeated shocks are delivered until cardioversion is achieved or three to four shocks at maximum defibrillator output, 360 joules, have been administered (Figs. 20–8 through 20–10). The pulse or

TABLE 20–5. Recommended Initial Energy Dose for Emergent Cardioversion*

Dysrhythmia	Energy Dose (joules)	Synchronized or Unsynchronized†
Ventricular fibrillation	200	Unsynchronized
Ventricular tachycardia	50	Synchronized
Paroxysmal supraventricular tachycardia	75	Synchronized
Atrial fibrillation	100	Synchronized
Atrial flutter	25	Synchronized

* Any dysrhythmia is treated as if it were ventricular fibrillation if there is no pulse.

† Unsynchronized cardioversion is used for hemodynamically unstable patients if synchronization process will cause delay in therapy.

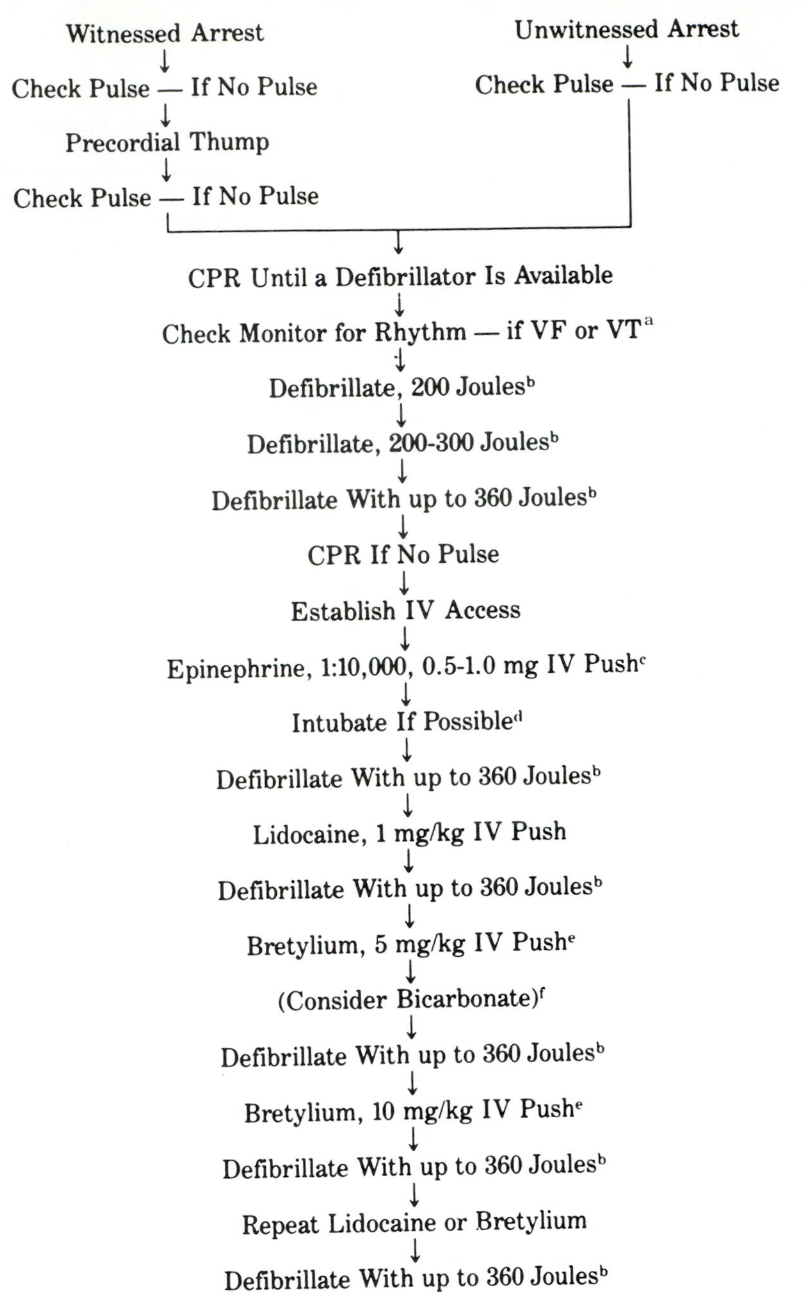

FIGURE 20–8. American Heart Association treatment algorithm for cardiac arrest due to ventricular fibrillation (and pulseless ventricular tachycardia). This AHA algorithm, as well as the others reproduced in this chapter, were developed to teach a generic and fundamental treatment plan for a broad range of patients. Some patients may require care not specified herein. This algorithm must not be construed as prohibiting such flexibility.

[a] Flow of algorithm presumes that VF (or VT) is continuing. [b] Check pulse and rhythm after each shock. If VF (or VT) recurs after transiently converting (rather than persisting without ever converting), use the energy level which has previously been successful for subsequent defibrillation. [c] Epinephrine is repeated every five minutes. The drug may be given via endotracheal tube in the absence of an IV line. Use of epinephrine as the first drug administered for VF refractory to defibrillation is empiric. Alternatively, lidocaine may be administered prior to epinephrine. [d] If tracheal intubation can be performed simultaneously with other maneuvers including chest compression, then the earlier it is accomplished the better. However, defibrillation is more important initially if the patient can be ventilated and oxygenated without intubation. [e] Alternatively, lidocaine may be repeated. [f] Value of sodium bicarbonate (dose titrated to neutralize base deficit calculated from arterial blood gas analysis) is questionable during cardiac resuscitation, and it is not recommended as routine therapy. (Reproduced with permission, from the Textbook of advanced cardiac life support. 2nd ed. Dallas: American Heart Association, 1987.)

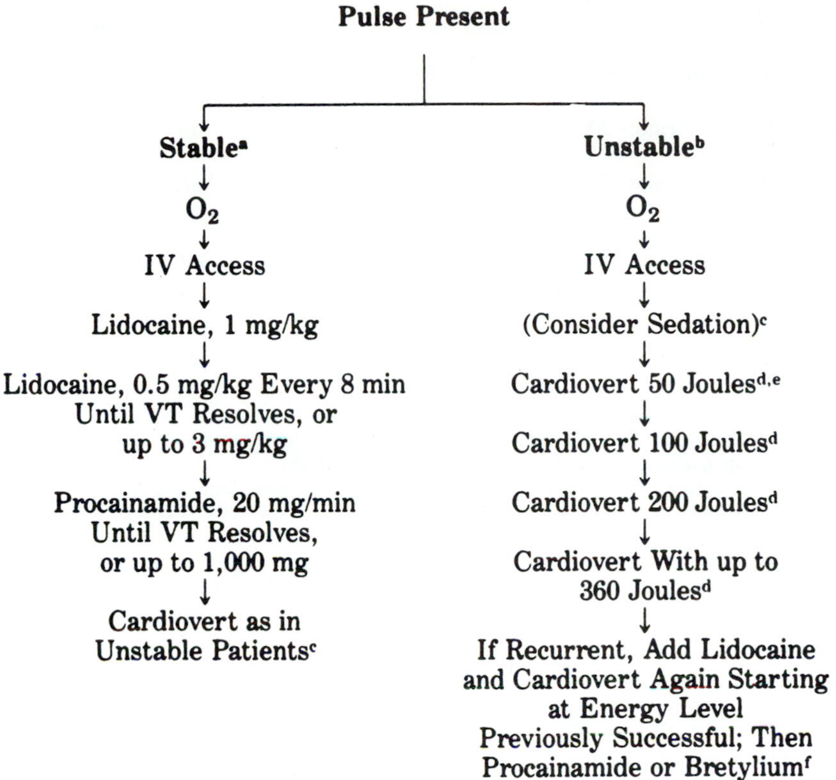

FIGURE 20–9. American Heart Association treatment algorithm for cardiac arrest caused by ventricular tachycardia.

[a] If patient becomes unstable at any time, move to "Unstable" arm of algorithm. [b] Unstable patients are recognized by signs of stupor, hypotension, pulmonary edema, or symptoms of angina or dyspnea. [c] Sedation, achieved by cautious administration of agents such as ultra–short-acting barbiturate, etomidate, propofol, or midazolam, may be considered for patients with mild signs and symptoms of hemodynamic compromise. It is associated with risks of regurgitation and aspiration, hypotension, and hypoventilation in all patients; it is not indicated in the presence of coma, pulmonary edema, or severe hypotension. [d] If coma, pulmonary edema, or severe hypotension persist, unsynchronized cardioversion avoids delay associated with synchronization. [e] Precordial thump may induce VF and is not recommendable. [f] If coma, pulmonary edema, or severe hypotension is present, use lidocaine followed by bretylium, if necessary. In all other patients, recommended drug order is lidocaine, procainamide, and then bretylium. (Reproduced with permission, from the Textbook of advanced cardiac life support. 2nd ed. Dallas: American Heart Association, 1987.)

ECG are reevaluated immediately after each shock.

When the rhythm disturbance persists after the first series of three to four shocks, efforts are directed at oxygenating the myocardium and enhancing its susceptibility to cardioversion (Figs. 20–8 to 20–10). These steps include increased ventilation, correction of metabolic abnormalities, and antiarrhythmic drug therapy specific to the dysrhythmia. In addition, chest compression and epinephrine are administered to pulseless patients in continuing cardiac arrest. Subsequent cardioversion attempts using maximum energy are delivered as two successive shocks, because diminished transthoracic resistance is observed after repeated shocks.

Defibrillation can be synchronized to the ECG in the presence of a rhythm with a QRS complex, such as VT or SVT (the QRS deflection can be sensed and discharge of the paddles timed accordingly). Synchronized defibrillation requires smaller electrical doses and avoids delivering a shock during the period of vulnerability immediately prior to the T wave, which can provoke VF. Unsynchronized cardioversion is used for the treatment of VF, whereas synchronized cardiov-

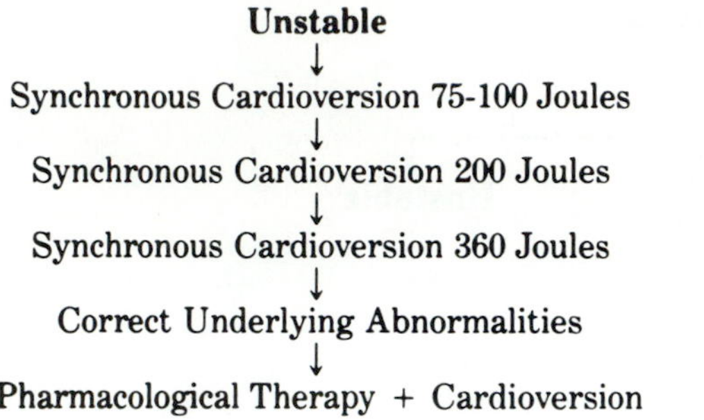

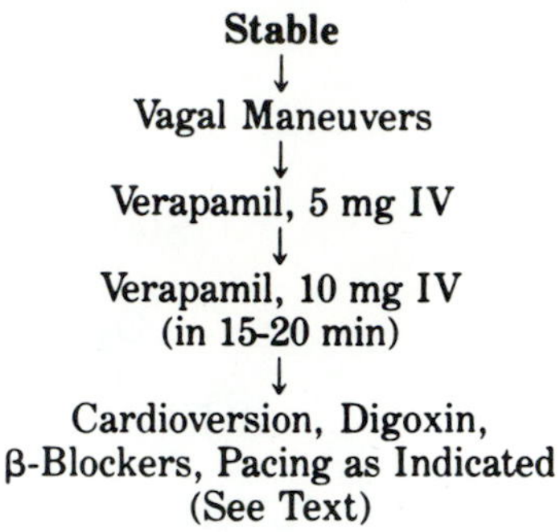

If conversion occurs but PSVT recurs, repeated electrical cardioversion is *not* indicated. Sedation should be used as time permits.

FIGURE 20–10. *American Heart Association treatment algorithm for cardiac arrest caused by paroxysmal supraventricular tachycardia (PSVT). Unstable patients are recognized by signs of stupor, hypotension, pulmonary edema, or symptoms of angina or dyspnea. Energy doses for synchronized cardioversion of supraventricular tachydysrhythmias other than PSVT are listed in Table 20–5. Lower doses of verapamil are used for elderly, anesthetized, or unstable patients. Verapamil-induced hypotension is treated with a vasopressor. Alternatively, adenosine (3 to 6 mg IV) may be used to terminate stable PSVT. (Reproduced with permission, from the Textbook of advanced cardiac life support. 2nd ed. Dallas: American Heart Association, 1987.)*

ersion may be used for termination of all other tachydysrhythmias. The synchronization mechanism is deactivated for defibrillation of VF because no QRS deflection exists and the paddles would not be discharged.

Precordial Thump

Precordial thump is a mechanical form of unsynchronized cardioversion that generates a small electrical current in the heart and occasionally converts acute tachydysrhythmias. A single thump is delivered to the sternum by the rescuer's fist. It may be administered to a monitored patient at the onset of VF or pulseless VT, or to an unmonitored patient without a pulse. If a single blow fails to restore a pulse or organized rhythm, basic life support measures are instituted until a defibrillator becomes available. The precordial thump is used only in the absence of the more effective defibrillator and only for pulseless patients, as induction of VF is possible.

Drug Therapy

In addition to epinephrine, antiarrhythmic drugs are administered for tachyarrhythmias during cardiac arrest to promote sustained cardioversion. Lidocaine and bretylium tosylate are equally effective during resuscitation from VF and pulseless VT. Lidocaine is the drug of choice because of its rapid effect (Fig. 20–8). Pharmacologic cardioversion of stable VT not requiring rapid electrical cardioversion is achieved with lidocaine or procainamide (Fig. 20–9).

Verapamil and adenosine are drugs of choice for pharmacologic cardioversion of SVT (Fig. 20–10). Beta-adrenergic antagonists and digoxin are not used initially because of lesser efficacy and longer onset time, respectively. These drugs, as well as procainamide, may be used to maintain a stable cardiac rate and rhythm following SVT termination. Table 20–6 is a summary of drug therapy during CPR.

SPECIFIC THERAPY OF CARDIAC ARREST DUE TO BRADYDYSRHYTHMIAS

Asystole is a lethal dysrhythmia, and severe bradycardias are life-threatening when the resulting heart rate is insufficient to generate effective cardiac output (usually less than 30 beats per minute). Extreme bradycardias, including heart blocks, may also be the progenitors of VF or asystole.

Table 20–6. CPR Pharmacology

Drug	Bolus Dose*	Infusion Rate	Remarks
BLS Drug Therapy			
Oxygen	100%		Never withhold; support ventilation as required
Epinephrine	1:10,000 (100 μg/ml); 10 ml (10–15 μg/kg) IV; 10 ml (1 mg) endotracheal		Repeat dose every 5 min May use peripheral IV if central venous route not available Avoid intracardiac injection
ACLS Drug Therapy			
CHRONOTROPES			
Atropine sulfate	0.3–1 mg IV or endotracheal		Total dose 2 mg
Isoproterenol		2–20 μg/min Titrate to effect	Beware of tachydysrhythmias and myocardial ischemia
ANTIDYSRHYTHMICS			
Lidocaine	1 mg/kg IV or endotracheal Repeat 0.5 mg/kg every 10 min as needed to total dose 3 mg/kg	2–4 mg/min Titrate	Use with caution in presence of high-grade AV block
Procainamide	100 mg IV Repeat every 5 min; loading dose 15 mg/kg	20–40 mg/min for loading infusion. Titrate 1–4 mg/min for maintenance infusion	Beware of hypotension and ECG toxicity
Bretylium tosylate	5–10 mg/kg IV Repeat dose every 15–30 min as needed to total dose 30 mg/kg	1–2 mg/min	Beware of postural hypotension, nausea
Propranolol	0.1–1 mg IV Titrate cautiously as needed to total dose 0.1 mg/kg		Beware of heart failure, bradydysrhythmias, and bronchospasm
Esmolol	0.1–1 mg/kg IV Titrate cautiously	25–200 μg/kg/min Titrate to effect	Beware of heart failure bradydysrhythmias, and bronchospasm
Verapamil	0.075–0.15 mg IV (max 10 mg) Repeat dose every 15–30 min as needed		Beware of hypotension; use with caution in presence of beta blockade, supraventricular conduction disease, heart failure May be used for rapid atrial fibrillation or flutter and PSVT
Adenosine	6–12 mg IV Repeat every 2 min up to two times		Inject rapidly For PSVT Not recommended for atrial fibrillation or flutter Beware of heart block, bronchospasm
INOTROPES			
Dopamine		Initial rate 2–5 μg/kg/min Titrate to effect	Beware of tachydysrhythmias and myocardial ischemia; Vasoconstrictor at 20 μg/kg/min
Dobutamine		Initial rate 2–5 μg/kg/min Titrate to effect	Beware of tachydysrhythmias and myocardial ischemia
Epinephrine	10–15 μg/kg for arrest situation 2–4 μg IV for hypotension, poor cardiac output	Initial rate 2–4 μg/min Titrate to effect	Beware of tachydysdysrhythmias and myocardial ischemia
Calcium chloride 10%	5–10 mg/kg IV Repeat dose every 10 min as needed		Central venous route preferable

(*Continued*)

TABLE 20–6. **CPR Pharmacology** *(Continued)*

Drug	Bolus Dose*	Infusion Rate	Remarks
VASOPRESSORS			
Norepinephrine		Initial rate 0.1–0.5 μg/kg/min Titrate to effect	Central venous route preferable
Phenylephrine	100–200 μg IV for hypotension	Initial rate 100–200 μg/min Titrate to effect	Central venous route preferable
Methoxamine	1–5 mg IV for hypotension		
VASODILATORS			
Sodium nitroprusside	50–100 μg IV	Initial rate 0.5 μg/kg/min Titrate to effect Maximum rate 8 μg/kg/min	May decrease Pa_{O_2}
Trimethaphan	1–2 mg IV	Initial rate 1–2 mg/min Titrate to effect	
Nitroglycerin	50–100 μg IV	Initial rate 0.5 μg/kg/min Titrate to effect	
Amrinone		Loading dose 0.75 mg/kg over 3 min, then 5–10 mg/kg/min Titrate to effect	

* Drugs are administered by bolus dose only to patients in cardiac arrest.

Emergent Cardiac Pacing

In instances of ventricular standstill due to acute complete heart block, activating an artificial pacemaker already in place is the best treatment. This is possible when a hospitalized patient is known to be at risk for development of complete heart block (for example, new conduction defect during anterior wall myocardial infarction, pulmonary artery catheterization in the presence of preexisting left bundle branch block, or emergency operations for a patient with syncope and trifascicular block on ECG). Pacemaker therapy becomes ineffective if delayed even minutes following cardiac standstill.

If a pacing wire is not already in place, external transcutaneous pacing electrodes are as effective as transthoracic pacing wires and offer fewer complications. Alternatively, repeated precordial thumps ("fist pacing") may be used for monitored acute ventricular asystole, provided each thump produces ventricular depolarization.

Drug Therapy

Epinephrine is the drug of choice for restoration of cardiac impulse formation and contraction in cardiac arrest due to asystole (Fig. 20–11). Drugs with predominantly beta-adrenergic actions, such as isoproterenol and dobutamine, are not used because coronary perfusion during CPR is diminished by beta-adrenergic-mediated peripheral vasodilation.

Atropine is used when bradycardia or heart block in the sinus or atrioventricular node produces hypotension (Fig. 20–12). Atropine-refractory bradycardia and second- or third-degree heart block occurring below the atrioventricular node are indications for drugs with beta-adrenergic activity (isoproterenol, dobutamine, dopamine, epinephrine) until a cardiac pacer is placed.

SPECIFIC THERAPY FOR CARDIAC ARREST DUE TO ELECTROMECHANICAL DISSOCIATION

A patient with an organized ECG pattern but no pulse or blood pressure has electromechanical dissociation (EMD). Electromechanical dissociation may be a terminal phenomenon, the result of extensive myocardial damage, or may be due to conditions which interfere with venous return to the

If Rhythm Is Unclear and Possibly Ventricular Fibrillation, Defibrillate as for VF. If Asystole is Present[a]

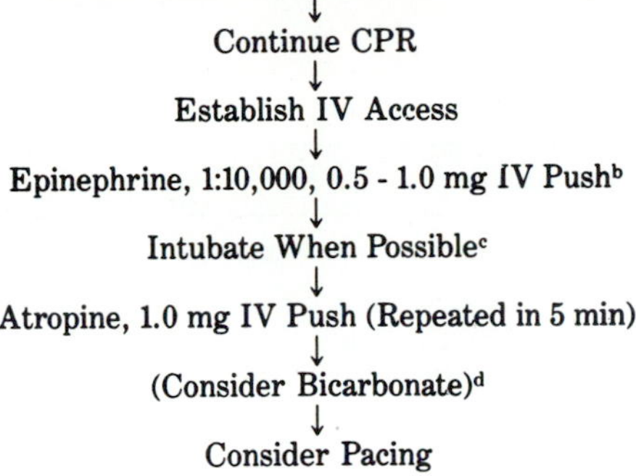

Continue CPR
Establish IV Access
Epinephrine, 1:10,000, 0.5 - 1.0 mg IV Push[b]
Intubate When Possible[c]
Atropine, 1.0 mg IV Push (Repeated in 5 min)
(Consider Bicarbonate)[d]
Consider Pacing

FIGURE 20–11. *American Heart Association treatment algorithm for cardiac arrest owing to asystole. For witnessed ventricular asystole in the presence of a rapidly applied external pacemaker, cardiac pacing is provided as initial therapy.*

[a] Asystole is confirmed by checking two ECG leads, paddle or ECG lead contact and cable connections, and oscilloscope gain adjustment to avoid improper therapy of VF or pulseless VT mistaken as asystole. [b] Epinephrine is repeated every five minutes. The drug may be given via endotracheal tube in the absence of an IV line. [c] If tracheal intubation can be performed simultaneously with other maneuvers (including chest compression), then the earlier it is accomplished the better. However, CPR and epinephrine are more important initially if the patient can be ventilated and oxygenated without intubation. [d] Value of sodium bicarbonate (dose titrated to neutralize base deficit calculated from arterial blood gas analysis) is questionable during cardiac resuscitation and it is not recommended as routine therapy. (Reproduced with permission, from the Textbook of advanced cardiac life support. 2nd ed. Dallas: American Heart Association, 1987.)

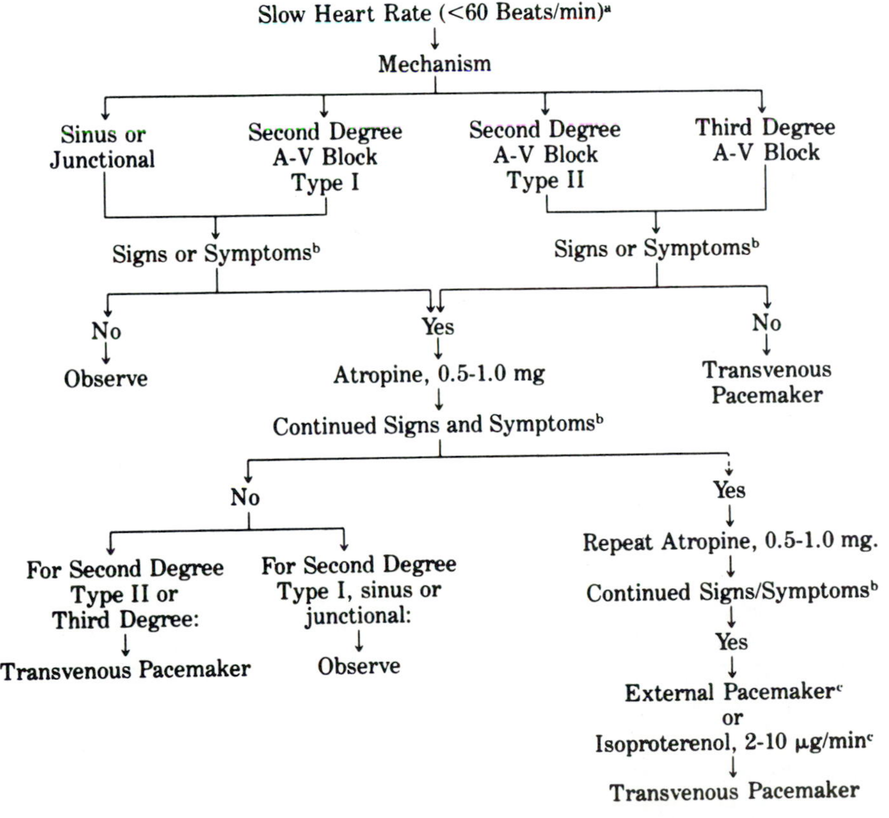

FIGURE 20–12. *American Heart Association treatment for algorithm for bradycardias.*

[a] Need for treatment is based on the site of conduction block and the patient's degree of hemodynamic compromise. [b] Signs: hypotension, altered sensorium, pulmonary edema, ventricular escape complexes or ischemia on ECG. Symptoms: angina or dyspnea. [c] Temporizing therapy prior to placing a transvenous pacemaker. Titrated infusion of epinephrine or dopamine may be used in lieu of isoproterenol to increase both heart rate and blood pressure. (Reproduced with permission, from the Textbook of advanced cardiac life support. 2nd ed. Dallas: American Heart Association, 1987.)

TABLE 20–7. **Special CPR Situations**

Cause of Arrest	Pathophysiology	Treatment
Trauma	Arrest due to massive blunt head and visceral injury, uncorrectable Reversible arrest caused by exsanguination, tension pneumothorax, cardiac tamponade, airway obstruction (due to loss of consciousness or airway injury) Associated cervical injuries, hypothermia	1. BLS with cervical spine precautions for airway opening 2. Rapid primary survey for reversible causes of arrest and specific treatment 3. See exsanguination, below 4. Consider thoracotomy for direct cardiac massage, treatment of pneumothorax and tamponade, clamping of aorta or pulmonary hilum
Exsanguination	Respiratory and cardiac arrest due to loss of cerebral and myocardial perfusion Chest compression ineffective in absence of venous return	1. Control hemorrhage 2. Restore blood volume via ≥2 large IVs with crystalloid solutions and O negative blood 3. BLS and ACLS as indicated; ACLS not effective until artificial circulation achieved
Electrocution	Primary apnea followed by secondary cardiac arrest due to hypoxemia, or Primary VF or asystolic cardiac arrest Associated burns, muscle destruction, myoglobinuria, bone fractures	1. Do not become a second victim! 2. Artificial ventilation as soon as possible 3. Chest compression and ACLS as indicated
Near-drowning	Submersion-induced asphyxiation followed by secondary cardiac arrest due to hypoxemia Full stomach due to swallowed water Pulmonary edema Hypothermia posible	1. Do not become a second victim! 2. Artificial ventilation as soon as possible; start mouth-to-mouth ventilation in water 3. Do not attempt to expel gastric water 4. Chest compression and ACLS as indicated
Hypothermia	Bradycardia, dysrhythmias, myocardial depression, coma, when T < 28°C Cardiac arrest due to VF or asystole Refractory to drugs, defibrillation, pacing until warmed Metabolic acidosis Diuresis	1. ECG monitoring 2. Dry patient 3. Core warming; IV fluids, heated inspired gas, warm lavage of pericardium, body cavities and viscera; cardiopulmonary bypass 4. BLS and ACLS as indicated
Carbon monoxide poisoning	Displacement of O_2 from hemoglobin, myoglobin, cytochrome binding sites by CO Airway obstruction due to unconsciousness, ventilatory depression Seizures Myocardial depression, dysrhythmias	1. BLS and ACLS as indicated 2. Ventilation with oxygen: CO elimination half-life 1.5 h in 100% O_2 at 1 atm; 0.5 h in 100% O_2 at 3 atm

heart or ventricular output: cardiac tamponade, tension pneumothorax, severe hypovolemia, or inhalational anesthetic overdose. Prompt treatment (pericardiocentesis, needle decompression of the pleural space, volume and vasopressor therapy, and discontinuation of the anesthetic) restores cardiac output. Massive pulmonary embolism with air or thrombus may also produce EMD.

When EMD cannot be reversed immediately, epinephrine enhances myocardial oxygen delivery during CPR and augments cardiac inotropy (Fig. 20–13). Calcium chloride increases contractility in patients with hypocalcemia and is useful in cases of cardiac arrest due to hyperkalemia, hypermagnesemia, and calcium channel blocker toxicity. See also Table 20–7.

Continue CPR
↓
Establish IV Access
↓
Epinephrine, 1:10,000, 0.5 - 1.0 mg IV Push[a]
↓
Intubate When Possible[b]
↓
(Consider Bicarbonate)[c]
↓
Consider Hypovolemia,
Cardiac Tamponade,
Tension Pneumothorax,
Hypoxemia,
Acidosis,
Pulmonary Embolism

FIGURE 20–13. American Heart Association treatment algorithm for cardiac arrest owing to electromechanical dissociation (EMD). Reversible causes of EMD (listed at bottom of algorithm) are considered immediately upon recognition of the condition, and specific therapy is provided before or simultaneously with drug administration and intubation.

[a] Epinephrine is repeated every five minutes. The drug may be given via endotracheal tube in the absence of an IV line. [b] If tracheal intubation can be performed simultaneously with other maneuvers including chest compression, then the earlier it is accomplished the better. However, CPR and epinephrine are more important initially if the patient can be ventilated and oxygenated without intubation. [c] Value of sodium bicarbonate (dose titrated to neutralize base deficit calculated from arterial blood gas analysis) is questionable during cardiac resuscitation and it is not recommended as routine therapy. (Reproduced with permission, from the Textbook of advanced cardiac life support. 2nd ed. Dallas: American Heart Association, 1987.)

Vascular Access

Peripheral arm veins are the first sites of vascular access during resuscitation because they are easily cannulated with few complications. Effective closed chest compression circulates drugs from peripheral venous sites, although circulation time is prolonged. It is inappropriate to withhold medications for subsequent administration through a yet unestablished central venous catheter when peripheral access is present.

Central venous drug administration reduces the time to onset of drug effect and is the ideal route when cardiac output is reduced. Central venous cannulation, most commonly via the internal jugular or subclavian vein, is performed if circulation is not restored following initial therapy and peripheral drug administration. Although femoral vein cannulation does not interfere with defibrillation, airway management, or chest compression, drug delivery by catheters lying below the diaphragm is unreliable because of poor flow in the inferior vena cava during closed chest compression.

Blind transthoracic intracardiac injection is the least desirable route of drug administration because of complications and the availability of safer alternatives for drug delivery.

Endotracheal Drug Administration

If intravenous access is delayed, most drugs can be instilled directly into the endotracheal tube, diluted to 10 cc in sterile saline. Onset is comparable to peripheral intravenous injection, but plasma concentrations are somewhat less and persist longer. The pressor effect of endotracheal epinephrine is one half to one third that of the intravenous route. Hyperventilation after endotracheal injection promotes dispersion of the drug.

Intraosseous Administration

Intraosseous administration of fluids and drugs can be used in pediatric patients when intravenous access cannot be achieved. The anterior surface of the tibia below the tibial tuberosity is pierced with a needle that is 18 gauge or larger. Volume expanders, blood, and drugs are flushed into the marrow cavity by gravity-fed or pressurized infusions. The rate of onset and dose response obtained by the intraosseous route is comparable to peripheral venous injection.

Acid-Base Therapy

Cardiopulmonary arrest results in a combined respiratory and metabolic acidosis. Intracellular acidosis causes depression of myocardial contractility, reduced myocardial and vasomotor responsiveness to catecholamines, a diminished threshold for the induction of VF, and increased energy dose requirements for cardioversion.

Acidosis in the first several minutes after cardiopulmonary arrest is due to carbon dioxide retention and correction is accomplished primarily by effective ventilation and artificial circulation. Surprisingly, intracellular acidosis and outcome from resuscitation are not improved by bicarbonate administration, despite correction of arterial pH. In part, this may be due to the CO_2 generated by the neutralization of acid by bicarbonate; poor cardiac output during CPR prevents elimination of this CO_2, which worsens acidosis. Other buffers that do not liberate CO_2 avoid respiratory acidosis but also fail to correct tissue intracellular acidosis, probably because of inadequate drug delivery to tissues.

No effective pharmacologic treatment is now available to correct metabolic acidosis during CPR; only improved tissue perfusion and pulmonary blood flow appear efficacious. Acidosis is best avoided by prompt therapy that restores native circulation and ventilation.

POSTRESUSCITATION LIFE SUPPORT

After resuscitation, the patient is evaluated to determine the degree of cerebral, cardiovascular, pulmonary, and renal function salvaged during BLS and ACLS, a well as the primary underlying cause of the cardiopulmonary arrest. If a primary condition can be identified, prompt definitive treatment may prevent recurrence of arrest.

The patient who is awake and breathing spontaneously after successful resuscitation is monitored in an intensive care unit for recurrence of cardiac arrest. A continuous prophylactic antiarrhythmic infusion, most commonly lidocaine, is indicated for 24 hours following resuscitation from VF and VT. Other supportive measures are needed for the patient who remains apneic or who has cardiovascular instability; these may include mechanical ventilation, pressors, inotropes, and other treatment for cardiogenic shock.

Support of cerebral function after global ischemic injury caused by cardiopulmonary arrest entails general measures which maintain cerebral oxygen delivery (e.g., avoiding hypotension, correcting hypoxemia) and control cerebral metabolic rate (e.g., preventing hyperthermia, treating seizures). Specific therapies such as hyperventilation, neuromuscular blockade, and large doses of barbiturates have not been shown to improve neurologic outcome from global cerebral ischemic injury. Corticosteroids, calcium channel blocking agents, and iron chelators remain controversial.

REFERENCES

Jaffe AS. New and old paradoxes. Acidosis and cardiopulmonary resuscitation. Circulation 1989; 80:1079–1083.

Paradis NA, Koscove EM. Epinephrine in cardiac arrest: A critical review. Ann Emerg Med 1990; 19:1288–1301.

Proceedings of the 1985 national conference of standards and guidelines for cardiopulmonary resuscitation and emergency cardiac care. Circulation 1986; 74:IV1–IV153.

Schleinen CL, Berkowitz ID, Traystman R, Rogers MC. Controversial issues in cardiopulmonary resuscitation. Anesthesiology 1989; 71:133–149.

Standards and guidelines for cardiopulmonary resuscitation and emergency cardiac care. J Am Med Assoc 1986; 255:2841–3044.

Textbook of advanced cardiac life support. Dallas: American Heart Association, 1987.

CHAPTER TWENTY-ONE

Cardiovascular Disease

The annual mortality from cardiovascular disease in the general population of the United States is greater than from all other diseases combined. Similarly, the leading cause of death after anesthesia and operations is perioperative cardiac morbidity, defined as myocardial infarction, unstable angina, congestive heart failure, or serious dysrhythmia. Hypertension accounts for 90 per cent of cardiovascular disease, followed by coronary artery disease, rhythm disturbances, peripheral vascular disease, cerebrovascular disease, congestive heart failure, and rheumatic heart disease. The prevalence of coronary artery disease may be underestimated, because 70 per cent of ischemic episodes in patients with coronary artery disease do not produce angina, and approximately 10 to 15 per cent of acute myocardial infarctions are silent.

Recent improvements in predicting patients at risk and in understanding the pathophysiology of myocardial ischemia have offered the prospect of reduced risk.

Determinants of myocardial oxygen demand ($M\dot{V}O_2$) include: (1) systolic wall tension, which is a function of aortic systolic pressure and left ventricular end-diastolic pressure and volume; (2) contractile state of the myocardium; and (3) heart rate (Table 21–1). Myocardial ischemia occurs when $M\dot{V}O_2$ exceeds critical coronary blood flow in patients with coronary artery stenosis. Under normal conditions, the coronary vascular bed autoregulates blood flow over a coronary perfusion pressure range of 60 to 130 mm Hg. During periods of ischemia, coronary vasodilator reserve is exhausted and coronary flow is dependent upon coronary perfusion pressure.

In addition to coronary perfusion pressure and degree of stenosis, other determinants of coronary blood flow include heart rate, status of the collateral circulation, coronary vasomotor tone, and intramyocardial compression forces, which vary during systole and diastole. Because of extravascular compression, only 20 to 30 per cent of left coronary artery flow occurs during systole. Intramyocardial compressive forces are less during systole in the thin-walled right ventricle and a greater percentage of right coronary flow (30 to 50 per cent) occurs during systole. Increases in heart rate not only increase myocardial oxygen consumption, but also result in decreased diastolic and collateral perfusion times and diastolic filling time.

Drugs used to treat myocardial ischemia reduce heart rate and myocardial contractility (beta blockers) and reduce coronary vasomotor tone (nitrates and calcium channel blockers). Treatment of congestive heart failure with diuretics, nitroglycerin, digitalis, and afterload reduction decreases ventricular wall tension and myocardial oxygen consumption. The reduction in left ventricular end-diastolic pressure results in an improvement in myocardial oxygen supply by reducing the transmyocardial gradient of blood flow also.

Oxygen delivery to the heart depends not only on coronary blood flow, but also on arterial oxygen

TABLE 21–1. Determinants of Myocardial Oxygen Supply and Demand

Oxygen Supply	Oxygen Demand
Coronary blood flow	Systolic wall tension
	Systolic aortic pressure
Oxygen transport	Left ventricular end-diastolic pressure
O_2 Saturation	Contractile state
Hemoglobin	Heart rate

content of the blood. The heart extracts oxygen maximally from the blood, so that increasing myocardial oxygen delivery depends on blood flow, hemoglobin concentration, and the hemoglobin saturation. Both supply and demand factors must be considered when managing a patient with cardiovascular disease during anesthesia and operation.

PREOPERATIVE EVALUATION

Preoperative evaluation of patients who might have coronary artery disease seeks to assess the patient in two ways. First, it is important to estimate the function of the heart by estimating its capacity as a pump (reflecting function of myocardium and valves), the stability of the rhythm, and the quality of the coronary circulation. Estimating pumping function can be as simple as documenting a history of good exercise tolerance—a patient who can easily climb a flight of stairs without chest pain or dyspnea is likely to have adequate myocardial reserve for the demands of anesthesia and operation. Patients who do not exercise (perhaps because of arthritis or other musculoskeletal problems), in whom the history is suggestive of cardiac disease, or who have suggestive findings such as cardiomegaly or nocturnal dyspnea, may need further testing to evaluate cardiopulmonary reserve. Noninvasive estimates of ejection fraction are often suitable tests for this purpose. The necessity of such testing depends in part on the planned operation: a patient scheduled for drainage of an infected finger performed under local anesthesia might not require such studies, whereas these studies would be needed before a major abdominal or thoracic operation.

Preanesthetic assessment for significant arrhythmias is based on the history (palpitations, fainting spells) and examination of the electrocardiogram (ECG) for heart block or arrhythmias. Should the ECG or the history suggest heart block, consultation with a cardiologist is appropriate. Prophylactic pacemakers are usually not required before anesthesia and operation except in those patients who already need them for routine activities.

Assessment of the functional status of the coronary circulation is difficult, because coronary artery disease often produces no symptoms. Studies have sought to identify risk factors to predict the likelihood of perioperative myocardial infarction. The results of these studies are sometimes contradictory, and risk factors that clearly imply severe coronary artery disease sometimes are not identified as statistically significant predictors of risk, probably because of the relatively small numbers of patients in the studies and the fact that treatment is not withheld. At present, it seems safe to include the following as preoperative findings that imply increased risk of myocardial infarction owing to coronary artery disease, listed in order from strongest to weakest predictors.

1. A history of a recent myocardial infarction warns of another in the perioperative period; the magnitude of the risk depends on the interval since the infarction. Perioperative myocardial infarction in the general population of patients occurs less than 1 per cent of the time; for a previous infarction more than six months previously 5 per cent; for infarctions three to six months previously, 10 to 15 per cent; for infarctions less than three months previously, 30 per cent. It is likely that these earlier figures represent overestimates, given current management. A small series of high-risk patients managed with intensive care and invasive monitoring experienced much better results than those described above. Although not logistically possible for all patients with coronary artery disease, this combination of aggressive monitoring and treatment appears to be of real value for patients who have major risk factors for perioperative cardiac morbidity.
2. Dipyridamole thallium scanning is sensitive (93 per cent) and specific (80 per cent) for detecting coronary artery stenosis and is superior to historical predictors and exercise stress testing for pre-

dicting a significant postoperative myocardial event in patients undergoing peripheral vascular operations; abnormal results suggest significant cardiovascular risks perioperatively.

3. A set of findings including Q waves on ECG, history of congestive heart failure, diabetes, history of angina, and myocardial infarction correlate with the risk of infarction. The presence of one or more of these five clinical variables is associated with approximately a fivefold increase in postoperative ischemic events.

4. Associated disease may suggest increased cardiac risk. Patients with peripheral vascular disease commonly have coronary artery disease also, as do patients with hypertension, diabetes, or histories of cigarette smoking.

Although controlled studies to prove that therapy improves outcome for these patients are lacking, the physiologic evidence is convincing enough to make it imperative to detect and treat angina, congestive heart failure, and hypertension preoperatively. High-risk patients with coronary artery disease may be candidates for coronary angioplasty or coronary artery bypass grafts before elective noncardiac operations, and must be evaluated for such perioperatively; consultation with a cardiologist is particularly valuable. It is clear that elective operations are best postponed until several months (usually at least six) after a myocardial infarction and for six weeks to three months after coronary artery bypass grafting.

Patients with significant carotid artery disease are at risk of stroke during and after anesthesia and operation. The greatest risk for stroke occurs in those with a history of transient ischemic attacks (TIA) and severe carotid artery obstruction (75 per cent or more occlusion) on angiography. These patients are treated surgically, but there are no convincing data that prophylactic carotid endarterectomy reduces the incidence of stroke in asymptomatic patients with carotid bruits.

Systemic hypertension is the most common form of cardiovascular disease. Hypertension is accompanied by structural changes that include smooth muscle hypertrophy in arteries and a decrease in the number of small arterioles peripherally, resulting in an increase in systemic vascular resistance. Initially, hypertrophy of the left ventricle allows the heart to maintain a normal cardiac output despite an increase in systemic vascular resistance. Eventually, the left ventricle becomes stiff and less compliant and cardiac output decreases in response to an increase in systemic vascular resistance, but this process often occurs over many years. Structural changes in the small arteries result in a greater change in luminal diameter and resistance for a given change in smooth muscle tone in hypertensive patients. These processes contribute to the marked lability in blood pressure that is evident in the untreated (or inadequately treated) hypertensive patient.

In addition to the heart, other organs are affected by chronic hypertension, including especially the kidney and brain. Structural changes in the walls of blood vessels, combined with alterations in circulating hormones (catecholes) and vasoactive substances (angiotensin), result in an increase in renal vascular resistance and impaired renal blood flow and function. Autoregulation in the cerebral vasculature is altered, resulting in a shift of the autoregulatory curve to the right; increased pressure is required to maintain flow to the brain. This autoregulation curve returns to near normal after treatment of the hypertension (see Chapter 30). Patients with chronic systemic hypertension need greater cerebral perfusion pressures than normal to maintain cerebral perfusion, and blood pressure must not be decreased rapidly to normotensive values because cerebral ischemia may result.

Antihypertensive medications, including beta blockers and clonidine, are continued until the time of operation because the rebound hypertension that occurs with the abrupt withdrawal of these drugs may lead to myocardial ischemia or infarction.

There are no large prospective studies of morbidity in treated versus untreated patients with hypertension scheduled for elective operation. However, effective treatment leads to a reduction in perioperative hemodynamic fluctuations. Further, patients who are hypertensive preoperatively have a greater incidence of neurologic deficit and mortality after carotid endarterectomy. Severe hypertension (diastolic blood pressure greater than 110 mm Hg) increases afterload and myocardial oxygen consumption, and may result in myocardial ischemia, infarction, congestive heart failure, and arrhythmias; it is associated with cerebral hemorrhage and progressive renal insufficiency also. Thus, there are many arguments favoring the control of blood pressure prior to elective operations, and for recommending that those with diastolic blood pressures of 110 mm Hg or greater receive additional treatment before proceeding with anesthesia and operation. Rapid intravenous treatment of hypertension is not recommended except in emergencies, because a sudden reduction in blood pressure to what may be considered "normal" blood pressures could precipitate ischemia in vital organs.

INTRAOPERATIVE MANAGEMENT

Regional versus General Anesthesia

Skillfully conducted regional anesthesia limited to an extremity produces no major physiologic alterations, yet blocks the pain that causes tachycardia and hypertension. Given adequate sedation, ventilation, and oxygenation, this is a very satisfactory form of anesthesia for patients at risk of myocardial infarction, pump failure, or arrhythmias.

The situation is less clear when spinal or epidural anesthesia is suggested as a panacea for the patient with cardiac disease who is to undergo a major operation. The anesthetics themselves can be expected to have mixed effects on myocardial oxygen balance: afterload and heart rate may decrease, but hypotension may threaten coronary perfusion pressure (a special hazard in aortic stenosis). Further, the hazards of postoperative pain, bleeding, and hypothermia remain when the effect of the regional anesthetic dissipates. Spinal or epidural anesthesia may be more useful when they are continued into the postoperative period for long-term pain relief (see Chapters 18 and 36), but at present, spinal or epidural anesthesia cannot by themselves be expected to solve the problems of managing patients with cardiac disease.

Effects of General Anesthetics

A number of studies have suggested that the technique used for general anesthesia has no effect on the incidence of myocardial infarction in patients with coronary artery disease. There are no large, randomized, prospective studies comparing outcome after general or regional anesthesia in patients with cardiovascular disease. Nonrandomized, prospective, and retrospective analyses, however, suggest that morbidity and mortality correlate with patient and surgical risk factors, and not the type of anesthesia.

Hypertension or hypotension may lead to myocardial ischemia, but tachycardia (heart rate 110 per minute or greater) appears to be a most reliable herald of ischemia. Beta blockers, with or without calcium entry blockers, are associated with decreased heart rate on arrival to the operating room and with a decreased incidence of perioperative myocardial ischemia. Calcium entry blocker therapy alone does not appear to offer a protective effect. Despite careful hemodynamic control, many perioperative myocardial ischemic events occur without associated hemodynamic abnormalities.

Of the inhalational anesthetics, halothane produces more myocardial depression than enflurane or isoflurane, whereas isoflurane has a greater effect on systemic vascular resistance; all reduce blood pressure when administered in clinical concentrations. The addition of nitrous oxide tends to increase systemic vascular resistance slightly, but arterial pressure is usually not changed owing to a corresponding decrease in cardiac output. However, the combination of nitrous oxide and a potent vapor has been used with great success for many years in those with cardiovascular disease, perhaps because the combination allows precise control of arterial pressure without excessive myocardial depression.

Of the intravenous anesthetics, thiopental and propofol produce a dose-dependent depressant effect on myocardial contractility, whereas etomidate produces minimal hemodynamic changes or alterations in myocardial function. However, successful induction of anesthesia in those with cardiovascular disease appears to depend on selection of the appropriate dose, rather than selection of a specific drug. Among the opiates, fentanyl and sufentanil provide hemodynamic stability and a favorable myocardial oxygen supply:demand balance. In larger doses, sufentanil can produce depression of myocardial contractility and must be used cautiously in patients with poor left ventricular function.

Drugs that act on normal coronary vessels to produce vasodilation may induce a "steal" phenomenon in those with coronary stenosis by promoting blood flow to normal areas of the myocardium and away from maximally dilated ischemic areas. Although there is evidence in animals that isoflurane may produce a coronary steal, this subject remains controversial. There may be a small subset of patients with stenosis of the collateral-supplying vessel who are at risk of isoflurane-induced coronary steal, but isoflurane is used frequently and successfully in patients undergoing coronary artery bypass grafting. Thus, isoflurane is clearly not contraindicated in those with coronary artery disease, but it is prudent to change to another anesthetic if myocardial ischemia occurs in a patient receiving isoflurane.

Intraoperative Monitoring and Detection of Ischemia

Monitoring the patient at risk of pump failure, whether from myocardial dysfunction or valve disease, includes the invasive monitoring of arterial pressure, filling pressures, and cardiac output. When left and right heart functions are likely to become dissociated, a pulmonary artery catheter is preferred over a right atrial catheter (see Chapter 6).

Monitoring for patients at risk of heart block or arrhythmias consists of employing an ECG lead that best reveals atrial activity (usually lead II).

Monitoring of patients at risk for myocardial ischemia relies on three premises. The first well-accepted idea is that even though such indicators of $M\dot{V}O_2$ as blood pressure and heart rate are carefully maintained near preoperative values, patients may still suffer unanticipated ischemia.

The second, more debated premise is that the occurrence of intraoperative myocardial ischemic events is correlated with the postoperative finding of myocardial ischemia. In a recent study of patients known to have coronary artery disease (or to be at high risk of it), Mangano found a greater incidence of postoperative than intraoperative ischemia by ECG monitoring (41 per cent versus 25 per cent); further, the occurrence of postoperative ischemia (almost all silent) was a significant predictor of postoperative adverse outcome, whereas the occurrence of intraoperative ischemia was not. This study was not designed to test the hypothesis that postoperative ischemia is a better predictor than intraoperative, and was halted when interim analysis of the data indicated that a potentially useful form of monitoring (postoperative ECG evidence of ischemia) had been discovered. It points out the importance of postoperative events, however, and reminds us that prevention of perioperative myocardial infarction does not end when the anesthesia is concluded successfully.

The third premise justifying special monitoring for patients with coronary artery disease is that when ischemia is detected, intervention can improve outcome. This has yet to be demonstrated in a controlled study, but is an intuitively appealing idea.

Techniques used to detect intraoperative ischemia include ECG, pulmonary vascular pressure monitoring, and transesophageal echocardiography. Radionuclear imaging, cardiomyography, coronary sinus catheters, and biochemical assays are used primarily as research tools.

Electrocardiographic evidence of ischemia has been defined as 1 mm or more of downsloping or horizontal ST-segment depression, greater than 2 mm of upsloping ST-segment depression or ST elevation of greater than 1 mm. Electrocardiographic changes consistent with ischemia occur in 18 to 74 per cent of patients with coronary artery disease undergoing noncardiac surgical procedures. Most of the changes are ST depression and 90 per cent of these occur in leads V_4 and V_5. Combining leads II, V_4, and V_5 increases the sensitivity for detecting ischemia to 96 per cent. The presence of left bundle branch block or digoxin therapy greatly impairs the use of the ECG for diagnosing ischemia.

Many monitors used in the operating room can be programmed for detecting and recording trends in ST-segment changes; their sensitivity is increased if the monitor is used in the diagnostic mode. On-line computer processing of multilead ECG is being developed, and advances in detection and interpretation of ST-segment and T-wave changes as well as arrhythmias are expected in the near future.

Pulmonary artery occlusion pressure can reflect increases in left ventricular end-diastolic wedge pressure due to stiffening of ischemic myocardium. Not only is pulmonary artery pressure monitoring invasive, it is not a sensitive monitor for detection of myocardial ischemia. Discrepancies up to 15 mm Hg have been noted between the pulmonary capillary wedge pressure (PCWP) and left ventricular end-diastolic pressure (LVEDP) during ischemia.

Pulmonary artery pressure and thermodilution cardiac output measurements obtained from a pulmonary artery catheter can be used to calculate some of the determinants of cardiac work, such as pulmonary vascular resistance (PVR), systemic vascular resistance (SVR), and right and left ventricular stroke work indices (RVSWI, LVSWI). Also, if the tip of the pulmonary artery catheter lies below the left atrium, the PCWP measurement is used to estimate LVEDP and to calculate coronary perfusion pressure (aortic diastolic pressure minus LVEDP). In patients with poor left ventricular function (ejection fraction less than 0.40 or with significant wall-motion abnormalities) changes in central venous pressure (CVP) do not predict changes in PCWP. Further, increased PCWP (more than 25 mm Hg) has been associated with a greatly increased risk of perioperative reinfarction. Thus, pulmonary artery catheter monitoring is not a sensitive monitor to detect myocardial ischemia, but in high-risk patients with cardiac disease it may improve care.

Transesophageal echocardiography (TEE) is used to measure regional ventricular wall-motion and wall-thickening changes to estimate ejection fractions, to detect intracardiac air, and to evaluate valvular function. Transesophageal echocardiography is the most sensitive monitor for myocardial ischemia. Sequential wall-motion and wall-thickening abnormalities occur earlier than ECG changes during myocardial ischemia, and a large fraction of wall-motion abnormalities occur without any changes in PCWP.

Intra-arterial blood pressure monitoring is commonplace in patients with cardiovascular disease, especially those with hypertension or associated pulmonary diseases, and in those undergoing operations that result in major hemodynamic alterations. Advantages include continuous recording of the blood pressure, and access for sampling of arterial blood for measurements including arterial blood gases, electrolytes, and hemoglobin levels. Indications for its use include uncontrolled hypertension, recent myocardial infarction or congestive heart failure, and expected moderate to severe fluctuations in blood pressure related to the operation.

Blood Pressure Control

Sudden severe increases in blood pressure increase afterload for the left ventricle producing an increase in wall tension and myocardial oxygen consumption. Although the normal heart tolerates mean arterial pressures of 120 mm Hg, in the failing heart, the increase in left ventricular end-diastolic pressure may exceed the arterial diastolic pressure resulting in a reduction in coronary perfusion and myocardial ischemia. Also, severe increases in blood pressure may produce congestive heart failure, arrhythmias, cerebral hemorrhage, and increase in blood loss during the operation. These and other factors argue for careful blood pressure control before, during, and after operation.

Patients are at risk of hypertension during (1) laryngoscopy and intubation, (2) skin incision, (3) sternotomy or craniotomy incisions and closures, and (4) during emergence. During these stressful periods, increased levels of circulating catecholamines and increased sympathetic nervous system activity are thought to be primarily responsible for the hypertension and tachycardia. Patients with inadequate blood pressure control preoperatively exhibit exaggerated responses to these stimuli.

To blunt the hypertension and tachycardia associated with laryngoscopy and intubation, a number of techniques have been used. Although narcotics alone do blunt the hemodynamic response to laryngoscopy and intubation, the large doses required may not be appropriate for most patients and operations (although ultra–short-acting drugs such as alfentanil hold promise for operations of moderate duration). When used in smaller doses in combination with induction agents such as sodium thiopental, these drugs reduce the total dose of thiopental and attenuate the response to laryngoscopy and intubation. Intravenous lidocaine (1 to 1.5 mg per kg) can be used to partially blunt this response. Also, pretreatment with antihypertensives including propranolol, labetalol, esmolol, clonidine, nifedipine, or enalapril may reduce the hemodynamic response to laryngoscopy and intubation. The choice of drugs depends on the patient, possible drug interactions, other concurrent diseases, whether a rapid sequence induction or awake intubation is required, and the proposed operation. For example, a large-dose narcotic technique may be useful for cardiac operations, whereas the same approach would be entirely inappropriate for a brief operation, even in the same patient.

Hypertensive patients not only demonstrate hypertension and tachycardia during periods of stress as described above, but they also have greater reductions in blood pressure in response to inhalational anesthetics, antihypertensive drugs, and sympathectomy associated with spinal or epidural anesthesia. Because of a contracted plasma volume secondary to the disease process, and perhaps owing to diuretic therapy or other dehydrating factors such as radiocontrast media or laxatives and enemas used for bowel preparation, hypertensive patients are often hypovolemic and require additional volume expansion on induction of anesthesia or before spinal or epidural anesthesia.

Intraoperative hypertension is usually treated by deepening anesthesia with inhalational anesthetics or narcotics; however, antihypertensives including nitroprusside, nitroglycerin, trimethaphan, esmolol, labetalol, propranolol, hydralazine, and sublingual nifedipine have been used. Because of the great incidence of coronary artery disease in patients having major vascular operations, nitroglycerin is often used for its coronary vasodilating effect in these patients. Although nitroprusside or isoflurane could produce a myocardial steal, these drugs are used successfully to treat intraoperative hypertension, often with improvement in signs of myocardial ischemia.

Intraoperative hypertension associated with an increase in intracranial pressure represents a specific problem, discussed in Chapter 30.

Intraoperative hypertension is best viewed a a sign of an underlying problem, not as a primary condition requiring antihypertensive therapy. Before treatment with an antihypertensive drug is begun, other causes of hypertension must be ruled out including light anesthesia, hypervolemia, hypercarbia, hypoxia, increased intracranial pressure, or unintended administration of vasoconstrictors.

Emergence from anesthesia is a critical time for a patient with a history of hypertension, coronary artery disease, myocardial dysfunction, or previous stroke. Sudden increases in blood pressure produce an increase in afterload for the left ventricle resulting in congestive heart failure, myocardial ischemia, cerebral hemorrhage, or surgical bleeding. Hypertension associated with emergence from anesthesia may be related to the abrupt discontinuation of inhalational anesthetics, especially if a narcotic has not been administered for pain on emergence. Careful titration of narcotics and other drugs such as labetalol, hydralazine, propranolol, esmolol, or sublingual nifedipine will blunt the hemodynamic response associated with emergence.

Intraoperative hypotension is an important predictor of perioperative cardiac morbidity. In the presence of severe coronary artery stenosis, decreases in arterial pressure may produce myocardial ischemia; the combination of hypotension and tachycardia is particularly devastating in this regard. Also, hypotension is associated with cerebral ischemia in patients with cerebrovascular disease, a history of hypertension, or during carotid endarterectomy operations.

Treatment of intraoperative hypotension includes volume expansion, treatment of bradycardia and other arrhythmias, and the use of vasopressors. Vasopressor therapy is usually a symptomatic treatment of a more fundamental problem; it is used primarily to gain time for definitive treatment and not as a substitute for other therapies. (There are exceptions to this rule. A patient with reduced ability to excrete extra sodium and water who becomes hypotensive after spinal anesthesia may be better treated with a short-term infusion of a vasoconstrictor than with intravenous saline.) Patients with coronary artery disease may not tolerate the increase in heart rate associated with indirect acting pressors such as ephedrine.

Pulmonary artery catheter monitoring allows measurements of PCWP and thermodilution cardiac outputs; together these data can be used to construct a Starling curve of cardiac function. The Starling curves for patients with reduced left ventricular function are depressed and shifted to the right (Fig. 21–1), indicating impaired pump function of the heart. These patients need greater filling pressures to maintain cardiac output.

Chronic congestive heart failure, systemic hypertension, excess catecholamine production, and hypothermia are associated with an increase in systemic vascular resistance and afterload for the left ventricle. Afterload reduction with sodium nitroprusside, nitroglycerin, hydralazine, calcium channel blockers, alpha-adrenergic antagonists, or angiotensin-converting enzyme inhibitors will result in an improvement in left ventricular performance. A decrease in systemic vascular resistance may be accompanied by tachycardia, especially if sodium nitroprusside or hydralazine are used. This response is blunted, however, in patients with a

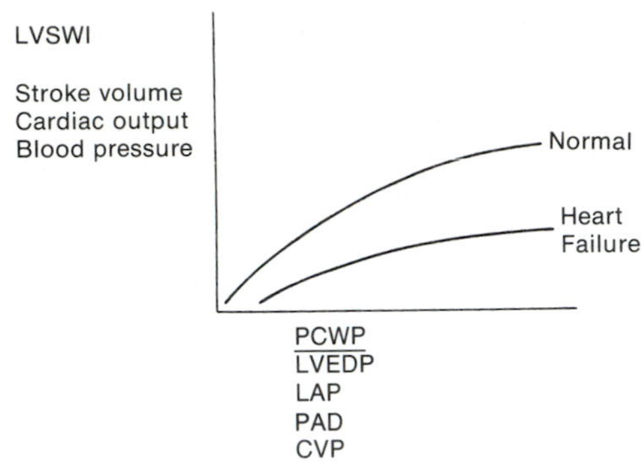

FIGURE 21–1. Ventricular function curves. On the abscissa are indices of muscle fiber length, of which left ventricular end-diastolic pressure (LVEDP) is the most closely related to left ventricular myocardial fiber length, and central venous pressure (CVP) the most distant. On the ordinate are indices of ventricular performance. The depressed or failing heart requires more preload to perform the same work, as shown by the performance curve displaced to the right. In clinical practice, blood pressure or cardiac output are related to CVP, pulmonary capillary wedge pressure (PCWP), or pulmonary artery diastolic pressure (PAD). If giving the patient additional fluid increases these indices of ventricular filling without improving blood pressure or cardiac output, the heart is presumed to have reached a flat portion of the function curve; inotropic therapy or reducing systemic resistance are indicated. (Reproduced with permission from Kaplan JA. Hemodynamic monitoring in cardiac anesthesia. 2nd ed. New York: Grune & Stratton, 1987:209.)

history of congestive heart failure or who are taking beta blockers. A reduction in ventricular wall tension will result in an improvement in endocardial blood flow as well as cardiac output. Some patients with a depressed Starling curve or reduced left ventricular performance may benefit from combined afterload reduction and inotropic support to enhance pump function, cardiac output, and myocardial perfusion.

POSTOPERATIVE CARE

After completion of the surgical procedure and discontinuation of the anesthetic, the patient is transferred to a recovery room or intensive care unit. High-risk patients (i.e., after open-heart operations, craniotomy, major vascular operations, or surgical procedures associated with large fluid volume replacement) are transported with the use of a portable hemodynamic monitor. Also, patients receiving infusions of vasoactive drugs or those at risk for major blood pressure fluctuations are monitored during transport because this is often a time when major hemodynamic abnormalities (hypertension, hypotension, tachycardia) occur.

The immediate postoperative period can be very stressful to the patient with severe cardiovascular disease. Hypertension and tachycardia occur following the discontinuation of inhalational anesthetics and the onset of pain. Hypothermia produces an increase in systemic vascular resistance, and shivering increases oxygen consumption radically. Other causes of postoperative hypertension include anxiety, reaction to an endotracheal tube, hypoxia, hypercarbia, hypervolemia, and withdrawal syndromes, especially following the abrupt discontinuation of preoperative drugs such as beta blockers, clonidine, or nitroprusside. With the few exceptions, the most important contributing factor to the development of postoperative hypertension is a history of hypertension preoperatively. Postoperative hypertension is usually brief in duration; 80 per cent of hypertensive events occur within 30 minutes of admission to the recovery room and end within three hours.

Postoperative hypertension may produce myocardial ischemia, infarction, congestive heart failure, arrhythmias, cerebral hemorrhage, or bleeding and disruption of vascular sutures. Approaches to treatment of postoperative hypertension include pain control with systemic narcotics, epidural or subarachnoid narcotics, and patient-controlled analgesia. In addition to pain, other causes of hypertension including hypoxia, hypercarbia, hypothermia, hypervolemia, and anxiety are treated before beginning intravenous antihypertensive therapy. Drugs used to control hypertension in the immediate postoperative period include sodium nitroprusside, nitroglycerin, trimethaphan, esmolol, labetalol, hydralazine, propranolol, or sublingual nifedipine. Nitroglycerin is recommended for patients with coronary artery disease because of its salutary effect on the coronary circulation.

Postoperative hypotension may decrease perfusion pressure to the heart, brain, or kidney and result in ischemia of these vital organs. Approaches to the treatment of hypotension are similar to those described under intraoperative blood pressure control.

Hypoxemia in the immediate postoperative period also increases the risk of cardiac complications and must be prevented as described elsewhere (see Chapters 22 and 25).

Conclusion

Despite recent progress in managing patients at risk for cardiac complications through careful hemodynamic control and the other measures described here, a significant number of patients suffer myocardial ischemia intraoperatively and myocardial infarction postoperatively. Progress will undoubtedly require increased understanding of the mechanisms of thrombosis and vessel spasm, and improvements in technology for detecting myocardial ischemia.

References

Eagle KA, Singer DE, Brewster DC, et al. Dipyridamole-thallium scanning in patients undergoing vascular surgery. JAMA 1987; 257:2185–2189.

Mangano DT. Perioperative cardiac morbidity. Anesthesiology 1990; 72:153–184.

Mangano DT, Browner WS, Hollenberg M, et al. Association of perioperative myocardial ischemia with cardiac morbidity and mortality in men undergoing noncardiac surgery. N Engl J Med 1990; 323:1781–1788.

Priebe HJ. Isoflurane and coronary hemodynamics. Anesthesiology 1989; 71:960–976.

Prys-Roberts C. Anesthesia and hypertension. Br J Anaesth 1984; 56:711–724.

Rao TK, Jacobs KH, El-Etr AA. Reinfarction following anesthesia in patients with myocardial infarction. Anesthesiology 1983; 59:499–505.

Shah KB, Kleinman BS, Rao TLK, et al. Angina and other risk factors in patients with cardiac diseases undergoing noncardiac operations. Anesth Anal 1990; 70:240–247.

Slogoff S, Keats AS. Randomized trial of primary anesthetic agents on outcome of coronary bypass operations. Anesthesiology 1989; 70:179–188.

CHAPTER TWENTY-TWO

ANESTHESIA AND RESPIRATORY DISEASE

The exchange of the respiratory gases between the atmosphere and pulmonary capillary blood is the most critical first step in the preservation of tissue Po_2 and metabolism. Disease processes that impair respiratory gas exchange also impair the exchange of anesthetic gases and vapors.

The goal of this chapter is to review the salient features of normal pulmonary gas exchange to develop a systematic approach to predicting the impact of pulmonary disease on respiratory and anesthetic gas exchange and provide a basis for clinical management. These principles will be used to describe the anesthesia management of patients with pulmonary disease, but not the management of thoracotomies, one-lung ventilation, or pulmonary lavage, which lie beyond the scope of this volume.

ANATOMY OF THE LUNG

The human lung consists of conducting airways and alveolated airways that are tightly coupled to the vascular supply. The conducting airways include the air passages of the nose, nasopharynx, and tracheobronchial tree down to the level of the terminal bronchioles. The best known quantitative description of the airway system is that of Weibel (1963). In the Weibel description, the airways of the lung consist of a series of branchings or bifurcations beginning at the tracheal carina such that the number of airways doubles with each generation of branching. Alveoli first appear at the level of the respiratory bronchioles (generation 17). Each successive generation incorporates more alveoli, leading to the alveolar ducts (generations 20 to 22) and terminating as alveolar sacs at generation 23. This organization and classification is summarized in Figure 22–1.

The pulmonary arterial blood supply to the lung is similarly organized. The pulmonary artery bifurcates within the mediastinum and divides successively as the vessels follow the course of the bronchial airways, eventually reaching the alveolated airways. The capillaries of the alveoli form a dense network between the layers of the alveolar membrane creating a rich, thin interface between the capillary blood and the alveolar gas. Returning pulmonary venous blood is collected by successive orders of converging vessels culminating in the pulmonary vein and left atrium.

PULMONARY VENTILATION

The Process of Ventilation

Pulmonary ventilation is the bulk flow (convection) of gas in and out of the lung. The conducting airways distribute inspired gas down to the res-

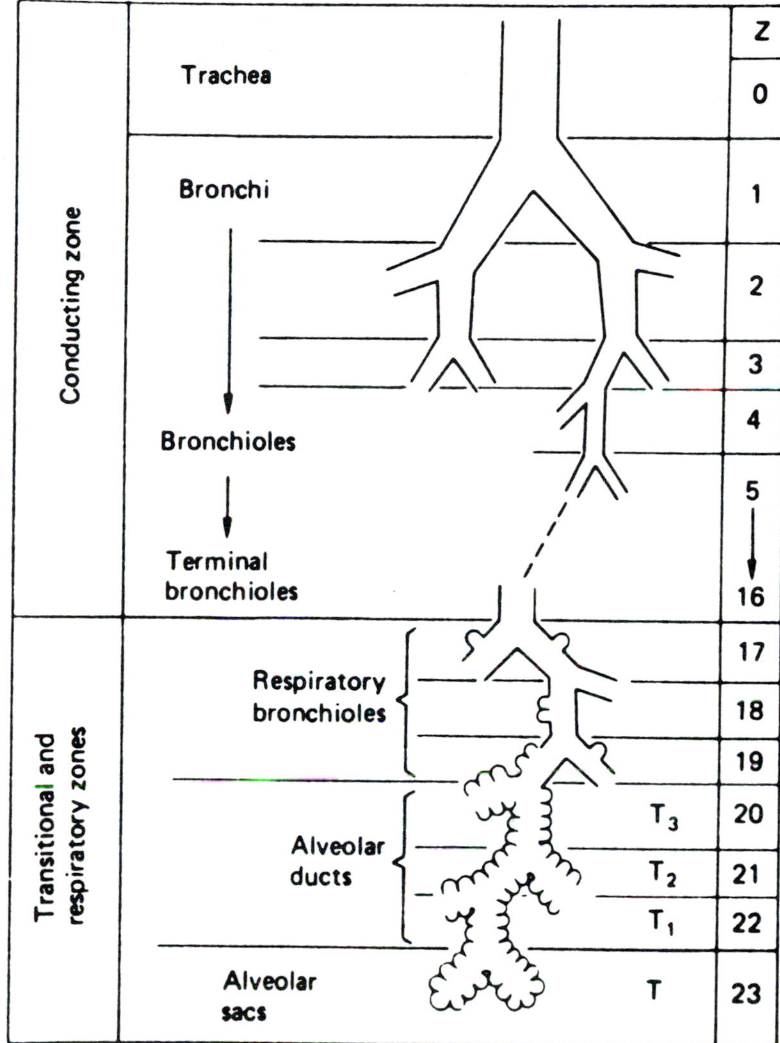

FIGURE 22–1. The airways of the human lung are organized into conducting and respiratory zones in a dichotomous branching system. The respiratory zone begins with the first alveolated airways at generation 17 (the respiratory bronchioles). (Reproduced with permission from Weibel ER. Morphometry of the Human Lung. Berlin: Springer-Verlag, 1984.)

piratory zone where gas exchange can take place in the alveolated airways.

In quantitative terms, the process of ventilation and gas exchange is shown in Figure 22–2. The expansion in total cross-sectional area of the lung with each successive generation causes gas velocity to decrease through each lung generation. For a typical inspiratory flow rate at rest of 200 ml per second (12 L per minute) the velocity of gas within the trachea will be approximately 100 cm per second (Fig. 22–2). As airway cross-section expands, convective velocity decreases until at generation 13 it is about 5 cm per second, approximately the diffusive velocity of O_2 at 37°C.

Within the alveolated airways beginning in generation 17, Figure 22–2 shows that the convective velocity of gas transport is much less than the diffusive velocity of O_2 (or CO_2). Within the terminal acinus (generation 23), the convective velocity is two orders of magnitude less than the diffusive velocity. This means that within the alveolated airways diffusion largely accounts for the exchange of gas between the freshly inspired tidal volume and the existing alveolar gas. Even when ventilation increases by a factor of ten during exercise (Fig. 22–2) diffusion predominates below generation 17.

For the purpose of understanding the gas transport process, the lung is divided into a number of volumes and capacities (Fig. 22–3). The total lung capacity (TLC) is the volume of gas contained within the lungs during a maximal inspiration. The

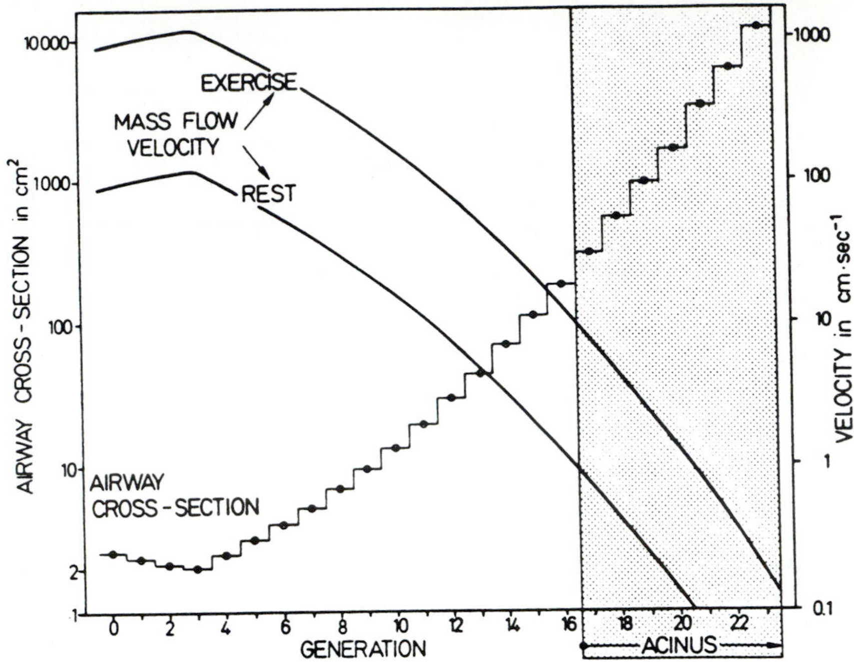

FIGURE 22–2. As total airway cross-section increases with airway branching, the convective velocity of inspired air decreases rapidly such that by generation 17 (stripped area) as fresh gas enters the acinus, the diffusive velocity of equilibration exceeds the convective velocity. By the time the fresh gas reaches 20-23, the speed of diffusion exceeds convection by one or two orders of magnitude. (Reproduced with permission from Weibel ER. The pathway for oxygen. Cambridge: Harvard University Press, 1984.)

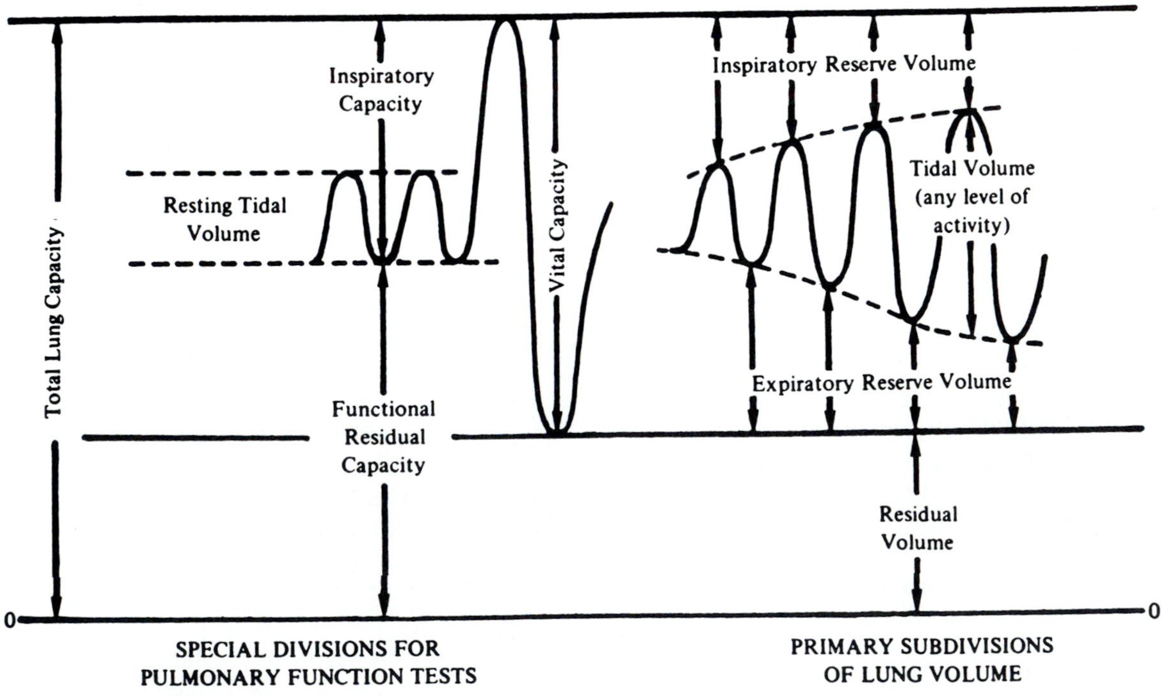

FIGURE 22–3. The total lung capacity (TLC) is subdivided into the residual volume (RV) and vital capacity (VC). Breathing takes place within the VC by increasing or decreasing the tidal volume (V_T). (Reproduced with permission from Biological Handbooks. Respiration and Circulation. Federation of American Societies for Experimental Biology, Chapter III, 1971.)

residual volume (RV) is the lung volume at maximal exhalation. Between TLC and RV lies the functional ability of the lung to move gas by convection. The vital capacity (VC) is the difference between TLC and RV. Within the VC, normal breathing takes place by the exchange of the tidal volume (V_T), which increases or decreases to accommodate the metabolic needs for O_2 uptake and CO_2 elimination. The volume of gas within the lung at the end of exhalation is the functional residual capacity (FRC). Minute ventilation ($\dot{V}_E$) is the total convective exchange per unit time (a function of V_T and respiratory breathing frequency [f]).

Combining the physical processes of convection and diffusion of Figure 22–2 with the lung volumes and capacities of Figure 22–3 yields a picture of the gas exchange process that is consistent with the anatomy of the lung and the physics of gas transport. At end-exhalation, the lung contains only FRC gas. During inspiration, V_T is inhaled creating a sharp interface between V_T and the FRC; the interface rapidly propagates down the conducting airways. As airway cross-section expands, and convective velocity decreases, the concentration differences across the V_T/FRC interface causes diffusive exchange to take place. CO_2 moves into the V_T from the FRC gas and alveolar blood vessels as O_2 moves from the V_T into the FRC and alveolar blood. The large cross-section available in the alveolated airways enhances this diffusive exchange so that equilibration is virtually complete over the course of a breath cycle in a normal person.

The Role of Compliance

During spontaneous ventilation, the convection of gas in and out of the lung results from expansion of the chest cavity by the diaphragm and muscles of the chest wall. In mechanical ventilation, convection is achieved by applying positive pressure to the airway, inflating the lungs and expanding the chest. Thus, the volume of gas moved in and out of the lung during mechanical ventilation at a given applied airway pressure is determined by the compliance of the lung and chest wall, as well as by the resistance to flow in the airways and the viscous resistance of the tissues of the lung and chest wall. The pressure-volume relationship of the lung in the chest cavity is shown in Figure 22–4. Compliance is the change in lung volume per unit of applied pressure. The nonlinear characteristic of the pressure-volume (compliance) curve, along with the larger volume excursion of the lower chest and diaphragm compared to the upper chest and apex of the lung, causes the base of the lung to receive a larger specific ventilation (ventilation volume per unit lung volume) than does the apex. In other words, compared to the apex, the base of the lung receives an excess of ventilation relative to its actual volume. Changes in static compliance of the lung and chest wall are reflected

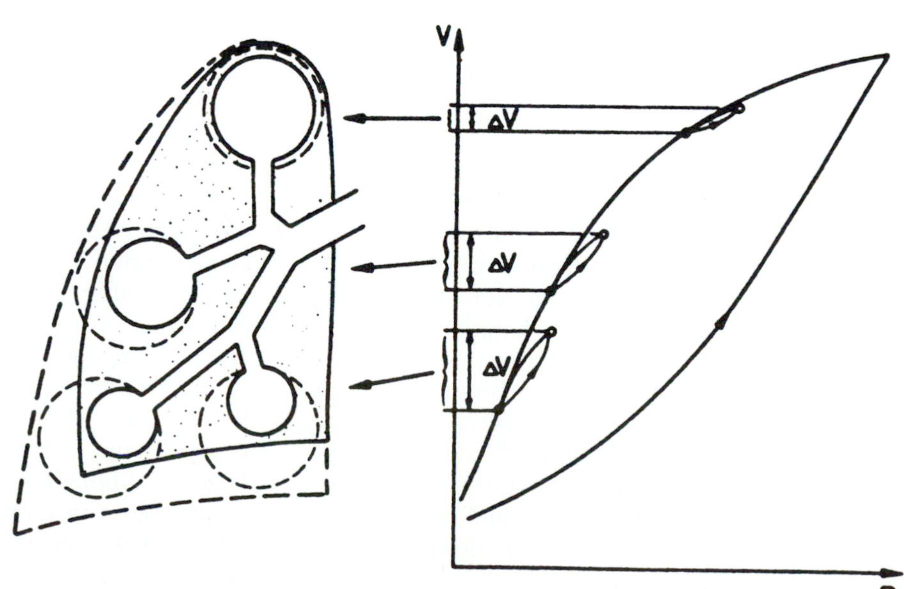

FIGURE 22–4. During quiet ventilation, the base of the lung receives a larger specific ventilation than the apex, owing to the greater expansion of the lower chest cavity and nonlinear pressure-volume curve of the lung and chest wall. (Reproduced with permission from Weibel ER. The pathway for oxygen. Cambridge: Harvard University Press, 1984.)

wall are reflected in the end-inspiratory airway pressure required for a given inspired volume.

The Role of Resistance

The pressure decrease that occurs along the airways during the process of ventilation is determined by the instantaneous flow rate multiplied by the air-flow resistance of the airways (Ohm's law). Thus any process that increases airways resistance will increase the pressure difference required for a given flow rate. In the case of spontaneous ventilation, an increase in airways resistance produces a more negative intrathoracic pressure on inspiration and an increased intrathoracic pressure on exhalation. This can be seen in a spontaneously breathing patient with central venous monitoring as a large respiratory excursion on the central venous pressure trace. In mechanical ventilation, during inspiration, a larger positive intra-airway pressure will develop for a given flow rate with an increase in airways resistance. During exhalation, a greater airways resistance is reflected in a lesser exhalatory flow rate for a given intrathoracic pressure.

Disease processes that decrease chest wall or lung compliance or that increase airways resistance, impair convective gas exchange. In these cases, gas will be distributed to the alveolated airways according to the distribution of the local airways resistances and compliances. To illustrate this point, a patient lying in the left lateral decubitus position for a right thoracotomy will have a larger fraction of V_T entering the right lung for a given applied airway pressure compared to the dependent left lung, owing to the large discrepancy in compliance between the two sides of the chest. In addition to this discrepancy in compliance, a patient with chronic bronchitis may accentuate this unequal ventilation by increases in airway resistance in the dependant lung through accumulation of secretions gravitating from the nondependant lung to the dependant lung.

Increases in local airways resistance at any level or any branch of the bronchial tree impair the convective transport of gas to all airways subtended by that branch. This is seen most dramatically in patients with chronic obstructive pulmonary disease where the distribution of pulmonary ventilation is very heterogeneous when viewed on a radionuclide ventilation scan.

PULMONARY PERFUSION

The Role of Blood Flow Distribution

Gas exchange between the capillary blood and alveolar gas occurs across the alveolar membrane. The quantity of gas exchanged between the blood and gas phase is determined by the difference between alveolar gas tension and mixed venous gas tension, the solubility of the gas in blood, and the blood flow. Just as the distribution of ventilation is not uniform throughout the lung, neither is the distribution of perfusion. In humans, blood flow is distributed in a vertical gradient from base to apex (Fig. 22–5). This gradient depends upon the difference between the hydrostatic pressure in the lung and the blood flow driving pressure in the pulmonary artery. Less flow reaches the apex of the lung because the pulmonary artery pressure is insufficient to drive blood to the apex of the lung under resting conditions. Conversely, the vascular hydrostatic pressure at the base of the lung is high relative to the apex, tending to distend the blood vessels and reducing the resistance to flow. Thus the pulmonary artery pressure drives blood flow preferentially through the base of the lung in a standing or sitting subject. This gravitational distribution of blood flow complements the distribution of ventilation, and as a result, blood flow and ventilation are fairly well (but not perfectly) matched (Fig. 22–6).

This proportional distribution of ventilation and blood flow (''V/Q distribution'') is maintained not only by the passive gravitational mechanisms described above, but by reflex pulmonary vasoconstriction responding to regional hypoxia called ''hypoxic pulmonary vasoconstriction'' (HPV). Many mechanisms combine to account for the disordered distribution of V/Q commonly seen among anesthetized patients, including abnormal posture, elevation of the diaphragm, decreased cardiac output, and inhibition of HPV by anesthetic agents. Studies of HPV in isolated lungs, intact animals, and humans do not all agree. However, it appears that the potent inhaled anesthetics and some direct-acting vasodilators (especially sodium nitroprusside) directly inhibit HPV in a dose-related fashion, although other concomitant changes such as decreases in cardiac output, which potentiate HPV, ameliorate this effect in patients. Intravenous anesthetic agents do not seem to inhibit HPV.

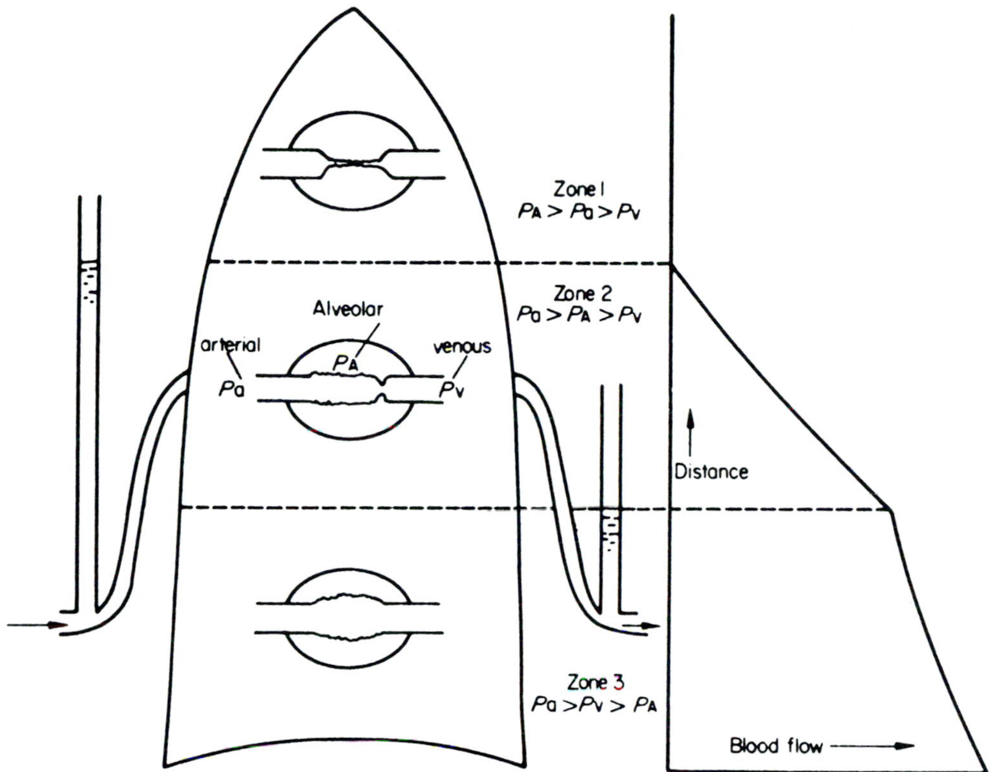

FIGURE 22–5. The vertical distribution of blood flow in erect humans is determined by the driving pressure in the pulmonary artery and the vertical hydrostatic pressure gradient within the vascular space of the lung. The apex is less well perfused than the base under resting conditions. (Reproduced with permission from West JB. Ventilation/blood flow and gas exchange. 3rd ed. Oxford: Blackwell Scientific Publications, 1977.)

Thus, it is possible (but not certain) that eliminating nitrous oxide and administering only a potent inhaled agent in oxygen might not produce the desired increase in arterial oxygen, if the patient suffers from atelectasis or is receiving one-lung anesthesia and requires active HPV to maintain a normal V/Q distribution.

The Transfer of Gas Between Blood and Alveolar Gas

Gas exchange across the alveolar membrane is governed by alveolar ventilation and perfusion. The transport process for a given gas is described by the mass balance between gas transported in blood and gas entering and leaving the lung in the pulmonary ventilation.

Many calculations in pulmonary physiology are derived from mass balance equations that are rooted in the law of conservation of mass. The most fundamental of these relate the net quantity of gas exchanged by ventilation to the quantities transported in blood (Fick's equation):

Amount of gas transported by arterial blood = Amount of gas delivered in the mixed venous blood + Amount of gas uptake (or elimination) by pulmonary ventilation.

$$\mathrm{Ca_g} \cdot \dot{\mathrm{Q}}_\mathrm{T} = \mathrm{C\bar{v}_g} \cdot \dot{\mathrm{Q}}_\mathrm{T} + (\mathrm{CI_g} - \mathrm{C\bar{E}_g}) \cdot \dot{\mathrm{V}}_\mathrm{E} \quad (1)$$

where $\mathrm{Ca_g}$ = arterial blood gas concentration (ml gas per ml blood)

$\mathrm{C\bar{v}_g}$ = mixed venous blood gas concentration (content)

$\dot{\mathrm{Q}}_\mathrm{T}$ = total pulmonary blood flow

$\mathrm{CI_g}$ = mean concentration of gas in inspired mixture

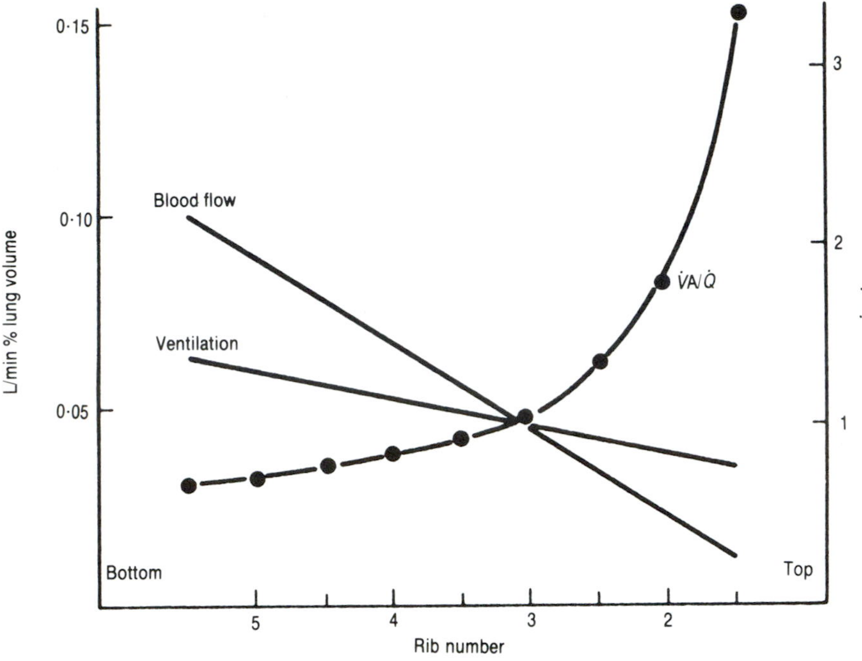

FIGURE 22–6. The distribution of ventilation-perfusion ratio ($\dot{V}/\dot{Q}$) in erect humans is the consequence of the independant distributions of ventilation and perfusion. The $\dot{V}/\dot{Q}$ is less than 1 in the base of the lung and increases vertically, becoming much greater than 1 at the apex. (Reproduced with permission from West JB. Ventilation/blood flow and gas exchange. 3rd. ed. Oxford: Blackwell Scientific Publications, 1977.)

$C\bar{E}_g$ = concentration of gas in mixed expired air

$\bar{V}_E$ = expired minute volume

The amount of gas transported by arterial blood is equal to the arterial blood gas concentration (content) multiplied by the total blood flow (QT or cardiac output). Similarly, the amount of gas transported by mixed venous blood is equal to the mixed venous content multiplied by QT. To increase the systemic arterial O_2 supply or reduce arterial CO_2 content, O_2 must be supplied and CO_2 eliminated by the lung. This uptake and elimination can only occur through blood vessels that come in contact with alveolar gas (blood flow through a ventilated acinus), or capillary blood flow (Qc). Mixed venous blood that does not participate in gas exchange is called shunt blood flow (Qs). QT is the sum of Qc and Qs and thus can be incorporated into the mass balance equation to yield:

$$Ca_g \cdot \dot{Q}_T = C\bar{v}_g \cdot (\dot{Q}c + \dot{Q}s) + (CI_g - C\bar{E}_g) \cdot \dot{V}_E. \quad (2)$$

These underlying concepts and equations are fundamental to pulmonary physiology and pathophysiology and provide the information necessary to calculate or derive virtually all of the relationships among ventilation, perfusion, and gas exchange.

Any disease process that interferes with the ventilation of perfused alveoli increases the apparent shunt and decreases the capacity of the lung to exchange gas. Similarly, redistribution of blood flow from well-ventilated acini to poorly ventilated acini also impairs gas exchange. Anesthesia and pulmonary pathology do both, and as a result anesthesia has a significant impact on gas exchange in patients with pulmonary disease.

DIFFUSION

Gas transport between pulmonary capillary blood and alveolar gas across the alveolar membrane occurs by the process of diffusion. Fick's law of diffusion relates the quantity of gas transported per minute ($\dot{V}g$) to the partial pressure decrease across the membrane (ΔP), the membrane thickness (ΔX) and area (A), and the diffusivity of the gas in the membrane (Dg):

$$\dot{V}g = Dg \times A \times \frac{\Delta Pg}{\Delta X}. \quad (3)$$

Fick's law states that the quantity of gas transported by diffusion ($\dot{V}g$) is equal to the diffusivity of the gas multiplied by the area and the partial pressure difference and divided by the membrane thickness. The measurement of carbon monoxide diffusion capacity in the pulmonary function laboratory combines D, A, and X into a single term (DL_{CO}), such that the diffusing capacity becomes:

$$DL_{CO} = \frac{\dot{V}CO}{\Delta P} . \tag{4}$$

Diffusing capacity is the ratio of gas uptake to the driving partial pressure difference.

Diseases that result in increases in functional alveolar membrane thickness (alveolar proteinosis, pulmonary edema) or reduce alveolar cross-section (pneumonia, pulmonary embolus, pneumonectomy) reduce diffusing capacity. A reduction in diffusing capacity becomes clinically important when it becomes the limiting factor in the exchange between alveolar gas and pulmonary capillary blood.

PULMONARY PATHOPHYSIOLOGY

Diseases of the lung and of other organ systems alter the physiology of gas exchange. Rational perioperative management of patients whose gas exchange has been altered by disease is based on an appreciation of the pathophysiology involved.

EXTRATHORACIC PATHOLOGY

Large space-occupying masses within the abdomen limit diaphragmatic excursion, and as a result limit convective gas transport, producing a form of restrictive lung disease. Large intra-abdominal neoplasms, ascites, hydramnios, normal pregnancy, or morbid obesity are typical examples. Patients with these conditions usually exhibit dyspnea on exertion or orthopnea, and may show evidence of hypoventilation (low arterial Po_2 and increased arterial Pco_2), even while fully awake. The use of sedative or narcotic drugs in these patients is dangerous unless arterial oxygen saturation and mental status are monitored closely. Such patients are not given premedicant depressant drugs until they reach the operating room or preparation area where they will be under close observation.

Patients with preexisting moderate to severe neuromuscular disease exhibit extrathoracic pathology also. Examples include patients with head or spinal cord injuries, increased intracranial pressure, myasthenia gravis, or Guillain-Barré syndrome. In these patients, there may be depressed respiratory control (neurologic) or impaired motor strength making them exquisitely sensitive to depressant drugs.

INTRATHORACIC PATHOLOGY

Extrapulmonary Pathology

Examples of extrapulmonary intrathoracic pathology with significant effects on gas transport include large mediastinal masses (thymoma, substernal thyroid tumors, hilar adenopathy), which produce large airway obstruction, pleural effusions, severe thoracic kyphoscoliosis, chest wall trauma (flail chest), and loss of neuromuscular control (phrenic nerve paralysis, high spinal anesthesia).

Pulmonary Pathology

The most common and troublesome problems with gas exchange occur in patients with preexisting pulmonary disease. Pulmonary diseases can be classified according to the functional organization of pulmonary physiology introduced in this chapter.

Diseases of the Conducting Airways

Management of upper airway obstruction at the level of the mouth, tongue, pharynx, or vocal cords is described in Chapter 13. Farther down the conducting airways one must consider tracheal stenosis (in patients with a previous tracheostomy), foreign bodies, severe tracheitis, acute bronchitis or bronchiectasis as conditions that may impair convective gas transport. It is critical that these patients be approached with a careful management plan to ensure airway security prior to the induction of general anesthesia.

Diseases of the Respiratory Airways

By far the most common airway diseases, however, occur in the small airways, and have their greatest impact when they involve the respiratory bronchioles. The classic examples are asthma and chronic obstructive pulmonary disease (COPD). Whereas these two diseases have totally different etiologies, they affect gas exchange similarly because the pathology acts in the same region of the airway system. Both produce expiratory obstruction in the small airways.

Deeper in the alveolated airways (generations 20 to 23) pathology tends to have less impact on convective gas exchange but a greater impact on diffusive transport. Pulmonary edema, alveolar proteinosis, and adult respiratory distress syndrome (ARDS) may alter pulmonary mechanics (reduced compliance or increased resistance), but in the early phases of the disease process the principle effect is impairment of alveolar or diffusional gas transport.

Diseases of Pulmonary Parenchyma and Vasculature

Diseases of the pulmonary parenchyma (silicosis or pulmonary fibrosis) affect lung mechanics through reductions in compliance and increases in tissue viscous resistance. The result is a restriction in pulmonary ventilation.

Finally our pathologic classification includes diseases of the pulmonary vasculature. These include pulmonary hypertension, vascular shunts (congenital heart disease or chronic liver disease) and pulmonary emboli.

PREOPERATIVE EVALUATION OF PULMONARY GAS TRANSPORT

The History

Preoperative evaluation of patients for anesthesia includes an assessment of the respiratory system. A history of cigarette smoking, dyspnea on exertion, or productive cough are all sought, along with significant exposure to occupational hazards, especially among asbestos workers, welders, miners, or fire fighters. A history of asthma (frequency, duration, and severity of attacks) is determined as well as the medication, dosage, and effectiveness of treatment.

The most effective functional assessment of pulmonary disease is exercise tolerance. Dyspnea at rest, orthopnea, or dyspnea on mild exertion indicate a severe respiratory impairment. Conversely, a patient with a long history of cigarette smoking who is able to walk more than a mile or climb several flights of steps without dyspnea has adequate function to meet perioperative demands.

Physical Examination

In examining the chest, look first at the shape of the chest and then at its motion. Increased AP diameter usually indicates chronic disease, an increased FRC, and a reduced VC. If the chest wall moves little or not at all with a deep inspiration, or the accessory muscles are used in quiet breathing, then the patient probably has little exercise capacity. Tachypnea at rest is also a sign of severe disease. Labored breathing or dyspnea in the semi-Fowler's position is usually indicative of an acute process and a severe impairment. The presence of intercostal or supraclavicular retraction, or paradoxical chest movement, is a sign of severe upper airway obstruction.

Percussion of the chest can reveal the tympanitic character and the limited diaphragmatic excursion characteristic of the emphysematous chest. Percussion may also reveal pneumothorax, pleural effusion, or lobar pneumonia.

On auscultation, breath sounds should be equal bilaterally from apex to base. Breath sounds are distant in moderate to severe emphysema, and often absent in the presence of a pneumothorax or pleural effusion. Rhonchi indicate small airways obstruction. Inspiratory wheezes may indicate the presence of a foreign body or secretions in conducting airways. Expiratory wheezes generally indicate increased resistance in the respiratory bronchioles due to COPD or asthma. The presence of rales that do not clear with coughing may indicate congestive heart failure (CHF), pulmonary edema, or an infectious process in the lungs.

Laboratory Data

THE CHEST FILM

Although routine preoperative chest films are of little value in healthy patients, the chest radiograph is the most useful laboratory indicator of the extent and character of pulmonary disease when there is a history suggesting respiratory problems. The hypertranslucency of COPD, or the increased hilar markings of CHF or early pulmonary edema, are often easily recognized early signs of the disease process. The absence of lung markings in the edge of the lung fields are indicative of pneumothorax, while the presence of opacities may reveal neoplasms, tuberculosis, a recent pulmonary embolus, or an infectious process.

THE ROOM AIR BLOOD GAS

The next most useful laboratory test is the arterial blood gas determination obtained while the patient breathes room air. A room air blood gas determination is obtained preoperatively in all patients with significant pulmonary disease (limited exercise tolerance, recent hospitalization for respiratory care, a requirement for chronic medication) or a recent history of CHF. In adult patients without pulmonary disease, Pao_2 decreases with age, ranging from 90 to 110 mm Hg in healthy young adults, to 70 to 90 in the elderly. A room air Pao_2 less than 70 indicates acute or chronic pulmonary disease. $Paco_2$ ranges from 35 to 45 mm Hg and is generally not age dependant. $Paco_2$ in excess of 45 at rest is indicative of either hypoventilation (respiratory depression) or CO_2 retention in a patient with severe pulmonary disease.

PULMONARY FUNCTION TESTING

The decision to obtain pulmonary function tests (PFTs) before anesthesia and operation is not a simple one. Even a patient with severe pulmonary disease might require no testing if it is anticipated that a peripheral operation will cause no impairment of ventilatory function. As with all other forms of testing, one must foresee that the results will alter management and outcome before ordering the test. Assessment of the results of bronchodilator therapy and more precise predictions of postoperative pulmonary function in patients scheduled for major abdominal or thoracic operations, especially pneumonectomy, provide the major indications for PFTs.

Pulmonary function tests quantify the nature and degree of functional impairment. The forced vital capacity (FVC) and forced expired volume in one second (FEV_1) are sensitive to restrictive and obstructive disease, respectively. The FVC is an index of the reserve available to increase the tidal volume. An FVC of 1.0 L or less is indicative of essentially zero reserve and severe disease. The FEV_1 is a measure of the ability to develop and sustain expiratory flow. Reduced FEV_1 indicates obstructive disease and a limitation of the ability to move gas out of the lung. An FEV_1 of less than 1 L represents severe disease.

The ratio of FEV_1 to FVC may help to differentiate obstructive from restrictive disease. In normal individuals approximately 85 per cent of the FVC can be exhaled in one second. In restrictive disease, FVC is reduced and as a result FEV_1 is also reduced; however, the patient with restrictive disease may still exhale 85 per cent of FVC in one second, indicating the absence of significant obstruction. Conversely, a young patient with acute asthma may have a near normal FVC but a reduced FEV_1, and as a result, a reduced FEV_1/FVC ratio indicating obstructive disease. Patients with COPD generally exhibit both restrictive and obstructive components. In COPD, FVC is reduced because the chest is in a state of chronic hyperinflation, with increased RV and FRC. This limits VC and constitutes a restrictive component of the disease. FEV_1 is also reduced in these patients as a result of their small airways disease and exhalatory obstruction. Generally, in COPD the obstructive component is greater than the restrictive component, so that the FEV_1/FVC ratio is decreased.

The presence of obstructive disease and its responsiveness to bronchodilator therapy can be evaluated using flow-volume loops. The flow-volume loop is a plot of inspiratory and expiratory flow versus exhaled volume (Fig. 22–7). It thus displays the ability of the patient to develop and sustain flow throughout the breath cycle. An expiratory obstructive pattern is revealed by the inability of the subject to develop or sustain a high expiratory flow for more than one third of the exhaled volume. If either the flow volume pattern or the FEV_1/FVC ratio improve following treatment with bronchodilators, then bronchodilatory therapy will aid perioperative management.

OTHER LABORATORY INVESTIGATIONS

More sophisticated laboratory data may be helpful in evaluating patients with specific pulmonary problems prior to operation. These include V/Q scans (radionuclide imaging), exercise studies, or split pulmonary function tests (PFTs of each lung independently) and are particularly useful in eval-

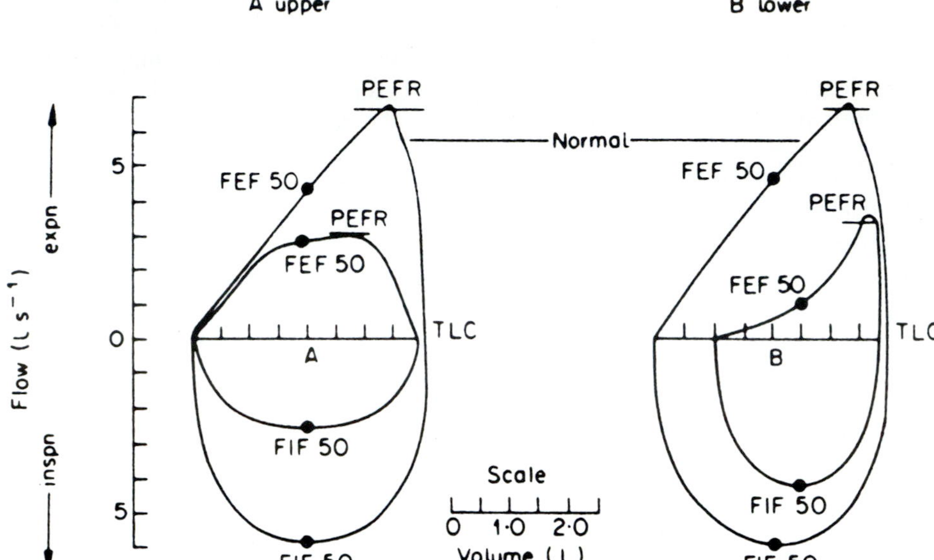

FIGURE 22–7. Maximum flow-volume loops for a healthy subject (outer loops), a patient with moderate obstruction to the intrapulmonary airways (inner right hand loop) and with obstruction to extrathoracic airways (inner left hand loop). PEFR is the peak-expiratory flow rate (the maximum that can be sustained for 10 ms). FEF_{50} and FIF_{50} are the forced-expiratory and inspiratory flow rates at the midpoint of the vital capacity. (Reproduced with permission from Cotes JE. Lung function: Assessment and application in medicine. 3rd ed. Oxford: Blackwell Scientific Publications, 1979.)

uating patients with pulmonary disease prior to pulmonary resection.

PREDICTING AND MANAGING PERIOPERATIVE RESPIRATORY FAILURE

Patients with preexisting pulmonary disease and little pulmonary reserve are at risk for pulmonary failure postoperatively. A major element in the success of modern surgery and anesthesia in caring for high-risk patients has been the successful management of postoperative ventilatory failure, making the prediction of perioperative respiratory failure and its prevention major concerns for the anesthesiologist.

Identification of the Risk Factors for Respiratory Failure

Anesthesia and operation provide many opportunities for compromised pulmonary function even in patients without pulmonary disease. The presence of preexisting pulmonary disease increases the likelihood of respiratory embarrassment in the perioperative period. By recognizing the factors that impair gas exchange, one can then manage patients with pulmonary disease with scrupulous care when these factors are present.

Pharmacologic Factors. Anesthetics and narcotics are central nervous system (CNS) depressants. In normal individuals, mild respiratory depression may mean the difference between a PaO_2 of 90 and a PaO_2 of 70, with little consequence. In patients with respiratory disease, mild respiratory depression may result in hypoxemia and desaturation because they normally operate close to the limits of their pulmonary reserve.

Similarly, mild residual paralysis from incompletely reversed neuromuscular blockade may have no detectable consequence in normal individuals, but may have disastrous results in patients with respiratory disease.

The use of beta blocking drugs intraoperatively for the management of hypertension must be approached with caution in patients with a history of CHF or bronchospastic disease.

Surgical Risk Factors. Operations on the upper airway (e.g., tonsillectomy, panendoscopy, resection of small tumors) may be no challenge to a patient with normal lung function. However, minor obstruction is a major problem for patients whose vital capacities are not much greater than their resting tidal volume.

Similarly, operations that interfere with ventilation because of pain or physical restriction (use of abdominal binders, or restrictive dressings to chest wall or upper abdomen) may create severe embarrassment to a patient with limited pulmonary reserve. Intracranial procedures (or head trauma) may also result in central respiratory depression requiring mechanical ventilatory support. The patient with respiratory disease is exquisitely sensitive to these factors.

Surgical or anesthetic complications such as pneumothorax or hemothorax from invasive monitoring procedures, or neck, chest, or flank incisions must be suspected early in patients who develop postoperative respiratory embarrassment. Patients with preexisting pulmonary disease decompensate quickly from these complications.

Intraoperative Management

The intraoperative management plan for patients with respiratory disease must consider the risk factors previously outlined. The choice of a specific technique (regional versus general anesthesia), agent, drug, or strategy is less important than the attention to detail once a plan has been selected. Regional anesthesia is not necessarily safer than general anesthesia in these patients because both techniques can produce respiratory embarrassment (regional anesthesia may result in high spinal or epidural anesthesia, inadvertent phrenic nerve block, or pneumothorax). As in most aspects of medicine, the choice represents a balance between providing appropriate operating conditions for the operation, patient comfort and acceptance, relative safety, and a minimum of postoperative residual effects.

In planning anesthesia management, patients at risk of postoperative ventilatory failure may be classified into two groups as shown below.

FUNCTIONAL IMPAIRMENT FROM DISEASE

1. *Mild*. Little or no functional impairment, no risk of unanticipated severe bronchospasm.
2. *Severe*. History of previous respiratory failure, sleep apnea syndrome, CO_2 retention preoperatively, less than twofold reserve in vital capacity.

SEVERITY OF OPERATION

1. *Mild*. Peripheral operations that do not impair diaphragm or chest wall function.
2. *Severe*. Thoracic or upper abdominal procedures; operations that produce neurologic or cardiovascular instability postoperatively.

Patients with mild disease scheduled for operations of mild severity require little in the way of extra precautions; those with severe disease scheduled for severe operations may require little precaution to avoid postoperative ventilatory failure, because it is almost inevitable that these patients will require mechanical ventilation postoperatively. Patients with mild disease undergoing severe operation, or those with severe disease undergoing mild operation can be managed without postoperative ventilatory failure under favorable circumstances, but these patients require special care and vigilance.

Premedicants are avoided if possible, or given in greatly reduced doses if needed. If the nature of the operation and the patient's mental state permit, then regional anesthesia offers several advantages over general anesthesia. First, pain is blocked with the least impairment of respiratory drive and diaphragmatic function. Second, a period of postoperative analgesia is guaranteed. However, high levels of spinal or epidural anesthesia can embarrass ventilatory function, making it important to control the level of anesthesia. Also, if excessive sedation is required, this may be worse for the patient than a well-conducted, light general anesthetic, because the associated respiratory depression can be managed by controlled ventilation intraoperatively, and it usually dissipates rapidly on emergence postoperatively.

Some operations (thoracic, high abdominal, some prone positions) so impair ventilatory function themselves that general anesthesia and endotracheal intubation are required to support respiratory function intraoperatively. Even in patients with significant respiratory disease, postoperative ventilatory failure is not inevitable after general anesthesia, provided that doses of narcotics, sedatives, muscle relaxants, and anesthetics are minimized and that the patient is not expected to support spontaneous ventilation until the effects of these drugs are gone.

Anesthesia management of patients with restrictive pulmonary diseases (kyphoscoliosis, muscle weakness, obesity, pregnancy) follows these general principles in a straightforward fashion. Unless challenged by major operation (thoracotomy), patients with mild restrictive disease usually retain enough ventilatory capacity to clear CO_2 postoperatively. Hypoxemia is caused by alterations in FRC and responds well to oxygen therapy. In more severe cases, simple measurements can predict postoperative ventilatory failure with some accuracy. Having measured the patient's vital capacity preoperatively, one can estimate that postoperatively it will be reduced only slightly by peripheral operations, but reduced to as little as one third the preoperative value by upper abdominal or thoracic operations. Patients usually suffer fatigue and ventilatory failure if their minute ventilations exceed 30 breaths per minute at tidal volumes of one half their vital capacities. If the predicted postoperative vital capacity is so small that this calculation does not yield a minute ventilation at least equal to the patient's preoperative minute ventilation, then postoperative ventilatory failure is predicted. In borderline cases, increasing postoperative vital capacity by relieving pain may alleviate the need for mechanical ventilation.

Management of patients with small airways obstruction (asthma, COPD) is more troublesome, as preoperative measurements cannot predict the extent of bronchospasm during and after operation. The history and, if needed, preoperative PFTs allow these patients to be classified into mild, moderate, and severe. Patients who have asthma or COPD but who enjoy good exercise tolerance, who have not suffered severe bouts of bronchospasm recently, and who do not require bronchodilators constantly, usually fare well. Likewise the management of those who come to the operating room for emergency operation with life-threatening bronchospasm is clear: immediate intubation, maximum doses of bronchodilators, and a period of postoperative ventilation are indicated. For patients with intermediate disease, the general principles outlined above reduce the chance of postoperative ventilatory failure.

Effective preoperative bronchodilator therapy and treatment of any airway infection are important before elective procedures. Stimulating the anesthetized airways of patients with asthma may provoke bronchospasm, which suggests that endotracheal tubes be placed or removed only when the airway is well anesthetized (with general or topical anesthetics). Regional anesthesia is often desirable, but high levels of motor block may impair the function of accessory muscles of respiration needed for active exhalation.

Patients with disorders of gas transport at the alveolar level who require anesthesia are managed according to the same principles employed in their care in the intensive care unit (ICU). These include close monitoring, increased F_{IO_2}, positive end-expiratory pressure (PEEP) as needed, and care to avoid fluid overload.

Patients with respiratory disease often have concomitant cardiovascular or renal diseases and are at a greater risk of developing pulmonary edema; their fluid management requires extra care. Indeed, patients with respiratory disease may require postoperative mechanical ventilation solely because of extensive surgical dissection and massive blood replacement.

Postoperative Management

Respiratory failure often makes its first appearance postoperatively. Complications developing in the immediate postoperative period may impair gas exchange directly (airway obstruction, fluid overload, and pulmonary edema), may restrict ventilation (pain, restrictive dressings), may reduce the patient's capacity to respond (CNS depression by narcotics or residual anesthetic gases, residual neuromuscular blockade), or may reduce the amount of available lung (lobectomy, pneumothorax or hemothorax). Consequently, patients with a number of risk factors and borderline pulmonary function require close monitoring in the immediate postoperative period, extending 24 to 48 hours or longer as necessary.

Epidural narcotics or patient-controlled analgesia (see Chapter 35) confer additional benefits to patients with respiratory disease. Control of pain is essential in promoting adequate ventilation postoperatively, especially after upper abdominal or thoracic procedures. The margin of safety between adequate pain relief and dangerous respiratory depression is significantly reduced in patients with pulmonary disease. Meticulous monitoring is required to assure that impending ventilatory failure is detected and dealt with early.

MONITORING GAS TRANSPORT INTRAOPERATIVELY

Modern anesthetic and respiratory equipment provides a wealth of information about gas exchange (see Chapters 5 and 6). It is important to chart initial data following induction of anesthesia so that changes that develop intraoperatively or postoperatively can be documented. This careful record provides early warning of deterioration in pulmonary function and saves time in arriving at the diagnosis (Table 22–1).

Monitoring Convective Transport

Once anesthesia has been induced and the airway secured, tidal volume (V_T), breathing frequency (f), minute ventilation (V_E), end-tidal CO_2 ($P_{ET_{CO_2}}$), and airway pressure are charted at regular intervals. Airway pressure includes peak airway pressure and plateau pressure. Plateau pressure is the airway pressure sustained during the inspiratory pause of the ventilator (i.e., at zero flow), and is an index of total lung and chest wall compliance. Increases in plateau pressure indicate a decrease in compliance which may be extrathoracic (use of high abdominal retractors, or compression of the chest wall), or intrathoracic (hemothorax, pneumothorax), or intrapulmonary (edema). Increases in peak airway pressure may indicate increased airway resistance owing to endotracheal tube obstruction, accumulation of secretions, blood or edema fluid in the airways, or a change in bronchial tone.

Evidence of bronchospasm or expiratory obstruction is reflected in the time required for complete exhalation and by the presence of expiratory wheezes. The time required for complete exhalation is found by examining the rate of filling of the bellows of the ventilator. If exhalation is incomplete, or complete just prior to the next inhalation, then insufficient time has elapsed for complete emptying. Increasing the expiratory time by increasing end-expiratory pause, reducing respiratory frequency, decreasing the inspiratory/expiratory the (I/E) ratio, or increasing inspiratory flow may overcome the problem. Bronchospasm is treated by deepening the level of anesthesia, adding a volatile agent with bronchodilatory properties (halothane, isoflurane), administering aerosols (beta-2 agonists), or infusing aminophylline (when the patient has a blood concentration of less than 10 μg per ml). Patients previously untreated with aminophylline require an initial loading dose of 5 mg per kg, administered slowly. All of these drugs must be used cautiously under general anesthesia to avoid tachyarrhythmias, which are potentiated by many anesthetics (aminophylline and halothane are especially arrhythmogenic). Bronchospasm under general anesthesia is common in patients with a history of asthma or COPD. Careful monitoring of airway pressure, breath sounds, and exhalatory time allows effective treatment before bronchospasm becomes intractable or life threatening.

TABLE 22–1. Monitoring During Anesthesia for a Patient with Lung Disease

- All patients
  - Breath sounds
  - Chest and upper abdomen movement
  - Airway pressure: peak, plateau
  - Ventilatory volumes: tidal volume, expired minute volume
  - Expired CO_2: end-tidal CO_2 and waveform
  - Peripheral oxygen saturation
- Moderate disease (exact choice of monitor depends on disease process)
  - Arterial blood gases
  - A-a D_{O_2} at $F_{I_{O_2}}$ 1.0
  - A-aD_{CO_2}
  - Apparent dead space
- Severe pulmonary disease, or combined cardiopulmonary disease
  - Pulmonary artery catheter: CVP, PCWP, CO
  - Pulmonary vascular resistance
  - Shunt fraction

Monitoring Pulmonary Perfusion

Pulmonary perfusion is normally monitored using a thermal dilution pulmonary artery (PA) catheter. Cardiac output (Q_T) measurements are very useful in patients with preexisting cardiac disease, pulmonary hypertension, or in procedures where large-volume intravenous infusions of blood or crystalloid are expected. Pulmonary artery systolic, diastolic, mean, and PA occlusion pressures may be recorded at intervals, along with calculated pulmonary vascular resistance (PVR).

$$PVR = [\text{mean PAP-PAOP}]/CO$$

Pulmonary vascular resistance is increased in patients with pulmonary hypertension, and may increase in patients with pulmonary emboli during anesthesia. An increase in PVR with an increasing arterial to end-tidal CO_2 difference ($Pa\text{-}ETDco_2$) is pathognomonic of pulmonary embolus.

Monitoring Gas Exchange

CO_2 TRANSPORT

Once a stable anesthetic depth has been attained, the minute ventilation and PET_{CO_2} are recorded regularly. In patients with pulmonary disease or in whom air embolus is a possible complication, arterial blood gas determinations reveal the $Paco_2$ associated with a given PET_{CO_2}. The difference between arterial and end-tidal CO_2 ($Pa\text{-}ETDco_2$) is an index of pulmonary function in general, and of alveolar dead space in particular. Alveolar dead space increases with pulmonary embolization (air, fat, or blood clots). Changes in $Pa\text{-}ETDco_2$ requiring a change in V_E or Fio_2 to maintain $Paco_2$ or Hbo_2 saturation indicate serious problems in gas exchange.

Physiologic dead space fraction can be calculated using the equation:

$$\frac{V_D}{V_T} = 1 - \frac{P\bar{E}_{CO_2}}{Pa_{CO_2}} \quad (5)$$

The Bohr dead space fraction substitutes PET_{CO_2} for $Paco_2$ in the above equation. Bohr dead space fraction does not include alveolar dead space and thus is insensitive to pulmonary embolic processes or decreases in pulmonary perfusion.

Unfortunately, mixed expired CO_2 ($P\bar{E}_{CO_2}$) is not generally available in clinical CO_2 monitors, in spite of the fact that the technology to monitor it is available on modern anesthetic machines. To overcome this problem, dead space fraction can be monitored indirectly by recording $\dot{V}_E$ with the associated $Paco_2$ or PET_{CO_2}. Assuming that CO_2 production remains unchanged, as is usual in anesthetized patients, if $\dot{V}_E$ must be increased to maintain a fixed $Paco_2$ (or conversely if $Paco_2$ increases while PET_{CO_2} decreases with a fixed $\dot{V}_E$), then CO_2 elimination has been impaired. Thus, observing $\dot{V}_E$ and arterial or end-tidal CO_2 measurements warns of changes in dead space fraction.

Dead space fraction increases if pulmonary perfusion is compromised, as when cardiac output decreases. When cardiac output declines, less lung is perfused; the unperfused lung becomes alveolar dead space. This almost routinely follows the induction of general anesthesia, when the dead space fraction increases from 25 to 30 per cent to 35 to 40 per cent and even higher in patients with respiratory or cardiac disease. Factors which augment this increase in alveolar dead space include increases in intrathoracic pressure or mechanical ventilation, which reduce venous return and cardiac output further.

OXYGEN TRANSPORT

Monitors that measure end-tidal CO_2 and peripheral oxygen saturation have not completely eliminated the need for measuring blood gases intraoperatively in patients with lung diseases. Changes in arterial Po_2 and arterial-alveolar tension differences occur before peripheral hemoglobin desaturation or obvious reductions in end-tidal CO_2. The measurement of Pao_2 as related to the PA_{O_2} or (more easily) the Fio_2 is a useful index of alveolar function in patients under anesthesia.

Use the alveolar gas equation to calculate alveolar PA_{O_2}:

$$PA_{O_2} = FI_{O_2}(PB\text{-}47) - PET_{CO_2}\left[FI_{O_2} + \frac{1 - FI_{O_2}}{R}\right] \quad (6)$$

FI_{O_2} = fractional inspired concentration of dry oxygen.

P_B = barometric pressure

47 = partial pressure of water vapor at 37° C

PET_{CO_2} = alveolar (or end-tidal) partial pressure of CO_2

R = respiratory quotient.

It is valuable to obtain the $P_{A-a}Do_2$ difference at $FIO_2 = 1.0$, because the term involving R drops out of the equation.

Normally, $PA\text{-}aDo_2$ while breathing 100 per cent O_2 is less than 50 to 100 mm Hg in anesthetized patients without pulmonary disease. A Pa_{O_2} of 150 mm Hg or less with an F_{IO_2} of 0.95 to 1.0 is a clear warning of severe O_2 transport impairment (a high shunt fraction [Q_S/Q_T]).

In patients with pulmonary or cardiac disease, pulmonary artery catheters are useful for monitoring central pressures, cardiac output, and systemic and pulmonary vascular resistance. The catheter also allows the calculation of Q_S/Q_T (using the mass balance shunt relationship of equation [2]), which is reflected in the $P_A\text{-}aD_{O_2}$. Despite the widespread use of pulmonary artery catheters in monitored patients, and the frequency of blood gas determinations, the calculation of shunt fraction remains neglected. The interrelationship of mixed venous, arterial, and expired gas tensions provides (through the mass balance equation) a clear picture of cardiopulmonary function in critically ill patients. For example, a decrease in Pa_{O_2} under conditions of unchanged ventilation or F_{IO_2} may reflect deterioration in lung function, a pulmonary embolus, a change in cardiac output, or the development of sepsis. Monitoring cardiac output and pulmonary arterial pressures is of help, but measuring mixed venous P_{O_2} and P_{CO_2} in conjunction with the other variables may help define the problem exactly.

Any of the foregoing monitoring techniques are valuable in caring for critically ill patients. Of the measurements described, those which receive less emphasis than they deserve in current practice are $Pa\text{-}AD_{CO_2}$, $P_A\text{-}aD_{O_2}$, and Q_S/Q_T, which are sensitive to changes in pulmonary or cardiovascular status. A systematic approach to monitoring alterations in ventilation and pulmonary blood flow, and the consequences on gas transport as reflected in mixed venous, arterial, and end-tidal gas measurements, provides early warning of developing problems and makes diagnosis more certain.

Summary

Improvements in clinical instruments incorporating microprocessors will allow, over the next decade, increasingly specific yet inexpensive monitors of gas transport. Familiarity with the structural organization and physiology of the lung, and the basic concepts of mass balance will aid the interpretation of these measurements to yield meaningful diagnoses and timely therapy.

References

Marshall BE, Longnecker DE, Fairley HB, eds. Anesthesia for thoracic procedures. Boston: Blackwell Scientific Publications, 1988.

Miller A, ed. Pulmonary function tests—A guide for the student and house officer. Orlando. Grune & Stratton, Harcourt Brace Jovanovich, 1987.

Weibel ER. The pathway for oxygen: Structure and function in the mammalian respiratory system. Cambridge. Harvard University Press, 1984.

West JB. Pulmonary pathophysiology—the essentials. 3rd ed. Baltimore: Williams & Wilkins, 1987.

CHAPTER TWENTY-THREE

HEPATIC AND RENAL DISEASE

PATIENTS WITH HEPATIC DISEASE

Patients with significant liver disease experience a markedly increased risk of dying after operation The 30-day postoperative mortality following open liver biopsy is reported as 31 per cent. To manage these patients successfully requires an understanding of the physiologic effects of hepatic dysfunction, and of the effects of anesthesia and operation on the liver.

Pathophysiology of Liver Disease

Hepatic diseases fall into three categories: obstructive and acute or chronic hepatocellular disorders. In obstructive disease, related to tumors or to gallstones, hepatic function is usually preserved. Operations are directed at restoring biliary tract patency; mortality and morbidity usually result from renal failure, sepsis, or hemorrhage.

Acute hepatic disease is usually viral, toxic, or thrombotic in origin. These patients come to operation only for emergency treatment of life-threatening illnesses or for orthotopic liver transplantation.

Chronic hepatic disease results from repeated bouts of acute hepatitis (alcohol) or deranged immune mechanisms (primary biliary cirrhosis, or chronic active hepatitis). Less commonly, inborn errors of metabolism (Wilson's disease, hemochromatosis) impair hepatic function. Cirrhosis is a final common pathway for chronic liver disease. Its pathological hallmarks (necrosis, fibrosis, and disordered architecture) cause disturbances of blood flow, lymph drainage, and bile passage.

HEPATIC BLOOD FLOW

The liver receives approximately 25 per cent of the cardiac output; two thirds of liver blood flow derives from the portal vein and one third from the hepatic artery. Because the portal blood is desaturated, the hepatic artery provides about half of the total oxygen requirement of approximately 1 ml per gm per minute. Although flow through the hepatic artery increases in response to diminished portal flow, the portal circulation does not compensate for decreases in hepatic arterial blood flow. This limited compensatory mechanism is further reduced in liver disease, increasing the risk of liver hypoxia.

Hepatic blood flow is affected by numerous factors related to both operation and anesthesia. It decreases in response to increased arterial P_{CO_2} and sympathetic tone. Positive pressure ventilation and positive end-expiratory pressure (PEEP) may increase hepatic venous pressure and decrease both cardiac output and hepatic blood flow; abdominal operations are associated with greater decreases in hepatic blood flow than are operations at other sites.

EFFECTS OF LIVER DISEASE ON THE CARDIOVASCULAR SYSTEM

Patients with severe liver disease typically have increased cardiac outputs, with decreased systemic vascular resistance owing in part to arteriovenous anastomoses thought to result from altered action and concentrations of estrogens. Despite cardiac outputs as great as 20 L per minute, perfusion of organs such as the liver and kidney may be inadequate, and functional intravascular volume is often inadequate.

Cardiomyopathy is likely if ethanol is the etiologic agent of hepatic failure. The combination of impaired myocardial performance and diminished, fixed peripheral vascular resistance particularly compromises these patients' abilities to cope with hypovolemia.

ALBUMIN SYNTHESIS

The healthy liver produces approximately 10 gm of albumin each day; its half-life is about 20 days. There may be no albumin deficiency in the first few days of acute liver failure, but hypoalbuminemia is a feature of severe chronic liver disease, especially in malnourished patients. Edema and ascites result, as do the expected aberrations in the pharmacokinetics of protein-bound drugs (see Chapter 7).

ASCITES

Three factors contribute to ascites production in patients with severe renal failure: the decreased oncotic pressure caused by chronic hypoalbuminemia; hepatic lymphatic obstruction owing to cirrhosis; and dilutional hyponatremia. Ascitic fluid accumulating under pressure in the abdomen has predictable pathophysiologic effects. The volume of distribution of hydrophilic compounds is increased, splanchnic capacitance is decreased, venous return and cardiac output are decreased, and the diaphragm is elevated, leading to atelectasis and V/Q mismatching.

The acute drainage of massive ascites is a necessary consequence of intra-abdominal operations, but cardiovascular collapse may result from sudden splanchnic vasodilation. Experience has shown that patients can tolerate this abrupt decrease in portal pressure provided blood volume is restored with intravenous fluids.

BILIRUBIN SECRETION

Bilirubin is a heme product culled by the reticuloendothelial system from hemoglobin and other hemoproteins. It is normally bound to albumin and conjugated by the liver and excreted in the bile. Even small bilirubin loads can overwhelm a hypoalbuminemic patient with diminished conjugating capacity. Unconjugated bilirubin unbound to albumin is toxic to mitochondria and causes an encephalopathy and kernicterus, in neonates. Increased serum concentrations of bilirubin and bile salts contribute to the constitutional symptoms and acute tubular necrosis of acute liver disease. Treatment of patients with hyperbilirubinemia consists of intravenous albumin or hemodialysis.

COAGULATION AND HEMATOLOGIC EFFECTS

Most soluble coagulation factors derive from the liver. Disorders of coagulation rapidly follow severe hepatic damage as the half-lives of some factors are short (Factor VII: 6 hours). Deficiency of the vitamin K-dependent Factors II, VII, IX, and X is linked to impaired bile secretion, as occurs in obstructive jaundice.

The liver is responsible for the clearance of activated coagulation products. A failure to extract these complexes leads to factor consumption and primary fibrinolysis. Important anticoagulant (antithrombins II and III, C1 inhibitor, alpha-2 antiplasmin, alpha-2 macroglobulin) and fibrinolytic factors are essential hepatic hemostatic products.

Platelet quantity and quality may suffer in liver disease. Normally, 30 per cent of circulating platelets may be found within the spleen, but up to 90 per cent are sequestered in hypersplenism accompanying portal hypertension. Intravascular coagulation consumes platelets, and uncleared dialyzable toxins disable platelets. Anesthetic management includes blood component therapy with platelets, fresh frozen plasma, cryoprecipitate, or vitamin K as dictated by laboratory studies (see Chapter 15).

Anemia in patients with hepatic disease is due to many factors. Bleeding is exacerbated by derangements of hemostasis. Effective erythropoiesis depends upon a normal liver for iron and heme transport with serum proteins such as haptoglobin, transferrin, and ceruloplasmin. Vitamin B_{12} is stored in the liver.

DRUG METABOLISM AND PHARMACOKINETICS

Although the pulmonary and renal parenchyma contribute, drug metabolism occurs chiefly in the liver; in patients with severe liver disease, diminished Phase I and II reactions increase the serum half-lives of many drugs. Other effects of liver disease also increase the efficacy of drugs: portosystemic shunts permit orally administered drugs to bypass the liver, thus reducing first-pass metabolism; hypoalbuminemia causes an increase in free plasma drug concentration. Other effects of liver disease require that drug doses be increased: ascites and increases in extracellular volume are associated with increased volumes of distribution for water-soluble drugs; gamma globulins are increased in most hepatic dysfunctions, so that drugs bound to these proteins have a larger volume of distribution.

GLUCOSE-GLYCOGEN METABOLISM

Despite the role of the liver in glycogen storage, fasting hypoglycemia is rare in liver disease; as little as 20 per cent of the hepatic parenchyma suffices for this function. Measurements of serum glucose ensure that hypoglycemia does not go unrecognized during anesthesia.

HORMONE METABOLISM

The hormonal abnormalities associated with hepatic dysfunction are multiple and complex. Estrogens, antidiuretic hormone, and thyroid stimulating hormone are all increased.

RENAL FUNCTION

Renal compromise owing to liver disease takes the form of impaired sodium and water handling, acute tubular necrosis, and hepatorenal syndrome. In cirrhosis and to a lesser degree in acute liver disease, the main defect is impaired excretion of salt and water, probably due to decreased effective circulating volume and renal blood flow. Regardless of salt intake, the urine in advanced liver disease may be almost free of sodium. There is a major increase in extracellular fluid, evident as ascites and edema.

Acute tubular necrosis occurs in patients with obstructive liver disease and with liver disease owing to hypovolemic shock, septic shock, and metabolic toxemia.

Hepatorenal syndrome is an unexplained progressive oliguric renal failure in patients with cirrhosis, hepatoma, or acute hepatitis. It resembles prerenal azotemia, which must be ruled out before making this diagnosis. Pathological examination reveals no consistent changes in the structure of affected kidneys, and transplanted kidneys from patients with hepatorenal syndrome have demonstrated normal function.

PULMONARY FUNCTION

Chronic hypoxemia in liver disease results from several causes. Intrapulmonary arteriovenous shunting may represent a significant fraction of the increased cardiac output, resulting in an increase in the shunt fraction (Q_s/Q_t). Increases in interstitial lung water from hypoalbuminemia and hyponatremia contribute to defects in O_2 diffusion. Ascites and pleural effusions produce a restrictive pulmonary disorder. Many patients with alcoholic cirrhosis also smoke heavily. Hypoxic pulmonary vasoconstriction is blunted by circulating vasodilator substances. The oxyhemoglobin dissociation curve is shifted rightward owing to increased 2,3-DPG concentrations, an effect that is offset by the respiratory alkalosis of chronic hyperventilation. Together, these effects make maintaining arterial oxygenation a major challenge in managing anesthesia for these patients.

NERVOUS SYSTEM

Hepatic encephalopathy is thought to result from accumulation of circulating toxic wastes normally cleared in the liver. Asterixis, somnolence, obtundation, and eventually coma are common neurologic signs. Ammonia has long been considered the cause, but there is no clear correlation between serum concentrations and symptoms. Other candidate molecules include mercaptans, octopamine, phenol, and short-chain fatty acids. The blood-brain barrier is thought to become more permeable in liver failure and intracranial pressure is often increased.

GASTROINTESTINAL SYSTEM

Malabsorption and inanition are common accompaniments of liver dysfunction. Cirrhosis increases portal resistance, engorging the portal circulation and promoting bleeding, especially from esophageal varices. Bacterial overgrowth predisposes the patient to encephalopathy from bacterial metabolic wastes. Peptic ulceration is a common, potentially fatal problem in cirrhotic patients.

Anesthetic Management in Severe Liver Disease

PREOPERATIVE EVALUATION

Preoperative assessment of the patient with liver disease seeks to determine the degree of impairment of liver function, the nature of the disorder, and the severity of the various sequelae described above.

For patients with disorders of mild severity, there may be no pathophysiologic consequences of the disease, as the liver possesses remarkable reserve; function can be normal in animals even after resection of up to 90 per cent of the liver. Because such patients (with subclinical or well-compensated liver disease) may develop postoperative liver failure, anesthesia management seeks to preserve remaining liver function.

For patients with severe liver disorders, thorough assessment allows the anesthesiologist to plan intraoperative care, as well as to seek to improve the patient's condition before operation. In consultation with the gastroenterologist and surgeon, the following measures can be undertaken to improve the condition of patients with severe liver disease:

1. Correct hypovolemia and electrolyte disorders.
2. Treat coagulopathy with vitamin K, soluble coagulation factors, and platelets.
3. Drain ascites as appropriate to relieve the effects of increased intra-abdominal pressure.
4. Control infection.
5. Sterilize the bowel with neomycin or inhibit bacterial urease with lactulose, to treat encephalopathy.
6. Treat anemia with packed red cell transfusions.
7. Monitor intracranial pressure and control cerebral edema.
8. Administer propranolol (if cardiomyopathy is not present) to decrease splanchnic blood flow and diminish portal hypertension.

PREMEDICATION

Sedative hypnotic premedication is not contraindicated in these patients but must be used with caution because of alterations in the blood-brain barrier, pharmacodynamics, and pharmacokinetics.

MONITORING

In advanced liver disease, invasive monitoring prior to induction of anesthesia is appropriate for any but the least invasive of surgical procedures. Coagulopathies are corrected before placing these cannulae.

CHOICE OF ANESTHETIC

Local anesthesia and monitored sedation or regional anesthesia may be used. Amide local anesthetics are poorly metabolized, requiring that succeeding doses after the first be reduced in amount. General anesthesia is often advisable because of the advantages of intubation and controlled ventilation in these patients.

MAINTAINING HEPATIC BLOOD FLOW

Preservation of the patient's remaining hepatocytes by maintaining hepatic blood flow and oxygenation is a major goal of anesthesia management in these patients. Since autoregulation of hepatic blood flow is compromised, careful attention is required to prevent hepatic cellular hypoxia.

As a rule, all anesthetics and anesthetic techniques lead to decreases in total hepatic blood flow or worsening of the ratio between hepatic oxygen supply and demand. The mechanisms include decreased cardiac output, increased splanchnic vascular resistance, arterial hypotension, or increased hepatic venous pressure. Although splanchnic flow decreases with all three volatile anesthetics now in use, isoflurane is less likely to produce hepatic cellular hypoxia. Opiates, barbiturates, benzodiazepines, relaxants, and spinal and epidural anesthesia reduce hepatic blood flow in proportion to decreases in blood pressure. Nitrous oxide limits F_{IO_2} and promotes bowel distension. The combination of isoflurane, oxygen, and small doses of narcotics seems at present to be the most rational choice for general anesthesia in patients with severe liver disease.

The conduct of anesthesia is as important as the choice of anesthetic, for both can influence hepatic oxygenation. Decrease in arterial blood pressure and cardiac output owing to positive pressure ventilation and PEEP will decrease hepatic blood flow. Hypocarbia diminishes hepatic blood flow, and respiratory alkalosis favors conversion of ammonium ion to ammonia, which more readily crosses the blood-brain barrier. Conversely, hypercarbia causes increases in sympathetic tone and decreases in hepatic blood flow; normocarbia is the best compromise for these patients.

Surgical site and position alter hemodynamics. The portal circulation, even in end-stage liver disease, is a low-pressure system (25 mm Hg). Gravity affects drainage, and positions that markedly increase abdominal or chest pressures can adversely affect hepatic blood flow.

FLUID MANAGEMENT

Colloidal solutions effectively restore intravascular volume to maintain urine output. Mannitol is preferred over furosemide, which exacerbates hypokalemic alkalosis. Either may further diminish intravascular volume.

AIRWAY MANAGEMENT

The patient with cirrhosis has an increased intragastric volume, with a decreased pH; ascites increases intra-abdominal pressure. Rapid sequence induction or awake intubation are indicated.

INTRAVENOUS ANESTHETICS

All of the intravenous agents used to induce anesthesia depend on the liver for their elimination. Although chronic abuse of alcohol confers tolerance to some anesthetics, cardiomyopathy and the alterations in pharmacokinetics described previously may accentuate the effects of normal doses in patients with cirrhosis. A general approach to the administration of drugs to patients with liver disease is to give the initial dose in small increments until the desired effect is achieved. Successive doses are given in reduced doses and only when indicated, as drug metabolism is likely to be impaired.

MUSCLE RELAXANTS

The choice of muscle relaxant, if needed, is predicated on the duration of the planned procedure. Although pseudocholinesterase production is decreased, the duration of effect of succinylcholine is not markedly prolonged. The nondepolarizing muscle relaxants are all acceptable for use. The increased volume of distribution requires larger initial doses. The duration of effect of atracurium is unaffected by liver disease, making it a good choice when immediate recovery of neuromuscular function is required after anesthesia.

TRANSMISSION OF HEPATITIS

Although precautions against transmission of viral illness are always appropriate, particular care is indicated in managing patients with liver disease, all of whom can be presumed to carry hepatitis virus.

Postoperative Hepatitis

After anesthesia and operation, some apparently healthy patients not exposed to blood products develop hepatitis. In a survey of 7600 healthy patients scheduled for elective operations, Schemel (1976) found 11 with preoperative liver disease by laboratory test. The operations were canceled for these 11 patients, and three went on to become jaundiced. Thus, in this population, between one in 2000 and one in 700 of healthy surgical patients developed liver disease, without anesthesia or operation. When a specific cause for postoperative jaundice cannot be found, the disease is sometimes attributed to the anesthetic, most often halothane, although there may be no distinctive chemical, immunologic, or microscopic signs of anesthesia-induced liver injury. Estimates of the incidence of severe hepatic dysfunction are given as one in 6000 to one in 20,000 halothane anesthetics. Because the incidence of this problem is much less than the incidence of hepatitis from other causes, and because good animal models are lacking, even the existence of the syndrome has been the subject of debate.

The proposed mechanisms include hepatic hypoxia, hypothetical toxic effects of reductive metabolites, or an autoimmune response to complexes of liver proteins and halothane metabolites. The available data do not implicate isoflurane; hepatitis is attributed to enflurane less often than to halothane; the incidence even after halothane is small, especially in children. Those at greatest risk appear to be middle-aged obese women, especially those who received repeated halothane anesthesia at intervals of a few weeks. There is no evidence that preexisting liver disease increases the risk of anesthetic-induced hepatitis, but it may be prudent to avoid halothane in a patient who has had halothane in the previous few months or who reports a history of unexplained hepatitis after anesthesia.

In evaluating a patient with jaundice or hepatic dysfunction after anesthesia, other causes are sought including obstructive jaundice, hemolysis, and viral hepatitis. The diagnosis of anesthetic-related hepatitis usually remains one of exclusion, however.

PATIENTS WITH RENAL DISEASE

Signs and symptoms of renal failure occur only after loss of 60 per cent of the 2 million nephrons. Conservative medical therapy suffices to treat renal insufficiency until only 10 per cent of the nephrons remain, at which time renal failure requires dialysis. The management of the patient with impaired renal function focuses on preserving remaining function, and altering therapeutic approaches to compensate for renal dysfunction. The patient with outright renal failure usually undergoes dialysis before operation; management focuses on avoiding derangements in fluid or electrolyte balance.

In addition, end-stage renal disease has effects on many organ systems that must be taken into account. These complications and their anesthetic implications are addressed here according to the component of renal function that is affected.

Renal Pathophysiology

The primary functions of the kidney are: (1) acid-base regulation, (2) water and fluid volume maintenance, (3) electrolyte balance, (4) hormone elaboration, and (5) excretion. To these ends, the kidneys normally receive about 25 per cent of the adult's cardiac output (renal blood flow is 1250 ml per minute) of which 10 per cent is filtered (glomerular filtration rate is 125 ml per minute). Although autoregulation normally keeps renal blood flow within narrow limits for a wide variety of mean arterial pressures, the functioning of the nephron is subject to neurohumoral regulation by antidiuretic hormone, aldosterone, renin, and catecholamines, all of which are secreted in response to the stress of operation.

In renal failure, the 50 mEq of hydrogen ion produced daily are not excreted; metabolic acidosis results. Acidemia exacerbates the hyperkalemia that usually coexists.

Patients with renal insufficiency often are unable to produce concentrated urine. Salt and water wastage with resultant hypovolemia occurs, especially when patients fast. As the ability to excrete water fails, the patient with oliguria or anuria depends upon dialysis to eliminate exogenous and endogenous water. Pulmonary edema and hypoxia may occur with modest infusions of volume.

The prominent disturbances of electrolyte balance are hyponatremia, hypocalcemia, and increased serum concentrations of chloride, potassium, phosphate, and magnesium ions. Patients with renal insufficiency who have not received dialysis may have potassium concentrations of 6 to 7 mEq per L; the chief electrocardiographic (ECG) findings are tall peaked T waves. Acute increases from this baseline hyperkalemia may be precipitated by respiratory acidosis, potassium sparing diuretics, or succinylcholine. When the serum potassium reaches 8 mEq per L, the PR interval becomes prolonged and the QRS complex widens. At concentrations greater than 9 mEq per L, the P wave disappears, and the QRS complex widens to a sine wave form. Supraventricular tachycardia, premature ventricular beats, and ventricular fibrillation occur.

Immediately treatment of hyperkalemia includes hyperventilation and the administration of glucose with insulin, and in life-threatening hyperkalemia, calcium to reverse the effects of potassium on excitable membranes. As succinylcholine increases serum potassium concentrations transiently by less than 1 mEq per L, it may be used for rapid sequence induction of anesthesia in these patients, provided that the serum potassium is not excessive before the succinylcholine is given.

Calcium is depleted in the syndrome of renal osteodystrophy. Patients suffer severe osteoporosis; care is required in moving them. Paradoxically, there may be metastatic calcareous deposits in patients with hyperphosphatemia. These deposits may affect essential tissues such as the cardiac conduction system. Hypocalcemia impairs myocardial contractility and potentiates hyperkalemia and ventricular irritability.

Effects on Other Organ Systems

CARDIOVASCULAR

Hypertension is an almost universal finding in renal insufficiency and renal failure. In many cases, renal failure is due to essential hypertension; in end-stage renal disease, increased renin excretion causes hypertension. Left ventricular hypertrophy results from hypertension and from increased cardiac output due to anemia. High output cardiac failure occurs in some patients with large arteriovenous shunts created for hemodialysis. Uremic pericarditis may cause tamponade.

Intravascular volume overload is often found in patients between dialysis treatments or those with oliguria. Volume depletion may result from polyuria or vigorous hemodialysis. Accelerated atherosclerosis and coronary artery disease associated with diabetes mellitus and hypertension commonly accompany severe renal disease.

HEMATOLOGIC

Anemia results from gastrointestinal bleeding, increased bleeding time, decreased erythropoietin secretion, and decreased red cell life span. The hematocrit may reach a nadir of 20 per cent, which has been demonstrated to decrease the blood/gas partition coefficient for potent anesthetic agents by up to 25 per cent, somewhat decreasing the time required for induction and emergence. Preoperative treatment is with recombinant human erythropoietin produced by *Escherichia coli*, or by transfusion with packed red blood cells with due attention to avoiding fluid overload. Patients adapt to chronic anemia; correction is based on the patient's responses to anemia and not an arbitrary goal based on a normal value for hematocrit.

There is a qualitative defect in platelet adhesiveness and aggregation, related to some dialyzable toxin(s). Transfusion of platelets is ineffective unless dialysis is performed also. In the absence of dialysis, platelet function can be restored with administration of 1-deamino-(8-D-arginine)-vasopressin (DDAVP), cryoprecipitate, or conjugated estrogens.

PULMONARY

Pulmonary edema results from volume overload and from the decreased oncotic pressure caused by proteinuria. Metastatic calcification occurs in pulmonary tissues, contributing to a diminution in diffusion capacity. Peritoneal dialysis restricts diaphragmatic motion, decreasing functional residual capacity.

GASTROINTESTINAL

Anorexia, hiccup, nausea, and vomiting are common in uremia. Gastrointestinal (GI) ulceration occurs in up to 25 per cent of patients with renal failure. Patients have increased gastric acidity and volumes, suggesting the use of appropriate precautions against aspiration of gastric contents, including preoperative cimetidine and metaclopromide, and rapid sequence induction or awake intubation of the trachea.

IMMUNE SYSTEM

Uremia impairs leucocyte chemotaxis. Immunity is further embarrassed by loss of humeral globulins in proteinuria and steroid treatments for some causes of renal failure. Sepsis is the major cause of death in patients with renal failure.

NERVOUS SYSTEM

Uremic toxemia presents as mental slowing, fatigue, and malaise and progresses to seizures, myoclonus, and coma if left untreated. Many patients receiving chronic hemodialysis suffer from depression or experience personality changes.

Peripheral sensory neuropathies usually affect the lower extremities; motor deficits occur less often. Dysautonomia occurs with severe disease and produces orthostatic hypotension, gastroparesis, or vomiting. Rapid sequence intubation is recommended for patients with vomiting or gastroparesis.

DIALYSIS

Dialysis controls volume overload, volume dependent hypertension, electrolyte imbalances, platelet defects, and acidosis (Table 23–1). Encephalopathy can be prevented and largely reversed. Red cell transfusion may be accomplished without volume change during hemodialysis. Dialysis does not improve renin-dependent hypertension, impaired immunity, anemia, hypoproteinemia, increased cardiac output, accelerated atherosclerosis, or GI ulceration.

Dialysis can provoke specific problems, with which the anesthesiologist must deal. Although dialysis therapy ameliorates the hemostatic defect of uremia, a bleeding diathesis is seen in up to 75 per cent of patients undergoing dialysis. Rebound heparinization has been recognized following hemodialysis, owing to the differences in the rates

TABLE 23–1. Effect of Dialysis on Physiologic Derangements in End-Stage Renal Disease

Improved by Dialysis	Not Improved by Dialysis	Caused by Dialysis
Volume dependent hypertension	Renin dependent hypertension	Accelerated atherosclerosis
Volume overload	Anemia	Rebound heparinization
Electrolyte imbalance	Increased cardiac output	Hypovolemia
Acidosis	Impaired immunity	Hypoproteinemia
Encephalopathy	Impaired wound healing	
Platelet dysfunction	GI ulceration	
Neuropathy	Hypoproteinemia	

of clearance of heparin and protamine after dialysis. In general, rebound heparinization is preferable to thrombosis of the hemodialysis shunt in patients who do not require operation. Rebound heparinization responds to protamine administration.

After vigorous dialysis, some patients suffer hypovolemia. This can be detected by questioning the patient about their weight and by testing for orthostatic hypotension. Lastly, hepatitis is endemic in patients with end-stage renal disease.

The Effect of Renal Failure on Drug Action

Clearance of water-soluble drugs and their metabolites is dependent upon renal excretion, a function which diminishes with loss of nephrons. Some drugs such as morphine and the benzodiazepines are metabolized to active compounds that accumulate in renal disease. The major metabolite of meperidine, normeperidine, accumulates to cause central nervous system (CNS) stimulation and seizures, particularly in children. Further, accumulated metabolites may compete with progenitor compounds for available protein binding sites, increasing the fraction of drug in the free active form.

Hypoalbuminemia commonly accompanies renal insufficiency owing to albuminuria in nephrosis. Patients with end-stage renal disease may lose up to 20 gm of albumin per day during peritoneal dialysis, and twice that if there is peritonitis. The effects of hypoalbuminemia have been described previously in this chapter and in Chapter 7.

Acidosis alters the relative equilibrium concentrations of some ionized drugs in circulation. Drugs with acidic pKa values are less ionized in acidosis, attain greater volumes of distribution, and have longer elimination half-lives.

Pharmacodynamics are altered in uremic patients because of toxic defects on the blood-brain barrier. Exaggerated CNS effects of some drugs can be anticipated. Prudence dictates careful incremental titration in these debilitated patients.

The Effect of Anesthesia on Renal Function

Inhalational anesthetics produce a dose-dependent reversible depression of renal function, as a result of reduced renal blood flow and glomerular filtration rate, although fluid administration produces diuresis (Table 23–2). The risk of permanent renal damage from inhalational anesthetics has been studied extensively since the recognition that metabolism of methoxyflurane released enough fluoride to cause nephrotoxicity. This was characterized by polyuria and inability to concentrate urine in response to antidiuretic hormone after 2.5 to 5 minimum alveolar concentration (MAC)-hours

TABLE 23–2. Effects of Volatile Anesthetics on Renal Function*

Agent	Urine Volume	Glomerular Filtration (%)	Renal Blood Flow (%)
Enflurane	Decreased	↓ 21	↓ 23
Halothane	Decreased	↓ 19	↓ 38
Isoflurane	Decreased	↓ 37	↓ 49

* (Adapted with permission from Bevan DR. Renal function in anaesthesia and surgery. New York: Grune & Stratton, 1979.)

of exposure to methoxyflurane. Nephrotoxicity was localized in the distal convoluted tubule and collecting ducts, where the response to antidiuretic hormone predominates.

Subclinical nephrotoxicity has been demonstrated in healthy volunteers following enflurane exposure for 9.6 MAC hours. Obesity and isoniazid therapy increase free fluoride release from enflurane. Patients with renal disease and some remaining renal function are not good candidates for enflurane anesthesia.

Anesthesia for Patients with Renal Disease

PREOPERATIVE EVALUATION

The preoperative evaluation of a patient with renal disease seeks to determine the patient's intravascular volume status, electrolyte balance, and renal function. In addition, depending on the severity of the renal failure, the systemic effects described previously are sought. Therapy for systemic disorders such as anemia, coagulopathy, fluid overload, or hyperkalemia is instituted preoperatively whenever possible. Patients maintained by dialysis require treatment within a day of elective operations.

PREMEDICATION

Sedative premedication is administered only in reduced doses. Premedication includes an H_2 receptor blocker and metaclopromide to reduce gastric acidity and volume.

MONITORING

Monitoring depends on the patient's condition. The site of vascular access for dialysis is protected from blood pressure cuffs or intravenous access, to minimize the chance of thrombosis or infection. If possible, arterial catheters are not used, to preserve future access sites. A bladder catheter is a source of urinary tract infection; it is used only if absolutely necessary, as in a long operation. In many patients, oliguria or anuria are well established and there can be no value to monitoring urine output. A central venous pressure cannula (usually) or a pulmonary artery catheter (rarely) is useful if the patient's blood volume is expected to change rapidly, as from severe bleeding. A nerve stimulator is essential if neuromuscular blockers are to be used.

POSITIONING

Careful positioning of the patient is required, as these patients may have little subcutaneous tissue and are subject to pressure-related tissue breakdown. As mentioned earlier, renal osteodystrophy makes fractures more likely. The presence of peripheral neuropathy may make the patient unaware of pressure on skin. The hemodialysis access sites should be available for monitoring (by palpation or Doppler flow meter) during the operation, and mechanical obstruction by the blood pressure cuff or positioning is avoided.

GENERAL ANESTHESIA

General anesthesia is often needed for these patients. Rapid intravenous induction, combined with cricoid pressure and immediate intubation of the trachea is advocated for uremic patients with evidence of dysautonomia or nausea and vomiting. However, these patients often have coronary artery disease, labile hypertension, or volume depletion, making the rapid induction of anesthesia more risky. Volume repletion, the use of a test dose of intravenous anesthetic, and a slower induction are prudent measures, if performed carefully. Succinylcholine is suitable, unless reason exists to avoid an increase in serum potassium of 1.0 mEq per L.

In patients with renal failure, excretion of pancuronium, d-tubocurarine, and metocurine is prolonged, making vecuronium and atracurium more suitable choices. Despite the theoretical advantages enjoyed by these drugs, careful monitoring and doses limited to the minimum needed are still required to avoid unwanted paralysis at the end of anesthesia. Reversal of neuromuscular blockade with anticholinesterase and anticholinergic drugs is feasible. These drugs have even longer durations of action in the presence of renal failure than do the nondepolarizing neuromuscular blocking drugs. Reports of late unopposed muscarinic effects (bradycardia, bronchospasm, and hypersecretion) have appeared, but these are not common problems.

Inhalational agents have an advantage over intravenous agents, as they are eliminated via the lungs and not the kidneys. Enflurane is avoided because of the rare possibility of nephrotoxicity from fluoride ion. The effects of small doses of intravenous drugs dissipate predictably, owing to redistribution. With large or repeated doses, effects may be prolonged, as renal elimination of the drugs and their metabolites is slowed.

REGIONAL ANESTHESIA

Regional anesthetic techniques are commonly employed in patients with end-stage renal disease. These hypertensive patients who cannot excrete sodium or free water may suffer hypertensive crises, pulmonary edema, or myocardial infarction when the effect of the anesthetic dissipates and vasoconstriction returns, exacerbated by pain. These patients are more prone to development of hypotension from autonomic neuropathy also. Acidemia predisposes to greater serum concentrations of local anesthetics with increased risk of toxicity. Earlier reports of a 40 per cent diminution in duration of brachial plexus block have been refuted subsequently. Arterial puncture during the block may result in hematoma in patients with uremic thrombocytopathy. However, nerve blocks offer potential benefits to patients having vascular access operations, as the accompanying sympathectomy improves flow in the limb and systemic hypotension is lessened.

REFERENCES

Brown BR Jr. Anesthesia in hepatic and biliary tract disease. FA Davis Co, 1988.

Gelman S, Dillard E, Bradley EL Jr. Hepatic circulation during surgical stress and anesthesia with halothane, isoflurane, or fentanyl. Anesth Analg 1987; 66:936–943.

Mazze RI, Calverley RK, Smith NT. Inorganic fluoride nephrotoxicity: Prolonged enflurane and halothane anesthesia in volunteers. Anesthesiology 1977; 46:265–271.

Priebe HJ, ed. The kidney in anesthesia. International anesthesiology clinics, vol 22. New York: Little, Brown & Co, 1984.

Schemel WH. Unexpected hepatic dysfunction found by multiple laboratory screening. Anesth Analg 1976; 55:810–812.

Strunin L, Davies JM. The liver and anaesthesia. Can Anaesth Soc J 1983; 30:208–217.

CHAPTER TWENTY-FOUR

Patients with Metabolic and Endocrine Disorders

Endocrine and metabolic disorders affect the function of almost every organ system, and thus are challenging problems for perioperative management. Patients with endocrine or metabolic diseases who are well compensated on medical therapy may require little more than routine anesthetic care, or the stress of operation may cause severe derangements. When the diseased endocrine gland is to be removed, surgical manipulation and removal may produce effects that must be anticipated. Occasionally, anesthetic agents themselves can have adverse effects in these patients; some drugs are contraindicated in certain disorders.

Thyroid

The thyroid gland produces tetraiodothyronine (thyroxine or T_4) and the more potent triiodothyronine (T_3). Circulating T_3 and T_4 are more than 99 per cent bound to serum proteins, especially thyroxine-binding globulin (TBG) and thyroxine-binding prealbumin (TBPA). However, the metabolic effect of these hormones is determined by the amount of free hormone available. In adults, circulating thyroid hormone regulates the basal rate of metabolism, oxygen consumption, and heat production.

The production and release of T_3 and T_4 from the thyroid are regulated by thyroid stimulating hormone (TSH), the production of which by the anterior pituitary is inhibited by circulating thyroid hormone and increased by thyrotropin releasing hormone (TRH), produced by the hypothalamus.

Free T_4 correlates with hypothyroidism or hyperthyroidism, but is difficult to measure, because it accounts for only about 0.5 per cent of the total T_4 present. Increased or decreased concentrations of thyroid binding globulin cause concomitant changes in the total amount of T_4 measured. Estrogens, infectious hepatitis, and genetic factors can increase the level of TGB; androgens, nephrosis, hypoproteinemia, and genetic factors can decrease the TGB. The T_3 resin uptake allows a correction for the effect of TGB on total T_4; T_3 resin uptake is directly proportional to the free fraction of thyroid hormone in the serum. If the total T_4 is increased but the resin uptake is decreased, the T_4 level is increased because of an increase in TGB and not excess free T_4.

Hyperthyroidism

The most common cause of hyperthyroidism is Graves' disease, an autoimmune disorder in which thyroid stimulating immunoglobulins (long-acting thyroid stimulator [LATS]) mimic the effect of thyroid stimulating hormone. Other causes of hyperthyroidism are toxic nodular goiters, subacute thyroiditis, and pregnancy (approximately 0.2 per cent of parturients).

The physiologic effects of hyperthyroidism are related to the increased metabolic rate and hyperdynamic state owing to the excess thyroid hormone (Table 24–1). The cardiovascular effects are due to sympathetic nervous system hyperactivity that occur despite normal levels of plasma catecholamines. This suggests that thyroid hormone sensitizes the adrenergic receptors to catecholamines. An extreme and life-threatening manifestation of hyperthyroidism is thyroid storm, due to a sudden discharge of thyroid hormones. The resulting systemic effects can mimic malignant hyperthermia and include hyperthermia, tachycardia, high-output congestive heart failure, and dehydration.

There are two approaches to pharmacologic therapy for hyperthyroidism. The first is to attenuate the production and release of T_3 and T_4. Propylthiouracil, methimazole, and potassium iodide are all used for this purpose. A second approach is to block the peripheral effects of thyroid hormone by using adrenergic antagonists. Beta antagonists are most commonly used, whereas sympatholytics such as reserpine and guanethidine are less commonly used. Lastly, glucocorticoids may be administered because they potentially facilitate the degradation of active hormone.

The stress of operation can cause severe hyperdynamic and hypermetabolic changes in the untreated or partially treated hyperthyroid patient. The best course is to render these patients euthyroid with medical treatment before operation, continuing antithyroid medication to the morning of operation. If this is not possible, beta-adrenergic antagonists are used to attenuate the cardiovascular manifestations of hyperthyroidism.

Table 24–1. Physiologic Effects of Hyperthyroidism

System	Effect
Cardiovascular	Increased cardiac output: heart rate, increased stroke volume, and increased ventricular contractility
	Widened pulse pressure with decreased sytemic vascular resistance
	Functional mitral insufficiency
	Mitral prolapse
	Atrial fibrillation
Pulmonary	Increased oxygen consumption
	Decreased vital capacity
	Increased residual volume
	FRC normal
	Decreased affinity of hemoglobin for oxygen
Renal	Polyuria
	Hypercalcemia and hypercalcuria
	Hypomagnesemia
Hepatic/GI	Increased gastric motility
	Increased LFTs (serum transaminases and alkaline phosphatase)
	Hepatomegaly and jaundice in extreme cases
Endocrine	Insulin antagonism by thyroid hormones causing exacerbation of diabetes mellitus
	Abnormal menstrual cycles
Hematologic	Pernicious anemia in 2 to 3 per cent of patients
	Platelet function and clotting system are normal
Other	Myopathy which may affect muscles of respiration
	Emotional lability and nervousness
	Ophthalmopathy in Graves' disease

It is prudent to minimize stress responses with adequate premedication and anesthesia. Drugs that may stimulate the sympathetic nervous system, such as ketamine and pancuronium are avoided. A nitrous oxide-narcotic technique may be an alternative to volatile agents, but incomplete inhibition of the sympathetic nervous system may precipitate a hyperdynamic reaction. Hyperthyroidism does not increase the minimum alveolar concentration (MAC) of volatile anesthetics in animals, yet in patients it may seem that the anesthetic requirement is increased, perhaps because the increased cardiac output retards the increase in the alveolar concentration of anesthetic, or the hyperactivity of the cardiovascular system is interpreted as representing inadequate anesthesia (Table 24–2).

If the operation is amenable to regional, spinal,

TABLE 24–2. **Anesthetic Considerations: Hyperthyroidism**

Period	Consideration
Preoperative	Achieve euthyroid state with antithyroid drugs Studies for airway compression Iodine 7 to 10 days prior to surgery in Graves' disease Give antithyroid drugs on morning of surgery Adequate premedication Avoid anticholinergic agents Have beta antagonist available
Induction	Thiopental has theoretical advantages Ketamine and pancuronium are avoided because of their sympathomimetic properties Ophthalmopathy requires appropriate eye care
Maintenance	Both volatile agents and balanced anesthesia have been used successfully and no technique has been proven superior Temperature must be monitored and cooling instituted as needed Be prepared to treat hypermetabolic state
Postoperative	If thyroidal surgery has been performed, airway obstruction may occur due to laryngeal nerve damage Patient is still at risk for sudden onset of a hypermetabolic state

or epidural anesthesia, these techniques are appropriate because of the sympathetic blockade produced. However, if the sympathetic blockade results in hypotension, treatment must be titrated carefully because of the potential sensitivity to catecholamines.

Hypothyroidism

Hypothyroidism usually is due to inadequate thyroid hormone secretion but rarely can occur from decreased peripheral sensitivity to the hormone. Inadequate secretion usually is due to idiopathic atrophy of the thyroid gland, autoimmune thyroiditis (Hashimoto's disease), radioiodine therapy or external radiation, thyroidectomy, replacement of thyroid tissue by tumor, or defective biosynthesis (which may occur after iodide, lithium, or sodium nitroprusside). Finally, tertiary hypothyroidism occurs if there is hypothalamic dysfunction.

The physiologic effects of hypothyroidism that are of greatest concern to the anesthesiologist are the depressed hemodynamic state and the changes in pulmonary physiology that can occur with hypothyroidism (Table 24–3). Because of the depressed hemodynamic state, hypothyroid patients may be sensitive to anesthetic agents that depress myocardial contractility or cause vasodilation. Similarly, the baseline alveolar hypoventilation and diminution of hypoxic and hypercapnic ventilatory drive make these patients sensitive to drugs that depress respiration. Amyloidosis may cause enlargement of the tongue and may hinder intubation. The changes in the coagulation system as well as increased capillary fragility predispose hypothyroid patients to increased bleeding. A rare

TABLE 24–3. **Physiologic Effects of Hypothyroidism**

System	Effect
Cardiovascular	Decreased cardiac output: decreased heart rate, decreased stroke volume, and decreased ventricular contractility Increased systemic vascular resistance with decreased cerebral, renal, and skin blood flow Abnormal systolic time intervals: increased preejection period; decreased left ventricular ejection time Pericardial effusions Defective baroreceptor reflexes
Pulmonary	Lung volumes are normal Decreased maximal breathing capacity Decreased hypercapneic and hypoxic drive Pleural effusions Enlarged tongue and thickened vocal cords
Renal	Decreased plasma volume Decreased GFR and creatinine clearance Increased ADH causing increased extracellular volume and hyponatremia
Hepatic/GI	Delayed gastric emptying and decreased intestinal motility Gastrointestinal hemorrhage Constipation
Endocrine	Enhanced norepinphrine production; epinephrine production normal Decreased cortisol production
Hematologic	Pernicious anemia in 12 per cent of patients Normochromic, normocytic anemia Abnormal platelet aggregability Decreased Factors VIII and IX
Other	Hypercholesterolemia Myxedema with slow wound healing Cold intolerance and hypothermia Delayed contraction/relaxation of muscles

TABLE 24–4. Hypothyroidism: Therapy

Therapy	Remark
T_4	0.15 to 0.2 mg per day is adequate replacement for most patients Converted to T_3 peripherally Half-life of 7.5 days with peak metabolic effect at 10 to 12 days Dose must be carefully titrated in patients with coronary disease
T_3	Used in patients who are severely hypothyroid Used when conversion of T_4 to T_3 is impaired

complication associated with profound hypothyroidism is myxedema coma. The constellation of signs and symptoms of myxedema coma include lethargy, hypothermia, bradycardia, and alveolar hypoventilation with hypoxemia. Hyponatremia with marked decreased free water clearance is often part of the syndrome.

The treatment of hypothyroidism is replacement of T_4 by administering levothyroxin (Table 24–4). Since T_4 is converted to T_3, there is generally no need to treat with T_3. The different organ systems respond to treatment at different rates, and myocardial function can improve in as little as two weeks, although effusions may take months to clear. Patients with coronary artery disease are treated with much smaller doses of levothyroxin, to avoid angina or even myocardial infarction. Only partial control of hypothyroidism is sometimes accepted because of this. Severe overt hypothyroidism or myxedema coma are treated with large doses of T_4, but in patients who are markedly depressed, the peripheral conversion of T_4 to T_3 may be impaired. In this case, T_3 is administered with care, because of the risk of myocardial infarction and sudden death.

The patient maintained in a euthyroid state with T_4 therapy presents no inherent anesthetic problems and may be treated in a routine manner. The usual daily dose of levothyroxine is given on the day of operation, even though the half-life of this drug is long. The overtly hypothyroid patient is at risk for severe hemodynamic, respiratory, and neurologic depression from anesthetic agents. As with hyperthyroid patients, the best course is medical treatment to attain the euthyroid state before elective operation is undertaken.

If emergency operation is required in the mildly hypothyroid patient, little or no premedication is given and appropriate steps are take to manage the delayed gastric emptying that may be present. There is a widespread clinical impression that hypothyroid patients are sensitive to anesthetic agents, not because of a decrease in MAC, but because of impaired distribution and metabolism of drugs and enhanced respiratory and circulatory depressant effects. Reduced doses of induction agents and volatile agents are recommended and inotropic agents and vasopressors must be readily available (Table 24–5).

Emergency operation in the severely hypothyroid patient requires consultation with an endocrinologist. Intravenous T_4 and T_3 may be administered, along with glucocorticoids. A slow emergence from anesthesia and postoperative mechanical ventilation can be anticipated.

PARATHYROID

Calcium homeostasis is regulated by three hormones: parathyroid hormone (PTH), secreted by the parathyroid gland; calcitonin, secreted by the thyroid gland; and vitamin D. The most important of these is PTH, the secretion of which is stimu-

TABLE 24–5. Anesthetic Considerations: Hypothyroidism

Period	Consideration
Preoperative	Achieve euthyroid state with thyroid replacement Studies for airway compression when goiter is present Give thyroid replacement on morning of surgery Little or no premedication if patient is not euthyroid Consider H_2 antagonist
Induction	Reduce the dose of induction agent Enlarged tongue and goiter may hinder intubation
Maintenance	Volatile agents and balanced anesthesia have been successfull Anesthetic requirement may appear to be reduced Temperature monitored, patient warmed Be prepared to treat hypotension
Postoperative	Reduced doses of sedatives and narcotics Airway obstruction may occur

lated by decreased serum ionized calcium levels and inhibited by increased ionized calcium levels. Parathyroid hormone stimulates bone resorption and renal tubular calcium reabsorption, both of which increase circulating calcium, and increases renal phosphate excretion, thereby decreasing serum phosphate levels.

Hyperparathyroidism

Primary hyperparathyroidism implies hypercalcemia resulting from the excessive secretion of PTH due to benign parathyroid adenomas (responsible for 90 per cent of disease), carcinomas (5 per cent), or hyperplasia of the parathyroid glands (5 per cent). The physiologic effects of hyperparathyroidism are related to hypercalcemia (Table 24–6).

When plasma calcium levels exceed 7.5 mEq per L, then action must be taken to decrease calcium levels. This is accomplished by increasing the urinary excretion of calcium with fluid loading and diuretics (Table 24–7). Mithramycin, a cytotoxic antibiotic, decreases serum calcium levels within 24 to 36 hours by inhibiting osteoclastic activity, but toxic effects include bone marrow depression and damage to the liver and kidneys. Hemodialysis can also be used to remove calcium in patients with renal failure.

Table 24–7. Hyperparathyroidism: Therapy

Therapy	Remark
Normal saline	Infused at a rate of 4 to 6 L per day Increases glomerular filtration rate Increases renal tubular clearance of calcium
Diuretics (furosemide ethacrinic acid)	Depress renal tubular reabsorption of calcium Thiazide diuretics are contraindicated
Phosphate	Increases rate of calcium uptake into bone Decreases calcium absorption in the intestine
Glucocorticoids	Reduce serum calcium by poorly understood mechanism Active in the kidney, intestine, and bone
Mithramycin	Used in acute management of severe hypercalcemia May cause thrombocytopenia, bone marrow toxicity, and hepatocellular necrosis
Calcitonin	Rarely used Decreases skeletal release of calcium

Table 24–6. Physiologic Effects of Hyperparathyroidism

System	Effect
Cardiovascular	Increased incidence of hypertension due to: Peripheral vasoconstriction combined with increased inotropy Renal tubular damage with increased renin Calcium-mediated release of vasoactive pressors Short QT interval with prolonged PR interval
Pulmonary	No effects
Renal	Decreased GFR with increased BUN and creatinine Nephrolithiasis and nephrocalcinosis
Hepatic/GI	Peptic ulcer disease in 2 to 10 per cent of patients Nephrolithiasis and nephrocalcinosis
Endocrine	No effects
Hematologic	Normal coagulation
Other	Diffuse osteopenia Muscle weakness and fatigability; worse in lower exremities Mental disturbances: depression and personality changes

The hypercalcemic patient may have concomitant hypomagnesemia, which predisposes the patient to arrhythmias. After volume loading and forced diuresis, the patient may suffer other electrolyte abnormalities, as well as hypovolemia. Overall, no specific anesthetic technique or drugs have proven superior for these patients. To maintain the serum calcium level in the normal range during operation, diuresis begun preoperatively is continued. There are physiologic reasons to expect that hypercalcemia can cause increased or decreased sensitivity to neuromuscular blocking agents; both increased sensitivity to succinylcholine and decreased sensitivity to atracurium have been reported. Thus, neuromuscular blocking agents are titrated to effect.

After parathyroid resection for hypercalcemia, the abrupt halt in parathyroid hormone secretion may lead to rapid remineralization of bone, with significant hypocalcemia or hypomagnesemia. Neuromuscular irritability with positive Chvostek's and Trousseau's signs may be the presenting features, but seizures, laryngospasm (hypocalcemia), and ventricular arrhythmias (hypomagnesemia) threaten life. The serum calcium concentration reaches its minimum several days after operation, but hypocalcemia may appear only hours after resection; examination for signs of hypocalcemia and measurements of the serum calcium are part of the recovery room care of these patients.

Hypoparathyroidism

In primary hypoparathyroidism, hypocalcemia results from decreased secretion of PTH, usually after surgical removal of the parathyroid glands (as during parathyroidectomy or as a complication of thyroid resection). Secondary hypoparathyroidism reflects resistance of peripheral tissues to the effects of PTH, resulting from the congenital defect pseudohypoparathyroidism, hypomagnesemia, chronic renal failure, gastrointestinal malabsorption, or anticonvulsant drugs.

The effects of hypocalcemia on neural and neuromuscular tissues depend in part on the rate with which the calcium concentration decreases. Thus, hypocalcemia occurring within 24 to 48 hours after parathyroidectomy may cause more severe problems than the same degree of hypocalcemia attained over many months. The effects of acute hypocalcemia are outlined in Table 24–8. Signs of hypocalcemia on physical examination include a positive Chvostek's sign (facial twitch after percussion of the facial nerve) or Trousseau's sign (carpopedal spasm provoked by a pneumatic tourniquet maintained at a pressure greater than systolic blood pressure for a few minutes), but these are not sensitive tests. Another sign of neuromuscular irritability is stridor from laryngeal muscle spasm, which must be treated immediately.

TABLE 24–8. Physiologic Effects of Hypocalcemia

System	Effect
Cardiovascular	Delayed ventricular repolarization and prolonged electrical systole resulting in: Increased QT interval, increased ST interval Potential 2:1 heart block and other ventricular dysrhythmias Potential atrial arrhythmias Congestive heart failure
Pulmonary	No effects
Renal	No effects
Hepatic/GI	No effects
Endocrine	No effects
Hematologic	Normal coagulation
Other	Neural irritability which may result in: Tetany Siezures Laryngospasm

TABLE 24–9. Anesthetic Considerations: Hypocalcemia

Period	Consideration
Preoperative	Administer intravenous calcium gluconate via continuous infusion to maintain serum calcium levels
Induction	There is no technique that is superior Titrate muscle relaxants to effect Measure calcium, treat with calcium gluconate
Maintenance	Avoid respiratory alkalosis Blood products containing citrate may worsen hypocalcemia
Postoperative	Monitor calcium levels If parathyroid surgery has been performed, recurrent laryngeal nerve damage may occur, causing airway obstruction

Whether hypoparathyroidism is chronic or acute, the diagnosis is confirmed by measuring serum calcium level. Treatment of hypoparathyroidism consists of calcium supplementation and vitamin D administration; in renal failure, dietary phosphate restriction or a phosphate binding antacid such as aluminum hydroxide is useful. Acute hypocalcemia resulting in tetany may include convulsions and laryngeal stridor. Treatment is with calcium gluconate given intravenously at 100 mg per minute to a total dose of 1 to 2 gm, followed by an infusion of calcium gluconate.

Before administering anesthesia to hypocalcemic patients, it is best to return the calcium concentrations to normal, because of the possibility of cardiac arrhythmias and hypotension. No anesthetic techniques or agents are specifically indicated for hypocalcemic patients. During operation, ionized calcium concentrations are maintained near the lesser normal values. Alkalosis worsens hypocalcemia; hyperventilation is avoided. Blood products containing citrate can decrease calcium levels and must not be administered too rapidly. Hypocalcemia may exaggerate hypotension due to volatile anesthetic agents (Table 24–9).

Adrenal Cortex

Over 25 different steroids are produced by the adrenal cortex, but they can be categorized into three types: glucocorticoids, mineralocorticoids, and sex hormones. The glucocorticoids affect body metabolism diffusely and are critical in mediating responses to stress. The mineralocorticoids are involved in maintaining fluid and electrolyte homeostasis.

Glucocorticoids

The most important glucocorticoid secreted by the adrenal cortex is cortisol, approximately 20 to 30 mg of which is produced each day. Cortisol's effects are diffuse and include the regulation of protein, carbohydrate, and lipid metabolism. Hemodynamic status is critically dependent on adequate circulating cortisol levels. Synthesis and secretion of cortisol are directly regulated by adrenocorticotropin hormone (ACTH), secreted form the anterior pituitary, which in turn responds to the hypothalamus. The hypothalamic-pituitary adrenal (HPA) axis regulates cortisol release in response to multiple stimuli, including plasma cortisol, which inhibits ACTH release, and corticotropin releasing factor secreted by the hypothalamus as part of the circadian rhythm and the stress response.

Glucocorticoid Insufficiency

Primary glucocorticoid deficiency (Addison's disease) occurs because of direct destruction of the adrenal cortex and includes decreases in all corticosteroids; secondary glucocorticoid deficiency reflects decreased ACTH secretion by the pituitary, and rarely includes aldosterone deficiency. The most common cause of secondary adrenal insufficiency is suppression of the HPA by glucocorticoids taken to treat a wide variety of diseases (Table 24–10).

The physiologic effects of adrenal insufficiency depend on the duration of the disease. Acute adrenal insufficiency may occur when a patient's adrenal gland cannot respond to stress, such as an operation, producing cardiovascular collapse and possibly death. The primary anesthetic consideration for hypoadrenal patients is to assure that adequate levels of cortisol are present in the perioperative period. Normally, cortisol secretion increases in response to stress; approximately 75 to 100 mg are secreted in the first 24 hours after operation, and up to 500 mg per day may be secreted under maximum stress. Patients who cannot respond to the stress of operation because of primary or secondary adrenal insufficiency require supplemental doses of corticosteroids. Although the relationship between perioperative hemodynamic collapse and depressed adrenal function is not well documented, the possible consequences are too devastating not to treat such patients with supplemental corticosteroids during operation.

Table 24–10. Physiologic Effects of Adrenal Insufficiency

System	Effect
Cardiovascular	Orthostatic hypotension Low voltage on EKG
Pulmonary	No effects
Renal	Increased ADH resulting in impaired water excretion Mild hyponatremia, normal potassium, and normal BUN
Hepatic/GI	Nausea and vomiting
Endocrine	Hypoglycemia
Hematologic	Anemia
Other	Weakness Increased ACTH, resulting in hyperpigmentation

Any patient who has recently received corticosteroids may have a suppressed HPA axis; the extent of the suppression depends on the duration and dosage of exogenous corticosteroid taken. Recovery of full adrenal function after withdrawal from steroids is inconsistant and may take up to a full year. Napolitano and Chernow provide criteria for choosing which patients to consider for perioperative steroid coverage. Patients who need perioperative steroid coverage include those who:

1. carry the diagnosis of primary or secondary adrenal insufficiency;
2. currently take steroids;
3. have been treated with steroids for a period exceeding one week in the past six months;
4. have signs or symptoms of hypoadrenalism;
5. are scheduled to undergo bilateral adrenalectomy.

Table 24–11. Properties of Commonly Prescribed Corticosteroids

Agent	Dose (mg)	Mineralocorticoid Potency*	Glucocorticoid Potency†	Duration of Action (hr)
Dexamethasone	0.75	0	25	72
Methylprednisolone	4.0	0.5	5	36
Prednisolone	5.0	0.8	4	24
Prednisone	5.0	0.8	4	24
Cortisol	20.0	1.0	4	8
Hydrocortisone	25.0	1.0	0.8	8
Cortisone	25.0	1.0	0.8	8

* The higher the number, the more likely the agent will cause metabolic alkalosis.
† The higher the number, the more likely the agent will cause suppression of hypothalamic corticotropin releasing factor (CRF) and pituitary adrenocorticotropic hormone (ACTH)
Adapted with permission from Chernow B. Critical care, state of the art. Fullertone: Society of Critical Care Medicine 1982; 3:1–52.

The characteristics of supplemental corticosteroids are summarized in Table 24–11. Ideally, the chosen dose is one that minimizes side effects but still prevents the possibility of hemodynamic compromise. A simple protocol includes 100 mg of hydrocortisone hemisuccinate intravenously preoperatively, 100 mg intraoperatively, and 100 mg postoperatively. However, this may overtreat many patients. The recommendations of Napolitano and Chernow take into account the anticipated severity of the operative stress (Table 24–12).

Table 24–12. Protocols for Patients who Require Supplemental Corticosteroids*

Situation	Steroid Coverage	Comments
Major surgery (elective)		
Preoperative	25 mg hydrocortisone hemisuccinate IV	Convert to equivalent oral corticosteroid preparation when gastrointestinal function returns and oral intake is tolerated. Continue to taper gradually until maintenance doses of daily oral corticosteroids are achieved.
Intraoperative	100 mg hydrocortisone hemisuccinate IV	
Postoperative	50 mg IV q8h next 24 hr: 25 mg IV q8h 2nd 24 hrs	
Major surgery (emergent) in patient with unknown HPA axis		
Preoperative	2 mg dexamethasone phosphate IV	Convert to hydrocortisone hemisuccinate as soon as test results are available. Continue to taper as outlined for elective major surgery.
Intraoperative	4 mg dexamethasone phosphate IV	
	Perform rapid ACTH stimulation test†	
Postoperative		
Minor surgery (elective)		
Preoperative	25 mg hydrocortisone hemisuccinate IV or IM	Convert to usual oral corticosteroid preparations when gastrointestinal function returns and oral intake is tolerated (1st postoperative day)
Postoperative	50 mg hydrocortisone hemisuccinate IV or IM	
Minor procedures		
Preoperative	Take usual oral corticosteroid dose	
Postoperative	Double the patient's usual oral corticosteroid dose and rapidly taper to routine maintenance dose	

* Reproduced with permission from Napolitano LM, Chernow B. Int Anesthesiol Clin 1988;26:226–232.
† Dexamethasone does not usually cross-react with plasma cortisol radioimmunoassay.
Abbreviations: HPA, hypothalamo-pituitary-adrenal; ACTH, adrenocorticotropic hormone.

Nearly any anesthetic technique may be used in the hypoadrenal patient who is adequately treated with corticosteroids. Etomidate is an exception, because it further depresses the HPA axis.

Glucocorticoid Excess

The most common cause of glucocorticoid excess is the administration of supraphysiologic doses as treatment for a number of diseases. Pathologic causes of hyperadrenocorticism (Cushing's disease) include pituitary adenomas, adrenal tumors, or ectopic ACTH production by extrapituitary malignancies, most commonly lung cancer. The physiologic effects of excess glucocorticoids are listed in Table 24–13. Medical therapy to inhibit the pituitary or the hypothalamic release of corticotropin-releasing factor (CRF) is not definitive, but may be used in the preoperative management of severely debilitated patients.

Cardiovascular and metabolic derangements are best treated preoperatively. The diabetes associated with excess corticosteroids may be exacerbated by surgical stress. The expected effects of obesity on gastric emptying and pulmonary function require special attention regarding anesthetic induction and postoperative ventilatory care. Muscle wasting may be associated with a reduced requirement for muscle relaxants. Because of the risk of pathologic fractures, careful attention to positioning the patient is necessary.

TABLE 24–13. Physiologic Effects of Excess Glucocorticoids

System	Effect
Cardiovascular	Hypertension
	Increased intravascular volume
	Increased sensitivity to catacholamines
	Predisposition to atherosclerosis
	Congestive heart failure
Pulmonary	No direct effects except functional effects of obesity
Renal	Alkalosis
Hepatic/GI	Ulcers
Endocrine	Increased gluconeogenesis and anti-insulin effects of glucocorticoids may cause diabetes mellitus
	Amenorrhea or oligomenorrhea
Hematologic	Increased erythrocyte volume and mass
	Decreased lymphocytes and eosinophiles; increased granulocytes
Other	Centripetal obesity
	Muscle wasting
	Demineralization of bone
	Poor wound healing and tissue friability
	Thin skin and easy bruisability
	Emotional lability

Mineralocorticoids

Aldosterone is the principal mineralocorticoid; it is regulated as part of the renin-angiotensin system. Aldosterone promotes reabsorption of sodium and excretion of potassium by the renal tubules.

Primary mineralocorticoid excess can arise from a solitary adrenal tumor, bilateral adrenal hyperplasia, or a tumor of the juxtaglomerular cells in the kidney. Increased sodium retention causes hypertension with increased diastolic pressures, but peripheral edema is rare. Hypokalemia can result in muscle weakness, and even intermittent paralysis. Treatment is empiric, and potassium supplementation and antihypertensives are the mainstays of therapy. Spironolactone is administered preoperatively to restore intravascular volume and electrolytes.

Mineralocorticoid deficiency is rare and usually results from overall decreases in adrenal function. Hyperkalemia is the most serious consequence, but patients may have hyponatremia and myocardial conduction defects also. The treatment is administration of fluorocortisol, a synthetic mineralocorticoid.

Anesthetic considerations revolve around maintaining normal fluid balance and electrolyte concentrations.

ADRENAL MEDULLA

The adrenal medulla produces the catecholamines epinephrine and norepinephrine. Although norepinephrine may be synthesized in peripheral autonomic nerve terminals, the final step in the synthesis of epinephrine takes place only in the adrenal medulla. Once secreted, the half-life of a catecholamine is less than one minute, because the hormone is quickly broken down on a single pass through the liver or kidney.

The disease of the adrenal medulla of greatest interest to anesthesiologists is pheochromocytoma, a catecholamine-producing tumor of the chromaffin tissue from which the adrenal medulla is derived. Ninety-five per cent of pheochromocytomas occur in the abdomen and 85 per cent are in the adrenal gland. The clinical manifestations of this disease are the result of excess catecholamine discharge (Table 24–14). Paroxysmal hypertension associated with diaphoresis, headache, tremulousness, and palpitations are frequent presenting symptoms.

Preoperative preparation of the patient with pheochromocytoma reduces the incidence and severity of perioperative cardiovascular problems; it is accomplished by adrenergic blockade. Prazocin, an alpha-1 antagonist, is superior (in theory) to phenoxybenzamine, a mixed alpha-1 and alpha-2 blocker, because the negative feedback loop mediated by the alpha-2 receptor is left intact. If tachycardia follows alpha blockade, beta-adrenergic antagonists may be given; beta blockade must never precede alpha blockade because myocardial failure could result. Some 20 to 30 per cent of patients may have a cardiomyopathy from sustained catecholamine release and these patients may be very sensitive to the myocardial depressant effects of beta-adrenergic antagonists. Labetolol has been used as the principal therapy for pheochromocytoma, but pulmonary edema has been reported after its use, possibly because its beta antagonist effect exceeds its alpha antagonist effect. Alpha-methyl-p-tyrosine (AMPT) inhibits the catecholamine synthetic pathway and can reduce catecholamine synthesis by 40 to 80 per cent. It has theoretical advantages, but side effects such as diarrhea, sedation, fatigue, neurologic changes, and muscle stiffness may limit its use (Table 24–15).

The administration of alpha antagonists may be continued up to the time of operation or may be withdrawn 24 to 48 hours preoperatively. There are two arguments against continuing alpha blockade up to the time of operation; (1) the localization of the tumor might be made difficult because of blunted hemodynamic responses to tumor manipulation, and (2) refractory hypotension may occur once the tumor is removed. However, withdrawal of an alpha antagonist may predispose the patient to cardiovascular instability. In practice, even fully blocked patients usually respond to direct manipulation of the tumor, and current diagnostic techniques easily identify the tumor site preoperatively; alpha blockers may be continued up until operation.

Invasive cardiovascular monitoring is required. The goal of anesthesia management is to block stressful stimuli and the responses to these stimuli. Intubation is not attempted until the patient is deeply anesthetized, usually with a narcotic combined with isoflurane or enflurane. Halothane is avoided because it sensitizes the myocardium to catecholamines. Because histamine release may cause catecholamine discharge, any drug that causes histamine release is avoided, as are drugs that activate the sympathetic nervous system,

TABLE 24–14. Physiologic Effects of Pheochromocytoma

System	Effect
Cardiovascular	Paroxysmal hypertension Myocarditis in 20 to 30 per cent of patients Congestive heart failure Arrhythmias Nonspecific EKG changes
Pulmonary	No direct effects
Renal	Decreased plasma volume
Hepatic/GI	Nausea and vomiting
Endocrine	Hyperglycemia
Hematologic	Increased hematocrit but normal red cell mass
Other	Nervousness and emotional lability

TABLE 24–15. Pheochromocytoma: Therapy

Therapy	Remark
Phenoxybenzamine	Alpha-1 and alpha-2 antagonist 18 to 24 hour duration of effect due to covalent binding of receptors Side effects: sedation, nasal congestion, orthostatic hypotension
Phentolamine	Alpha-1 and alpha-2 antagonist Shorter duration
Prazosin	Selective alpha-1 antagonist May cause less tachycardia than nonselective alpha antagonists
Beta antagonist propranolol atenolol	Must never be given unless alpha blockade is complete Given when tachycardia exacerbated by alpha blockade May cause congestive heart failure when myocardial dysfunction is already present

such as pancuronium and ketamine. Succinylcholine may also stimulate sympathetic activity, and is usually avoided. Vecuronium is an excellent choice for neuromuscular blockade because it has minimal effects on hemodynamics.

Sodium nitroprusside is an appropriate vasodilator and antihypertensive because of its rapid onset and offset. The seemingly more logical choice, phentolamine, is subject to tachyphylaxis, and its longer duration of action may make treatment of hypotension difficult after excision of the tumor. Manipulation of the tumor provokes hypertension, but once the blood supply to the tumor has been isolated, hypotension is common. Hypotension is treated with volume expansion and an infusion of a vasopressor if needed. Fluid therapy is usually monitored by pulmonary vascular pressures, because the patients are susceptible to myocardial dysfunction from chronic catecholamine stimulation.

DIABETES MELLITUS

Type I diabetes is associated with an absolute deficit of insulin and almost always requires exogenous insulin for control. These patients are at risk for ketosis. Type II diabetes is often associated with peripheral resistance to insulin, but these patients have normal levels of circulating insulin. The effects of longstanding diabetes are listed in Table 24–16.

TABLE 24–16. Physiologic Effects of Diabetes Mellitus

System	Effect
Cardiovascular	Autonomic neuropathy resulting in: Orthostatic hypotension Resting tachycardia and insensitivity to atropine and propranolol Masked angina and silent myocardial infarction Increased incidence of hypertension, ventricular dysfunction, and cardiomegaly
Pulmonary	Impaired respiratory response to hypoxemia in patients with significant autonomic neuropathy
Renal	Renal insufficiency due to diabetic nephropathy
Hepatic/GI	Delayed gastric emptying
Endocrine	No effects
Hematologic	No effects
Other	Retinopathy Neuropathy affecting peripheral and autonomic nerves

TABLE 24–17. Anesthetic Considerations: Well-Controlled Diabetic Mellitus

Period	Consideration
Preoperative	Start dextrose-containing IV on morning of surgery at 100 to 150 ml per hr Give one half to two thirds the patient's usual dose of intermediate-acting insulin; Hold any short-acting insulin Consider H_2 antagonist
Induction	Consider rapid sequence induction
Maintenance	No technique superior Administer dextrose-containing IV solution throughout the surgical procedure For long procedures, measure serum glucose intraoperatively and treat with intravenous insulin as needed
Postoperative	Monitor serum glucose and continue dextrose-containing IV solutions

The operative management of the diabetic patient is based on the preoperative assessment. Type II diabetics are unlikely to develop ketoacidosis, and the main goal is to maintain normal blood glucose concentrations throughout the procedure. Type I diabetics are assessed to assure that they do not have ketoacidosis. Secondary manifestations of the diabetes such as autonomic dysfunction, renal insufficiency, coronary artery disease (silent myocardial ischemia is prevalent), and hypertension must be fully assessed. Oral hypoglycemic agents may be continued until the evening before operation, remembering that some of them may produce hypoglycemia for up to 48 hours.

Regimens for control of the insulin-dependent diabetic vary from the simple to the complex. There is little evidence to document that one is superior in terms of metabolic control or overall outcome. A conventional approach for the well-controlled fasting diabetic is outlined in Table 24–17.

The most important aspect of anesthetic management for diabetic patients is maintaining glucose homeostasis. This is accomplished by providing adequate carbohydrate to prevent proteolysis, lipolysis, and ketoacidosis, and providing insulin to maintain blood glucose levels near normal. Because diabetic patients may have gastroparesis, measures to reduce the risk of regurgitation and aspiration are prudent, but a rapid sequence induction is not necessary in all patients.

The effects of modern anesthetic agents on blood glucose concentrations and insulin release are probably not significant in clinical management. For example, in vitro studies with halothane and enflurane have shown concentration-dependent suppression of glucose-stimulated insulin release. This implies that hyperglycemia may be exacerbated during anesthesia with these agents, but these actions are not profound. Other mechanisms also may cause intraoperative hyperglycemia such as changes in sympathetic tone, and increases in glucagon and cortisol level; thus, the recommendation for intermittent monitoring of blood glucose before, during, and after operation seems most appropriate.

OBESITY

The effects of obesity on multiple organ systems must be taken into account in anesthetic management. The physiologic effects of obesity are outlined in Table 24–18. What seems to be hypertension may represent only a small blood pressure cuff; increased systemic vascular resistance is a common finding, however. Physiologic changes of respiration include increased oxygen consumption and carbon dioxide production. Functional residual capacity and vital capacity are decreased because the abdominal contents limit excursion of the diaphragm. Pulmonary compliance is reduced and the work of breathing is increased. These changes are accentuated in the supine position. Arterial oxygen tension is decreased, presumably secondary to ventilation-perfusion abnormalities with hypoventilation of dependent lung fields. Both obstructive and central sleep apnea syndromes are associated with obesity and imply a dangerous sensitivity to respiratory depressants.

Table 24–19 outlines the anesthetic considerations for the obese patient. Obese patients must be considered at risk for aspiration of gastric contents because of an increased incidence of gastroesophageal reflux and hiatal hernia, as well as increased gastric volume, acidity, and pressure. Therefore, preoperative administration of H_2-receptor blockers and metachlopramide are often appropriate, along with a rapid sequence induction or awake intubation (see Chapter 13).

The pulmonary defects in obesity can result in

TABLE 24–18. Physiologic Effects of Obesity

System	Effect
Cardiovascular	Hypertension, increased SVR
	Increased total blood volume
	Increased cardiac output but normal cardiac index
	Ventricular dysfunction with congestive heart failure in morbid obesity
	Predisposition to atherosclerotic vascular disease
Pulmonary	Decreased vital capacity, inspiratory capacity and functional residual volume
	Increased oxygen consumption and carbon dioxide production
	Mechanical dysfunction of chest and diaphragm
	Obesity hypoventilation syndrome
Renal	Increased sensitivity to fluoride-induced nephrotoxicity
Hepatic/GI	Increased gastric pressure
	Increased incidence of gastroesophageal reflux and hiatal hernia
	Increased incidence of gallbladder disease and incidence of fatty liver
Endocrine	Glucose intolerance or exacerbation of diabetes mellitus
	Increased cortisol production
	Menstrual irregularities
Hematologic	No effects

TABLE 24–19. Anesthetic Considerations: Obesity

Period	Consideration
Preoperative	Administer H_2 antagonist
	Prepare for potentially difficult intubation
Induction	Consider rapid sequence induction, awake intubation
	Assure complete preoxygenation
Maintenance	There may be increased biotransformation of halogenated agents
	Use oxygen concentrations no less than 50 per cent
	If oxygenation is a problem, apply PEEP with care and increase oxygen concentration as needed
Postoperative	Extended postoperative monitoring is indicated if obesity hypoventilation syndrome is present
	Vigorous chest physiotherapy, supplemental oxygen

severe oxygen desaturation, even with positive pressure ventilation and positive end-expiratory pressure (PEEP), which has variable effects. Inspired oxygen concentrations of 50 per cent or greater may be required to prevent hypoxemia.

Fatty infiltration of the liver and abnormal liver function tests are common. Whether this enhances hepatotoxicity from anesthetic agents is unclear, but case reports suggest that hepatic dysfunction after halothane anesthesia is more common in obese women.

Spinal and epidural techniques may be technically difficult, and it may be appropriate to reduce doses, just as in pregnancy. In the supine position, an obese patient with impaired intercostal muscle function from such a block may suffer ventilatory failure; supplemental oxygen and cautious use of sedatives and narcotics is required. The choice between regional and general anesthesia depends on the details of the individual case, but it is apparent that major conduction anesthesia (spinal or epidural) is not necessarily superior to general anesthesia in these patients.

REFERENCES

Brown BR, ed. Anesthetics and the obese patient. Contemporary anesthesia practice series. Philadelphia: FA Davis, 1982.

Cork RC, Vaughan RW, Bentley JB. General anesthesia for morbidly obese patients—an examination of postoperative outcomes. Anesthesiology 1981; 54:310.

Napolitano LM, Chernow B. Int Anesthesiol Clin 1988; 26:226–232.

Vaughan RW, Bauer S, Wise L. Volume and pH of gastric juice in obese patients. Anesthesiology 1975; 43:686.

CHAPTER TWENTY-FIVE

PEDIATRIC ANESTHESIA

Infants and children requiring anesthesia present unique challenges for the anesthesiologist. This chapter presents an approach to the management of these challenges.

PEDIATRIC PHYSIOLOGY

The essential features of physiologic function that form the basis of rational anesthesia management of children are presented here to serve as a foundation for the subsequent discussions of pharmacology and clinical care.

Pulmonary and Cardiovascular Systems

FETAL CARDIOPULMONARY DEVELOPMENT

At 16 weeks of gestation, the tracheobronchial tree has achieved 16 branching generations ending in the terminal bronchiole, the distal growth center for development of the essential functional pulmonary unit, the acinus. If, through disease, genetic effect, or the pressure of a space-occupying lesion (e.g., a diaphragmatic hernia) the lungs fail to develop all 16 branches by this stage, then pulmonary hypoplasia results.

At 24 weeks the pulmonary capillaries come into closer approximation with the primitive alveolar saccules, and the type II alveolar epithelial cells begin to secrete an immature form of alveolar phospholipid lining that can function as a surfactant at a gas-liquid interface. The potential for alveolar gas exchange with pulmonary capillary blood thus begins. The diffusion barrier for oxygen, the matching of capillary flow with the alveolar epithelial membrane and alveolar gas, the stability of the alveoli, and the central control of breathing remain inadequate for effective spontaneous and unsupported ventilation in most infants until at least 28 weeks gestation.

At birth, the total lung volume, crying vital capacity, and functional residual capacity (FRC) are all significantly less per unit body mass than they are at over 7 years, but especially less when compared to the infant's metabolic needs and alveolar ventilation. Thus, the average FRC of 30 ml per kg of a normal newborn is only somewhat less than the mean adult value of 34 ml per kg, but the ratios of FRC to alveolar minute ventilation differ greatly (newborn 0.23; adult 0.56), indicating a much greater reserve volume of gas in the lung of the adult in relation to alveolar ventilation (Table 25–1).

CARDIOPULMONARY ADAPTATION TO EXTRAUTERINE LIFE

The fetal cardiovascular system, well established by the eighth week of gestation, performs admirably with the placenta as the organ of fetal external gas exchange. The flow patterns depicted in Figure 25–1, a parallel circuit, must adapt to

TABLE 25–1. Pulmonary Function (Mean Values)

	Newborn	Adult
Body weight (kg)	3	70
Cal/kg/hr (large calories [Kcal])	2	1
Oxygen consumption ($\dot{V}O_2$) (ml/kg/min)	7.0	3.5
CO_2 production ($\dot{V}O_2$) (ml/kg/min)	5.5	3.0
Expired minute volume ($\dot{V}_E$) (ml/kg/min)	200–210	90–100
Tidal volume (V_T) (ml/kg)	6	6
Respiratory rate (f) (breaths/min)	35–60	15–20
Anatomic dead space (D_S) (ml/kg)	2.5	2.0
Physiologic dead space-tidal volume ratio (D_{S_p}/V_T)	0.3	0.3
Alveolar ventilation (V_A) (ml/kg/min)	130	60
Total lung capacity (TLC) (ml/kg)	63	82
Vital capacity (VC) (ml/kg)	35	70
Functional residual capacity (FRC) (ml/kg)	30	34
FRC/$\dot{V}_A$	0.23	0.56
Tracheal internal diameter (mm)	4	16
Tracheal length (mm)	57	120

(Adapted with permission from Fisher BJ, Carlo WA, Doershak CF. Pulmonary function from infancy through adolescence. *In* Scarpelli EM, ed. Pulmonary physiology: fetus, newborn, child, adolescent. 2nd ed. Philadelphia; Lea and Febiger, 1990:429.)

increased pulmonary blood flow at birth, accompanied by closure of the ductus arteriosus and foramen ovale, resulting in a series circuit. The central feature in this adaptation consists of an abrupt and substantial reduction in the pulmonary vascular resistance of the fetal circuit, which allows only ten per cent of the right ventricular output to flow through the lungs in utero.

The cardiac output of the newborn meets changing metabolic demands primarily by adjustments in heart rate, because the relatively stiff ventricular walls limit the ability to vary stroke volume. A reduction in heart rate greater than 20 to 30 per cent below normal levels for age in a newborn or young infant (i.e., a rate less than 100 beats per minute), invariably causes a reduction in cardiac output.

The principal differences in the blood of the fetus compared with that of the older infant are the presence of fetal hemoglobin and relatively small concentrations of 2,3-diphosphoglyceraldehyde (2,3-DPG) in the red cells. Fetal hemoglobin binds oxygen more readily than does adult hemoglobin; this is characterized by a left-shifted oxyhemoglobin dissociation curve (Fig. 25–2). Combined with lesser 2,3-DPG levels, this favors uptake of oxygen in the placenta (or lung) but results in lesser volumes of oxygen unloaded in the peripheral tissues at physiologic capillary oxygen tensions.

Failure of the newborn to establish adequate alveolar ventilation or pulmonary blood flow causes persistent acidemia and hypoxemia, and, in turn, causes opening of the ductus and pulmonary vasoconstriction, increased pulmonary vascular resistance, diminished pulmonary blood flow, and a decrease in the left atrial pressure below that in the right atrium, opening the foramen ovale. Fatal asphyxia ensues unless this cycle is interrupted quickly by controlled alveolar ventilation with oxygen.

The integrated control of breathing is not well developed even in the full-term newborn (37 to 42 weeks gestation). Over 70 per cent of preterm newborns experience periodic breathing, with nearly half of these suffering prolonged apneic episodes accompanied by bradycardia and arterial hemoglobin desaturation well below 90 per cent. The development of ventilatory control parallels the gestational (or postconceptual) age from 25 weeks, when protracted apnea with severe hypoxemia nearly always occurs if the fetus is born, through 40 weeks when apnea causing serious hypoxemia rarely occurs.

CARDIOPULMONARY DEVELOPMENT IN THE NEONATE AND INFANT

The neonate (age 1 to 28 days) and infant (age 1 to 12 months) undergo cardiopulmonary development that strengthens considerably their abilities not only to meet basic metabolic needs but to withstand infection or trauma (such as that incurred in surgical operations). These include the following:

1. Maturation of the integrated central control of ventilation.
2. Continued expansion of total lung volume.
3. Stiffening of the thoracic wall to provide outward tethering of transpulmonary forces that help maintain small airways.
4. Maturation of the diaphragm and chest wall

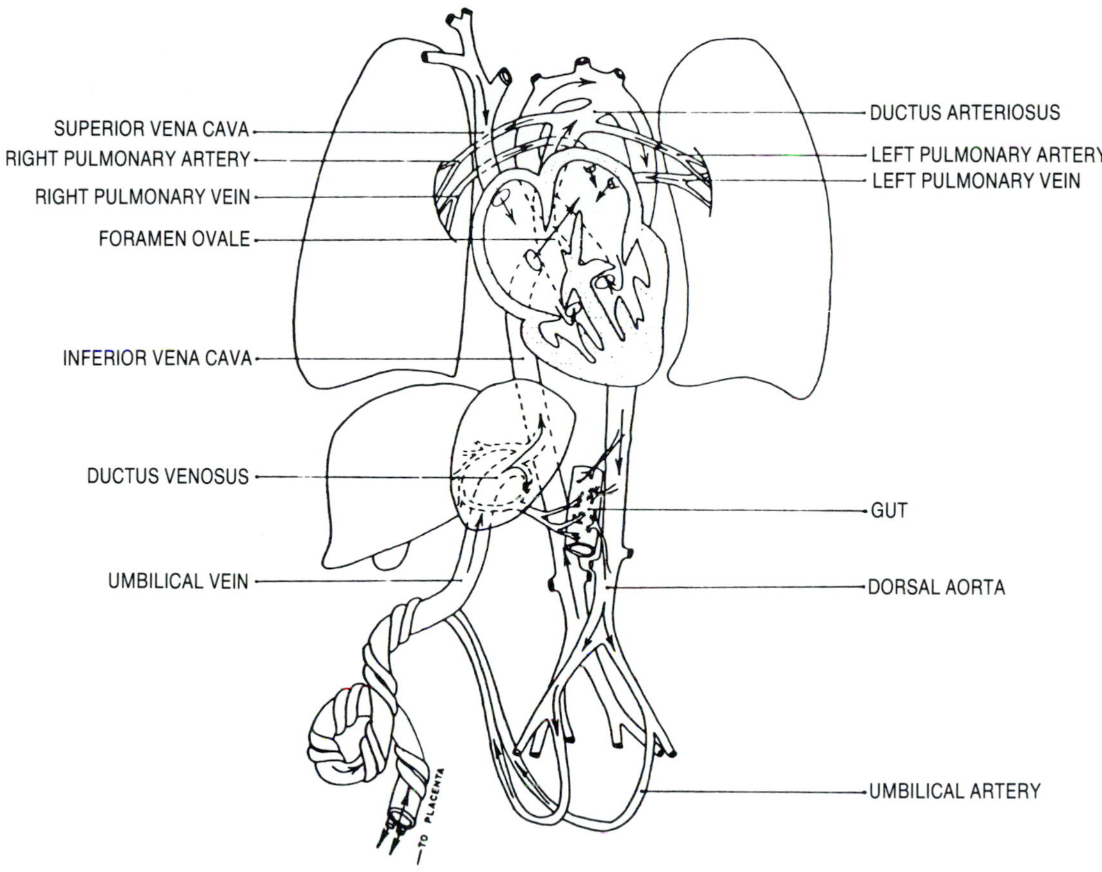

FIGURE 25–1. Schematic representation of the fetal circulation (not to scale). (Reproduced with permission from Avery ME. The lung and its disorders. Philadelphia: WB Saunders. 1964.)

Table 25–2. Normal Arterial pH, Blood Gas Tensions, Hematocrit (Mean ± SD)

	Age				
	1 hr	*24 hr*	*1–24 mo*	*Child*	*Adult*
pHa	7.33	7.37 (.03)	7.40 (.03)	7.39 (.02)	7.40 (.03)
Pa_{CO_2} (mm Hg)	36 (4)	33 (3)	34 (4)	37 (3)	39 (5)
Base excess (mEq/l)	−6.0 (1)	−5.0 (1)	−3.0 (3)	−2.0 (2)	0.0 (2)
Pa_{O_2} (21% O_2) (mm Hg)	63 (11)	73 (10)	—	95 (4)	95 (4)
Hematocrit (vol %)	53 (5)	55 (7)	35 (2.5)	38 (2)	45 (4)

Adapted with permission from Koch G, Wendel H. Adjustment of arterial blood gases and acid base balance in the normal newborn infant during the first week of life. Biol Neonate 1968;12:136–161. Levison H, Featherby EA et al. Arterial blood gases, alveolar-arterial oxygen difference, and physiologic dead space in children and young adults. Am Rev Resp Dis 1970;101:972.

Albert MS, Winters R. Acid-base equilibrium of blood in normal infants. Pediatrics 1966;37:728–732.

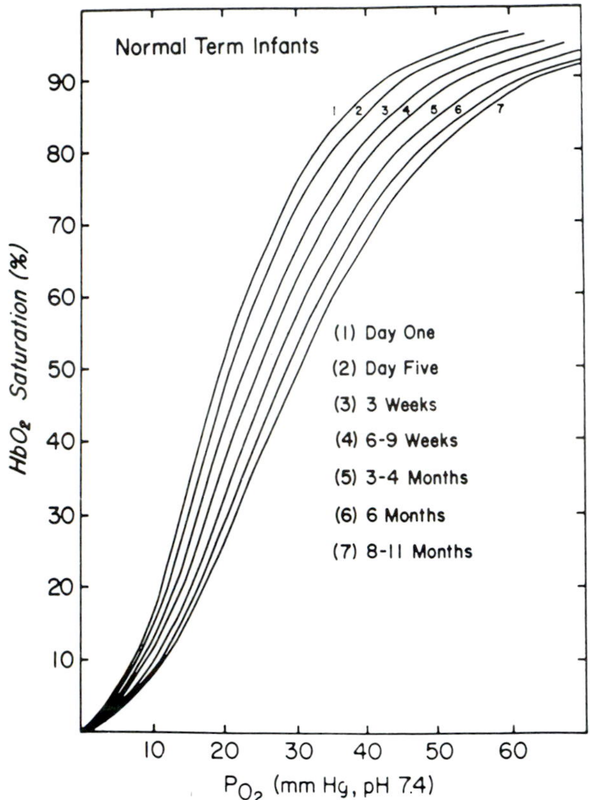

FIGURE 25–2. The P_{50} on day 1 of 19 mm Hg shifts to 30 mm Hg at 11 months of age. (Reproduced with permission from Smith CA, Nelson NM. Physiology of the newborn infant. 4th ed. Springfield: CC Thomas, 1976.)

muscles to increase the power available for breathing and coughing.

6. Continued reduction in pulmonary vascular resistance.

7. Thickening of the left ventricular wall relative to the right ventricle.

8. Stroke volume increases and heart rate decreases (Fig. 25–3).

9. Physiologic anemia reaches its nadir at 12 weeks, but by age 6 months fetal hemoglobin is replaced and total hemoglobin concentration is well above 10 gm per dl.

Thus, by the end of infancy at 12 months of age, the cardiopulmonary system approaches that of the adult (Table 25–2, Figs. 25–3 and 25–4). Maturation continues throughout childhood and adolescence until functional adulthood at age 15 (Table 25–3).

Central and Autonomic Nervous Systems

A detailed review of nervous system development lies beyond the scope and purpose of this chapter; the features significant to anesthesia management include the following:

1. The newborn brain constitutes 12 per cent of the body weight and receives approximately 34 per cent of the cardiac output compared with the adult, whose brain represents 2 per cent of body weight and receives about 14 per cent of the cardiac output.

2. The newborn's blood-brain barrier is far more permeable than that of the older child or adult to molecules that are lipid soluble (for example, bilirubin and barbiturates).

3. The fetus, by the time of viability (24 to 25 weeks gestation), responds to noxious stimuli with facial grimaces as well as significant cardiovascular and metabolic changes, indicating probable perception of pain.

TABLE 25–3. Normal Cardiovascular Function (Mean and Range or SD)

	Age				
	1–30 days	*1–24 mo*	*2–6 yr*	*7–13 yr*	*14–30 yr*
Heart rate (beats/min)	125 (100–190)	120 (80–160)	100 (80–120)	90 (70–110)	80 (55–95)
Systemic arterial pressure (mm Hg)	73 (8)	96 (30)	90+ (2x age) to age 14 yrs.		
	50 (5)	66 (25)	60+ (2x age) (adult level)		
Cardiac output (ml/kg/min)	200–250	170–200	150–170	100–140	90–115

Adapted with permission from Behrman RE, Vaughan VC. Nelson's textbook of pediatrics. 12th ed. Philadelphia: WB Saunders, 1979:1100–1101.

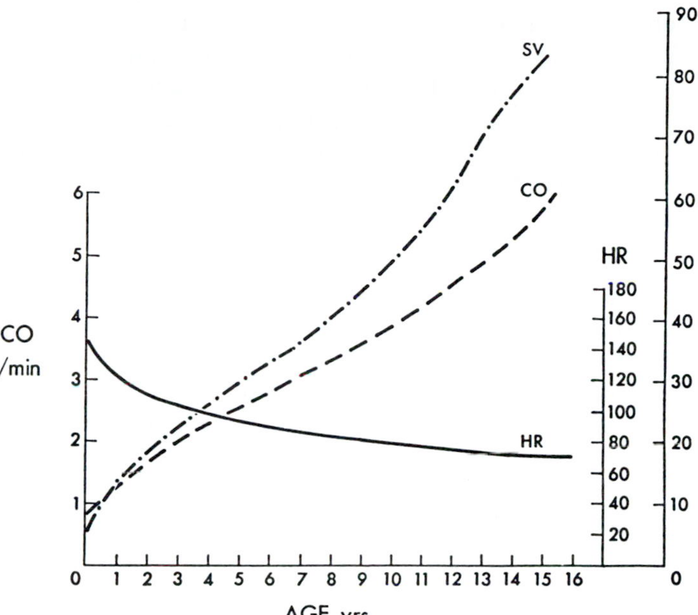

FIGURE 25–3. *Postnatal changes in cardiac output (CO), heart rate (HR) and stroke volume (SV) from birth to 16 years. (Reproduced with permission from Rudolph AM. Congenital heart disease. Chicago: Year Book Medical Publishers, 1974.)*

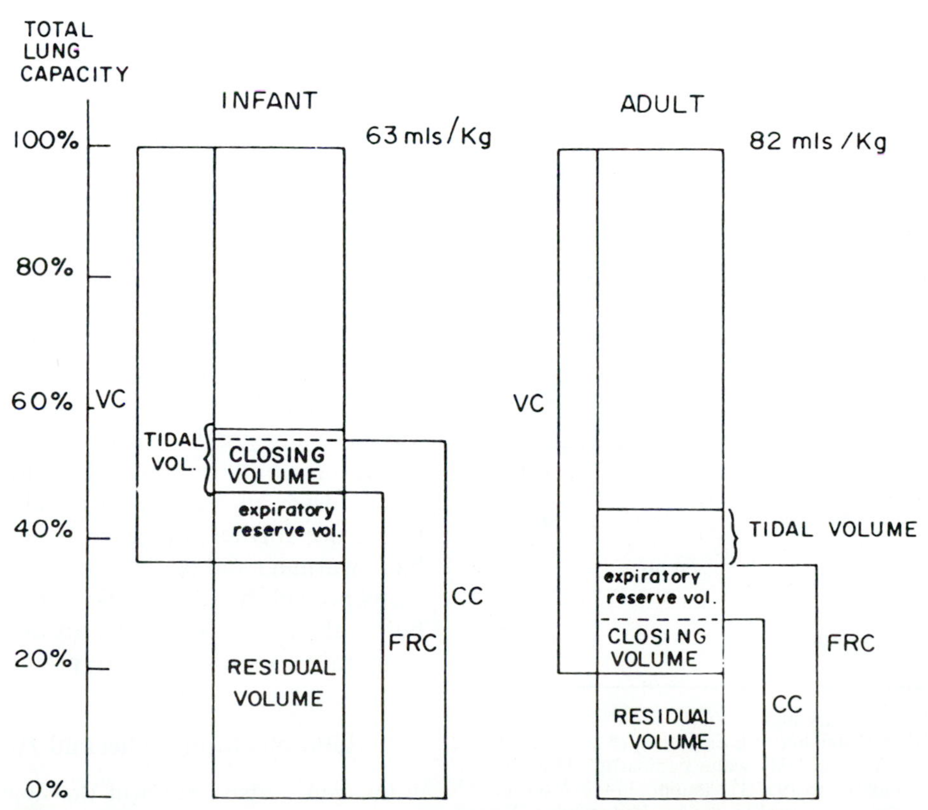

FIGURE 25–4. *Lung volumes in the infant and adult. (Reproduced with permission from Smith CA, Nelson NM. The physiology of the newborn infant. 4th ed. Springfield: CC Thomas, 1976.)*

4. At term, the parasympathetic nervous system appears to be well developed, but sympathetic functions do not seem to fully mature until four to six months of age. The bradycardic response to hypoxemia characteristic of the newborn and its attenuation by atropine illustrates the parasympathetic predominance of reactions to this as well as other major autonomic stimuli, such as laryngoscopy.

Whether the infant's responses imply the perception of pain remains conjectural. The issue seems moot, because if only nitrous oxide analgesia is used, the ensuing hyperglycemia and systemic arterial hypertension may place the infant at an increased risk of intracranial hemorrhage. Thus, the anesthesiologist ordinarily seeks to prevent these manifestations of the stress response as well as the possible perception of pain by providing sufficient anesthesia.

Renal System and Fluid Balance

Despite apparent structural maturity, the kidney of the preterm or term newborn is not functionally mature. Glomerular filtration rate, renal blood flow, the tubular maximum for p-aminohippuric acid, and maximal concentrating ability increase with advancing postconceptual age (Table 25–4).

The preterm newborn exhibits renal function that is far less effective than that of the term newborn, but with striking improvement by age 6 months; renal function approaches that of an adult by 12 months. The preterm infant is ill equipped to conserve or excrete sodium in response to acute sodium deprivation or excessive load. Also, the concentrating ability of the preterm newborn kidney during water deprivation or excess loss reaches only 35 per cent, and that of the term newborn only 50 per cent, of adult levels. However, the term newborn's capacity to dilute urine following an excessive water load approaches adult levels by age 6 weeks, but remains reduced in the preterm infant for many weeks or months.

TABLE 25–4. Normal Basal Fluid Volumes and Characteristics (Range or Mean ± SD)

	Age		
	1–30 days	*1–24 mo*	*2 yr–Adult*
Urine volume (ml/kg/hr)	1–4	1–4	1–4
Urine osmolality (mOsm/L)	100–600	50–1400	50–1600
Extracellular volume (% body wt)	42 (6)	34 (4)	25
Blood volume (ml/kg)	80–90	70–75	65–70

Data from Behrman RE, Vaughan VC. Nelson's textbook of pediatrics. 12th ed. Philadelphia: WB Saunders, 1979:230, 1311. Friis-Hansen B. Changes in body water compartments during growth. Acta Paediatr Scand 1957;110 (suppl):36–42. Mollison PL. Blood transfusion in clinical medicine. Philadelphia: FA Davis, 1967:145.

The newborn's total body water contributes 70 to 75 per cent of its body mass compared with 50 to 60 per cent in the child and adult. Extracellular water constitutes over half of the total body water—or roughly 40 to 45 per cent of body mass in the newborn—decreasing rapidly over the first few postnatal days to approximately 30 to 33 per cent of body mass. The extracellular fluid compartment appears to remain proportionately similar throughout infancy, thereafter declining gradually to approximately 20 per cent of body mass in the older child and adult. Blood volume, a component of the extracellular fluid compartment, varies with age in relation to body mass from approximately 90 ml per kg in the preterm and 80 ml per kg in the term newborn, to 70 to 75 ml per kg in the infant and child and 65 to 70 ml per kg in the adult (Table 25–4).

Water requirements and their variability in preterm neonates differ considerably from those in term neonates, infants, and older children or adults. The preterm infant, especially if less than 1500 gm birth weight, has immature skin and an exceptionally great ratio of surface area to body mass, resulting in unusually large evaporative water losses in relation to metabolic rate; these losses are further increased by exposure to ambient warmers and phototherapy units. These concerns prevail in larger preterm and full-term newborns also, but to a lesser extent because their evaporative losses are more predictable.

Metabolism and Thermal Homeostasis

Oxygen consumption in the newborn averages 5 ml per kg per minute on day one, increasing to 7 to 8 ml per kg per minute by day 7; this increased oxygen consumption persists throughout infancy, declining gradually in later childhood and thereafter to adult levels of 3 to 4 ml per kg per minute.

Metabolism drives minute ventilation and cardiac output, which in infants are double the values observed in older children. Both increased ventilation and increased cardiac output are achieved by increased rates of activity (breaths or beats per minute) (Tables 25–1 and 25–3). Thus, minute volume in the infant is approximately 200 ml per kg per minute with a frequency of 35 to 60 breaths per minute, compared to 90 ml per kg per minute with a frequency of 15 to 20 breaths per minute in the adult. Cardiac output averages 200 ml per kg per minute at heart rates of 100 to 190 beats per minute in the newborn and 100 ml per kg per minute with heart rates of 55 to 95 in the adult. Similarly, basic resting caloric requirements of the newborn are more than double those of the older child and young adult (120 versus 35 to 50 Kcal per kg per day). Responses to cold environments increases metabolic activity even further.

Pediatric Pharmacology

The commonly used anesthetics, muscle relaxants, narcotics, and other adjuvant drugs differ in their pharmacokinetics and pharmacodynamics in the newborn and infant as compared to the older child and adult. The following are the major variations that concern the anesthesiologist:

1. The greater volumes of total body water and of the extracellular fluid compartment in the newborn and infant result in substantially greater volumes of distribution for drugs.
2. The brain, heart, liver and kidneys constitute 18 per cent of the body weight of the newborn but only 5 per cent in the adult, so that a relatively larger fraction of a dose of an inhaled or injected drug is distributed to these organs rather than to muscle or fat.
3. Neonates, especially if born preterm, have significantly lesser plasma protein levels, with predictable pharmacokinetic results.
4. Lipid-soluble drugs diffuse more readily into the neonatal brain because of the permeability of the neonatal blood-brain barrier.
5. Most hepatic enzyme systems involved in microsomal drug metabolism are either inactive or immature unless induced by exposure to a drug such as phenobarbital.
6. The lesser glomerular filtration rate causes slower elimination of most drugs and their metabolites.

Pediatric Anesthesia Equipment

Anesthetic and airway equipment, as well as vascular cannulae, infusion sets, and monitoring devices must be appropriate for the size of the infant or child requiring anesthesia.

The two popular breathing systems for infants and small children (under 25 kg) are the various modifications of the Mapelson D system and the circle absorber system (see Chapter 5). The Mapelson modification most widely used over the past decade has been the Bain system, in which the fresh gas flows through an inner tube that lies inside the expiratory tube, through which warm expired gas flows. These pediatric partial rebreathing systems waste large volumes of gases and vapors because of the need for large total flows to clear CO_2. The cost of the newer volatile anesthetics has led to a return to the circle absorber systems, with modifications including small-bore delivery system tubing, a 0.5 to 1.0 L rebreathing bag and pediatric bellows for the mechanical ventilator.

For the infant under age one year, unless undergoing anesthesia for a brief procedure, it is best to intubate the trachea to ensure airway patency. Pediatric laryngoscope blade configurations vary, but the most widely employed in the United States is the Miller series (Miller-0 for small newborns). The Miller-0 and Miller-1 blades are available with a cannula paralleling the light tubing along the side of the blade and a proximal nipple attachment for continuous oxygen flow (2 L per minute) during laryngoscopy; this simple device reduces the likelihood of hypoxemia in infants undergoing tracheal intubation.

Uncuffed Magill and Murphy polyvinylchloride tubes in conventional shape and in angled configurations for procedures involving the head and neck constitute the most commonly employed pediatric tubes in the United States today. Cuffed tubes have not proven necessary for most patients under age eight years. By that age, the funnel shape of the laryngeal and cricoid structures found in younger children no longer persists, and the internal diameter of the trachea approximates the largest internal diameter of the glottis, requiring a cuffed tracheal tube.

MANAGEMENT BEFORE THE INDUCTION OF ANESTHESIA

Preanesthetic Evaluation

A number of age-related considerations affect the preanesthetic evaluation of the pediatric patient. The spectrum of common pediatric diseases and abnormal conditions differs considerably from that in the adult. Younger patients cannot give their own medical history, so this must be obtained from one or both parents. Some toddlers cooperate reluctantly or cry during a physical examination. The persistent and vigilant anesthesiologist, nonetheless, can obtain virtually all the required information by maintaining awareness of the following points and conducting a thorough preanesthetic interview and evaluation.

Children over six months of age vary in their emotional responses to a proposed anesthetic and operation. Despite the brevity of the preanesthetic visit, the anesthesiologist can attempt to gain the confidence of the infant or child and establish rapport with the parents prior to any physical examination of the patient.

The pediatric preanesthetic physical examination emphasizes the upper airway, lungs, and heart. Small nares, purulent rhinitis, adenoid and tonsillar hypertrophy, or a small mandible with a protruding maxilla frequently herald the development of upper airway obstruction after premedication or anesthetic induction. Children older than six years may have loose deciduous teeth that could be dislodged by an oropharyngeal airway or laryngoscope.

Many syndromes peculiar to patients of pediatric age have anesthetic implications. When confronted with a child with such abnormalities, one can consult a textbook on pediatric anesthesia for a table listing these syndromes and their anesthetic problems (see References).

Prematurity (birth at less than 37 weeks after conception) predisposes the patient to anemia, as well as postoperative apnea and bradycardia. A hemoglobin nadir of 11 $\pm$ 2 g per dl occurs at two to three months of age in the infant born at full term. In prematurely born infants weighing less than 1.2 kg at birth, the expected minimum hemoglobin is 7.7 g per dl. As with adults, these levels of anemia are no threat to life during ordinary operations.

An upper respiratory infection (URI) occurs an average of five times per year in pediatric patients, and persists up to ten days. In adults, mucus clearance remains impaired for up to a week, and pulmonary mechanics remain abnormal for up to five weeks after symptoms have cleared. Otherwise healthy children demonstrate no detrimental effects from anesthesia given during a URI. However, wheezing and rales during preoperative evaluation indicate lower airway disease, which contraindicates elective anesthesia.

Patients who could be infectious from exposure to an exanthem have their operations postponed to prevent them infecting other patients; if their operation cannot be postponed, they must be isolated from others in the hospital.

Many children manifest functional heart murmurs that have no physiologic significance. Functional murmurs sound soft and do not radiate; they can be difficult to differentiate from organic murmurs at a single examination. When an anesthesiologist detects such a murmur, confirmation of the diagnosis with the parent (tact is required: the parent may not be aware of the murmur) or directly with the pediatrician is advisable. If the implications of a murmur seem uncertain, consultation with a pediatric cardiologist should be obtained.

Preanesthetic Preparation

PREOPERATIVE REASSURANCE

Many children, including some adolescents, psychologically regress under the stress of anesthesia, operation, and separation from parents. Some children develop disturbing psychological changes manifested by nightmares, enuresis, and temper tantrums. Various approaches have served to minimize the unpleasant aspects of hospitalization, including (1) eliminating intramuscular injections; (2) preoperative puppet shows and a visit with an anesthesiologist; and (3) minimizing the length of time the child is separated from parents by having the parents present during anesthesia induction and by performing the operation on the day of admission. One of the most effective measures—yet sometimes one of the most difficult to achieve—is for the parents to demonstrate confidence and cheerfulness. Many parents have difficulty hiding their fears and tensions and transmit them to the child. During the preanesthetic visit with the parents, away from children who are old enough to understand, the parents are counseled about this as well as about the risks of anesthesia for their child.

PREANESTHETIC MEDICATION

The numerous regimens and drugs advocated for preanesthetic sedation of the pediatric patient testify to the lack of an overall solution. In younger patients, tachycardia often is desirable, atropine therefore remains the parasympatholytic agent commonly used in pediatric patients. Doses are twice those used in adults, but the drug is as effective given by mouth as intramuscularly (IM) (Table 25–5). Scopolamine can substitute for the atropine (in the same dose), providing additional preoperative sedation, but it will significantly increase the incidence of emergence delirium. Glycopyrrolate does not produce tachycardia and induces such an intense antisialagogue effect that children complain of pharyngeal soreness for up to seven hours.

Sedation and analgesia can be achieved with barbiturates or benzodiazepines combined with narcotics in flavored oral preparations that infants and children find acceptable. We favor an oral premedication consisting of atropine, meperidine, and pentobarbital or diazepam (Table 25–5). Inpatients receive pentobarbital and the greater dose of meperidine; outpatients receive diazepam and the lesser dose of meperidine.

TABLE 25–5. Drugs for Preanesthetic Sedation

Age (months)	Inpatient	Outpatient
0–6	Atropine IM or PO	Atropine PO
6–12	Atropine + pentobarbital IM or PO	Atropine + diazepam PO
Over 12	Atropine + pentobarbital + narcotic IM or PO	Atropine + diazepam + narcotic PO
	Dosage	
	Atropine	≤4 kg: 0.04 mg/kg IM or PO >4 kg: 0.02 mg/kg, minimum 0.16 mg, maximum 0.6 mg IM or PO
	Scopolamine	0.02 mg/kg IM or PO
	Pentobarbital	4 mg/kg IM or PO, maximum 100 mg IM (one injection)
	Morphine	0.1 mg/kg IM, maximum 10 mg IM
	Meperidine	1 mg/kg IM; 1.5 mg/kg PO in outpatients; 3 mg/kg PO in inpatients
	Diazepam	0.2 mg/kg PO

The narcotic and belladonna drugs can be mixed and given with one injection.

PREOPERATIVE FASTING

We recommend that children abstain from solid food and milk for 12 hours prior to induction of anesthesia. This fasting interval is based on the frequency of recovery of milk from the stomachs of infants after tracheal intubation. In contrast, the rapid turnover of body water in young infants predisposes them to dehydration. Recent studies demonstrate that children drinking up to 240 ml of clear liquids (depending on body size) two hours prior to anesthetic induction have gastric residual volumes and acidity no different than those fasting for 4 to 12 hours. We therefore offer clear liquids until two hours prior to induction of anesthesia.

INTRAOPERATIVE ANESTHETIC MANAGEMENT

Selection of Anesthetic Agents and Adjuvant Drugs

Pediatric anesthesiologists use most of the common anesthetic agents and techniques. Halothane and isoflurane have replaced narcotics as the basal anesthetic agent over the past decade in the healthy infant, but fentanyl remains the agent of choice in sick infants with cardiopulmonary instability. Nitrous oxide remains the most common carrier gas. Pancuronium and vecuronium have replaced curare. The tachycardia of pancuronium particularly benefits neonates whose cardiac output depends predominantly on heart rate. We advise the use of a written list of the appropriate weight-adjusted doses of the drugs used during the anesthetic (Table 25–6), including the common

TABLE 25–6. Intravenous Drug Dosages in Infants During Anesthesia

Adjuvant Drugs	Newborn	Infant
Atropine	0.04 mg/kg (≤4 kg)	0.02 mg/kg (>4 kg), minimum 0.16 mg IV
d-Tubocurarine		
Initial	0.3 mg + 0.3 mg increments to effect	0.6 mg/kg
Maintenance	25% initial total dose	25% initial dose
Vecuronium	0.1 mg/kg initial dose	0.1 mg/kg initial dose
Maintenance	15% initial dose	15% initial dose
Pancuronium		
Initial	0.05 mg + 0.05 mg increments to effect	0.1 mg/kg
Maintenance	20% initial dose	20% initial dose
Metocurine	0.4 mg/kg initial dose	0.4 mg/kg initial dose
Maintenance	25% initial dose	25% initial dose
Atracurium	0.4 mg/kg initial dose	0.4 mg/kg initial dose
Maintenance	25% initial dose	25% initial dose
Succinylcholine	2 mg/kg	1 mg/kg
Neostigmine	0.07 mg/kg	0.07 mg/kg
Thiopental (2.5%)	4 mg/kg	4 mg/kg
Ketamine	2 mg/kg	2 mg/kg
Fentanyl	1–2 μg/kg	1–2 μg/kg
Morphine	0.1–0.2 mg/kg	0.1–0.2 mg/kg

Cardiovascular Drugs	*Dosage*
Sodium bicarbonate	1–3 mEq/kg (depending on pHa and base excess)
Calcium chloride (10%)	10–12 mg/kg
Calcium gluconate (10%)	15–60 mg/kg
Epinephrine	
Initial*	1–10 μg/kg/min
Maintenance	0.1–2.0 μg/kg/min
Isoproterenol†	0.1–2.0 μg/kg/min
Dopamine‡	1–20 μg/kg/min
Dobutamine	2.5–10 μg/kg/min
Furosemide	0.5–1.0 mg/kg
Lidocaine (1%)	1.0 mg/kg

* Start with a low dose; double the dose periodically until desired effect is achieved or maximum dose is reached.

† Dilute in syringe to 1 or 10 μg/kg/ml; give with calibrated syringe pump.

‡ Dilute in syringe to 10 or 100 μg/kg/ml; give with calibrated syringe pump.

emergency drugs; those most likely to be used are prepared in appropriate syringes before induction of anesthesia.

Induction

Rapid, unthreatening anesthetic inductions minimize psychological trauma to the pediatric patient. We allow the child some control of the situation, including the choice of sitting in the anesthesiologist's lap, being held by the circulating nurse, or sitting or lying on the operating room table. A soft, caring and reassuring voice combined with firm, honest direction of events despite the child's hesitation improves the child's confidence in most instances. Distracting the child with a story that involves the sensations the child may experience during the induction helps allay anxiety. In the healthy child, we often apply monitoring devices and cannulate a vein after inducing unconsciousness.

INHALATION INDUCTION

Halothane enjoys a clear superiority as an inhalation induction agent. Disguising the odor of the mask and initial gas flow with a drop of a common liquid food flavoring, such as those found in grocery stores, makes the mask more acceptable to most children. Doubling the halothane concentration every two to four breaths while the patient breathes spontaneously without assistance minimizes the duration of the induction.

Other inhalational agents present difficulties in inhalation induction. Enflurane and isoflurane are more pungent and disagreeable than halothane. Laryngospasm occurs in 5 per cent of isoflurane inductions, and seizures occur in 7 per cent of children anesthetized with enflurane.

INTRAVENOUS INDUCTION

Intravenous induction agents offer a practical means of achieving rapid induction of anesthesia in the neonate and infant and of reducing psychological trauma in older children who refuse the mask. Thiopental requirements are increased in the infant under 12 months (ED_{50} 6 to 7 mg per kg), but the onset of unconsciousness appears more rapidly in infants because of their greater brain blood flow. The considerations involved in using ketamine in infants and children are the same as in adults.

OTHER METHODS OF INDUCTION

Other methods of inducing anesthesia include rectal methohexital (20 to 30 mg per kg), a method particularly suitable for children 6 to 36 months old. Induction times with this method range from 4 to 22 minutes, averaging 8 minutes. However, 8 per cent of patients are not asleep 15 minutes after administering the drug, and 8 to 13 per cent of the patients defecate, producing unknown and sometimes inadequate absorption of the drug.

Airway Management

Managing the pediatric upper airway and ventilating the lungs by mask requires different skills than in the adult. Unintentional pressure from the third and fourth fingers can force the tongue against the palate. The fingertips of the hand holding the mask must be kept on bony surfaces. The second finger, applied to the posterior surface of the symphysis menti, applies anterior pressure to pull the mandible forward. Similarly, the third or fourth finger, applied to the posterior aspect of the mandibular ramus, pushes the mandible forward, lifting the tongue off the posterior pharynx.

Tracheal intubation demands technical finesse, especially in the infant. The minimal working space in the infant's oropharynx requires precise technique: the tongue is swept well to the left by the laryngoscope blade with the handle of the laryngoscope at 45 degrees to the ceiling to keep the tongue behind the blade and to put the blade and larynx in the same axis.

Because of their greater oxygen consumptions and smaller functional residual capacity, infants develop arterial hemoglobin desaturation more readily than do adults during apnea. Prior ventilation of the lungs with 100 per cent oxygen for one minute prevents desaturation during a subsequent 30- to 60-second period of apnea. Insufflation of oxygen down the side of an Oxyscope laryngoscope blade may substantially increase the duration of apnea tolerated without desaturation.

The appropriate endotracheal tube size varies with the patient's age; the recommendations in Table 25–7 represent averages. Once the calculated size reaches 6.5 mm internal diameter (ID), we suggest using a cuffed endotracheal tube 0.5 mm ID smaller than the calculated size to avoid excessive tracheal gas leaks. An appropriate size tube allows an air leak at 10 to 40 cm H_2O peak static inflating pressure.

A history of prolonged tracheal intubation, tracheostomy, laryngeal stridor, or laryngotracheitis (croup) suggests the possibility of a narrowed subglottic tracheal diameter. These children require an endotracheal tube at least 0.5 mm ID smaller than usual.

Table 25–7. Age and Dimensions of Endotracheal Tubes

Age of Patient	Internal Diameter* (mm)	Connector† (mm)	Minimum Length‡ (oral) (cm)
Preterm	2.0–2.5	3.0	10–11
0–3 mo	3.0	3.0	11–12
3–7 mo	3.5	4.0	13
7–15 mo	4.0	4.0	14
15–24 mo	4.5	4.5	15–21
2–10 yr	(Age[yr] + 10)/4		
10–15 yr	6.0–7.5 cuffed	6.0–8.0	21–23
Adults	7.5–9.0 cuffed	8.0–10.0	24–26

* *Average* uncuffed tube size for age. Occasionally a size 0.5 ID smaller or larger is required in normal patients. Tubes are labeled with internal and external diameters in millimeters.

† Tapered, 15-mm male at machine end. Size refers to internal diameter at tube end.

‡ For nasal tubes, add 2–3 cm.

Maintenance of Anesthesia

INHALATION AGENTS

The average minimum alveolar concentration (MAC) of halothane increases from 0.87 per cent in the term newborn to 1.2 per cent at one month and remains at that level until six months, then declines to approximately 0.95 per cent at 12 months and 0.9 per cent at three years of age (Fig. 25–5). The reasons for these alterations in potency with age remain unclear. In the younger infant, the 30 per cent increase in dose requirement is accompanied by a greater susceptibility to systemic arterial hypotension at effective anesthetic levels of halothane (end-tidal concentrations of approximately 1.5 to 2.0 MAC). Whether these findings represent a hazard to the infant because of impaired blood flow to vital organs remains uncertain.

There are similar age-dependent variations in MAC for isoflurane (Fig. 25–6). Isoflurane in healthy term neonates and older infants is associated with less bradycardia or hypotension than is halothane.

Enflurane offers two advantages over halothane: a greater threshold for tachydysrhythmias and better abdominal muscle relaxation. Its car-

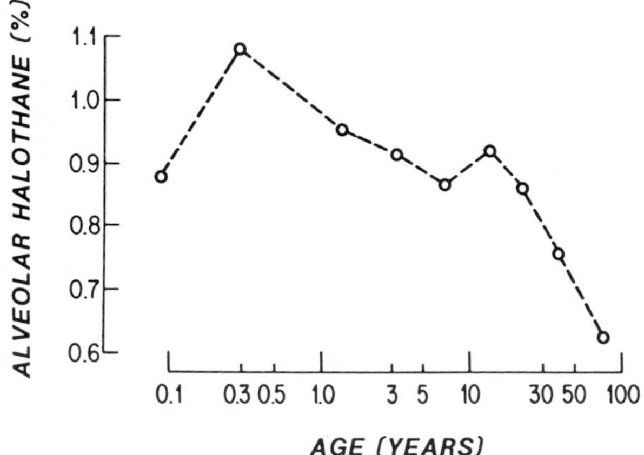

FIGURE 25–5. Minimum alveolar concentration (MAC) of halothane versus patient age. Note the higher requirements in infants and teenagers. Neonates have lower requirements than older infants. (Adapted with permission from Ryan JF, et al., eds. A practice of anesthesia for infants and children. New York: Grune and Stratton, 1986.)

diovascular depressant effects and its tendency to cause twitching and even seizures in greater anesthetic concentrations limit its use, however.

NARCOTICS

Narcotic anesthesia, usually supplemented by muscle relaxants, nitrous oxide, and minimal concentrations (less than 0.5 per cent) of halothane or isoflurane, offers special advantages to the sick infant whose cardiovascular system may be severely impaired by anesthetic concentrations of the potent volatile agents. The drug most often used is fentanyl by intermittent bolus injection of 1 to 2 μg per kg to total dose of 10 to 20 μg per kg. Postoperative management includes short-term mechanical ventilation (4 to 24 hours) to assure safe recovery from narcotic effects.

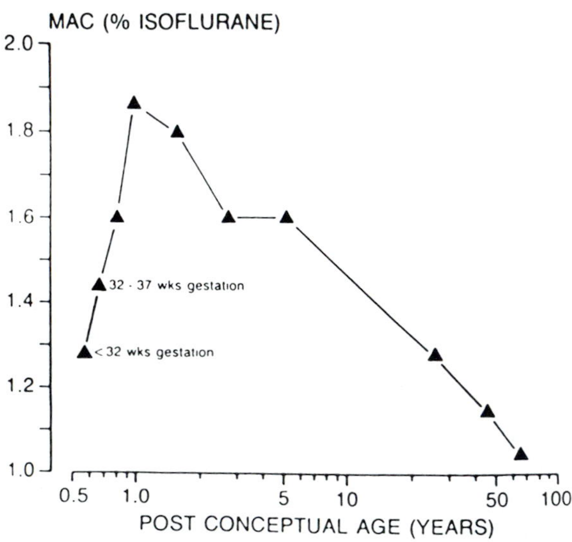

FIGURE 25–6. The MAC of isoflurane and postconceptual age. Values for postconceptual age were obtained by adding 40 weeks to the mean postnatal age for each age group. The MAC of isoflurane in preterm neonates is significantly less than in full-term neonates and older infants 1 to 6 months of age (P<0.005). (Reproduced with permission from LeDez KM, Lerman J. Anesthesiology 1987; 67:301.)

Narcotic antagonists, though effective immediately in many of these infants, have not eliminated the need for mechanical support of ventilation. Thus, narcotic anesthesia is reserved for infants undergoing major procedures who are expected to be candidates for intensive observation for up to 24 hours after anesthesia. This caveat does not apply to the use of narcotics to supplement inhalation agents, as in the use of fentanyl in doses of 1 to 3 μg per kg, or morphine in doses of 0.1 to 0.2 mg per kg. The elimination half-life of morphine in neonates (13 hours) and presumably in younger infants greatly exceeds that of older children and adults (2 hours).

RELAXANTS

In healthy term and older infants, nondepolarizing muscle relaxants can be given in the usual doses, but variability in duration of effect seems to be greater, and onset of action appears to be more rapid. The similarity in effective dosage over the age range occurs because the greater sensitivity of the immature myoneural junction of the infant to nondepolarizing relaxants is offset by the larger volume of distribution of the drugs. Infants require intravenous doses (in mg per kg) similar to those for adults when atropine and neostigmine are used for reversal of neuromuscular blockade. The effective intravenous dose of succinylcholine is 1 mg per kg.

Pediatric patients apparently experience fewer problems with intraoperative awareness than do adults. In healthy patients, 70 to 75 per cent N_2O in oxygen allows sufficient oxygen. Morphine in 0.05 to 0.10 mg per kg increments provides good intraoperative pain relief which extends into the postoperative period. Fentanyl in equipotent doses of 0.5 to 1.0 μg per kg also gives good intraoperative pain relief. Some pediatric anesthesiologists avoid narcotics in infants less than 6 to

12 months old, especially if they have a history of prematurity or apnea and bradycardia.

Monitoring

Observation of the patient and the rational use of monitoring devices greatly enhances the safety of anesthesia in infants and children. Minimum monitoring guidelines call for the same monitors in infants and children as in adults (see Chapter 6), although interpretation of these monitors may vary with age. For example, normal blood pressure is different in neonates and young infants than in adults (Table 25–3).

Rectal or esophageal temperature monitoring readily detects hypothermia in infants. Axillary temperature may increase in malignant hyperthermia earlier than does core temperature.

Most neonates and young infants undergoing intracavitary procedures benefit from an intra-arterial catheter for monitoring of blood pressure and changes in blood electrolytes. The radial artery of the full-term newborn accepts a 22-gauge catheter inserted either percutaneously or by cutdown (without ligating the artery). Aggressive flushing of a radial arterial catheter must be avoided because this can cause cerebral emboli. Less accessible, but perhaps safer, are the dorsalis pedis and posterior tibial arteries in the foot. The temporal and, in the newborn, umbilical arteries can be used but are associated with cerebral emboli or renal hypertension respectively.

A central venous pressure catheter in the right atrium can be useful for evaluating adequacy of blood replacement in patients experiencing major blood loss. Pulmonary artery catheters are seldom indicated because right and left heart functions are rarely dissociated in pediatric patients undergoing noncardiac operations. Urine output in the infant can be measured accurately with a small volume urometer provided the tubing remains unkinked and all the urine flows into the urometer. Similarly, surgical suction lines used in infants are short and flow into calibrated traps.

Temperature Control

The environmental temperature of many operating rooms is between 20 and 22°C; this temperature is at the margin of the healthy newborn infant's ability to thermoregulate, requiring a threefold increase in oxygen consumption to maintain body temperature. Thermal stress also increases plasma catecholamines, causing pulmonary and systemic vasoconstriction and metabolic acidemia that may precipitate a return to a fetal circulatory pattern, especially if the neonate cannot increase cardiopulmonary function to meet the raised metabolic demand.

Maintaining the body temperatures of neonates and young infants, even for short superficial procedures, requires a multifaceted approach. An overhead radiant warmer during induction and emergence, raising the operating room temperature, placing a plastic bag between the patient and the OR table sheets, placing the intubated patient's head and limbs in plastic sandwich bags, and covering the remainder of the patient with an adhesive plastic drape or reflective blanket all serve to minimize the patient's loss of heat to the environment. A servo-controlled circulating water blanket, and heated and humidified anesthetic gases provide the heat needed to maintain an infant's core temperature, even when a body cavity is open.

Intraoperative Fluid Therapy

The daily requirements of neonates and children for fluids and nutrition were established in 1957 (Table 25–8A and B). Of the commercially available intravenous fluids, one-quarter normal (0.2 per cent) saline most closely resembles the obligatory fluid losses of the neonate. Anesthesiologists and surgeons have tended to use this hypotonic maintenance fluid for third-space replacement and postoperative treatment, but this can produce hyponatremia. Because neonates readily handle the added sodium, most pediatric anesthesiologists now use lactated Ringer's solution for maintenance fluid replacement. We seek to administer

TABLE 25–8A. Maintenance Fluid Requirements (Oral or Parenteral)

Wt. (kg)	ml/kg/hr	ml/kg/24 hr
<10	4	100
10–20	40 + 2 ml/kg >10 kg	1000 + 50 ml/kg >10 kg
>20	60 + 1 ml/kg >20 kg	1500 + 20 ml/kg >20 kg

Requirements increase with fever or other causes of increased metabolism.

TABLE 25–8B. Fluid Replacement Therapy

"Third-space" replacement:
 Lactated Ringer's solution 3–10 ml/kg/hr during operation depending on operative site; reevaluate when total dose reaches 40 ml/kg.
Colloid replacement in lieu of blood if hematocrit ≥36 [newborn], or ≥30 [older infant, child]:
 Fresh frozen plasma and/or 5% albumin in lactated Ringer's (10–20 ml/kg)
Blood replacement
 Estimated blood volume (EBV)
  90–100 ml/kg premature newborn
   90 ml/kg newborn
   70 ml/kg child, adult male
   65 ml/kg adult female
 Acceptable arterial hematocrit (Hct_a)
  ≥36% if <52 wk postconception
  ≥30% if ≥52 wk postconception
 Allowable blood loss (ABL) calculation (Hb_i = initial Hct; Hb_t = target Hct):
  $ABL = EBV \times (Hb_i - Hb_t)/Hb_i$
 Replace ABL ≤10 ml/kg with lactated Ringer's
 Replace ABL >10 ml/kg with 5% albumin in lactated Ringer's or fresh frozen plasma
 Replace blood losses >ABL with blood to maintain Hct_a
Technique
 Warm fluids and blood
 Use calibrated syringe pump for maintenance fluids
 Use manual syringe injection for colloid and blood

Adapted with permission from Holliday MA, Segar WI. Maintenance need for water in parenteral fluid therapy. Pediatrics 1957;19:823–828. Furman EB. Intraoperative fluid therapy. Int Anesthesiol Clin 1975;13(3):133–147. Grogono AW. Albumin extravasation during surgery. Br J Anaesth 1976;48:929–930. Gross JB. Estimating allowable blood loss: corrected for dilution. Anesthesiology 1983;58:277–280.

eight hours of maintenance fluids to patients in the operating room and postanesthetic care unit so that they are not required to drink shortly after anesthesia.

Third-space losses in the pediatric patient resemble those in adults (Table 25–8B). However, preterm infants or neonates with a diaphgramatic hernia or congenital heart disease may not tolerate large volumes of third-space fluid replacement without developing interstitial pulmonary edema. The normal pediatric cardiovascular system handles acute variations in blood volume of up to 10 per cent. This permits "priming" neonates and young infants with up to 10 ml per kg of blood before a bloody surgical procedure begins, especially when the blood loss will be difficult to measure, such as in craniectomies for craniosynostosis. All of the problems of multiple blood volume transfusions appear to occur earlier in neonates and young infants, perhaps because the rate of infusion, in ml per kg per minute, tends to be greater in smaller patients than larger ones. Hyperkalemia and hypocalcemia often develop during rapid transfusion in infants and children, whereas dilutional coagulopathies occur infrequently.

Emergence

Emergence ordinarily occurs more rapidly in neonates and young infants than in adults for the same reasons that induction is more rapid. As in adults, tracheal extubation during the excitement stage of emergence may result in laryngospasm. The initial treatment of laryngospasm consists of constant positive airway pressure with forward mandibular thrust and extension of the occipitoatlantal joint to relieve residual supraglottic soft tissue obstruction. For hypoxemia with an oxygen hemoglobin saturation below 85 per cent, but before the onset of cyanosis or bradycardia, we advocate intravenous succinylcholine, 0.1 mg per kg; inspiratory efforts against a closed glottis can cause severe pulmonary edema in an otherwise healthy patient of any age.

Because young infants cannot cooperate or follow verbal commands, alternative means of assessing recovery from neuromuscular blockade are used. One common sign, the flexion of the hips with the raising of one or both legs from the operating table corresponds to an inspiratory pressure of −35 cm H_2O. Since hypothermia delays recovery of neuromuscular function following reversal of nondepolarizing muscle relaxants, reversal of the effects of neuromuscular blockers is not attempted unless the patient's core temperature is at least 35°C.

POSTANESTHETIC CARE

The special problems of the pediatric patient recovering from an anesthetic require a recovery room staffed with nurses who are experienced in dealing with children and equipped with pediatric equipment. Children require more psychological care than do adults because they are not capable of understanding the strange new environment. Even experienced nurses occasionally have difficulty determining if patients are crying because they are in pain, are hungry, or want their parents.

Postanesthetic prolonged apnea (≥15 seconds) occurs in an average of 37 per cent of infants born at less than 37 weeks gestation because of immaturity of respiratory control. This apnea, often with bradycardia and hypoxemia, may occur at up to 60 weeks of gestational age, but it is most common and severe in the infant under 44 weeks postconceptual age. Infants born at term occasionally manifest immature respiratory control or sudden infant death syndrome as late as 15 months after birth, but this seems unrelated to anesthesia.

Mild hypoxemia presents the most common problem observed in the pediatric acute care unit, yet delivering increased inspired oxygen to the child is frequently complicated by the child's lack of cooperation. Therefore, we monitor all patients in the recovery room with pulse oximeters. Because neonates and young infants are more at risk for apnea and bradycardia than older children, we monitor patients less than six months of age with an electrocardiogram and impedance apnea alarm system.

Emergence delirium occurs frequently in pediatric patients over two years of age, with a peak incidence of 13 per cent between the ages of three and nine years. Scopolamine premedication increases the incidence of emergence delirium, as does the lack of narcotics. Morphine, 0.05 to 0.10 mg per kg, or fentanyl, 0.5 to 1.0 μg per kg, effectively treats emergence delirium.

Postextubation subglottic edema (croup) occurs occasionally in patients between one and eight years of age. Humidity, aerosolized racemic epinephrine by mask every one half to two hours, and intravenous hydration usually relieve the partial airway obstruction. The value of corticosteroids in the treatment of this entity remains unproven.

In neonates and young infants, hypothermia frequently causes apnea, intense peripheral vasoconstriction, and metabolic acidosis from the metabolism of free fatty acids liberated during nonshivering thermogenesis. The pediatric recovery room must be equipped to rewarm cold patients and maintain the body temperatures of small infants. Overhead radiant warmers or circulating warm air blankets are effective.

REGIONAL ANESTHESIA

Regional anesthesia in infants and children provides the advantages of reduced requirements for other anesthetic agents and excellent postoperative analgesia. It also exposes patients to the risks of both a general anesthetic and a regional technique, because infants and children usually will not hold still if awake during an operation under regional block.

Local anesthetic agents, given in usual doses by body weight, exhibit efficacy and toxicity in neonates and infants similar to those seen in older children and adults. Because of small body mass, it is often necessary to use dilute solutions of local anesthetics to avoid overdose, however.

Pediatric axillary nerve blocks are administered under general anesthesia, without the use of paresthesias for placement. Rather, the transarterial (using a 25-gauge needle) or nerve stimulator approaches are used. As much as 1 ml per kg of 0.25 per cent lidocaine, or 0.5 ml per kg of 0.50 per cent bupivacaine (2.5 ml maximum) with 1:200,000 epinephrine may be used.

The absence of fat over the sacrum of infants and children makes caudal anesthesia technically easy. However, in the infant the dural membrane may be as close as 1 cm to the sacrococcygeal ligament. Therefore, in pediatric caudal blocks the needle is not advanced into the sacral canal; rather, the caudal canal is approached as if it were the lumbar epidural space, using loss of resistance. Caudal anesthesia is appropriate for most operations below the umbilicus. A dose of 1 ml per kg of 0.25 per cent bupivacaine with 1:200,00 epinephrine produces a T10 level. Decreasing the concentration to 0.125 per cent bupivacaine decreases the incidence of motor block and is particularly appropriate for ambulatory patients. Children may be discharged home after caudal anesthesia, provided no motor lock is present and they can walk without assistance and without postural hypotension. Voiding prior to discharge is not necessary.

For herniorrhaphies, wound infiltration or ilioinguinal and iliohypogastric nerve blocks with 1 mg per kg (maximum 10 ml) per side of either 0.25 per cent or 0.125 per cent bupivacaine provides effective postoperative pain relief. The block is performed by inserting a 22-gauge needle perpendicular to the skin one child's finger-breadth from the anterior iliac spine along a line connecting the spine and the umbilicus. The needle is advanced until the internal and external oblique fascial planes have been pierced or until the needle strikes the inner table of the iliac crest. Two thirds of the local anesthetic is injected here and the remainder is injected as the needle is withdrawn, leaving a skin wheal to block the perforating branches of T11 and T12.

The neonatal spinal cord ends at L3; by the end of the first year of life, the end of the cord is found at the adult position of L1. The neonatal dural sac ends at S3, rising to S1 by one year, also. Lumbar epidural blocks therefore are done at L4-5 or L5 to S1, using pediatric epidural kits. We use a dose of 0.5 ml per kg of 0.25 per cent bupivacaine with 1:200,000 epinephrine. Preservative-free narcotics can also be instilled via this route.

Penile nerve blocks provide postoperative pain relief after circumcision and hypospadias repair. There are several techniques, but we prefer to inject 1 mg per kg of bupivacaine (the total dose diluted to a volume appropriate to the child's anatomy) without epinephrine in the midline just caudad to the symphysis pubis. The needle is inserted in the midline at the base of the penis and advanced off the symphysis in increments, similar to "walking off" a rib in an intercostal nerve block.

Spinal anesthesia in neonates is becoming increasingly popular for the preterm infant requiring herniorrhaphy who is at risk for postoperative apnea. Because the spinal cord extends to L3 in neonates, the lumbar puncture is performed at L4-5 or L5 to S1. Placing the patient in the sitting position makes the block technically easier to perform and increases the success rate. Spinal anesthesia produces very little hemodynamic change in neonates, so the intravenous cannula may placed in the lower extremity after the block is established. Because extreme flexion of the neonatal neck produces airway obstruction, the neonate's head must be supported while the block is being introduced.

The dose of tetracaine for spinal anesthesia is 0.4 mg per kg in 0.04 ml per kg of 10 per cent dextrose. Epinephrine increases the duration of the block from 60 minutes to 95 minutes. Because the doses are so small, the dead space volume of the spinal needle must be measured and that volume (0.05 to 0.10 ml) must be considered in the volume the patient receives.

ANESTHESIA FOR THE NEONATE

The details of the anesthetic management of a neonate (zero to 28 days of age) lie beyond the scope of this text. The anesthesiologist who does not specialize in neonatal care may be required to prepare a newborn for emergency transport or for anesthesia and operation. The common lesions threatening the life of a neonate and their major associated clinical problems are outlined in Table 25–9.

Preparation of a sick neonate for transfer to a referral center or to an operating room aims at stabilizing the cardiopulmonary system, body temperature, metabolic functions (including correction of birth asphyxia) and providing energy substrates to meet immediate metabolic needs. A

TABLE 25–9. Surgical Lesions of the Neonate and Their Anesthetic Problems

Lesion	Problems
Airway obstruction Choanal atresia Pierre Robin syndrome Neoplasm Laryngeal stenosis	Asphyxia arrest, aspiration pneumothorax
Diaphragmatic hernia and eventration	Asphyxia, shock, hypoplastic lungs, pulmonary vascular hypertension, gastric distention, congenital heart disease, pneumothorax, small abdomen
Esophageal atresia and tracheoesophageal fistula (TEF)	Pneumonitis, gastric distention (TEF), airway secretions, cogenital heart disease, possible inability to ventilate lungs after gastrostomy (TEF)
Lobar emphysema	Air trapping, mediastinal shift
Congenital heart disease	Asphyxia, cardiac failure, shock, pulmonary vascular hypoperfusion, pulmonary edema
Omphalocele, gastroschisis	Hypothermia, acidosis, shock, asphyxia, hypovolemia, congenital heart disease
Intestinal atresia	Regurgitation
Pyloric stenosis	Dehydration, aspiration, electrolyte derangement
Gastrointestinal perforation, peritonitis, other obstruction (volvulus, intussusception)	Hypovolemia, distention, shock aspiration, sepsis hypoventilation
Incarcerated hernia, imperforate anus, megacolon	Fluid deficit/loss, occult blood loss
Sacrococcygeal teratoma	Massive blood loss, prone position during operation, hypothermia

TABLE 25–10. Stabilization of Vital Systems in the Neonate

Clear airway
Oxygen to achieve Pa_{O_2} 50–70 mm Hg
Decompress stomach
Warm to 37°C (colon), 36°C (skin over liver)
Establish intravenous route
  Plastic cannula (24 gauge or larger)
  Percutaneous, cutdown, umbilical vein
Correct acidosis of pHa <7.30
Ventilate if Pa_{CO_2} >50 mm Hg
Correct dehydration
  Insensible losses
  Gastrointestinal losses
  Other losses
Correct hypovolemia: Ringer's lactate, albumin, plasma; packed RBCs or whole blood if Hct <36%
Correct hypoglycemia (<40 mg/dl): 15% dextrose in water, 1 ml/kg IV
Arterial cannula—radial, temporal, umbilical

protocol for this is outlined in Table 25–10, and appropriate drug dosages are given in Table 25–6.

ANESTHETIC MANAGEMENT OF AMBULATORY PEDIATRIC PATIENTS

Pediatric patients are particularly good candidates for ambulatory procedures because they are generally healthy, because children emerge from anesthesia more rapidly than do adults, and because they benefit greatly from the psychological support of a familiar environment. Stable physical status 3 patients are also suitable, even if they have a tracheostomy in place and are mechanically ventilated at home, provided that the family is capable of providing the special needs of these children.

Healthy full-term infants born at 38 weeks gestation or later are suitable ambulatory surgery patients if they are at least four weeks postnatal *and* 44 weeks postconception at the time of their anesthetic. Prematurely born infants become suitable candidates after they attain 60 weeks of postconceptual age and have not required an apnea monitor for one month.

COMPLICATIONS OF ANESTHESIA

Over the past 40 years the anesthesia-related mortality for infants and children has decreased from 1:600 cases to less than 1:1000 cases when all types of patients are included, and to approximately 2:100,000 cases for elective anesthesia in ASA physical status 1 or 2 patients in major pediatric centers. In an excellent prospective, multi-institutional study in France of 40,240 anesthetics administered to children under age 15 years (of whom 5 per cent were infants under one year), only one death occurred, which resulted from unrecognized postanesthetic respiratory depression. The incidence of cardiac arrest overall was 3:10,000 cases; in the infants the incidence was 2:1000 cases, whereas that in children age 1 to 14 years was 2:10,000 cases, a tenfold difference. The overall incidence of major complications possibly caused by anesthesia was 7:10,000 cases.

Pain is the most frequent complication following anesthesia; it is best treated by narcotics given before emergence from anesthesia or by a regional anesthetic. Prevention of pain ordinarily requires less total drug than does treatment once pain becomes intense.

Nausea and vomiting affect 10 to 20 per cent of children recovering from anesthesia. Challenging the patient postoperatively with clear liquids increases the incidence of postoperative nausea and vomiting. We no longer require children to drink and retain clear liquids as a condition for discharge home, but encourage them to ingest clear liquids up to two hours prior to anesthesia induction. Combined with the administration of intravenous fluids, this assures adequate hydration. This approach has reduced the incidence of nausea and vomiting by more than half compared with forced postoperative drinking.

Postintubation subglottic edema has been discussed previously (see *Postanesthetic Care*).

Nightmares, enuresis, and recall of separation from parents or of anesthesia induction by mask as terrifying events were reported over 30 years ago as sequelae of anesthesia and operations in children. Comparable data describing the sequelae of modern pediatric anesthesia practice with the type of preparations and sedation discussed above have not been published. By investing time and understanding in the preanesthetic relationship with the child and parents, the anesthesiologist can minimize the incidence and degree of this psychic trauma.

REFERENCES

Cook DR, Marcy JH. Neonatal anesthesia. Pasadena: Appleton Davies, 1988.
Gregory G, ed. Pediatric anesthesia. 2nd ed. New York: Churchill Livingstone, 1989.

Kurth CD, Spitzer AR, Broennle AM, Downes JJ. Postoperative apnea in preterm infants. Anesthesiology 1987; 64:483–488.

Motoyama EK, Davis PJ, eds. Smith's anesthesia for infants and children. 5th ed. St. Louis: CV Mosby, 1990.

Ryan JF, Todres ID, Cote CJ, Goudsouzian NG. A practice of anesthesia for infants and children. New York: Grune & Stratton, 1986.

Scarpelli EM, ed. Pulmonary physiology—fetus, newborn, child, adolescent. Philadelphia: Lea and Febiger, 1990.

Schecter NL, ed. Acute pain in children. Pediatr Clin North Am 1989; 36:781–1052.

Tiret L, Nivoche Y, Hutton F, Desmonts JM, Vourc'h G. Complications related to anesthesia in infants and children. Br J Anaesth 1988; 61:263–269.

CHAPTER TWENTY-SIX

OBSTETRIC ANESTHESIA AND PERINATOLOGY

> The application of anaesthesia to midwifery involves many more delicate problems than its mere application to surgery. New rules must be established for its use, its effect on the action of the uterus, upon the state of the child and upon the puerperal state of the mother.
>
> JAMES YOUNG SIMPSON, 1848

GENERAL CONSIDERATIONS

As Simpson pointed out a century and a half ago, anesthesia care for parturients entails issues beyond those involved in caring for surgical patients. Because almost all anesthetic drugs cross the placenta, one anesthetizes two patients at once. Opioids, sedatives, local anesthetics, inhalation anesthetics, and, to some extent, neuromuscular blockers must all be given in minimal effective doses to avoid deleterious effects on the fetus, the progress of labor, or the intrauterine environment. The minimum alveolar concentration (MAC) of inhalation anesthetics is decreased by 25 to 40 per cent in parturients, perhaps because of increased circulating levels of progesterone and endorphins; this is another reason to minimize the doses of anesthetic drugs in parturients.

The obstetric patient is unlike the usual patient scheduled for an elective operation. Her stomach usually contains food, or acid of pH less than 2.5, increasing the risk of aspiration pneumonia, still the leading cause of maternal anesthetic mortality. Emergencies such as fetal distress, maternal hemorrhage, uterine rupture, and prolapsed cord demand immediate anesthesia and delivery to ensure both maternal and neonatal survival. Vaginal delivery necessitates an alert, cooperative mother who can assist the forces of labor by bearing down in the second stage. Medical conditions such as diabetes mellitus, heart disease, and endocrine disorders are aggravated by pregnancy, whereas other disorders may be caused by pregnancy, such as preeclampsia-eclampsia and the coagulopathies which accompany abruptio placentae, intrauterine fetal death, and amniotic fluid embolism. The newborn may require specialized medical care as well.

PHYSIOLOGIC ALTERATIONS OF PREGNANCY AND THEIR IMPLICATIONS FOR ANESTHESIA CARE

Although by definition pregnancy is not a pathologic state, the marked physiologic changes it entails require attention in managing anesthesia.

Respiration

In pregnancy, generalized swelling and capillary engorgement of the upper airway, larynx, and tracheal bronchial tree make airway obstruction more likely; the hazards of trauma and further edema from laryngoscopy and tracheal intubation are worsened as well. Placement of a nasal airway can result in nosebleed. Because of laryngeal edema, endotracheal tubes one size smaller than usual are appropriate, especially in teenage mothers and those with preeclampsia-eclampsia.

In the normal mother at term, vital capacity is unchanged and total lung capacity is decreased by only 5 per cent, owing to elevation of the diaphragm. Functional residual capacity is reduced by 15 per cent, which speeds the uptake of the insoluble inhalation anesthetics. At term, minute ventilation is increased approximately 40 per cent; during labor without adequate pain relief, minute ventilation increases further, reaching three times normal, which speeds considerably the uptake of the soluble inhalation anesthetics. Hyperventilation leads to respiratory alkalosis and compensating metabolic acidosis. At term, basal metabolic rate is increased by 15 per cent and oxygen consumption, for a given amount of work, by 20 per cent or greater. This increase in oxygen requirement, combined with a diminished functional residual capacity, adds to the risk of maternal hypoxia.

Circulation

The maternal blood volume at term is increased by 35 to 40 per cent, 1200 to 1500 ml; 500 ml of this increase is contained in the uterus and is expressed into the circulation when the uterus contracts at delivery. As the average blood loss in vaginal delivery or cesarean section seldom exceeds 500 or 1000 ml, respectively, transfusion with blood or colloid solutions is rarely necessary in an uncomplicated delivery. Although in normal pregnancy the total red blood cell mass is increased, there is a much greater increase in plasma volume, explaining the diminished hematocrit of pregnancy. With proper diet, the hematocrit rarely decreases below 35 per cent.

Measured in the lateral decubitus position, maternal cardiac output (CO) reaches 140 per cent of normal at the end of the first trimester. It remains at this level until it decreases near term. With onset of labor, CO again increases 40 per cent or more and does not return to normal until two weeks postpartum.

Blood pressure normally is not increased in pregnancy, because of peripheral vasodilation. The heart rate increases by approximately 10 to 15 beats per minute. During uterine contractions, CO and blood pressure both increase; blood pressure is best measured in the interval between contractions. Effective analgesia decreases but does not eliminate these circulatory responses to contractions. Elevation of the diaphragm causes the heart to appear enlarged on both physical examination and chest x-ray. Benign systolic heart murmurs and left axis shift by electrocardiogram may appear as pregnancy progresses.

Assuming the supine position during the second half of pregnancy produces partial or complete obstruction of the vena cava and aorta by the gravid uterus, decreasing venous return to the right heart and producing symptoms of circulatory insufficiency in 10 to 15 per cent of patients. Even in the absence of maternal symptoms, decreased uteroplacental perfusion may cause fetal distress. Women who do not show signs of caval compression compensate by means of collateral circulation through the perivertebral plexus and vasoconstriction in the lower extremities. The engorged perivertebral veins are more easily entered during epidural block, making accidental intravenous injection of toxic amounts of local anesthetics more likely.

Given the effects of caval compression, the sympathetic blockade induced by spinal or epidural block can result in cardiovascular collapse. In 80 per cent of supine gravidas, spinal anesthesia with sensory levels at T8 or higher reduces the blood pressure enough to compromise uteroplacental circulation (systolic pressure decreased by 30 per cent or to a value less than 100 mm Hg). Prophylaxis and therapy for caval obstruction consist of left uterine displacement, which is accomplished by placing the patient in the left lateral decubitus position, by displacing the uterus to the left manually, or by placing a wedge or inflatable device beneath the patient's right flank (Fig. 26–1). During the second half of pregnancy, it is best for the patient to avoid the supine position; during labor and delivery or cesarean section, left uterine displacement is maintained until birth.

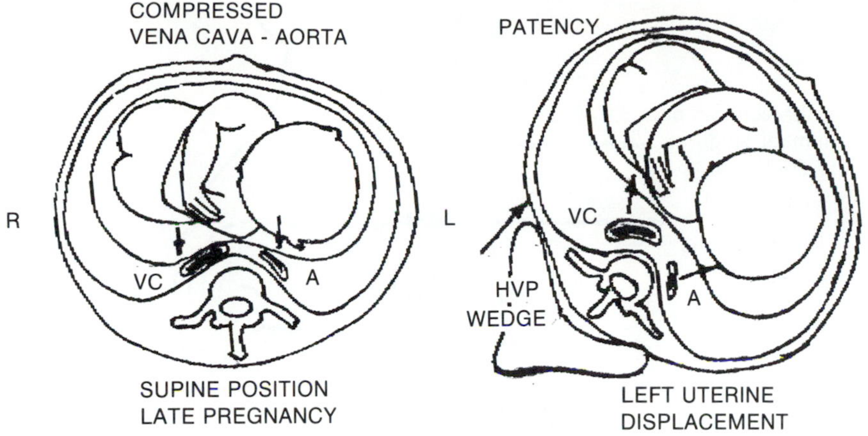

FIGURE 26–1. Left uterine displacement employing a hip wedge. R, right; L, left, VC, vena cava; A, aorta.

Gastrointestinal Tract

Both the volume and the acidity of the contents of the stomach are increased during pregnancy. Gastric emptying time is prolonged by labor, apprehension, pain, and displacement of the stomach by the uterus, which repositions the gastroduodenal junction and creates a functional hiatal hernia. Also, the enlarged uterus and the lithotomy position increase intragastric pressure. Together, these changes subject the sedated or unconscious parturient to a greater risk of pulmonary aspiration of gastric contents. The interval from the last meal to induction of general anesthesia is of little value in determining the risk of aspiration in the gravid patient.

A major component of aspiration pneumonia is Mendelson's syndrome, or acid aspiration pneumonitis, which occurs when the aspirate has a pH of less than 2.5 Animal studies support the idea that reducing the acidity of stomach contents can decrease the pulmonary damage following aspiration. Clear antacids such as sodium citrate are preferred because the insoluble antacids such as magnesium or aluminum salts themselves cause severe lung damage when aspirated. Thirty ml of a clear antacid given only minutes before induction usually increases gastric pH above 4.0 for over an hour. The H_2 blockers, cimetidine or ranitidine, will reliably decrease both gastric acidity and volume, but require 60 to 90 minutes after oral intake for optimal effect. For elective operations under general anesthesia, these medications are given orally the night preceding and two hours before induction of general anesthesia; in an emergency situation when given intramuscularly or slowly by the intravenous route, they will maintain the decreased gastric acidity following the oral clear antacid. Metoclopramide is a potent antiemetic that increases both gastric emptying and gastroesophageal sphincter tone without affecting gastric pH and is often used in conjunction with the H_2 blockers.

Reducing gastric acidity provides little protection against aspiration of solid material, which can be even more devastating than acid aspiration. The best protection against aspiration in the parturient is to ensure consciousness with intact protective airway reflexes. If consciousness is lost or laryngeal reflexes are compromised, the lungs must be protected by cricoid compression of the esophagus, followed by rapid tracheal intubation. Induction of general anesthesia in the lithotomy position is avoided.

The Parturient

Pain During Labor and Delivery

The pain of labor and delivery includes two components (Fig. 26–2). Visceral pain is caused by dilation and effacement of the cervix during uterine contractions, and possibly by uterine ischemia; somatic pain represents stretching of the vagina and perineum during the descent of the fetus. Although visceral pain dominates the first stage of labor and somatic pain the second, there is considerable overlap.

The pain of cervical dilation and effacement is referred to the lower abdomen, between umbilicus

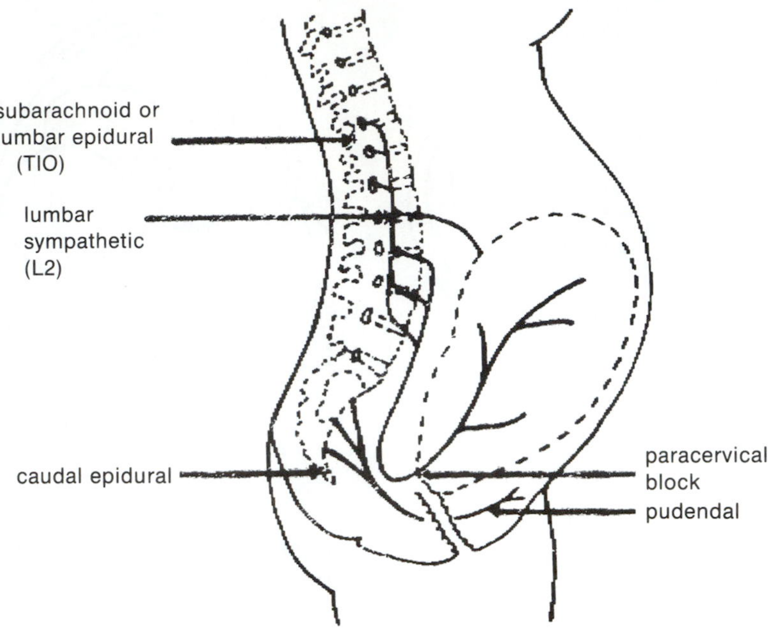

FIGURE 26–2. Sensory pathways and sites of injection in obstetric regional anesthesia. Visceral pain from cervix and uterus is blocked by paracervical blocks, bilateral lumbar sympathetic blocks at L2, and segmental peridural block of T10 to L1. Somatic pain from perineum is blocked by pudendal nerve blocks, saddle (subarachnoid) block, or low caudal peridural block. All labor pain is abolished by a modified saddle (subarachnoid), lumbar peridural, or caudal peridural block extending from T10 to L5. (From Gutsche BB: Analgesia and anesthesia for childbirth. In Reeder SJ, et al. Maternity nursing. 14th ed. Philadelphia: JB Lippincott, 1980. Modified from Bonica JJ: Principles and practice of obstetric analgesia and anesthesia. Philadelphia: FA Davis Co, 1967:492.)

and pubis, and to the lower back. Early in labor, this may be perceived only as pressure; as contractions strengthen, the pain intensifies and is referred to hips and thighs. These sensations are mediated by small, unmyelinated nerve fibers that pass from the cervix through the pelvis and hypogastric plexuses to enter the sympathetic chain at L3 to L5, reaching the dorsal root ganglia and spinal cord via the white rami communicantes of T10 to L1.

Somatic or vaginal pain dominates the second stage of labor and begins as the presenting part descends through the vagina, usually at about 8 cm dilation of the cervix in a primagravida. Initially, this is perceived as a need to defecate, but with further descent the mother has an uncontrollable urge to bear down, thus activating accessory forces of labor. Somatic pain is conveyed primarily via the pudendal nerves to dorsal nerve roots S2 to S4. Interrupting somatic pain with conduction anesthesia eliminates the urge to bear down.

Contractions produce labor pains when intrauterine pressure exceeds 30 mm Hg, but the degree of pain experienced varies greatly among parturients. Prenatal education, a supportive partner, and the helpful attitudes of nurses and physicians can reduce the discomfort experienced.

Providing Pain Relief

The ideal form of analgesia for labor and delivery embraces several goals:

1. Satisfactory pain relief for the mother.
2. Little interference with the progress of labor.
3. Minimal risks to either mother or fetus.
4. Provision of satisfactory conditions for the particular delivery involved.
5. Early interaction between mother and newborn, preferably in the delivery room.

No one technique of analgesia or anesthesia meets all of these criteria in all instances. Combinations of techniques, modified to meet circumstances, are the rule.

Nonpharmacologic Methods of Analgesia

Nonphamacologic methods of analgesia for labor and delivery include acupuncture, hypnosis, and "prepared childbirth." Acupuncture, not used by classic Chinese practitioners for labor and delivery, produces at best limited and unpredictable analgesia. Hypnosis likewise results in variable degrees of analgesia from none to complete, as patients differ greatly in their abilities to achieve a state of trance. Natural or prepared childbirth is based on the premise that prenatal education, encouragement by spouse and labor-floor personnel, and the use of breathing and relaxation exercises will reduce or eliminate the need for medication. Succcss is unpredictable, and many women require some form of pharmacologic analgesia as labor progresses.

Pharmacologic Methods of Analgesia

Pharmacologic techniques that provide pain relief in parturition can be divided into four categories:

1. Systemic medication for analgesia and sedation, using opioids, tranquilizers, or ketamine.
2. Analgesia with subanesthetic concentrations of inhalation agents.
3. General anesthesia, now seldom used for vaginal delivery.
4. Regional anesthetic techniques.

Just as do patients before surgical procedures, pregnant women who are to undergo anesthesia require evaluation and counseling by an anesthesiologist. When circumstances do not allow individual prenatal consultation, the anesthesiologist can speak to groups of mothers in a prenatal course, thereby allaying fears and creating realistic expectations for obstetrical anesthesia. When the parturient arrives in the labor suite, before she has severe discomfort, the anesthesiologist visits her to evaluate her condition, discuss plans for anesthesia, and obtain informed consent.

All patients receiving drugs for pain relief require monitoring of vital signs throughout labor, in the delivery room, and during postpartum recovery. Trained labor-floor nurses in constant attendance can perform these functions, provided that an anesthesiologist is immediately available. During delivery, an anesthesiologist attends mothers who are given analgesics or anesthetics. Parturients given analgesics or anesthetics also require a 16- or 18-gauge intravenous catheter to allow for hydration, transfusion, or the rapid administration of anesthetics or drugs as needed.

SYSTEMIC MEDICATIONS

Parenterally administered drugs, usually opioids, are often given to control pain and anxiety in the first stage of labor. In uncomplicated labors in which episiotomy is not required, systemic medications alone may provide adequate analgesia throughout labor and delivery. Frequent intravenous administration of small doses is preferred, because of predictable pharmacokinetics. As equianalgesic doses of different opioids cause similar degrees of respiratory depression, choice among opioids is dictated by their duration of action. Long-acting opioids, such as morphine, largely have been abandoned. Meperidine, still the most frequently used opioid in obstetrics, is being replaced by the agonists-antagonists, such as butorphanol and nalbuphine. Patient controlled analgesia (PCA) is becoming more widely used for pain control during labor.

Although careful testing reveals some impairment of neonatal neurobehavioral function after even small doses of opioids, deficiencies persist only for a day or two and do not affect subsequent neonatal feeding, weight gain, or development. Opioid-induced respiratory depression is rapidly antagonized by naloxone both in mother and newborn. Because naloxone given before delivery may cause vomiting, hypertension, and extreme discomfort, naloxone is not given to any but the most depressed parturients and is reserved for the newborn. If the mother has used opioids for a long period, her habituated newborn may suffer opioid withdrawal if given naloxone.

Tranquilizers, including the antihistamines, phenothiazines, benzodiazepines, and butyrophenones, have been given with opioids to provide sedation, to allay anxiety, and to diminish nausea and vomiting. Their use has diminished as most women choose to be awake and alert for delivery and as the widespread use of regional anesthesia has made more evident the disadvantages of tranquilizers. In the presence of pain, tranquilizers given alone may lead to confusion and delirium. The drugs rapidly cross the placenta; they may depress neonatal muscle tone, respiration, and temperature regulation, and are without effective antagonists. Barbiturates and scopolamine, popular several decades ago for sedation and amnesia (twilight sleep), are rarely used in modern obstetrics.

Ketamine, a dissociative anesthetic, is a potent analgesic against somatic pain. Small intravenous doses (0.25 mg per kg) yield profound analgesia and amnesia lasting from two to five minutes; with such small doses, consciousness is retained while hallucinations and unpleasant dreams are uncommon. Ketamine is most useful in providing rapid onset of analgesia of a short duration for spontaneous vaginal delivery, vacuum extraction, or forceps delivery. Total doses larger than 1 mg per kg may cause loss of consciousness and increased uterine tone in the mother, and respiratory depression and muscle rigidity in the newborn.

INHALATION ANALGESIA

The inhalation of subanesthetic concentrations of anesthetics provides analgesia for vaginal delivery. John Snow first described a technique using chloroform. Advantages include rapid onset of analgesia, maintenance of protective airway reflexes, absence of significant maternal and neonatal depression regardless of duration of analgesia, little effect on uterine activity or the urge to bear down, and rapid maternal recovery. These advantages obtain only when the mother remains awake and responsive to command. Drawbacks of the technique include the potential for delirium and excitement (second stage of anesthesia), and the need for constant supervision to avoid unconsciousness. Self-administered inhalation analgesia for the first stage of labor has been largely abandoned in the United States because of the hazards of unsupervised use of anesthetics. Continuous administration of 30 to 50 per cent nitrous oxide usually provides effective analgesia for the latter part of labor, delivery, and postpartum examination. Forceps delivery is often possible with inhalation analgesia, if supplements such as small doses of ketamine, local anesthetic infiltration of the perineum, or pudendal block are added.

GENERAL ANESTHESIA

General anesthesia is rarely appropriate for vaginal delivery. Because it results in loss of maternal bearing down, induction must be delayed until birth is imminent. In addition to increasing the likelihood of pulmonary aspiration, forceps or vacuum extraction deliveries, and newborn depression, general anesthesia denies the mother the birth experience and delays bonding. In the past, general anesthesia at greater than two MAC of a potent inhalation agent (halothane 1.5 to 2 per cent) was used to inhibit uterine contractions, either to terminate tetanic contractions or to allow intrauterine manipulation for removal of a retained placenta. If required, uterine relaxation is now more rapidly and safely produced with intravenous tocolytics, such as beta-2 agonists, nitroglycerin and magnesium sulfate, or with inhalation of amyl nitrite.

The most valid indication remaining for general anesthesia during vaginal delivery occurs when the mother becomes physically uncontrollable during delivery. Anesthesia management is similar to that described later for cesarean section.

REGIONAL ANESTHESIA

Of the many techniques of regional anesthesia described for labor and delivery, only local infiltration of the perineum, bilateral pudendal nerve block, subarachnoid block, and epidural block, including both the lumbar and caudal approach, are now in common use. Bilateral lumbar sympathetic block at L2, except in rare instances, offers no advantage over segmental epidural block at T10 to L1. Paracervical block has been abandoned largely because of the unpredictable occurrence of fetal bradycardia accompanied by fetal acidosis and even death. In the vaginal delivery of a dead fetus, paracervical block is useful in eliminating pain arising from cervical dilation and uterine contraction. It also provides excellent analgesia for postpartum curettage or repair of a cervical laceration.

Bilateral Pudendal Nerve Blocks. These blocks are usually performed before delivery by the obstetrician, using a transvaginal or a transcutaneous approach with the mother in lithotomy position. Most of the somatic pain associated with stretching of the vagina and perineum is eliminated, but because the overlapping innervation of the perineum by the ilioinguinal nerve and the genital branch of the genitofemoral nerve remains intact, the urge to bear down is not abolished. The block provides complete anesthesia for episiotomy and repair, and is usually sufficient for low forceps delivery; supplementation with inhalation analgesia is required for mid-forceps application. The blocks require 8 to 10 ml of 1 per cent lidocaine or the equivalent on each side. Onset usually occurs within five minutes. Pudendal block is not associated with maternal or fetal side effects, nor does it impede the progress of labor.

Subarachnoid Block. Either a true saddle block from L5 to S5, or a modified saddle block extending from T10 to S5 is useful for delivery. Saddle blocks are usually done with the subject sitting, using a hyperbaric solution of tetracaine, bupivacaine, or lidocaine. For true saddle block, lumbar puncture is performed at the L4-L5 or the L5-S1 interspace, using 3 to 4 mg of tetracaine, 4 to 5 mg of bupivacaine, or 25 to 30 mg of lidocaine. The patient remains sitting for two to three minutes after the injection. Adequate anesthesia is provided for forceps application and episiotomy, without abolishing uterine pain.

Modified saddle block (T10) is accomplished by injecting 5 to 6 mg tetracaine, 6 to 8 mg bupivacaine, or 40 to 50 mg lidocaine at L3-4 and keeping the patient sitting for only 30 seconds. Not only does this block yield profound perineal analgesia, but the resultant T10 sensory level gives complete uterine pain relief, allowing cervical and uterine manipulation. The addition of 0.2 to 0.3 mg of epinephrine or 0.5 to 1.0 mg of phenylephrine prolongs tetracaine analgesia to three hours or more, which makes this block useful for analgesia for the latter part of the first stage of labor. Onset of analgesia is rapid, permitting injection just before delivery, making this an excellent choice when analgesia is required for urgent vaginal delivery in which forceps or vacuum extraction may be indicated.

Severe hypotension may appear within a minute following injection; it is best prevented as described previously for the supine hypotensive syndrome, by left uterine displacement and rapid intravenous infusions. Treatment includes these measures and the intravenous injection of 10 to 15 mg of ephedrine or mephentermine. Drugs used successfully in other patients to treat hypotension following regional anesthesia, such as norepinephrine, methoxamine, phenylephrine, dopamine, or dobutamine, restore maternal blood pressure but have been shown in animal studies to compromise uterine blood flow; they are best avoided. Recently, small doses of phenylephrine (20 to 40 μg) given intravenously in uncomplicated human pregnancies had been found as effective as ephedrine in restoring blood pressure after subarachnoid block, with no adverse effects on the fetus.

Although subarachnoid block abolishes the mother's bearing-down reflex, this can be be overcome by coaching her to push during contractions. In occiput transverse or posterior presentations, saddle block allows manual, forceps or vacuum rotation, or simply delivery in the posterior presentation over a large episiotomy.

Of all patients undergoing subdural puncture, gravid women have the greatest incidence of headache. This complication is best avoided by choosing a 25- or 26-gauge needle, and facing the bevel to the side so as to split and not sever dural fibers. The 24-gauge Sprotte pencil-point needle, or a 29-gauge needle passed through an introducer also produce few headaches. Adequate postpartum hydration (at least 3000 ml per day, oral or intravenous) and use of a tight abdominal binder when the patient is upright may reduce the incidence and severity of headache. Although widely recommended in the past, keeping the patient supine in bed for a fixed period of time after lumbar puncture is of no benefit in decreasing the incidence of headache (see Chapter 18).

Continuous Lumbar Epidural Analgesia. Continuous lumbar epidural analgesia has largely supplanted all other types of analgesia for vaginal delivery, as it provides an essentially pain-free labor and delivery without measurable neonatal depression. Epidural block is usually begun during the active phase of labor when pain occurs, usually at 5 to 6 cm cervical dilation in the primagravida or at 4 to 5 cm in the multipara; anesthesia may begin earlier if the patient experiences severe pain. Epidural block is also useful for trial of labor, as for an attempted vaginal birth after cesarean section (VBACS). An epidural to a T10 sensory level does not block signs of uterine dehiscence, but provides excellent analgesia for the trial of labor. Should the trial fail, the level of anesthesia can be raised to the required T4 level needed for cesarian section. After the epidural catheter has been inserted at L2-3 or L3-4 and the results of giving a small test dose are satisfactory (see Chapter 18), the anesthetic is begun with a total of 10 to 12 ml of 0.125 to 0.25 per cent bupivacaine, 1 to 1.5 per cent lidocaine, or 2 per cent chloroprocaine. This produces a T10 sensory level that blocks visceral pain from cervix and uterus.

Anesthesia is maintained by repeated injections or continuous infusion of a dilute local anesthetic solution, such as 0.125 per cent bupivacaine, at a rate of 10 to 12 ml per hour. Later, the somatic pain of vaginal stretching is alleviated by injecting 10 to 14 ml of an anesthetic solution of the same or greater concentration. Placing the patient in the sitting position during this injection does not improve the quality of the perineal analgesia. This injection provides a pain-free second stage as well as satisfactory conditions for delivery and episiotomy repair.

Lumbar epidural block for labor is a major anesthetic undertaking, requiring frequent monitoring of maternal vital signs, fetal heart rate, and uterine contractions. Because the mother loses the sensation of uterine contraction, continuous monitoring of those contractions is required when labor has been induced or augmented with oxytocin. Hypotension after epidural block is slower in onset than that following subarachnoid block, but can be just as severe. Like spinal anesthesia, epidural anesthesia abolishes the urge to bear down; the mother can be coached to bear down effectively with contractions.

Continuous Caudal Block. Although formerly popular in obstetric anesthesia, this method has largely been replaced by continuous lumbar epidural block, which is more reliable, easier to perform, requires only about one half to two thirds the amount of local anesthetic, and can be reliably extended to permit cesarean section. The caudal approach may be useful in patients in whom a lumbar epidural anesthetic is not feasible.

Anesthesia for Cesarean Section

The incidence of cesarean delivery has increased over the past two decades from less than 10 per cent to nearly 20 per cent of all deliveries. Despite a modest increase in maternal morbidity, cesarean delivery is associated with a marked decrease in neonatal mortality and morbidity compared with that accompanying a difficult vaginal delivery or intrauterine manipulation. Cesarean section may be performed as an elective procedure, as an urgent procedure (10 to 15 minutes) when progress of labor ceases or when there is evidence of a deteriorating intrauterine environment, or as an emergency procedure that permits no delay because of extreme fetal distress, a prolapsed umbilical cord, or maternal hemorrhage.

Anesthetic techniques for cesarean section fall into three categories: (1) regional anesthesia with spinal or epidural block, (2) general anesthesia, and (3) local infiltration.

REGIONAL ANESTHESIA

Regional anesthesia is often preferred because of freedom from neonatal depression and decreased risk of maternal pulmonary aspiration. In addition, the mother remains awake and can share in the birth experience. Although regional techniques take time to perform (making them most suitable to elective cesarean section), they are also feasible for urgent operations in the hands of a skilled operator; subarachnoid anesthesia can even be used for emergency cesarian section if the mother's condition permits. Contraindications to regional anesthesia include uncorrected maternal hypovolemia, infection at or near the site of spinal or epidural injection, septicemia, neurologic abnormality, severe coagulopathies, or the mother's refusal.

Subarachnoid or epidural block to at least the T4 sensory level provides satisfactory conditions for cesarian section. In the past, T6 sensory levels were considered adequate for cesarean section, but briefer operations carried out through a high classical uterine incision were the rule. The low cervical incision now popular requires additional time, more abdominal retraction, and extra-abdominal repair of the uterus, requiring a high sensory level (T4 to T2) to minimize the visceral pain associated with these maneuvers. Subarachnoid block with hyperbaric tetracaine 8 to 11 mg (or hyperbaric bupivacaine, 12 to 15 mg, or hyperbaric lidocaine, 65 to 80 mg) usually provides these levels.

Severe maternal hypotension follows almost immediately such high subarachnoid blocks unless left uterine displacement and fluid loading with at least 15 ml per kg of balanced salt solution precede the block. The incidence of hypotension can also be reduced by giving prophylactic ephedrine, either 50 mg intramuscularly ten minutes before the block, or 10 to 25 mg intravenously immediately following subarachnoid injection. If hypotension develops nevertheless, left uterine displacement, volume expansion, and ephedrine in 10 to 15 mg intravenous doses are effective treatments.

Because of the slower onset of hypotension and the diminished threat of headache, lumbar epidural block is often preferred over subarachnoid block for cesarean section. Onset of complete analgesia requires 15 to 20 minutes, depending on the local anesthetic chosen, but this need not hinder skin preparation or draping, and rarely delays skin incision. From 20 to 25 ml of 1.5 to 2 per cent lidocaine (or 0.5 per cent bupivacaine or 3.0 per cent chloroprocaine) usually produce an adequate T4 sensory level. Two thirds to three quarters of the initial dose are given at the first evidence of receding block.

The addition of 1:200,000 to 1:400,000 epinephrine to the local anesthetic solution, rarely contraindicated, both prolongs and intensifies the block and decreases initial maternal blood concentrations of the local anesthetic, without producing adverse effects on either uterine or placental blood flow. Because large doses of local anesthetic are used in the epidural space for cesarean section, accidental rapid intravascular injection of the drug is almost certain to produce convulsions and at times cardiac arrest, particu- Therefore, the total dose required is given in increments, pausing at least two minutes between each 5- to 6-ml dose and observing for signs and symptoms of toxicity. Because maternal deaths have followed accidental intravascular injection of 0.75 per cent bupivacaine, this concentration is no longer recommended for the obstetric patient. However, accidental rapid intravenous injection of equivalent amounts of lesser concentrations of bupivacaine produces similar results.

If the operation is not required for fetal distress and the mother's oxygenation and circulatory status are satisfactory, delays between the induction of anesthesia and uterine incision do not harm the newborn when spinal or epidural block is employed, allowing the surgeon to use careful techniques of dissection. A delay of more than three minutes between uterine incision and delivery may be associated with neonatal depression and acidosis.

GENERAL ANESTHESIA

General anesthesia is indicated in the true emergency situation to reduce delays in delivering the infant, when a mother prefers or requires this method, or when regional anesthesia is contraindicated. Several aspects of general anesthetic management require emphasis.

As described above, parturients are at special risk for aspiration pneumonitis. Clear antacids, metaclopromide, and H_2 blockers are helpful and rapid sequence induction and immediate intubation are required, unless the patient's airway anatomy is such as to require awake intubation. In fact, except in the most unusual circumstances, present standards of practice forbid general anesthesia without intubation for a gravid patient at any time after the first trimester.

When general anesthesia is given, neonatal depression is worsened by delays between induction and uterine incision, and by delays between uterine incision and delivery. Nothing is gained by delaying delivery to allow redistribution of drugs in fetal tissues. The condition of the infant is also improved by maintaining left uterine displacement and by providing the mother with an inspired oxygen concentration of at least 60 per cent before delivery, which appreciably increases neonatal oxygenation at birth.

Because only a minimal depth of general anesthesia is necessary to provide sufficient analgesia and amnesia before delivery, induction requires either thiopental 4 mg per kg or ketamine 1.0 mg per kg, usually not exceeding a total dose of 250 mg or 75 mg, respectively. Maternal awareness is prevented by maintaining end-tidal concentrations of two thirds MAC of a potent inhalant such as 0.5 per cent halothane, 0.75 per cent isoflurane, or 1.0 per cent enflurane. Following delivery, the nitrous oxide concentration can be increased, small amounts of narcotics, thiopental or other sedatives may be given intravenously, and the volatile agent continued in the concentrations given above, to decrease the requirement for neuromuscular block, without impairment of uterine contractions.

Both depolarizing and nondepolarizing neuromuscular blockers cross the placenta in varying degree. Full blocking doses of nondepolarizing neuromuscular blockers given before birth may cause neonatal weakness.

LOCAL INFILTRATION

Local infiltration is rarely employed today, except when competent anesthetic care is not available. It is time consuming and requires large amounts of local anesthetic. Because it does not produce complete analgesia, the patient may require heavy sedation or general anesthesia.

Intraspinal Narcotics for Obstetric Anesthesia

Intraspinal narcotics have assumed a major role in obstetric anesthesia (see also Chapters 10 and 36) because they produce excellent analgesia with no motor or sympathetic block. Epidural injection of narcotics alone results in limited analgesia that is usually inadequate for the first stage of labor, and always requires supplementation for delivery and episiotomy repair. However, fentanyl (50 to 75 μg) or morphine (3.5 to 5.0 mg) placed in the epidural space following cesarean section provides excellent postoperative analgesia lasting 2 to 4 hours or up to 24 hours, respectively.

Adding fentanyl to the local anesthetic solutions used for epidural analgesia speeds the onset of anesthesia and prolongs the duration. Fentanyl 50 to 100 μg added to the local anesthetic significantly decreases visceral discomfort and improves the quality of the epidural block for cesarean section. Adding 50 μg of fentanyl to dilute solutions of local anesthetics, such as 0.125 per cent bupivacaine, results in equivalent levels of sensory analgesia, but far less motor block than is produced by more concentrated solutions of local anesthetic alone. In a continuous epidural infusion, a solution of fentanyl 1 to 2 μg per ml and 0.0625 per cent bupivacaine infused at 10 to 12 ml per hour maintains excellent analgesia with minimal motor block.

Subarachnoid injection of either 25 to 50 μg fentanyl or 0.25 to 0.5 mg morphine alone or in combination results in a faster onset of more profound analgesia than does epidural administration. Combined with pudendal blocks for delivery, subarachnoid morphine provides satisfactory (although not complete) analgesia for labor and vaginal delivery with no sympathetic and minimal motor block. The addition of 15 to 20 μg fentanyl or 0.15 to 0.2 mg morphine to the local anesthetic used in spinal anesthesia for cesarean section both improves the quality of the block and provides excellent postoperative analgesia. Doses of intraspinal fentanyl less than 100 mg have not been associated with adverse effects on the newborn.

The side effects of intraspinal narcotics and their treatment are described in Chapter 36. They are no more severe in women who have just given birth than in other patients and are easily managed by limiting doses, carefully observing patients, and the appropriate use of small doses of naloxone.

PREECLAMPSIA AND ECLAMPSIA

The special management of difficulties such as breech presentations or twin births, parturients with intercurrent diseases such as diabetes, and the diseases such as abruptio placentae which complicate pregnancy, is beyond the scope of this chapter. However, preeclampsia and eclampsia are common and affect strongly planning for anesthesia. Of obscure origins, but involving decreased placental perfusion and excesses of angiotensin, renin and aldosterone, the syndrome becomes evident in the second half of pregnancy. Proteinuria, hypertension, and often edema characterize preeclampsia, which progresses to eclampsia when convulsions occur. Other findings include depressed renal function, coagulopathy, hyperreflexia, and fetal distress.

Although these hypertensive patients retain water and gain excessive weight, they are functionally hypovolemic with a contracted intravascular space. As do other hypertensive patients, preeclamptic parturients respond with exaggerated hypertension to painful stimuli, intubation, and vasoconstrictors, and with exaggerated hypotension to the vasodilating effects of general anesthetics and spinal or epidural anesthesia. Because it blocks sympathetic responses to pain and has minimal ill effects on the fetus, epidural anesthesia is a good choice for labor and delivery, whether vaginal or cesarean, but several precautions are required for safety. Before an epidural puncture, impaired coagulation must be ruled out by testing. Generous fluid loading will prevent catastrophic hypotension, but a central venous or pulmonary artery catheter may be needed to guide fluid replacement. Because placental perfusion is already compromised, even small decreases in blood pressure may not be tolerated, and close fetal monitoring is a necessity. Lastly, because these patients may overreact to vasopressors, small doses are used at first.

When administering general anesthesia, as for an emergency cesarean operation, the use of muscle relaxants is complicated by the magnesium sulfate the patients receive. Magnesium potentiates both depolarizing and nondepolarizing muscle relaxants, which nevertheless can be used safely if given in reduced doses with careful monitoring.

DRUGS USED IN OBSTETRICS THAT AFFECT ANESTHETIC MANAGEMENT

Drugs obstetricians use to enhance or retard labor, or to treat preeclampsia-eclampsia have im-

TABLE 26–1. Obstetric Drugs Affecting Anesthetic Management

Drug	Use	Side Effects/Interactions	Avoidance/Treatment of Side Effects
Oxytocin (synthetic) (10 to 30 units/L IV)	Induce/augment labor Minimize postpartum blood loss	Vasodilation, decreased blood pressure Sinus tachycardia, increased CO Rare ST-T changes Antidiuresis and water retention	Avoid concentrated bolus infusion i.e., 10 units IV Instead mix in IV bag 10 to 30 units and run rapidly
Ergot derivatives (0.2 mg IM)	Stimulate uterine contractions	Hypertension, nausea, agitation Severe hypertensive interaction with vasopressors	Avoid IV injection or slowly fractionate IV injection Prefer IM injection
Prostaglandins ($F_2\alpha$:250 μg IM q 20	F_2: Stimulate cervical ripening	Increased lung resistance	Administer IM or subcutaneously
	F_2: Potent uterine contraction stimulant Postpartum atony	Nausea, vomiting, temperature elevation F_2:α: Hypertension, uterine rupture, DIC	Do not give IM or intramyometrial
Beta-2 agonists	Inhibit or arrest preterm labor Relax uterus for external version Treat hyperactive or tetanic uterine contractions	Maternal and fetal tachycardia Hypotension, increased cardiac output, nausea, vomiting, tremor Postpartum uterine atony Cardiac arrhythmias, maternal hypokalemia, hyperglycemia Pulmonary edema associated with steroid therapy, and rapid hydration Risk of arrhythmia during general anesthesia	Some suggest preferable to wait 1 hr if possible before proceeding to anesthesia for cesarean In an emergency, ethrane preferred over halothane Hypokalemia and hyperglycemia do not require therapy
Magnesium	Preeclampsia-eclampsia and preterm labor inhibition	Competes with calcium at the neuromuscular junction, may result in muscle weakness, respiratory embarrassment or rarely cardiac arrest Addition to all neuromuscular blockers	After full induction dose of succinylcholine, use nondepolarizers sparingly if at all, twitch monitor recommended Risk of postoperative hypoventilation Do not treat magnesium weakness with calcium

portant systemic effects which must be taken into account when planning anesthesia management. These drugs and their important effects are summarized in Table 26–1.

Perinatology

The anesthesiologist must be familiar with perinatology so as to manage the mother's anesthetic and to resuscitate the newborn when needed. Close observation of the fetus before and during labor permits early diagnosis of asphyxia and expeditious delivery. Fetal monitoring takes two forms: physical monitoring (fetal heart rate) and, less often used, biochemical monitoring (fetal blood pH).

BIOPHYSICAL MONITORING

Recent studies of neonatal outcome have raised questions about the value of electronic fetal heart rate monitoring, which may be no better than auscultation of the fetal heart by persons well trained in evaluating uncomplicated labor. The technique is still commonly employed in managing high-risk pregnancies. Fetal heart rate is determined either from the fetal electrocardiogram (ECG) obtained from an electrode placed on the presenting part of the baby, or from an ultrasound Doppler device placed on the mother's abdomen. Uterine contractions are likewise monitored either directly, via a catheter inserted through the cervix into the uterine cavity, or indirectly via a tocodynamometer, a pressure-recording device placed on the ab-

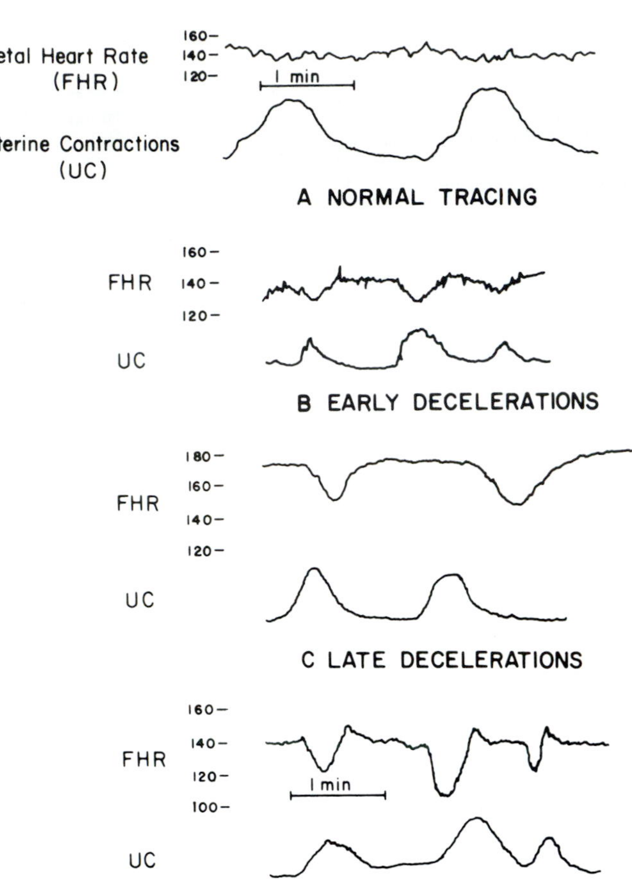

FIGURE 26–3. Bioelectronic monitoring of fetal heart rate (FHR) and uterine contractions (UC).

domen. A continuous, simultaneous tracing of fetal heart rate and uterine contractions is recorded on paper (Fig. 26–3).

The normal fetal heart rate is 120 to 160 beats per minute, with a normal variability (measurable only from the fetal ECG) that includes both short-term (up to 5 beats per minute) and long-term (up to 15 beats per minute) changes (Fig. 26–3A). Absence of this variability is ominous and indicates fetal acidosis unless it can be attributed to other causes, such as prematurity, maternal fever, or the use of drugs such as opioids, tranquilizers, anticholinergics, magnesium, and some local anesthetics.

Decreases of fetal heart rate (called "decelerations" by obstetricians) and their relation to uterine contractions provide clues to fetal health. Three basic types have been described:

1. *Early uniform deceleration* is the mirror image of uterine contraction: it begins and ends with contraction, and the nadir of the fetal heart rate corresponds to peak contraction (Fig. 26–3B). Compression of the head and not acidosis or fetal distress produces these changes. Although abolished by anticholinergics, early uniform deceleration do not require treatment.

2. *Late uniform deceleration* resembles early deceleration but is out of phase with contractions: the fetal heart rate does not begin to decrease until after the start of the contraction, reaches its slowest rate after the peak of intrauterine pressure has passed, and does not return to baseline until the contraction has ceased (Fig. 26–3C). This pattern implies uteroplacental insufficiency associated with fetal acidosis, hypoxia, and distress, and, often, the need for expeditious delivery. Uteroplacental and intervillous circulatory insufficiency may result from aortocaval compression, maternal hypotension, or rapid or prolonged uterine contractions that can be corrected, with the resulting improvement in fetal health reflected in the tracing.

3. *Variable deceleration* is the most common

type, occurring in over 50 per cent of labors. Although associated with uterine contractions, bradycardia is irregular, and occurs at various times throughout contractions (Fig. 26–3D). These decelerations accompany umbilical cord compression and stimulation of baroreceptor reflexes, and are thought to represent increases in vagal tone. Unless they are prolonged beyond 30 seconds, are associated with bradycardia of less than 70 beats per minute, show loss of fetal heart-rate variability, or have an increased baseline heart rate, they are usually benign. Changing the maternal position often lessens or abolishes this pattern.

Evaluation of the high-risk pregnancy before labor and employing external noninvasive fetal monitoring has been useful. The non stress test employs changes in fetal heart rate as associated with spontaneous movements or contractions in a healthy fetus. The contraction or oxytocin stress test monitors heart rate in relation to oxytocin-induced contractions, stimulated at a rate of three every ten minutes. Late uniform decelerations occurring in over half of the contractions indicate a compromised fetal environment and the need for expeditious delivery, usually by cesarean section.

A more comprehensive antepartum biophysical fetal profile incorporates the non stress test and four variables determined by ultrasonic imaging: (1) breathing movements; (2) gross body movements; (3) muscle tone; (4) amniotic fluid volume. Each of the five items is scored 0 or 2. A total score of 8 or 10 characterizes a normal fetus, a score of 4 or 6 suggests chronic asphyxia, while a score of 0 or 2 is indicative of severe chronic asphyxia and the need for prompt delivery.

BIOCHEMICAL MONITORING

Biochemical monitoring of the fetal blood pH during labor often complements electronic fetal monitoring. A sample of fetal capillary blood is taken from the presenting part via an endoscope inserted through the vagina into the cervix. A capillary blood pH of greater than 7.25 is considered normal, 7.21 to 7.25 is considered equivocal, and below 7.21 is considered acidotic, signaling fetal distress.

CARE OF THE NEWBORN IN THE DELIVERY ROOM

Birth is associated with transient neonatal asphyxia, which is spontaneously overcome by most newborns. Moderately or severely depressed neonates require prompt and effective therapy to aid in a rapid adaptation to extrauterine life and to prevent neurologic, circulatory, respiratory, and gastrointestinal problems.

From birth until the upper airway is cleared, the newborn's head is maintained below the level of the torso, in the sniffing position. The mouth and posterior pharynx are quickly cleared of secretions. Nasal suction and aspiration of gastric contents, often associated with bradycardia and further depression, are delayed until adequate respiration, circulation, and reflex activity are present. With the airway ensured, normal respiration usually appears. Gently slapping the soles of the feet encourages breathing, crying, and lung expansion; more vigorous forms of stimulation are traumatic, dangerous, and not effective. Should the neonate remain dusky or cyanotic despite normal respirations, oxygen is given via a tight-fitting face mask until color improves. Gentle assistance to breathing may prove helpful.

Immediate evaluation of a newborn is best accomplished by use of the Apgar score assessed at one and five minutes (Table 26–2). Resuscitation is not delayed until the one-minute score is ascertained. If the neonate does not respond to initial routine treatment, or if the one-minute score is less than 7, resuscitation is begun by following established guidelines (the "ABCs") of cardiopulmonary resuscitation (see Chapter 33).

Neonates remaining apneic, gasping, or with inadequate respirations require positive pressure ventilation. With the head in a sniffing position and an oral airway in place, ventilation is immediately attempted using a mask and breathing bag and oxygen concentrations in excess of 50 per cent, at 25 to 40 breaths per minute. Adequacy of ventilation is assessed by ascultation of the lungs. Although pressures up to 60 cm H_2O initially may be required to expand the newborn's lungs, lesser pressures may provoke gasping followed by a normal breathing pattern. If the lungs cannot be expanded or if the fetal heart rate remains below 100 beats per minute beyond 30 seconds, the trachea is intubated, followed by positive pressure breathing with oxygen. Unless pulmonary aspiration of meconium is suspected or heart sounds are absent, bag and mask ventilation precedes intubation, as this is frequently successful in initiating respirations and in improving oxygenation without the

TABLE 26–2. **The Apgar Score***

Sign	Score 0	1	2
Heart rate	Absent	<100 beats/minute	>100 beats/minute
Respiratory effort	Absent	Irregular, slow, gasping	Regular, rhythmic
Muscle tone	Limp	Some flexion of extremities	Active motion
Reflex response to stimulation	None	Grimace	Vigorous cry
Color	Pale, completely cyanotic	Body pink, extremities cyanotic	Completely pink

* The Apgar score at one minute is indicative of the degree of depression at birth. A score of 7 to 10 indicates minimal or no depression, 3 to 6 indicates moderate depression, and 0 to 2 indicates severe depression requiring vigorous resuscitation. The five-minute Apgar score suggests the severity of depression and the effectiveness of resuscitation.

delay and vagal responses associated with related to laryngoscopy. Ventilation is continued until breathing becomes regular and respiratory exchange adequate.

The fetus may aspirate meconium in utero, but more frequently aspiration occurs just after birth, causing mechanical obstruction, chemical pneumonitis, and even death. When the fetus is delivered through thick meconium in a vertex presentation, the obstetrician thoroughly clears the baby's oral and nasal pharynx by suction before delivery of the shoulders. If, at birth, the neonate does not breathe at once or if signs of respiratory obstruction are evident, tracheal intubation is performed immediately, but no attempt is made to begin positive pressure ventilation. Instead, meconium is aspirated by applying negative pressure directly to the tracheal tube. Tracheal suction may be required several times before adequate ventilation is possible.

A neonate born through meconium and breathing immediately is first given oxygen; laryngoscopy and intubation follow, to determine whether meconium is present below the cords. If meconium is found in the trachea, the cycle of oxygenation by mask, laryngoscopy, and tracheal suction via the endotracheal tube is repeated until no more meconium can be removed. If meconium is aspirated from the trachea, the baby is transferred to a neonatal intensive care unit (ICU) for appropriate intensive care under the direction of a neonatologist.

The newborn's heart rate rarely fails to increase to over 100 beats per minute when ventilation and oxygenation are established. Should cardiac arrest occur or the heart rate remain less than 100 beats per minute after adequate ventilation, closed chest cardiac compression at 120 per minute is begun and the trachea intubated, if this has not yet been accomplished. Positive pressure breathing is at the rate of one breath for every fifth chest compression. The sternum is compressed 1.5 to 2 cm at its midpoint, as illustrated in Figure 26–4; compression continues until a heart rate above 100 per minute is maintained. Elevation of the legs may improve venous return.

Severely depressed neonates inevitably suffer marked metabolic acidosis, requiring correction before the transition to neonatal circulation occurs. This is accomplished with 2 mEq per kg of sodium bicarbonate solution prepared by diluting the usual bicarbonate solution (7.5 or 8.4 per cent) with an equal volume of preservative-free water. The solution is injected into the umbilical vein over a two-minute period and repeated in three to five minutes, if there is no improvement. Further doses of bicarbonate are not given without first ascertaining serum electrolyte values, osmolality, and acid-base status. Bicarbonate administration causes an increase in Pa_{CO_2}, which requires enhanced ventilation. Hyperosmolar bicarbonate solutions have been implicated in the development of intracerebral hemorrhages, especially in the premature neonate. The doses recommended present little risk compared with the hazard of untreated metabolic acidosis.

A poor response to therapy suggests an intravascular fluid deficit, which can be treated with 10 ml per kg of balanced salt solution, or lesser amounts of 5 per cent albumin, packed red blood cells, or whole blood, depending on the hematocrit. Failure of the heart rate to respond to these

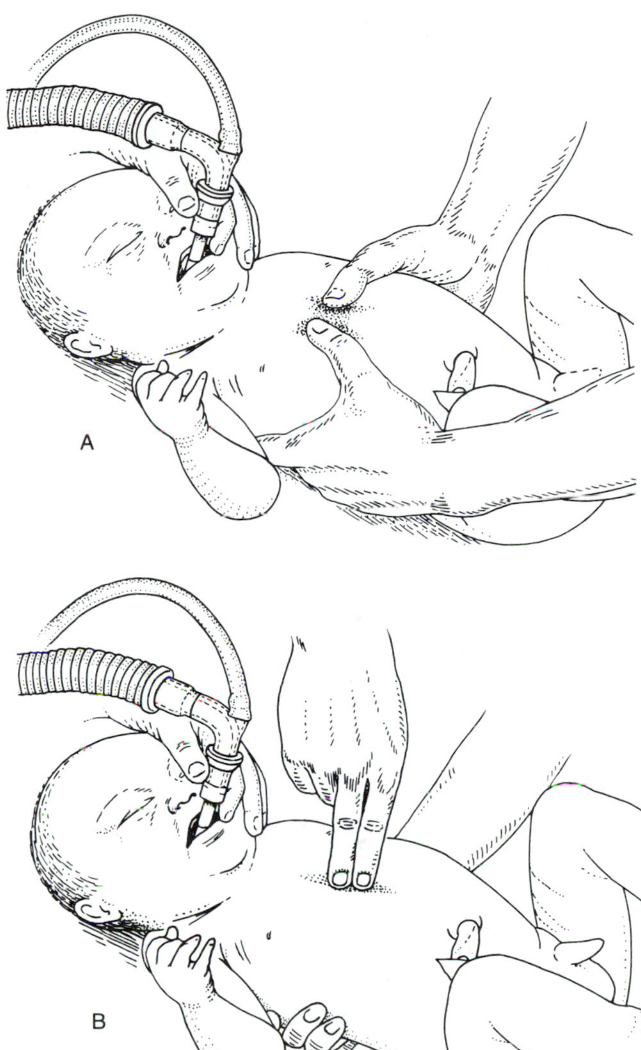

FIGURE 26–4. *Two methods of closed chest cardiac compression of the neonate.*

A, The two-thumb technique, in which the remainder of the fingers are interlocked behind the upper back. Note that the pressure is applied on the upper sternum just above the midline. Also note the continued ventilation of the neonate via an endotracheal tube.

B, The two-finger technique using the index and middle fingers of one hand. The other hand of the resuscitator is placed under the upper back to serve as a hard surface.

measures prompts the use of cardiac stimulants such as epinephrine (0.2 ml per kg of a 1:10,000 solution), calcium gluconate (1 to 2 ml per kg of a 10 per cent concentration), or both, given through an umbilical venous catheter and not by direct cardiac injection.

If opioids given to the mother have depressed the newborn's respiration, naloxone, 10 μg per kg, is given intravenously or intramuscularly. Because depression can recur when the effect of the naloxone dissipates, close observation is required. If respiratory depression does not respond to naloxone, there must be a cause other than opioids for the respiratory depression. If chronic maternal narcotic abuse is suspected, naloxone must be withheld from the neonate because it may cause sudden and disastrous withdrawal.

Its relatively large body surface area and inability to shiver render the neonate particularly vulnerable to rapid cooling. To prevent hypothermia, the infant is dried immediately and then placed fully exposed under a suitable warmer, protected from drafts. A newborn must never be placed naked on a metal surface, which serves as a heat sink.

Moderately or severely depressed neonates require pediatric evaluation and care in an intensive care facility. These babies frequently experience apneic episodes, respiratory distress, convulsions, and hypothermia, and may be unable to accept oral feedings. They may require monitored oxygen supplementation and ventilatory support.

APPRAISAL

Anesthetic management of the parturient is both demanding and different from that of a surgical patient. Conditions surrounding labor and delivery are often uncontrollable. The physiologic changes of pregnancy alone predispose even healthy parturients to such hazards as hypoxia, anesthetic overdose, hypertension, hypotension with regional anesthesia, and pulmonary aspiration. Management of anesthesia for delivery at the conclusion of high-risk pregnancies is even more challenging.

Today, many mothers and fathers wish to play an active role in delivery, helping make even more popular continuous epidural block, which has become the dominant form of obstetrical analgesia. The anesthesiologist who cares for the woman giving birth must put aside the comfortable routines of the operating room, but in return gains immeasurable satisfaction from playing an important role in the lives of parents and infant.

REFERENCES

Abboud TK, Shakuntala N, Murakawa K, et al. Comparison of the effects of general and regional anesthesia for Cesarean section on neonatal neurologic and adaptive capacity scores. Anesth Analg 1985; 64:996–1000.

James FW III, Wheeler AS, Dewan DM. Obstetric anesthesia: The complicated patient. 2nd ed. Philadelphia: FA Davis, 1988.

Moore TR, Key TC, Reisner LS, Resnik R. Evaluation of the use of continuous lumbar epidural anesthesia for hypertensive pregnant woman in labor. Am J Obstet Gynecol 1985; 152:404–412.

Shnider SM, Levinson G. Anesthesia for obstetrics. 2nd ed. Baltimore: Williams & Wilkins, 1987.

CHAPTER TWENTY-SEVEN

Geriatric Patients

Unless specifically restricted to obstetrical or pediatric patients, every anesthesiologist eventually becomes a subspecialist in geriatric medicine. Population demographics demonstrate unequivocally that elderly Americans, already numbering more than 20 million, are the fastest growing component of our society. With aging comes age-related disease, much of it responsive to surgical treatment. Typically, 25 per cent or more of patients undergoing surgery are 65 years of age or older. These patients require appropriate adjustments of their anesthetic, perioperative, and chronic pain management therapies. The sections which follow introduce the physiology of aging, the essentials of age-related disease, and their relevance to the design, execution, and outcome of anesthetic management.

Concepts of Gerontology

Determining the chronologic age at which people become "elderly" has always been an inexact process. Attempts to establish physiologic age using biologic markers of aging have yet to provide a useful alternative except, in some cases, to assess the effectiveness of experimental "anti-aging" therapies. Traditional descriptors of agedness are derived from estimates of *life expectancy*, a statistical term that describes the average number of years of life which remain to members of a specific population. These estimates assume stable environmental and socioeconomic conditions. The relative agedness of a population can then be quantified by determining what portion of society has more (or less) than a given number of years of life remaining. This approach still requires arbitrary division of a population into two or more subgroups.

Life span is a more idealized, biologic parameter. It describes maximal obtainable age; at approximately 110 to 115 years, human life span has not changed, as far as can be determined, throughout recorded history. To use an engineering analogy, life *span* is the "design life," or theoretical useful lifetime, of biological machinery. It is a goal realized only in an optimal and benign environment. In contrast, life *expectancy* is an empirical measure of functional longevity under realistic conditions, a "mean time between failures (MTBF)" applied not to equipment, but to people.

The concepts of life span and expectancy are not, unfortunately, of great utility in clinical practice, since under these circumstances individuals and not whole populations are of greatest concern. Conventional guidelines simply assume that the "geriatric" era begins at age 65 and continues until death. This senescent segment of adulthood can be further subdivided: those aged 65 to 74 years ("elderly"), 75 to 84 years ("aged"), or 85 years and older ("very old").

If free of disease, the active elderly person maintains a normal daily routine without major changes in lifestyle, although these individuals may instinctively adjust their level of physical activity to meet reduced capabilities. As one becomes aged, however, limitations in musculoskeletal strength, coordination, balance, and quickness require dramatic alteration in daily routine. In the discussion that follows, the terms elderly and geriatric will be used as they are most commonly employed—as synonyms for patients 65 years of age or older.

STUDIES OF AGING

Age-related changes that are not universal, or those in which severity or magnitude do not increase in direct proportion to advancing age, probably represent age-related disease, rather than the physiologic process of aging. Organ system function is also influenced by daily physical activity, genetic background, gender, and by exposure to environmental factors and chronic drug therapy. Increased awareness of factors other than age that may alter organ function in an elderly patient population has improved our understanding of the effects of aging on physiologic systems.

Cross-sectional clinical or experimental studies measure physiologic variables simultaneously in groups of young and elderly subjects. Easy to design and execute, these studies do not reliably exclude patients with subtle manifestations of age-related disease. In addition, cross-sectional studies fail to identify cohort-specific factors such as genetic background, nutritional deficiencies, or exposure to environmental contaminants which may have selectively and permanently altered organ system function in one of the two groups under study.

In contrast, *longitudinal* studies require investigators to obtain repeated measurements over a long period of time in an aging population. Each subject provides individual control values for comparison with subsequent measurements. Some subjects eventually manifest signs of age-related disease; when they do, they are excluded from the study, leaving behind a smaller study group free of defined disease. Although difficult and expensive to organize, longitudinal studies have made it clear that much age-related impairment of function of concern to anesthesiologists reflects disease rather than aging itself. Consequently, the details of experimental studies purporting to demonstrate effects of aging are of great importance; new data require substantial revision of the "conventional wisdom" regarding age-related changes in pharmacokinetics and cardiovascular physiology.

DEFINITION OF AGING

Aging is defined only in conceptual terms; the mechanism responsible for this phenomenon at biochemical or cellular levels remains undiscovered. Current hypotheses propose that aging may reflect a loss of capacity for nucleic acid synthesis or the inadequate scavenging of free-radical molecular species. Whatever the precise lesion, aging is a universal, progressive process that produces changes in both the structure and the function of tissues and organs during the adult and later years of life span.

Several corollaries of aging are also now well established. First, the peak of physical (somatic) maturation and organ system functional capacity occurs not in the second decade of life, but nearer the age of 30 years. In addition, most organ systems appear to be well maintained in health throughout the middle years. However, function declines rapidly in the eighth decade and beyond. Although at one time aging was thought to produce a simple, linear decline of all capacities with advancing years, the actual function of integrated organ systems changes in a complex manner. In addition, individual aging rates vary considerably, even in the absence of disease.

Those elderly patients who maintain functional capacities greater than usual are said to be "physiologically young." In contrast, when function declines early, patients are referred to as "physio-

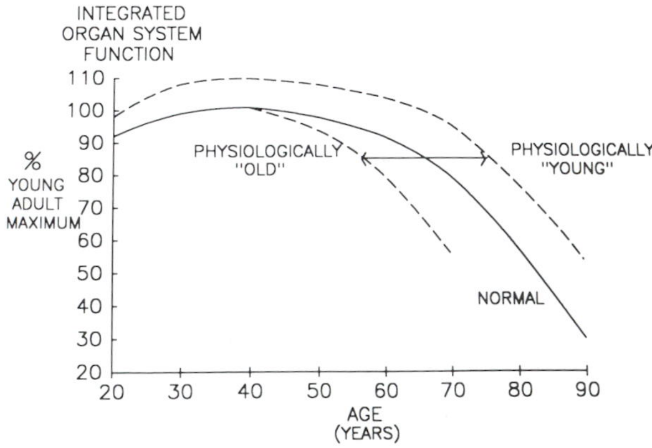

FIGURE 27–1 *Variability in the rate at which organ system function changes with increasing age explains the presentation of patients as physiologically "young" or "old."*

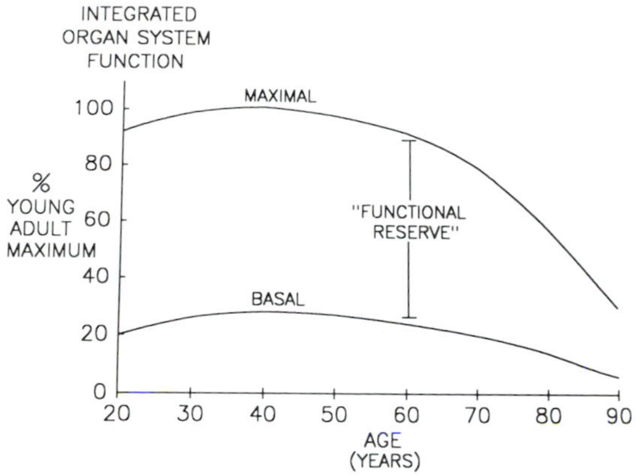

FIGURE 27–2 Age-related decline in organ system "functional reserve," defined as the difference between basal and maximal levels of function.

logically old" (Fig. 27–1). Estimating the relative physiologic age of geriatric patients during the preanesthetic evaluation assists not only in predicting outcome, but also in designing the anesthetic.

Maximal organ system capacity at all ages in healthy patients is greater than basal requirements. The difference between maximal capacity and basal levels of function represents *functional reserve*, used to meet the demands imposed by trauma, disease, surgery, and convalescence. Objectively assessed using various exercise or stress tests, functional reserve is progressively and significantly impaired in elderly patients (Fig. 27–2). Evidence of severely compromised cardio-respiratory reserve remains the most reliable predictor of poor outcome in a geriatric patient.

Cardiopulmonary Function

Cardiopulmonary function responds to physical activity and to the metabolic demands of the individual as a whole. Vigorous exercise or shivering may increase systemic oxygen consumption fivefold or more. Classic data suggesting that aging produces an irreversible reduction of resting cardiac output are not supported by more recent studies of fit and active elderly subjects in whom metabolic demands for cardiopulmonary function are maintained.

The modest decreases in resting cardiac index seen in most elderly subjects, largely resulting from a lower resting heart rate, are appropriate responses to the decreased metabolic requirements for oxygen that age imposes through muscle and major organ atrophy. Cardiac function itself is not the factor which limits cardiac index. The rates of myocardial shortening and ventricular pressure generation, two indices of myocardial contractility, remain uncompromised in healthy elderly subjects, at least under submaximal demand.

Aging does impose progressive limitations upon maximal heart rate. It also compromises the cardiac response to intense adrenergic stimulation and inotropic drugs. Although the elderly clearly suffer reduced maximal cardiac output and aerobic capacity, there are numerous individuals over 80 years old who retain sufficient capacity to work or compete as athletes.

Short-term demands for increased cardiac output appear to be met in the elderly patient largely by increased left ventricular diastolic volume and augmented preload; baroreflex-mediated changes in heart rate are reduced. The reduced compliance of the aged ventricle narrows the margin between inadequate filling pressure and volume overload making more critical the management of the rapid variations in central blood volume that are common during anesthesia and operation. Small decreases in venous return during positive pressure ventilation or surgical hemorrhage compromise stroke volume and may subsequently produce arterial hypotension. In contrast, rates of intravenous infusion which seem modest in young adults may nevertheless produce surprisingly large increases in atrial and pulmonary pressures in elderly patients, disrupting the balance of forces which control lung water. These acute stresses on cardiovascular and pulmonary function may precipitate iatrogenic pulmonary edema in elderly patients.

Aging also causes loss of arterial elasticity, with progressive stiffening of the arterial tree. These changes in vascular structure reduce the ability to store hydraulic energy, thereby increasing impedance and requiring greater cardiac work, leading to age-related hypertrophy of the left ventricular wall. Increased systolic and modestly reduced diastolic blood pressures yield a corresponding increase in arterial pulse pressure. The "overshoot" seen on radial artery waveform tracings and the discrepancy between invasive and cuff blood pressures increases progressively with age as the elasticity of large arteries decreases. Although more exaggerated in patients with established atherosclerotic disease, widening of arterial pulse pressure is a reflection of aging itself: it has been demonstrated even in populations where hypertensive vascular disease is virtually unknown.

Loss of tissue elasticity also appears to be the primary mechanism by which age exerts its effect on pulmonary function. Replaced by fibrous connective tissue, lung elastin content declines with advancing age. Consequently, even without disease, elderly patients experience emphysema-like increases in lung compliance. The changes are not uniform, impairing the match of ventilation and perfusion, increasing physiologic shunt and reducing the PaO_2. In the absence of disease, pulmonary functional reserve is adequate to maintain full oxygen saturation under most circumstances, although PaO_2 is significantly lower in elderly than in young adult patients before, during, and after surgery (Fig. 27–3). Elderly surgical patients require extra oxygen, particularly after abdominal surgery or drugs which depress respiration, including sedatives given for procedures done primarily under local or regional anesthesia.

Age-related loss of elastic tissue also produces progressive loss of lung recoil, enlarging residual volume (Fig. 27–4). Diminished tethering effects allow closing capacity (i.e., the lung volume at which small airway closure occurs) to decrease to within the range of lung volumes normally used for tidal breathing. With the breakdown of alveolar septae and a progressive reduction in the surface area available for gas exchange, aging increases both anatomic and alveolar dead space, impairing the efficiency of carbon dioxide excretion. There

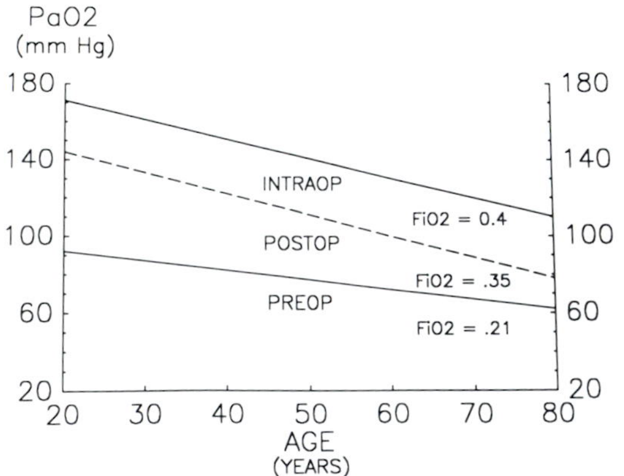

FIGURE 27–3 Preoperative, intraoperative, and postoperative arterial oxygenation all decrease progressively with increasing age, reducing the safety margin between ambient and minimally acceptable levels of arterial oxygen saturation.

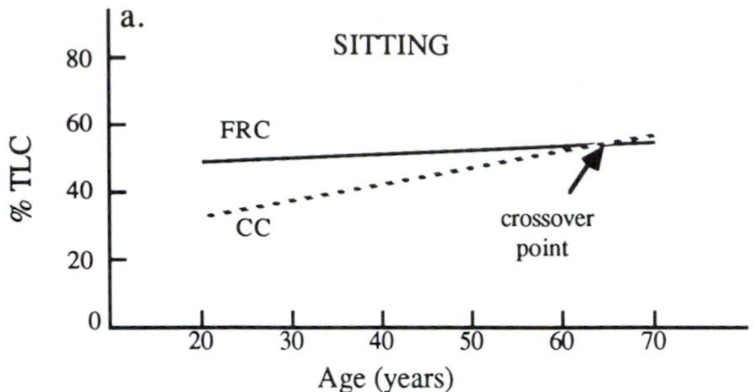

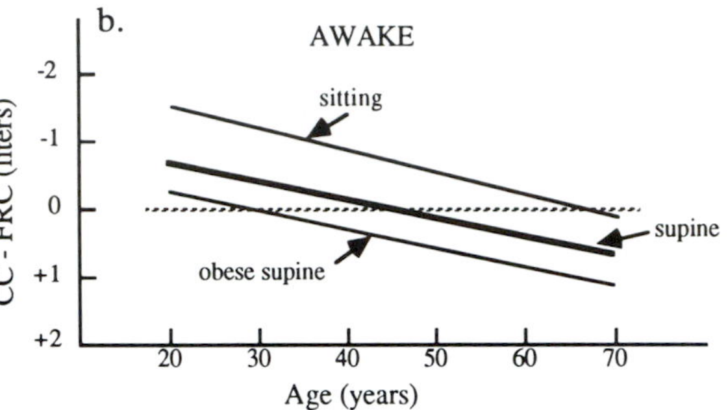

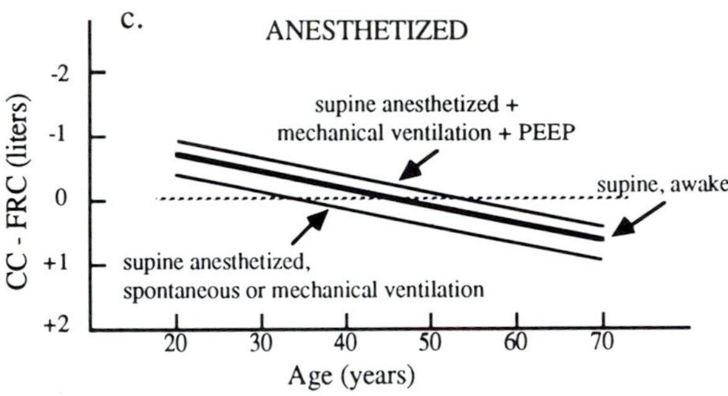

***FIGURE 27–4** Closing capacity (CC) and functional residual capacity (FRC) change with age in supine adults. CC and FRC change with age, posture, and anesthesia. It is suggested that gas exchange is progressively impaired as CC exceeds FRC, and these figures are based on data relevant to this hypothesis. Panel a, both FRC and CC increase with age because the elastic recoil of the lung is reduced. CC increases at a greater rate than FRC, and in the awake, sitting subject, CC = FRC (crossover point) at 65 years of age.*

Panel b, the difference, CC-FRC, is plotted against age, first for the sitting subject from panel a and then for a subject in the supine position. The cephalic movement of the diaphragm with the supine posture decreases the FRC but does not alter CC, so that the crossover point, when CC is greater than FRC, moves down to approximately 45 years. In obese subjects, the reduction of FRC is exaggerated further, and the crossover point is here shown at 30 years, although this is better expressed as a function of the weight-height relation.

Panel c, in anesthetized subjects, the difference between CC and FRC is worsened, unless PEEP is applied. (Reproduced with permission from Marshall BE. Pulmonary ventilation. In Marshall, BE, Longnecker, DE, Fairley HB, Eds. Anesthesia for thoracic procedures. Boston: Blackwell Scientific Publications, 1988:39–72.)

is no evidence of abnormal moment-to-moment regulation of ventilation or of altered sensitivity to small changes in carbon dioxide in healthy, alert subjects. However, elderly individuals respond less vigorously to hypoxia or hypercarbia and therefore require closer monitoring until completely recovered from anesthetics, analgesics, and other depressants.

HEPATORENAL FUNCTION

The primary effects of aging on hepatic physiology appear to be largely quantitative, not qualitative. Aging is associated with a marked reduction in liver size: one third of normal hepatic tissue mass in the young adult atrophies by the age of 80 years (Fig. 27–5). Splanchnic blood flow is reduced in proportion to hepatocellular attrition; thus, relative perfusion is maintained, but liver blood flow falls markedly when measured either in absolute terms or as a fraction of cardiac output. In effect, there is an age-related redistribution of perfusion.

Although plasma concentrations of transaminase and hepatic microsomal enzyme activity in elderly subjects are comparable to those of young adults, bromsulphalein (BSP) retention test results usually approach the upper limit of "normal" in the seventh decade of life. This test of overall hepatocellular capacity generally remains slightly abnormal even in healthy older patients. Although adequate to meet normal demands for coagulation factors and other specialized proteins, total hepatocellular synthetic activity is significantly reduced, and may be easily overwhelmed under conditions of maximal stress and surgical intervention. As they age, women more than men appear to maintain normal ranges of hepatic clearance for many drugs, especially the benzodiazepines. Women also may remain more susceptible to hepatic enzyme induction, especially with chronic cigarette smoking.

In the elderly patient, mild atrophy of renal parenchymal and cortical tissue is associated with a dramatic reduction in tissue vascularity. Total renal blood flow decreases by about 10 per cent, and glomerular filtration rate (GFR) by about 8 ml

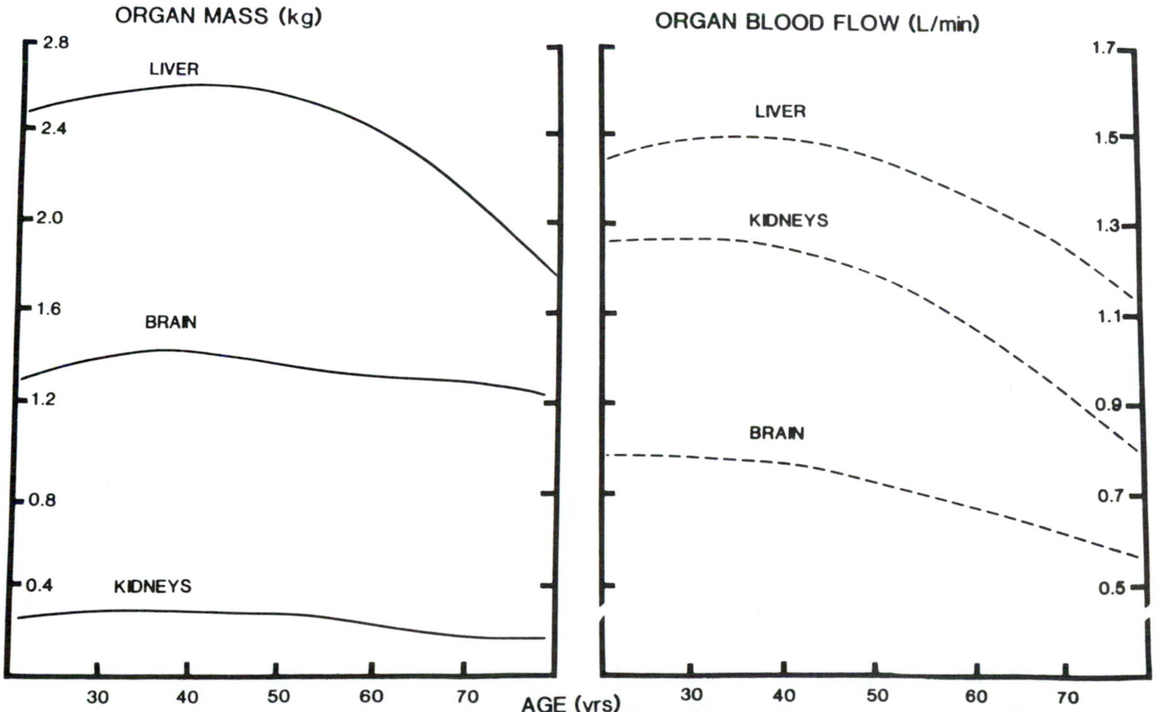

FIGURE 27–5 There are significant age-related changes in the tissue mass and blood flow of liver, brain, and kidney.

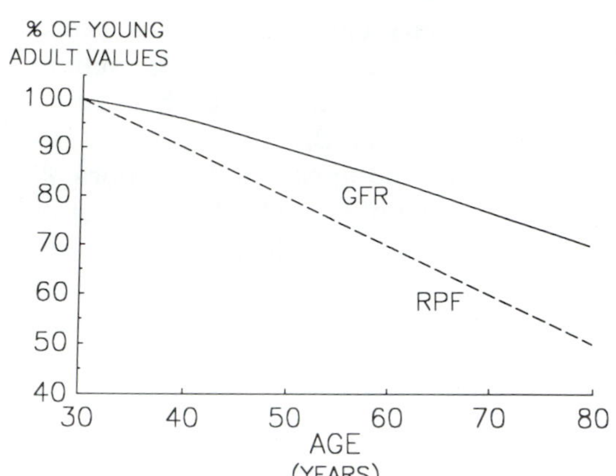

FIGURE 27–6 Age-related decline in glomerular filtration rate (GFR) and renal plasma flow (RPF). Data were obtained from longitudinal studies in which all patients showing evidence of renovascular disease were excluded.

per min per 1.73 m^2 during each decade of the middle adult years. Glomerular filtration rate declines somewhat more slowly than renal plasma flow (Fig. 27–6), because of compensatory increases in filtration fraction. Loss of nephron units is accelerated by age-related glomerular sclerosis, which produces anatomic continuity between the normally distinct afferent and efferent arterioles.

Aging reduces skeletal muscle mass and creatinine load. Serum creatinine in elderly patients may remain at levels normal for young adults, even though GFR decreases with age. Basal renal function is sufficient to avoid uremia, but functional reserve is reduced; elderly patients require careful preoperative preparation and intraoperative fluid and electrolyte management. Diminished thirst, poor diets, and diuretics make dehydration a more likely finding preoperatively in elderly patients. Responsiveness to antidiuretic hormone (ADH) and sodium conservation are impaired by aging, factors that also limit the capacity of elderly patients to respond to perioperative salt and water shifts.

Metabolism and Body Composition

The progressive loss of skeletal muscle mass and selective atrophy of metabolically active tissues in brain, liver, kidney, and other vital organs steadily reduce the metabolic requirements of healthy aging subjects. Resting body heat production decreases by about 15 per cent between young adulthood and senescence. A comparable reduction in heat production has been demonstrated intraoperatively: with increased heat loss due to less effective thermoregulation, elderly patients' body temperature decreases more than twice as fast as that of young adults.

Elderly patients have a progressive decrease in the ability to handle an intravenous glucose challenge. Age-related loss of skeletal muscle may contribute to this phenomenon, because these tissues normally provide storage for carbohydrates. Age-related glucose intolerance reflects either impairment of insulin function or antagonism of the ef-

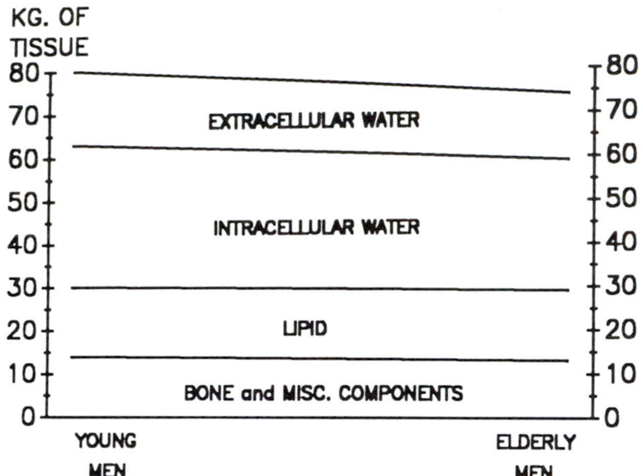

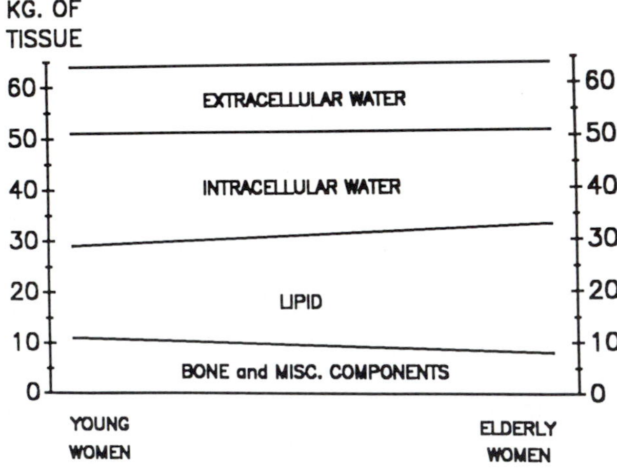

FIGURE 27–7 Typical changes in body composition for men and for women which occur by the age of 80 years, compared to those values measured in young adults. Aging produces atrophy of skeletal muscle mass with a corresponding contraction of intracellular water.

fects of this hormone. Insulin secretion itself appears to remain normal in both timing and magnitude.

By the age of 80 years, most elderly individuals gain about 12 kg of adipose. After moderate increases in the fourth, fifth, and sixth decades of life, total body weight falls rapidly, ultimately returning to or below young adult values because of an 8 kg loss of skeletal muscle mass and a 20 per cent reduction of total body water. However, despite the clinical impression that aging produces circulating hypovolemia, recent data obtained from healthy elderly subjects demonstrate that plasma and extracellular fluid volumes are actually well maintained. The essential factor in maintenance of circulating blood volume is daily physical activity. Virtually all of the age-related change in body water is limited to intracellular compartments (Fig. 27–7).

Aging increases the ratio of lipid to total body water in both sexes. This increases the steady-state distribution volumes for anesthetics and for other lipid-soluble drugs, while reducing the size of the hydrophilic compartment for neuromuscular blocking drugs and other highly charged molecules.

Central Nervous System Function

Age-related changes in the nervous system have direct consequences for the planning of anesthetics for elderly patients. Among the most important effects of age on the nervous system is the selective attrition of cerebral and cerebellar cortical neurons. There is exaggerated neuronal loss within the thalamus, locus ceruleus, and basal ganglia, areas normally involved in the synthesis of dopamine, catecholamines, serotonin, and other brain neurotransmitters. The susceptibility of the elderly to the side effects of the dopaminergic-blocking or anticholinergic drugs such as droperidol and scopolamine may be due to age-related reductions in neurotransmitter concentrations.

The intrinsic mechanisms by which the brain closely couples regional neuronal electrical activity, cellular metabolism, and blood flow appear to remain intact in the aged. Likewise, autoregulation of cerebral blood flow in response to changes in blood pressure, and cerebrovascular responsiveness to carbon dioxide remain active in the absence of disease or acute intracranial pathology. Because of the slight decline in the density of neuronal elements relative to the less active supporting components of the brain tissue, standard indices for cerebral blood flow and oxygen consumption (both traditionally expressed per 100 gm of brain tissue) exhibit a slight parallel decline with advancing years. Total brain mass is reduced by 30 per cent or more, however, and therefore absolute brain blood flow decreases markedly (Fig. 27–8), especially in the neuron-rich gray matter.

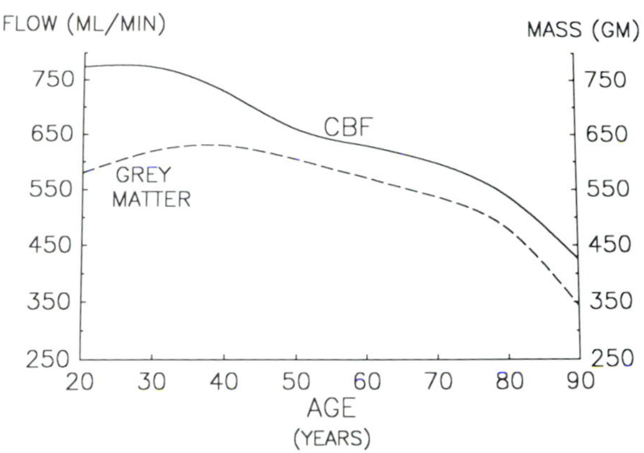

FIGURE 27–8 *Age-related changes in cerebral blood flow (CBF, solid line) occur largely as a consequence of neuronal attrition in grey matter (dashed line).*

Aging produces marked simplification of synaptic interconnections between neurons in cortical and some subcortical areas. There is deterioration of complex mental functions that rely upon short-term memory, visual and auditory reaction time, and other manifestations of "fluid intelligence." Even minimal perioperative sedation may produce amnesia or disorientation for surprisingly long periods of time in elderly patients, a special problem in those scheduled for outpatient surgery.

Aging increases thresholds for virtually all forms of perception including vision, hearing, touch, joint position, sense, smell, and temperature. These changes are so consistent and universal that objective measurements of summed sensory deficits may have value as biological markers of aging. Both central processes and degenerative changes within specialized end-organs contribute to what is, in effect, an age-related process of progressive deafferentation.

In contrast, complex afferent information such as pain continues to undergo extensive processing and modification within the central nervous system. Therefore, age-related deafferentation does not itself guarantee the elderly patient reduced postoperative pain. In fact, the more imminent threat of death or incapacitation may cause an elderly patient to experience more intense discomfort than might a young adult. Consequently, one cannot simply withhold from aged patients treatment for pain and anxiety out of concern for drug-induced complications. Instead, therapy must be individually adjusted to each patient's requirements.

PERIPHERAL NERVOUS SYSTEM

Aging produces a loss of peripheral nerve fibers. Both afferent and efferent nerve conduction velocities decrease progressively. Impairment of corticospinal transmission may also contribute to the increased time required from intention to onset of voluntary motor activity observed in elderly subjects. Fine muscle control and the ability to maintain postural steadiness also decline by the age of 80 years.

Reduced protoplasmic transport within motor nerve axons also deprives aging skeletal muscle of essential myotrophic support. Consequently, there is a loss of muscle mass and proliferation of skeletal muscle motor end-plate structures beyond their usual distribution immediately beneath the nerve terminal itself. These extrajunctional cholinoceptors may reduce the effectiveness of competitive nondepolarizing neuromuscular blocking agents, producing a subtle increase in initial dose requirement. Overall, the effect of aging on peripheral nerve and skeletal muscle is one of progressive disseminated neurogenic atrophy. In many elderly patients, however, lifelong habits of exercise and physical activity can maintain skeletal muscle strength surprisingly well.

Sympathoadrenal pathways, like the rest of the peripheral nervous system, are subject to age-related neuronal attrition and increased fibrosis. Adrenal tissue mass also decreases about 15 per cent by the age of 80 years. Nevertheless, plasma concentrations of epinephrine and norephinephrine are actually greater in elderly than in young adults, both at rest and in response to exercise-induced stress. Because autonomic end-organ responsiveness is markedly impaired by aging, the increased levels of plasma catecholamines are usually not clinically apparent unless abruptly suppressed. In effect, a "hyperadrenergic state" counterbalances the reduced effectiveness of aging autonomic end-organs. It represents a compensatory mechanism that partially restores the effectiveness of autonomic homeostasis.

Reduced autonomic end-organ responsiveness probably reflects a change in the quality, rather than a reduction in the quantity, of adrenoceptors. Receptor affinity for both beta-adrenergic agonists and antagonists declines with increasing age. Elderly patients have lesser increases in heart rate following isoproterenol, epinephrine, or atropine than do young adults, yet they also require greater doses of propranolol or esmolol in order to achieve effective receptor blockade. These changes in adrenoceptor function may be magnified further by reduced adenylate cyclase activity within the cell itself.

Whatever the precise site or mechanism, age-related changes in autonomic responsiveness im-

TABLE 27–1. Anesthetic Implications of Age-Related Physiologic Changes

Physiologic Change	Anesthetic Implications
Reduced central nervous system reserve	Decreased anesthetic requirement; prolonged residual depression
Neuronal atrophy in peripheral nervous system	Impaired autonomic responsiveness; slight increase in nondepolarizer dose requirements
Reduced renal blood flow, tissue loss	Reduced ability to handle salt and water loads; delayed excretion of many drugs
Reduced hepatic blood flow, tissue loss	Reduced rates of hepatic drug biotransformation; predisposition to coagulopathy
Decreased cardiac reserve, reduced ventricular compliance	Limitation of maximal cardiac output; intolerance of rapid changes in preload
Loss of pulmonary elasticity	Impaired matching of ventilation and perfusion, increased oxygen gradient
Decreased immune responsiveness	Susceptibility to stress-related infection and sepsis
Reduced skeletal muscle mass	Decreased heat production; relative glucose intolerance; increase in body lipid fraction

pose severe constraints upon the abilities of elderly subjects to maintain stable arterial blood pressures during the hemodynamic disruptions associated with anesthesia and operation. Hemodynamic variables normally subject to autonomic control are underdamped and less efficiently regulated. Baroreflex responsiveness, the vasoconstrictor response to cold stress, and beat-to-beat heart rate responses following postural changes in elderly subjects are less rapid in onset, lesser in magnitude, and less effective in stabilizing blood pressure than those of young adults. Intraoperative and postoperative extremes of arterial hypotension and hypertension are more frequent, more severe, and more often require treatment than those that occur in younger adults (Table 27–1).

CLINICAL PHARMACOLOGY

Elderly patients often require lesser doses of anesthetic drugs than do the young, but the explanations for this are often unclear. Changes in organ function and body composition imposed by aging affect both the pharmacokinetics and pharmacodynamics of drugs used in anesthesia. When short-acting anesthetics are injected intravenously, it may not be possible to completely distinguish between these two processes. Concentrations of drugs change so rapidly and in such a complex manner that the traditional two-compartment pharmacokinetic model describes poorly the early-phase relationships between drug dose, drug concentration, and drug effects.

More complex pharmacokinetic models have been used in an attempt (Fig. 27–9) to determine whether age-related increases in apparent drug potency represent actual enhanced tissue sensitivity to drug effects or the predictable consequences of plasma drug concentrations that are greater than expected. Elderly patients, however, have more variability in cardiac output and its subsequent distribution to peripheral tissues than do young adults. Consequently, much of the research re-

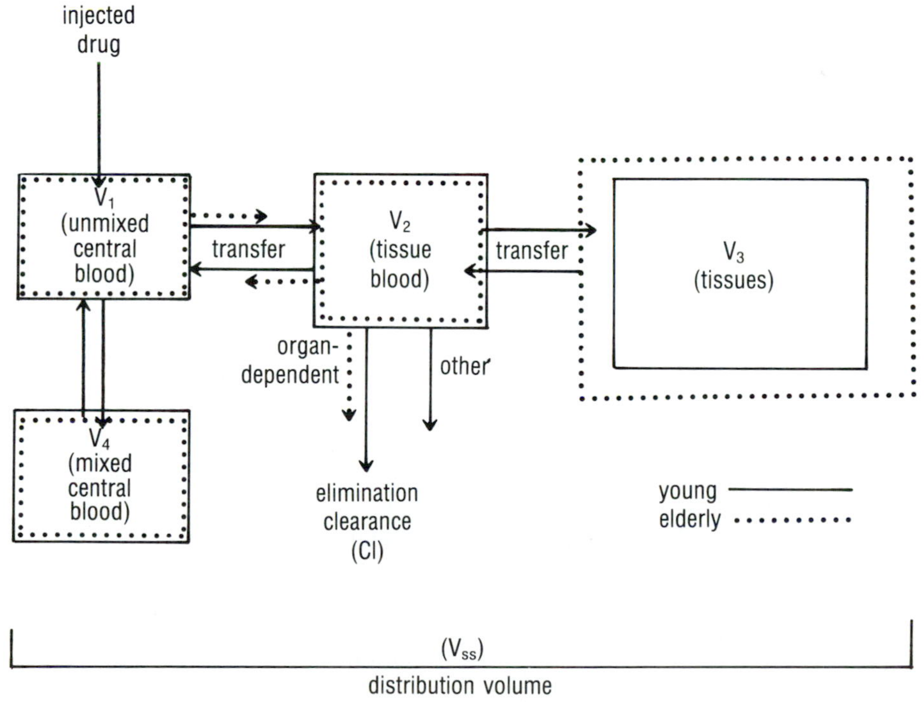

FIGURE 27–9 A proposed "four-compartment" pharmacokinetic model used to assess early-phase drug distribution in elderly subjects. High initial plasma concentrations of intravenous drugs may be due to delayed transfer from central to peripheral blood volume. Organ-dependent clearance is reduced, and the relative distribution volume of lipophilic drugs is increased in the elderly patient.

garding age-related changes in clinical pharmacology is noticeably inconsistent, and in some cases, actually contradictory.

Minimum alveolar concentrations (MAC) for inhalational anesthetics provide an index of drug requirement that is particularly useful for assessing the general effects of age on pharmacodynamics. The MAC is determined under steady-state conditions, avoiding some of the complex and unresolved pharmacokinetic uncertainties described above. Extensive experience with a wide variety of inhalational agents shows that beginning at the third decade of life, anesthetic requirement decreases by about 30 per cent over the next four or five decades (Fig. 27–10).

Data for narcotics, barbiturates, and benzodiazepines are much less consistent; it remains unclear whether the apparent age-related increase in their potency is real or simply reflects poor drug mixing within the central circulation. Interpretation of data is further confounded by difficulty in defining anesthetic end points. Complex analysis of the processed electroencephalogram (EEG) suggests that aging increases brain sensitivity to narcotics, but not to barbiturates or to etomidate. Clinical experience suggests a more generalized and more consistent reduction in dose requirement in elderly patients for virtually all drugs that depress the central nervous system.

Doses of the neuromuscular blocking drugs are changed little by the process of aging itself. Slightly impaired neuronal mobilization of acetylcholine is probably offset by increases in end-plate cholinoreceptor concentration. Consequently, the dose required initially to produce nondepolarizing neuromuscular blockade with pancuronium, vecuronium, curare, or atracurium is either unchanged or increased only slightly. The dynamics and the efficacy of antagonism or "reversal" of nondepolarizing neuromuscular blockade by neostigmine or by edrophonium are also unchanged. Pharmacokinetic factors in the elderly often prolong the duration of these drugs' clinical effects, but the choice of reversal agents, not patient age, determines the speed and completeness of return of neuromuscular function following a given level of blockade.

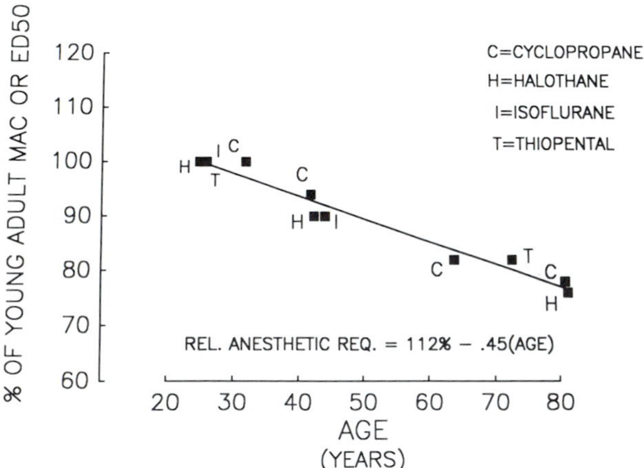

FIGURE 27–10 *Consistent linear age-related decline in relative anesthetic requirement (MAC or ED_{50}) for cyclopropane (C), halothane (H), isoflurane (I), and thiopental (T) in unsedated human subjects suggests a fundamental physiological mechanism rather than pharmacologically unique explanations.*

In contrast, succinylcholine dosage requirements are determined primarily by the available circulating mass of plasma cholinesterase, a quantity that reflects both cholinesterase concentration and plasma volume. Age appears to have little effect, although some elderly men reportedly have unexpectedly low levels of cholinesterase activity due to subclinical hepatocellular attrition, and may therefore experience prolonged blockade following the usual dose of this drug.

The pharmacokinetics of most intravenous anesthetics are dramatically altered by age. Elimination half-life ($t_{\frac{1}{2}}\beta$), the time required for a 50 per cent reduction of plasma drug concentration, is proportional to the rate of drug clearance and inversely proportional to the volume in which the drug is distributed. Aging impairs the clearance of virtually all drugs requiring hepatic or renal elimination and aging increases the fraction of total body weight which is lipid, increasing the distribution volume for lipid-soluble molecules. The elimination half-lives of almost all intravenous anesthetics, narcotics, and adjuvants is thus prolonged in the elderly.

In contrast, a few drugs such as atracurium and succinylcholine do not depend primarily upon renal or hepatic mechanisms for their biotransformation or elimination. Consequently, their durations of effect change little in the elderly patient.

With the possible exception of meperidine, reduced drug binding to plasma and tissue proteins reported to occur with advancing age is probably not pharmacokinetically important. Drug interactions and drug side effects may, however, occur

TABLE 27–2. Adjustments of Anesthetic and Adjuvant Drugs in Elderly Patients

Drug Group	Adjustment Needed
Potent inhalational agents	Decrease inspired concentration, allow more time for emergence
Barbiturates, etomidate, (?) propofol	Small to moderate decrease in initial dose; smaller maintenance doses
Narcotics	Marked decrease in initial dose; anticipate increased duration of effect (except fentanyl)
Local anesthetics for spinal/epidural anesthesia	Small to moderate decrease in segmental dose requirement; anticipate prolonged effect and urinary retention
Benzodiazepines	Modest decrease in initial dose; anticipate marked increase in duration (except midozolam)
Succinylcholine	None
Nondepolarizing relaxants	Same or slight increase in initial dose; anticipate increased duration (except atracurium)
Neostigmine, edrophonium	No change in dose; prolonged effect
Atropine	Increased dose requirement; anticipate central anticholinergic syndrome
Adrenergic agonists	Increased doses

with greater frequency and severity in elderly patients. Chronic disease and the hospitalization of elderly patients also encourages polypharmacy, further aggravating the chance for drug-induced complications (Table 27–2).

ANESTHETIC MANAGEMENT AND OUTCOME

Overall perioperative mortality increases with advancing age, beginning in the third decade of life. Assuming competent standards of practice, epidemiologic data suggest that anesthetic outcome reflects the physical status of the patient, not the age (Fig. 27–11). *Age-related disease*, not age itself, is primarily responsible for the progressive increase in morbidity and mortality characteristic of the elderly surgical patient population. Aging and accelerated loss of organ system functional reserve, however, may increase the risks for patients over the age of 85 years, or when there is multiple organ system dysfunction.

Perioperative outcome is also largely determined by the site of operation and the urgency of the procedure. Adequate time for diagnosis, treatment, and preparation of the anesthetic plan decreases the rate and the severity of complications. Two thirds of a geriatric surgical population summarily "cleared" for major surgery by consultants nevertheless demonstrate mild to severe functional deficits when evaluated with invasive monitoring which permits measurement of cardiopulmonary function. Less than 15 per cent of these patients are physiologically normal. One third of the deficits discovered represent profound abnormalities such as congestive heart failure and marked hypoxemia, factors known to be highly predictive of subsequent perioperative morbidity and mortality.

There is no single best anesthetic for elderly patients, but specific complications may be more commonly associated with one form of anesthesia than with another. For example, thromboembolism is more common after hip surgery with general anesthesia than with regional techniques. Nevertheless, when overall outcome is determined over a period that encompasses both immediate and delayed sequelae (a period of at least 30 days), the choice of anesthetic agent or technique per se does

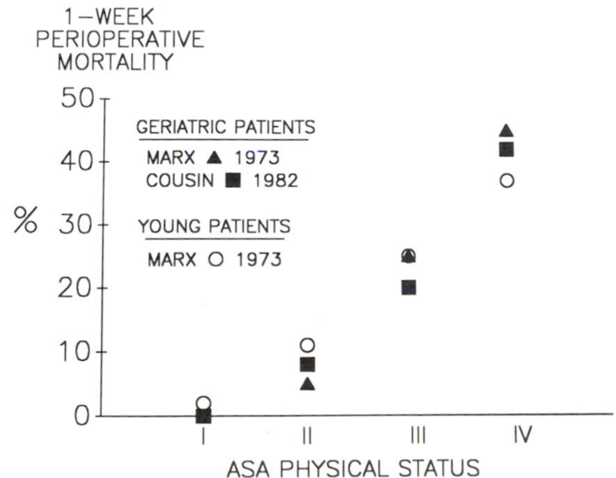

FIGURE 27–11 For any given physical status (PS) category, overall perioperative mortality is essentially the same for young as it is for elderly adults in typical metropolitan hospital surgical population with a large component of traumatic injury and emergency surgery. (Data originally published in large-scale studies reported in 1973 and 1982.)

not appear to be a major determinant of outcome. Numerous retrospective and prospective clinical studies have arrived at this conclusion: there are no significant differences in perioperative survival or major morbidity attributable specifically to the anesthetic agent selected. In particular, neither regional nor general anesthesia have yet been shown to provide the safest anesthetic for an elderly patient.

A few principles unique to the design of the anesthetic plan for elderly patients have emerged from consideration of geriatric physiology. The goal of prompt and complete postoperative recovery of mental function, a major concern with elderly patients who may already exhibit deteriorating mental ability, is compromised in direct proportion to the pharmacologic complexity of the anesthetic routine. If a cold operating room produces hypothermia, awakening is delayed, perhaps because of the direct depressant effects of hypothermia, or the reduced rates of drug clearance. Even when anesthetic management is appropriate and surgical convalescence uncomplicated, the return to preoperative mental status after prolonged general anesthesia may require five to ten days.

The neurophysiologic and pharmacologic mechanisms responsible for this subtle but prolonged disruption of the nervous system remain unknown. The most common cause of failure to emerge promptly from anesthesia is the use of too much or too many anesthetic agents! For example, the use of intravenous sedation has been shown to retard the rapid recovery of mental function that otherwise occurs in elderly patients after spinal or epidural anesthetic.

Sedation may also lead to profound and prolonged disorientation in elderly patients, and can aggravate a preexisting situational psychosis. Although "sundowning" and other types of diffuse abnormal mentation are assumed to reflect latent organic brain dysfunction in elderly patients, they also occur, at least in part, because of deficient care. To remain oriented, elderly patients require increased sensory input and environmental cues that are often absent in a hospital setting. Feelings of dependency, loss of self-confidence, and the despair for the future that concern many elderly surgical patients worsen matters too.

Even the physical management of elderly patients requires some specific adjustments. Aged skin and bones are fragile. Joints are stiff and the range of motion is limited, requiring gentle and expert routine care if traumatic injury from improper positioning, bandaging, or enforced inactivity are to be avoided. In elderly surgical patients, bleeding diatheses, hypercoagulable states, and a predisposition to bacterial infection appear more likely than in younger adults, especially if sustained sympathoadrenal stress responses occur during protracted recovery.

Therefore, an anesthetic plan that includes postoperative epidural sympathectomy and analgesia may be of special value, eliminating the long periods of inadequate relief of postoperative pain sometimes imposed upon geriatric patients because of fears of narcotic side effects. For reasons detailed above, perioperative management of fluids, metabolic state, electrolytes, and temperature must be meticulous. Aged patients do not require fundamentally different anesthetic management than do younger patients. They do require a higher standard of preparation, sensitivity, and vigilance.

Reference

Avram MJ, Krejcie TC, Henthorn TK. The relationship of age to the pharmacokinetics of early drug distribution: The concurrent disposition of thiopental and indocyanine green. *Anesthesiology* 1990;72:403–411.

DelGuercio LRN, Cohn JD. Monitoring operative risk in the elderly. *JAMA* 1980;243:1350–1355.

Hanowell LH, Boyle WA III. Perioperative care of the hemodynamically unstable geriatric patient. *Int Anesthesiol Clin* 1988;26:156–168.

Krechel SW, ed. Anesthesia and the geriatric patient. Orlando: Grune and Stratton, 1984: 252.

Morrison RC. Hypothermia in the elderly. *Int Anesthesiol Clin* 1988;26:124–133.

CHAPTER TWENTY-EIGHT

Outpatient Anesthesia

Outpatient surgery accounts for more than half of the operations performed in the United States. It has become popular because patients believe it allows them greater control over their business and personal lives and because third-party payers find it reduces costs. The evolution of day surgery units has in many instances placed anesthesiologists in the role of "gatekeeper" for surgical outpatients, because they are in the best position to determine whether a patient is an acceptable day surgery unit (DSU) candidate. This chapter discusses patient selection and preoperative preparation, intraoperative anesthetic management, postanesthetic care, and follow-up for those undergoing outpatient surgery.

Patient Selection, Evaluation

The range of surgical procedures performed on outpatients now includes almost any that do not involve opening the cranium, chest, or abdomen, that do not produce major physiologic changes, and that do not require intense postoperative care. Discharge from DSU depends primarily upon recovery from anesthesia rather than from the operation; the anesthesiologist often determines the appropriateness of an individual patient for an outpatient surgical procedure. Such patients are usually classified as ASA physical status 1 or 2, but in many instances patients of ASA physical status 3 with stable systemic diseases are excellent candidates. On occasion, patients classified as ASA physical status 4, with appropriate preoperative evaluation and preparation, can have satisfactory outpatient surgical experiences. Other factors that affect the decision regarding outpatient surgery are included in Table 28–1.

Morbid obesity raises concerns about ventilation and airway management, pain management, and the patient's ability to walk postoperatively. Asthma is often cited as a contraindication to outpatient anesthesia and operation, but a well-controlled asthmatic patient may undergo general anesthesia safely in the DSU. Both the patient and the surgeon must understand that hospitalization may be required if an acute asthma attack occurs. Physical or mental handicaps may make it impossible for a patient to receive adequate perioperative care outside of a skilled nursing facility. In general, the deciding question in assessing the appropriateness of an ambulatory surgery unit is whether the patient could be cared for more safely in a hospital than at home after the operation.

Some operations are not appropriate for a DSU. Extensive blood loss or physiologic shifts of large volumes of fluid require prolonged postoperative observation and hydration. When postoperative pain requires parenteral narcotics, special arrangements must be made to administer them safely at home. In recent years, freestanding recovery centers, nursing homes, and home nursing services have offered longer-term (24 to 48 hours) post-

TABLE 28–1. Outpatient Anesthesia: Patient Selection

Patient

1. *ASA Physical Status* (1, 2, possibly 3, rarely 4): there must be no substantial risk of a postoperative complication (MI, respiratory failure) that could be ameliorated by care in the hospital.
2. *Reliability, compliance:* the patient and partner must follow directions for postoperative care.
3. *Discharge situation:* a capable person must watch and help the patient at home after operation. The place in which the patient will live, whether apartment, hotel room or nursing home, must be suitable for the care prescribed.
4. *Age:* only specific health problems, not age itself, rule out day surgery for the elderly. Premature infants at risk of apneic episodes are not candidates for discharge on the day of surgery; infants born at term must be older than 4 weeks postnatal and older than 42 weeks gestational to undergo same-day surgery.

Procedure

1. Physiologic derangements produced by the operation itself must not require hospital care.
2. Blood loss must not be so great as to require transfusion (although autologous transfusion has been used for outpatient plastic surgery procedures).
3. Postoperative pain must be controlled with safe doses of opioids.
4. There can be no risk of airway obstruction.
5. The potential complications of the procedure must not immobilize the patient.

operative recovery care. The incidence and severity of complications that are due to the operation may also require inpatient management. Surgical procedures likely to produce postoperative bleeding, airway compromise, or vertigo are best performed where postoperative hospitalization is available.

Even if the patient and the procedure are amenable to outpatient management, the discharge environment must be suitable. Patients who have received anesthesia suffer impairments in cognitive and motor functions. They need assistance in traveling home and must be accompanied by a responsible adult after the operation.

Preoperative evaluation before a day surgery operation is identical to that preceding any operation, but the patient may not be available in person for the preanesthetic visit, and the anesthesiologist must assure that the criteria for DSU admission are met (Table 28–1). Necessary laboratory studies and basic information about the patient's medical and anesthetic history are best obtained prior to the day of operation, so that significant abnormalities may be investigated, additional data may be obtained from consulting physicians, and the most efficient use may be made of both the patient's time and the DSU's facilities. Healthy patients may need only to complete a screening questionnaire (or respond to questions put by a health evaluation computer program), deferring the physical examination until the day of admission. Alternatively, the patient scheduled for a day surgery procedure may visit a preanesthetic evaluation clinic, as described in Chapter 3. An interview by the anesthesiologist in person or by telephone can clarify the available options for anesthetic management, allay anxiety, and provide realistic expectations regarding the day of operation and postoperative recovery.

The laboratory tests required for a given patient are determined by the patient's health and the proposed operation (Chapter 3), whether the patient is scheduled to go home on the day of operation or to stay overnight. Experience in day surgery units and the desire to make patient evaluation more efficient in these units has contributed to present efforts to eliminate unnecessary testing.

Patients scheduled for day surgery procedures receive special instruction before coming to the day surgery unit. Patients are advised as to when they can eat before operation, and what, and the medications they can take on the day of operation. There must be a clear understanding of arrangements for transportation home, the need for an adult to care for the patient after operation, the degree of pain and immobility to be expected, the pain medication that will be prescribed, and any other measures needed postoperatively. Written instructions and an agreement signed by the patient and the person briefing the patient improve compliance.

ANESTHETIC MANAGEMENT

Preoperative Preparation

Patients who require medication daily, particularly for cardiac or pulmonary disease, are directed to take their prescribed doses on the morning of operation. Scheduling insulin-dependent diabetics early in the morning simplifies their care. Those receiving long-acting insulin receive one third to one half their usual dose, along with a glucose-containing intravenous solution. When the patient has recovered from anesthesia and can retain solid food without nausea or vomiting, the remainder of the morning dose of insulin may be administered. An alternative method of managing insulin requirements is useful when anesthesia and operation are unlikely to cause nausea. The patient takes no insulin before operation and treats the postoperative period as if he had just arisen in the morning, administering the normal dose of insulin postoperatively and resuming a normal meal schedule.

Attempts to ensure that patients have empty stomachs at the beginning of anesthesia have resulted in preoperative restriction of food and liquids for eight hours or longer in adults before elective operations. Recent studies have questioned the usefulness of this restriction, particularly for fluids. Ingestion of fluids by healthy inpatients up to two hours preoperatively does not appear to increase gastric volume as compared to that of patients who have fasted for several hours. On the other hand, patients who fast from evening until a scheduled operation the next day report thirst and hunger and are often found to be hypoglycemic when they arrive in the operating room. When risk factors are absent (impaired gastric emptying caused by pain, diabetes, opioids, pregnancy, obesity, or hiatal hernia), aspiration of gastric contents is a rare complication the incidence of which probably is not reduced by prolonged fasting. A conservative recommendation is that healthy adult patients scheduled for elective outpatient surgery fast for six hours before anesthesia.

Although results vary among studies, more outpatients than inpatients arrive in the operating room with stomach contents of pH less than 2.5 or volume greater than 25 ml, and thus are considered to be at risk for acid aspiration pneumonitis. Although these findings invite the routine prescription of histamine-2 (H_2) blockers, soluble antacids, or metoclopramide to reduce gastric acidity and volume in DSU patients before operation, this practice has not become popular. At present there is no evidence that the use of these agents would decrease the already small incidence of aspiration pneumonitis in these patients. The rare adverse side effects of H_2 blockers and metoclopramide also make it inadvisable to prescribe these drugs routinely for healthy DSU patients who do not suffer the risk factors listed previously.

Practice regarding premedication of outpatients varies widely; some centers use no premedication, while others premedicate patients routinely. Midazolam in small doses seems to delay discharge from the recovery room little, but in general, premedicants are withheld to reduce the chance of delayed awakening. Factors influencing this decision include patient age, type and duration of operation, patient expectations, and the availability of a preoperative area to accommodate and monitor sedated patients. The DSU where patients are admitted to a bed and observed there for two hours preoperatively and four hours postoperatively is more likely to administer routine premedication than the unit in which patients walk to the operating room within an hour of their admission and are discharged as soon as possible postoperatively.

Pediatric patients often benefit from preanesthetic medication designed to allay anxiety, induce drowsiness, and minimize secretions, particularly when an inhalation induction is planned. Some physicians prescribe oral premedication for children, eliminating dreaded preoperative injections (see Chapter 25); emergence and postoperative recovery do not appear to be affected adversely by its use.

Anesthetic Agents and Techniques

Any anesthetic agent or technique may be safely used in the DSU, as long as overdose and slow emergence are avoided. Determining factors include patient choice, surgical requirements, patient age and physical status, duration of drug action, and requirements for postoperative care. The special goal of outpatient anesthesia is to allow rapid recovery from the immobilizing effects of anesthesia and operations, yet to leave the patient as comfortable as possible during the transition from recovery in the DSU to recovery at home. This condition is often described as "street fitness," a misnomer that implies greater cognitive and motor ability than usually exist in the postoperative period.

More important than the choice of drugs in achieving this goal is the judgment of the person administering the anesthetic. Even agents soluble in tissue or with long durations of action allow early recovery if they are used in small doses and are discontinued early enough. Nevertheless, for day surgery patients, the best sedatives, hypnotics, opioids, muscle relaxants, and anesthetics are those with pharmacokinetic properties that promise the most rapid offset of effect.

LOCAL ANESTHESIA/ MONITORED ANESTHESIA CARE

The combination of local anesthesia and monitored anesthesia care with sedation (MAC) offers safety and early discharge for those outpatient surgical procedures and patients suited to these techniques. Local anesthetic may be administered by the anesthesiologist in the form of local infiltration of the operative site or field block, or it may be administered by the surgeon at the sterile field. The physical and the emotional comfort of the patient is attended to by the anesthesiologist (Table 28–2). Patients respond quite favorably to such attention and often voice their appreciation in the postoperative follow-up call.

Patients' responses to sedative drugs are variable. Each administration is a titration, with respiratory depression and airway obstruction indicating that too much drug has been given, and the patient's anxiety indicating too little drug. Adequate sedation may be identified by a patient's calm demeanor, slurred speech, slowed heart rate, or reduced blood pressure. The benzodiazepines, particularly midazolam, have assumed a major role in intraoperative sedation of day surgery patients. These drugs allay anxiety and produce some degree of amnesia. Individual responses vary widely: 1 to 10 mg of midazolam may be needed for a 70-kg patient. Repeated administration of 0.5 to 1 mg intravenously every two to five minutes until the patient's eyes close spontaneously usually provides adequate anxiolysis and amnesia. When the patient asks to remain more aware, or when the patient must remain more alert because of bleeding in the airway or to cooperate with the surgeon, smaller doses of sedative are used and the patient is provided more constant verbal assurance.

Table 28–2. Features of Monitored Anesthetic Care

1. Minimize patient exposure prior to and during prepping and draping.
2. Arrange pillows and warm blankets for comfortable positioning.
3. Administer appropriate drugs in small increments to allay anxiety, reduce perception of pain, and produce amnesia, without causing the patient to lose consciousness ("conscious sedation").
4. Converse with the patient, offering reassurance and asking about the patient's needs.

Opioids, particularly fentanyl, are commonly part of monitored anesthesia care. Narcotic analgesics administered prior to the injection of local anesthesia (50 to 100 μg of fentanyl two to five minutes before injection) often increase the patient's comfort. Infusions of short-acting narcotics allow precise control of depth of sedation and permit rapid recovery, but also carry the risk of overdose if almost constant attention to the delivery of the drug lapses. Meperidine in small doses (12 to 50 mg) controls shivering and provides postoperative analgesia.

Ultra–short-acting barbiturates are sometimes added to the pharmacologic regimen of monitored anesthesia care to provide hypnosis and sleep, but these must be used with great caution. A 25 to 100-mg dose of thiopental infused two minutes prior to a brief major stimulus (injection of local anesthetic, dilatation of the uterine cervix) effectively blunts patient discomfort during this period. However, barbiturates potentiate the respiratory depressant effects of opioids and other sedatives, and must be administered with great care to avoid apnea or upper airway obstruction. Small doses of ketamine (0.1 to 0.5 mg per kg) can be used in place of opioids to supplement benzodiazepines with less risk of ventilatory depression, but at an increased risk of dysphoria. A controlled infusion of propofol (approximately 50 to 150 μg per kg per minute) is more expensive than midazolam but provides easily controlled, rapidly reversible sedation.

GENERAL ANESTHESIA

General anesthesia in the DSU must meet all the requirements of any successful general anesthetic, yet allow the patient to go home promptly after the surgical procedure. Less soluble inhaled anesthetics, intravenous agents with short durations of action, or ones for which pharmacologic antagonists are available are popular. The inhalation induction of anesthesia is employed primarily (in children) to avoid intravenous cannulation while the patient is awake. For most patients, anesthesia begins with thiopental or methohexital, although large doses of either of these agents contribute to postoperative lethargy. Consequently, propofol is gaining popularity as both an induction and a maintenance agent for brief outpatient surgical procedures. Use of etomidate as an induction agent has been limited because it is associated with postoperative nausea, and because of concerns about suppression of adrenal function.

Indications for endotracheal intubation are identical in outpatients and in hospitalized surgical patients (see Chapter 13). One must weigh the risks of airway obstruction, hypoventilation, or passive regurgitation and subsequent aspiration against the risks of hypertension, tachycardia, sore throat, hoarseness, or dental or laryngeal damage attributable to intubation.

The choice of agents for maintenance of general anesthesia in outpatients is determined by patient factors, surgical requirements, and the viewpoint of the anesthesiologist. The proponents of "balanced" anesthesia argue that the use of relatively large doses of narcotic analgesics, muscle relaxants, and small doses of inhalation anesthetics allows a more rapid return to consciousness. Others feel that the administration of narcotic analgesics to patients who are expected to walk within a few hours of their operations increases the incidence of postoperative nausea and vomiting. As a rule, compared to those receiving opioids as part of the anesthetic, patients who receive greater concentrations of inhaled agents instead can be expected to awaken somewhat more slowly, but to make a better recovery of cognitive function by several hours after operation, if they have not received narcotic analgesics in the recovery room. To promote rapid awakening, new volatile agents that are insoluble in blood, such as desflurane, are being investigated. However, the limiting factor preventing discharge from the recovery room is often not somnolence, but nausea and vomiting.

Many DSU procedures are superficial and require no muscle relaxation, so that muscle relaxants often are used only for intubation, for which succinylcholine remains a good choice because of the brevity of its action. The shorter-acting nondepolarizing neuromuscular blockers, atracurium and vecuronium, are preferred when muscle relaxation is needed in longer surgical operations. Although overall postoperative muscle pains occur less often when nondepolarizing muscle relaxants are used, in at least one study, day surgery patients reported similar pain after vecuronium and after succinylcholine.

SPINAL AND EPIDURAL ANESTHESIA

Spinal and epidural anesthesia are sometimes used in ambulatory surgical patients. However, more time may be required to perform a spinal or epidural block than to begin general anesthesia, and the patients may run prolonged postoperative courses, too. Postural hypotension from residual sympathetic blockade and slow return of sensory and motor function may delay discharge. Spinal or epidural anesthesia may contribute to difficulty voiding; in most day surgery units patients are required to urinate before leaving.

Whereas recent studies show that patients need not remain supine after dural puncture to avoid headache, a patient living far from the DSU may find it difficult to return for care. The incidence of incapacitating postdural puncture headache has been reported to be as great as 18 per cent in ambulatory surgical patients. Such a complication rate may be accepted in certain patients if choosing spinal anesthesia avoids some other more serious complication, but these situations are uncommon. Short-acting local anesthetics, such as procaine or lidocaine without epinephrine, are appropriate for brief procedures when early recovery is expected.

Epidural anesthesia has been proposed as an effective alternative to spinal anesthesia. However, larger doses of local anesthetic are required, increasing the risk of systemic toxicity. Should dural puncture occur, the likelihood of headache is great because of the size of the needle used. Commonly used agents for epidural anesthesia in outpatients include 2-chloroprocaine, procaine, lidocaine, or mepivacaine.

Regional anesthesia with minimal or no sedation may be advantageous in the elderly, in whom residual effects of general anesthesia or heavy sedation may last for days, because of the decreased rate of drug clearance. However, a brief general anesthetic that employs only the least amounts required of the shortest-acting agents can produce nearly as little postoperative impairment as does a regional anesthetic.

REGIONAL NERVE BLOCK

Regional nerve block or field block provides profound analgesia with minimal physiological derangement. Periorbital and retrobulbar block are performed for ophthalmologic surgery. The brachial plexus may be blocked using either the axillary or interscalene approach, but the supraclavicular approach is less suitable because of possible pneumothorax. Intravenous perfusion blocks (Bier blocks) are easily performed and provide adequate analgesia for many brief procedures on the hand and wrist. The potential for sudden release of large amounts of local anesthetic into the systemic circulation detracts from the popularity of this technique. Blocks of the inguinal region for hernia repair and blocks of the wrist and ankle for work on the hand and foot are relatively easily performed and are accepted by most patients. Prolonged blocks in the surgical outpatient impair postoperative mobility and increase the risk of inadvertent injury in the affected area. Avoiding local anesthetics with long durations of action decreases the likelihood of such occurrences.

Postanesthetic Course

Ambulatory surgery patients remain in the care of skilled medical personnel for a much shorter time than do inpatients who progress from a recovery room to a surgical ward. Whereas the complications after anesthesia are the same in outpatients and inpatients, the consequences of complications that may be only minor for inpatients can be major for outpatients, because they may delay or prevent discharge. Such complications are best avoided, if possible, and special efforts must be made to identify postoperative problems and reduce their impact.

Nausea, vomiting, and postoperative pain are the most common management problems in the DSU recovery room. In addition to the physical discomfort, retching and vomiting may pose a risk to suture lines, thus increasing the risk of postoperative bleeding and hematoma. Many factors contribute to postoperative nausea, including narcotic analgesics, patient movement with subsequent motion sickness, middle ear disturbances, inhalational anesthetics, the surgical procedure, and postoperative pain. Drugs ranging from anticholinergics (atropine), to pressors (ephedrine), to major and minor tranquilizers have been administered to decrease nausea. Other drugs (nitrous oxide, alfentanil) are sometimes avoided, with the same goal.

Given the multitude of factors contributing to nausea and vomiting postoperatively, and the sedative or dysphoric side effects of most antiemetics, it is not surprising that no single drug regimen has been invariably effective. A good choice at present is droperidol, which is given during the operation in small intravenous doses (0.125 to 0.5 mg in adults); antiemetic effects are significant, with tolerable levels of postoperative sedation.

After outpatient operations, which patients and their surgeons may view as minor, patients may be surprised to experience pain. Pain management for these patients begins with preoperative education by the surgeon, anesthesiologist, and nursing staff, so that the patient can anticipate the potential for discomfort and the plans for its relief.

Life-threatening complications of anesthesia are most commonly related to the airway or the cardiovascular system. Airway or respiratory problems may develop over several hours postoperatively, especially when the operation has been in the airway or when airway injury has occurred during the course of the anesthetic; prolonged periods of postoperative observation are required when airway compromise is possible. Perioperative cardiovascular disturbances (hypertension, hypotension, myocardial ischemia, arrhythmias, or bradycardia) are becoming more common as older and less healthy patients are managed in day surgery units. Consultation with specialists in other disciplines may be needed to determine the potential severity of a perioperative incident and whether the patient must be observed overnight in the hospital.

Most symptoms that occur during the recovery room stay are part of the normal recovery process and require only reassurance. Careful preoperative preparation combined with gentle and caring reassurance postoperatively is preferable to pharmacological treatments that might delay the return home.

Discharge from the DSU

Before discharge, outpatients are expected to reach a level of function that includes return of vital signs to baseline, and, in most cases, walking, voiding, and tolerating oral fluids. Some patients are ready for discharge when they arrive in the recovery room; others may require several hours of care before they can go home safely. Duration of recovery may be affected by both anesthesia and operation. Factors considered in assessing readiness for discharge are listed in Table 28–3.

Assessment of respiratory function includes depth and frequency of respiration, as well as patency of the airway. There must be no residual effects of muscle relaxants, and the respiratory depression associated with narcotics must be acceptable. The complications of airway instrumentation such as sore throat, hoarseness, and lip, tooth, and gum injury must also be assessed and recorded.

The term "stability of vital signs" is a euphemism for adequate cardiovascular and pulmonary function. In the postoperative period, patients ready for discharge must exhibit blood pressures and pulse rates within approximately 15 per cent of the preoperative values. Arrhythmias, chest pain, or other evidence of myocardial ischemia must be resolved and must be determined not to pose a threat to the patient's well-being. Attention to adequate hydration is particularly important in the ambulatory surgical patient to avoid hypovolemia and hypotension.

The surgical outpatient accompanied by an appropriate companion must be oriented to his surroundings, but need not be remarkably alert at the time of discharge, particularly if postoperative pain has required narcotic analgesics.

The rare patient who remains hypothermic in the recovery room is not a candidate for discharge. Most DSU procedures are brief enough that the patient's body temperature does not decrease more than 1.5 to 2.5° C. Persistent hypothermia delays recovery, provokes shivering, and increases myocardial oxygen demand; it must be treated successfully before discharge.

Mobility, rather than the ability to walk per se, is required for discharge. The patient may not be able to walk because of the operation but must be able to move from wheelchair to car and from car to a comfortable place within the home.

Postoperative bladder distention is an inconvenient and uncomfortable complication of operation and anesthesia. Patients who can urinate prior to leaving the recovery room are less likely to experience this complication at home. Most patients who receive adequate fluids in the perioperative period experience an urge to void prior to meeting other criteria for discharge. Those patients who have received adequate intravenous fluids, have not had an operation likely to interfere with their ability to urinate, and who have felt no need to do so, may be discharged from the DSU with specific instructions to seek care for urinary retention if they have not voided within six hours of the end of the operation.

TABLE 28–3. Discharging Day Surgery Unit Patients After Operation

Respiration
Maintains patent airway unassisted
Acceptable degree of respiratory depression
No threat of swelling or hematoma in airway
Cardiovascular
Heart rate and blood pressure near preoperative values
Hypovolemia corrected with IV fluids
Central nervous system
Orientated to person, place, and time
May doze, but must awaken easily
Adequate vision
Surgical site
No more than expected swelling and drainage
No more than expected pain
Temperature
No hypothermia
Nausea
Acceptable severity of vomiting
No threat of dehydration
Evening follow-up phone call scheduled
Mobility
Able to sit
Transfer bed to chair and back with one assistant
Walks, unless prevented by the operation
Bladder
Voids, or is asked to call if has not voided in 6 hours

Prior to discharge, patients and their escorts are again reminded of what to expect in terms of postoperative limitation of activity, pain management, and potential for delayed complications of anesthesia and operation. Postanesthetic follow-up, usually by means of a telephone call or postcard questionnaire, provides a means of identifying problems, documenting safe recovery, and monitoring the quality of the care provided.

Extremes of Age

The management of anesthesia for elderly patients is described in Chapter 27; in the day surgery unit, these principles apply equally. Stringent evaluation for discharge and careful arrangements for postoperative care are important to success. The principles of pediatric anesthesia management given in Chapter 25 govern care of these patients in the DSU.

In summary, successful outpatient anesthesia requires an appropriate patient undergoing a surgical procedure that allows recovery at home, with minimal risk of life-threatening complications. The recovery and return home are aided by choice of anesthetic techniques and agents that minimize postanesthetic complications and by careful preoperative preparation of the patient and the companion who accompanies the patient home.

REFERENCES

Patel RI, Hannallah RS. Anesthetic complications following pediatric ambulatory surgery: A 3-year study. Anesthesiology 1988;69:1009–1012.

Wetchler BV, Anesthesia for ambulatory surgery. 2nd ed. Philadelphia: Lippincott, 1991.

White PF, ed. Outpatient anesthesia. New York: Churchill Livingstone, 1990.

Young ML, Conahan TJ. Complications of outpatient anesthesia. Semin Anesthesia 1990;9:62–68.

CHAPTER TWENTY-NINE

Managing the Desperately Ill Patient:
Trauma and Shock

One of the most challenging tasks in modern medicine lies in the acute operative management of the critically ill patient. Advances in the technology of medicine and the blurring of distinctions between the operating room and the intensive care unit have made care of the critically ill an important part of anesthesia practice. Patients whose operative mortality would once have been considered prohibitive, such as the octogenarian cardiac surgical patient, the septic liver transplant patient, or the multiply injured accident victim, now undergo operation and survive.

These patients present several challenges to the anesthesiologist. They arrive for emergency operations at unusual hours, with full stomachs, and near to or in shock. Underlying physical processes differ, but the principles of anesthetic management of all desperately ill patients are similar. The anesthesiologist must ensure adequate oxygen supply to critical organs while providing anesthesia during the surgical procedure. Successful treatment requires expertise in physiology, familiarity with a wide variety of drugs, technical facility, and the ability to react quickly to rapidly changing circumstances.

Shock

The common end point in many critically ill patients is shock, in which the metabolic needs of the body's tissues are not met by the circulation. This definition intentionally avoids reference to normal or abnormal hemodynamics or tissue metabolism. Shock occurs in the presence of a normal, increased or decreased cardiac output or blood pressure, and may be absent with profound decreases in blood pressure or cardiac output (as during cardiopulmonary bypass with hypothermia).

Traditional definitions have differentiated between warm and cold shock, with sepsis or anaphylaxis representing the former, and hemorrhage, trauma, or cardiogenic shock the latter. Characteristic hemodynamic patterns have been described for each of these syndromes. The term warm shock implies an increased cardiac output and reduced peripheral resistance. Cold shock suggests impaired cardiac output and increased peripheral resistance. A problem with the use of such terms is the tendency for shock patterns to overlap or change over time: myocardial depressant sub-

TABLE 29–1. Differential Diagnosis of Shock

Type	Etiology	Manifestations
Septic	Disseminated infection	Vasodilation, ↑ cardiac output*, fever
Spinal	Cervical cord lesion, spinal anesthesia	Vasodilation, neurologic deficits
Anaphylactic	Hypersensitivity (toxin, sting, drug)	Vasodilation, bronchospasm
Cardiogenic	Cardiomyopathy, ischemia, valvular lesion	Vasoconstriction, ↓ cardiac output
Hemorrhagic	Blood loss	Vasoconstriction, bleeding site†
Hypovolemic	Dehydration (diuretics, sweating)	Vasoconstriction, ↓ urine output, ↓ skin turgor
Traumatic	Tissue and organ injury, blood loss	Traumatic injuries
Endocrine	Adrenal, thyroid, pituitary insufficiency	Variable depending on hormone deficiency
Vascular	Pulmonary emboli, venous or arterial thrombosis	↓ Cardiac output

* In the initial stages, output may decrease in late sepsis.
† May be internal and occult rather than external.

stance is a circulating factor found in septic shock that can depress cardiac output even in the presence of decreased systemic vascular resistance (Table 29–1).

Lactic acidosis from anaerobic metabolism, decreasing urine output owing to renal hypoperfusion, and respiratory failure are early indicators of shock. Adult respiratory distress syndrome (ARDS), disseminated intravascular coagulation (DIC), acute tubular necrosis (ATN), and multisystem organ failure (MSOF) are later sequelae of sustained tissue hypoxemia.

An understanding of the balance between oxygen demand, consumption, and delivery in shock is critical to its management. Oxygen demand is the volume of oxygen required by the tissues to supply metabolic needs. Oxygen consumption refers to the actual oxygen uptake by the tissues. There may be a discrepancy between demand and consumption. In cyanide toxicity, for example, cellular oxygen consumption is quite reduced, despite normal demand, because cyanide poisons the mitochondria and blocks oxidative phosphorylation. If oxygen demand is greater than oxygen consumption, anaerobic metabolism and lactic acidosis result. Oxygen delivery is a function of arterial oxygen content and cardiac output. It represents the blood-borne oxygen that is available for consumption by the body (Table 29–2).

Decreases in hemoglobin concentration, arterial oxygen saturation, or cardiac output proportionately decrease oxygen delivery. Note that decreases in arterial oxygen saturation, rather than in the partial pressure of oxygen in arterial blood, affect delivery. Hemoglobin is 100 per cent saturated and oxygen delivery is essentially equal, whether PO_2 or 80 or 500 mm Hg (except in cases of severe anemia when plasma-borne oxygen becomes significant). Changes in patient temperature, activity, acid-base balance, stress level, injury, or the development of sepsis can change the oxygen demand and consumption. The balance between supply and demand determines the patient's response to shock. The goal of supportive therapy in shock is to provide sufficient oxygen delivery to allow maximal tissue oxygen consumption, meeting tissue oxygen needs and thereby improving survival.

Anesthetic management of critically ill patients is complicated by the complex interplay between the primary disease and the operative and anesthetic interventions used in its treatment. Thiopental was termed the "ideal form of euthanasia" after its use as a sole anesthetic agent at Pearl Harbor resulted in deaths among the wounded. The profound hemodynamic alterations in these pa-

TABLE 29–2. Oxygen Delivery and Consumption

Oxygen delivery (ml/min)	= blood O_2 content (ml O_2/dl blood) × cardiac output (dl/min)
	= (1.34 × Hb × $Sa{O_2}$) × cardiac output (L/min) × 10
	= 1000 ml/min
Oxygen consumption	= (oxygen delivered by arteries) − (oxygen returned by veins)
	= 1.34 ($Sa{O_2}$ − $S\bar{v}{O_2}$) × Hb × cardiac output (L/min) × 10
	= 250 ml/min

tients were unrecognized, as was the fact that the usual thiopental dose can be lethal in a bleeding casualty patient.

HEMORRHAGE AND SHOCK

Hemorrhage is the form of shock most familiar to the anesthesiologist. Its recognition and management are intrinsic to anesthetic practice. Acute loss of 15 per cent of the blood volume of a healthy unanesthetized adult (Class I hemorrhage), is well tolerated and may produce only a slight tachycardia. Class II hemorrhage, or the loss of 15 to 30 percent of the blood volume, can be diagnosed by the presence of tachycardia, a narrow pulse pressure, anxiety, and abnormal capillary refill. The diastolic component of the blood pressure often increases because of an increase in circulating catecholamines. Class III hemorrhage (the acute loss of 30 to 40 per cent of the blood volume) is accompanied by tachycardia, tachypnea, anxiety, and systolic hypotension. Any blood loss greater than 40 per cent represents immediately life-threatening Class IV hemorrhage; signs include marked tachycardia, hypotension with a narrow pulse pressure, depressed mental status, and profound oliguria (Table 29–3).

The anesthesiologist must recognize that the patient has lost blood, and determine either that hypovolemia can be corrected before beginning anesthesia (always the preferable course) or that the rate of hemorrhage is so fast that correction is not possible without immediate operation to control bleeding. Once one of these two strategies has been chosen, decisions about the timing and route of volume resuscitation, appropriate hemodynamic monitors, preparation and use of blood products, and choices of agents for induction and maintenance of anesthesia can be made.

Bleeding patients usually appear pale, with cool or clammy extremities. Agitation, confusion, and combativeness are signs of inadequate cerebral perfusion. By seeking to provoke orthostatic hypotension in the patient on the operating table, one can estimate the degree of intravascular volume depletion. In this test, the blood pressure and the pulse are recorded in the supine position and after one minute in the 45-degree head-up position. If the systolic blood pressure decreases by more than 10 mm Hg or the pulse increases by ten or more beats per minute, the patient suffers from orthostatic hypotension, indicating an intravascular volume deficit exceeding 1 L in a normal adult.

These patients have increased sympathetic nervous system activity, with tachycardia, vasoconstriction, and myocardial stimulation. The most pressing concern in their treatment is the prompt repletion of intravascular volume. The placement of large, short intravenous cannulae (16 or 14 gauge or even 8 French) permits rapid administration of replacement solutions. Each lost ml of blood requires 3 to 4 ml of crystalloid solutions, 1 to 2 ml of colloid solutions, or 1 ml of blood for replacement (see Chapter 15). Although the choice of colloid or crystalloid solutions still generates

TABLE 29–3. Hemorrhagic Shock*

Class	Signs and Symptoms	Treatment
Class I hemorrhage (loss of < 15%) EBL = 750 ml	Minimal tachycardia normal BP, capillary refill	Crystalloid
Class II hemorrhage (Loss of 15–30%) EBL = 750–1500 ml	Tachycardia, narrowed pulse pressure, delayed capillary refill	Crystalloid
Class III hemorrhage (Loss of 30–40%) EBL = 1500–2000 ml	Tachycardia, change in mental status, decreased systolic pressure	Crystalloid
Class IV hemorrhage (Loss of > 40%) EBL > 2000 ml	Marked tachycardia, very narrow pulse pressure, depressed mental status	Crystalloid plus blood

* Modified with permission from Beecher HK, Simeone FA, Burnett CH, Shapiro SL, Sullivan ER, Mallory TB. The internal state of the severely wounded man on entry to the most forward hospital. Surgery 1947; 22:642.

TABLE 29–4. **Induction Drugs in Shock**

Drug	Dose Range*	Side Effects
Thiopental	0.5–3.0 mg/kg	Myocardial depression, vasodilator, lowered ICP
Ketamine	0.5–2.0 mg/kg	Sympathomimetic, minimal respiratory depression, may enhance O_2 uptake
Etomidate	0.1–0.3 mg/kg	Hemodynamic stability, lowers ICP, adrenal suppression
Midazolam	0.05–0.4 mg/kg	Good amnestic, may lower SVR and cause tachycardia
Propofol	0.5–4.0 mg/kg	Pain on injection, myocardial depression, lowers SVR
Fentanyl	1–25 μg/kg	No myocardial depression
Sufentanil	0.1–5.0 μg/kg	Profound analgesia
Alfentanil	10–100 μg/kg	Respiratory depression

* Appropriate dose varies widely, but the lesser doses are recommended in critically ill or hypovolemic patients.

controversy, crystalloid solutions are inexpensive, give satisfactory results in healthy patients, and may have beneficial effects on renal perfusion. Red cell transfusions are necessary in Class III or IV hemorrhage, where oxygen delivery is seriously impaired by the loss of hemoglobin.

Patients with moderate blood loss (10 to 20 per cent) who may appear to be in little distress before anesthesia, may suffer catastrophic cardiovascular collapse following a standard dose of thiopental or an inhaled anesthetic. Anesthetic agents may directly depress the heart, but the abolition of compensatory reflex responses to hypovolemia is the major cause of hypotension after anesthesia in these patients. Positive pressure ventilation impedes venous return, particularly when venous pressure is already decreased. Fluid resuscitation prior to induction of anesthesia is essential to prevent profound decreases in cardiac output and blood pressure.

Rapid sequence induction of anesthesia with intravenous agents (Table 29–4) is often needed for bleeding patients, as they are presumed to be at risk for aspiration of stomach contents. Diminished blood volume and the greater fraction of the total cardiac output directed to the brain and heart both accentuate the effect of intravenous anesthesia. Thiopental, despite is mild depressant effects on the heart, may be used safely in greatly reduced doses (0.5 to 1.5 mg per kg, depending on the patient's condition). Propofol causes hypotension, probably owing both to a decrease in vascular resistance and to myocardial depression. Midazolam is used infrequently in this country for hemodynamically comprised patients, but is a preferred agent in Europe. It is a mild myocardial depressant when used alone. Two drugs often used in hypotensive patients are etomidate and ketamine. Etomidate causes minimal myocardial depression, and virtually no change in heart rate, preload or afterload. Its major drawback lies in its ability to suppress the adrenal axis, and therefore the endocrine response to stress.

Ketamine is the only induction agent with stimulatory effects on the cardiovascular system, causing an increase in heart rate and central sympathetic output. There is also some recent laboratory evidence that ketamine can improve survival in hemorrhagic shock, possibly by improving capillary perfusion in regional tissue beds. Patients in severe shock can still become severely hypotensive after even small doses of ketamine.

The potent inhalational agents, halothane, enflurane, and isoflurane can be used for the maintenance of anesthesia. They cause dose-related myocardial depression and impair sympathetic reflexes as well; patients tolerate only small amounts of anesthetic until intravascular volume is returned to normal. Nitrous oxide may be used provided oxygen saturation, and therefore oxygen delivery, is not diminished.

The cardiovascular actions of the nondepolarizing muscle relaxants determine their use in these patients. Curare and atracurium may cause the release of histamine, and can cause hypotension when given rapidly in large doses in the presence of hypovolemia. Vecuronium has little effect on hemodynamics and is often preferred for this reason. Pancuronium is vagolytic and may be preferred if tachycardia is acceptable.

The use of pressors such as phenylephrine or ephedrine is a temporizing measure during volume replacement. The goal of volume replacement is adequate oxygen delivery; pressors increase blood pressure and maintain flow to heart and brain at the expense of blood flow not only to the skin, muscles, and splanchnic circulation, but to the kidneys as well.

In the awake patient, vital signs and mental status are monitors of organ perfusion, while in the anesthetized patient, invasive monitors are often appropriate. Urinary output of greater than 0.5 ml per kg per hour is consistent with adequate renal perfusion. In uncomplicated cases, good urinary output generally indicates an adequate cardiac output.

An arterial catheter is helpful, but not mandatory in the management of pure hemorrhagic hypotension. While it permits immediate monitoring of the blood pressure during induction, difficulties in obtaining access to the arterial circulation must not delay surgical intervention. The shape, respiratory variation, and amplitude of the arterial waveform provide information about the patient's intravascular volume status, vascular resistance, and cardiac ejection. An arterial catheter also provides ready vascular access for monitoring of hemoglobin, electrolytes, blood gases, and pH, all of which may be abnormal during shock and resuscitation (Table 29–5).

Central venous catheters are used in the hemorrhaging patient to monitor central venous pressure (CVP), to infuse vasoactive agents into the central circulation, or for volume infusion. Although the CVP best reflects filling of the right side of the heart, and is a poor estimate of left ventricular preload, trends in the CVP can guide volume replacement.

The pulmonary artery catheter (PAC) allows measurement of left sided filling pressures, cardiac output, and calculation of systemic vascular resistance. Placement and interpretation of data from a pulmonary artery catheter requires more time than central venous access, and the incidence of complications is greater.

Central venous monitoring is preferred to pulmonary artery monitoring in hemorrhagic shock in the absence of coexistent cardiac disease or the need for vasoactive infusions. Volume resuscitation is adequately monitored by trends in the CVP. Changing the CVP catheter to a Swan-Ganz catheter is appropriate if the CVP is greater than 15 mm Hg and the blood pressure remains inadequate.

CARDIOGENIC SHOCK

Like hemorrhagic shock, cardiogenic shock is a variant of cold shock (low output). The lesion, however, is not that of insufficient intravascular volume (preload), but of inadequate stroke volume. Anesthesiologists care for these patients after acute myocardial infarction and during emergency cardiac transplantation, repair of acute valvular rupture, or revascularization (Table 29–6).

Patients in cariogenic shock are cool, clammy, and tachypneic. They prefer the head-up position (because of excess lung water), and are often unable to assist in positioning themselves on the operating room table. Having no myocardial reserve, they tolerate myocardial depressants poorly, including inhaled or intravenous anesthetics. Of the

TABLE 29–5. Monitoring in Shock

Monitor	Indication	Use in Shock
EKG	Standard OR monitor	Arrhythmia, ischemia
$ETCO_2$	Standard OR monitor	Adequacy of ventilation
Pulse oximetry	Standard OR monitor	Arterial O_2 saturation
Urinary catheter	All forms of shock	Indicative of renal perfusion
Arterial catheter	All forms of shock	Immediate blood pressure measurement, blood gas analysis; Hb, electrolyte analysis
Central venous catheter	Uncomplicated hemorrhage, dehydration, trauma	Cardiac preload monitoring, vasoactive infusions, volume repletion
Pulmonary arterial catheter	Cardiogenic shock, septic shock, anaphylaxis	Indirect indicator of LV preload, measures cardiac output, SVR
Mixed venous oximetry	All forms of shock	Indicates balance between O_2 supply and demand

TABLE 29–6. Cardiogenic Shock

Type	Signs and Symptoms	Treatment
Cardiomyopathy	Fatigue, congestive failure, high SVR, low CO	Diruetics, afterload reduction, inotropic support
Cardiac ischemia	Angina, reversible EKG changes	Nitrates, lower HR, sedation
Aortic stenosis	Syncope, angina, congestive failure, high SVR, low CO	Maintain SVR, increase preload, lower HR
Aortic regurgitation	Congestive failure, angina, low SVR	Increase HR, preload, lower SVR, maintain contractile state
Mitral stenosis	Atrial fibrillation, pulmonary edema, pulmonary hypertension	Lower HR, increase preload, maintain SVR
Mitral regurgitation	Congestive failure, pulmonary hypertension	Maintain or raise HR, lower SVR, maintain preload

intravenous sedative-hypnotic agents, midazolam or etomidate are the least likely to have significant hemodynamic effects. Ketamine has been used, but it increases myocardial oxygen demand.

Combinations of large doses or narcotics, muscle relaxants, and oxygen have emerged as the anesthetic regimen of choice where myocardial compromise exists. The synthetic narcotics, such fentanyl and sufentanil, cause minimal changes in myocardial contractility, myocardial oxygen consumption, and vascular resistance, and provide the greatest stability during the induction and maintenance of anesthesia.

Nitrous oxide and the potent inhaled anesthetics cause myocardial depression in a dose-related manner. They are unsuitable as sole anesthetics in cardiogenic shock but may be used cautiously as components of balanced anesthesia. Isoflurane depresses cardiac output less than enflurane or halothane because of its vasodilating effects, but has been implicated in causing coronary steal.

There are a variety of ways in which the anesthesiologist can alter blood pressure, pulse, and cardiac output. Each approach differs in its effect on coronary perfusion and myocardial oxygen consumption (Table 29–7).

Drugs are employed to improve cardiac performance by modifying the reflex responses to decreased cardiac output. Tachycardia and volume retention (which increases preload) are compensatory responses that support cardiac output in the failing heart. Arterial vasoconstriction, however, preserves blood pressure at the expense of cardiac output. Judicious afterload reduction with agents such as sodium nitroprusside or trimethaphan allows the heart to function on a more favorable Starling's curve and can enhance stroke volume without decreasing blood pressure.

Afterload reduction is not tolerated in severely ill patients, and intraoperative inotropic support is often necessary. Dopamine, epinephrine, dobutamine, and amrinone are common choices. The first two are endogenous sympathetic hormones, the third a synthetic sympathomimetic, and the last inhibits intracellular phosphodiesterase (Table 29–8).

At lesser rates (2 to 5 μg per kg per minute), dopamine infusions act primarily on renal and splanchnic dopaminergic receptors to increase organ perfusion. In the middle range (5 to 10 μg per kg per minute), beta-adrenergic effects pre-

TABLE 29–7. Myocardial Oxygen Consumption (MV_{O_2}) After Hemodynamic Interventions

Intervention	Effect on Cardiac Output	Effect on MV_{O_2}	Effect on Coronary Perfusion
Increased afterload (vasoconstrictor)	↓	↑	↑
Increased preload (volume)	↑	↑	↓
Increased pulse (pacing, beta-1 agonist)	↑	↑	↓
Inotropic support (Ca^{++}, beta-2 agonist)	↑	→, ↑ *	→
Decreased afterload (vasodilator)	↑	↓	↓

* Phosphodiesterase inhibitors have inotropic properties, but do not change myocardial oxygen consumption.

TABLE 29.8. **Inotropic Agents and Vasopressors**

Agent	Dose (Adults)	Agonist Effect
Endogenous catecholamines		
Dopamine (DA)	1–3 μg/kg/min	Renal, splanchnic
	3–10 μg/kg/min	Beta
	>10 μg/kg/min	Alpha
Norepinephrine (NE)	2–20 μg/min	Mixed alpha and beta
Epinephrine (EPI)	1–2 μg/min	Beta
	2–10 μg/min	Mixed alpha and beta
	>10 μg/min	Alpha
Synthetic catecholamines		
Dobutamine (DB)	2–20 μg/kg/min	Beta
Isoproterenol (ISO)	0.5–20 μg/min	Beta
Noncatecholamines		
Calcium	0.25–1 gm	Increase inotropy
Ephedrine	5–10 mg	Releases NE
Phenylephrine	10–500 μg/min	Alpha
Metaraminol	20–500 μ/min	Releases NE
Methoxamine	1–5 mg	Alpha
Digoxin	0.5 mg increments	Inhibits Na/K pump
Amrinone	0.75–3 mg/kg (load)	PDE inhibitor
	5–10 mg/kg/min infusion	Increases cAMP
Glucagon	1–5 mg	Increases cAMP

dominate, primarily effecting cardiac stimulation. Alpha-adrenergic receptors are stimulated at rates greater than 10 μg per kg per minute, causing peripheral vasoconstriction. Epinephrine also has markedly different effects at different infusion rates. At 1 to 2 μg per minute it is primarily a beta-adrenergic agent, between 2 to 10 μg per minute it is mixed alpha and beta, and above 10 μg per minute, alpha-adrenergic effects predominate. Dobutamine is a synthetic beta-1 and beta-2 agent, causing both increased inotropy and peripheral vasodilation. Each of these agents bind to specific cellular receptors and cause increased cyclic adenosine monophosphate (cAMP), which modulates intracellular calcium movement. Amrinone increases cAMP by inhibiting phosphodiesterase. It has positive inotropic effects and causes peripheral vasodilation.

The intra-aortic balloon pump (IABP) provides a mechanical means of supporting the failing heart, both by enhancing coronary perfusion and decreasing left ventricular afterload. The IABP acts sequentially with the left ventricle. The left ventricular assist device (LVAD) and the mechanical heart are alternatives that are occasionally employed as bridging devices while awaiting a suitable heart for transplantation. They act in parallel with the failing left ventricle.

The monitoring devices routinely used for intraoperative management of patients in cardiogenic shock vary among institutions, depending on available technology and expertise. Transesophageal echocardiography and mixed venous oximetry, for example, are new devices in use at a small number of centers.

The use of a urinary catheter is routine as a general measure of organ perfusion. Temperature is monitored with rectal, esophageal, nasal, or (rarely) tympanic membrane probes.

Patients in cardiogenic shock are monitored with arterial and pulmonary artery catheters. The performance of the failing left ventricle is evaluated with serial cardiac output determinations and pulmonary artery diastolic (PAD) or occlusion pressures (PAOP). Therapy is titrated to enhance oxygen delivery by following trends in the cardiac output, arterial oxygen saturation, and hemoglobin.

A cardiac index greater than 2.0 to 2.2 L per minute per m^2 is usually consistent with adequate systemic perfusion. The index is determined by averaging several successive output determinations and dividing the result by the body surface area. Consistent technique, with the output measurement at the end of exhalation, will minimize error. Although thermodilution cardiac output values are inaccurate in the presence of significant tricuspid regurgitation, shunts, or inaccuracies in injectate temperature or volume, reproducible results are the rule. The systemic vascular resistance (SVR) is derived by calculation (see Chapter 6). The value of the pulmonary artery catheter in the management of the patient in shock is in the titration of volume therapy, inotropic state, and afterload to obtain a desirable balance of cardiac output, blood pressure, SVR, and oxygenation.

The oxygen saturation of mixed venous blood ($S\bar{v}O_2$) from the pulmonary arterial port of the PAC is a measure of systemic oxygen balance. $S\bar{v}O_2$ decreases with anemia, decreased cardiac output, arterial oxygen desaturation, or increased oxygen consumption. Normal $S\bar{v}O_2$ is between 60 to 75 per cent. Values greater than 75 per cent are consistent with a wedged PAC, hypothermia, left to right shunt, sepsis, or cell poisoning from cyanide. Values less than 60 per cent are consistent with cardiac decompensation, less than 50 per cent with lactic acidosis, and less than 20 per cent with permanent cellular damage owing to asphyxia. Continuous monitoring of mixed venous oxygen saturation is possible with fiberoptic technology, and used in some institutions for all cardiac surgical cases.

The newest technological advance is the transesophageal echocardiogram. Use of this device allows visualization of the left ventricle, regional wall motion, and evaluation of valvular function. It can assist in directing volume therapy, diagnosing regional ischemia, or inotropic support.

SEPTIC SHOCK

Septic shock typifies warm shock: there is peripheral vasodilation, with decreased systemic vascular resistance. In the early hours of the syndrome, heart rate and cardiac index increase and the blood pressure decreases. Recent research has shown that despite the increase in cardiac index, the ventricle dilates, stroke volume remains the same, and as a result, ejection fraction decreases. The dilated, compliant left ventricle responds well to increases in preload, and volume therapy is generally the first step in treatment of septic shock. Some patients develop a progressively decreasing cardiac index owing to myocardial depression, while others continue a hyperdynamic pattern (Table 29–9).

Sepsis is not purely a disturbance in cardiovascular physiology; virtually all organ systems suffer from some derangement in blood flow or function. Central nervous system effects are manifested by confusion, lethargy, or obtundation. Adult respiratory distress syndrome can develop from sepsis, and hyperpnea with respiratory alkalosis is an early manifestation. Decreases or redistribution in renal blood flow can cause oliguria or anuria. Cholestasis and increased transaminase values indicate hepatic dysfunction.

Although early treatment of the primary disorder with antibiotics or an operation to eliminate the infection is of paramount importance, sepsis is a toxic process that often takes 48 to 72 hours to respond to treatment. During those hours, support of vital organ perfusion is the goal of therapy.

The coincident development of sepsis and ARDS was recognized as early as 1950. Owing to concerns about exacerbating ARDS, physicians were reluctant to infuse fluids to support blood pressure in hypotension. As a result, many septic patients were given inadequate volume support. Routine use of invasive monitoring has led to recognition of the characteristic capillary leak, systemic vasodilation, and reduced left ventricular preload of untreated sepsis. Aggressive volume

TABLE 29.9. Septic Shock

Phase	Signs and Symptoms	Treatment
Early: increased cardiac output	Peripheral vasodilation, tachypnea, fever, hypotension, decreased resistance, high output	Antibiotics and drainage, maintain intravascular volume, vasopressors
Late: decreased cardiac output	Vasoconstriction, myocardial depression, multisystem organ failure (ARDS, renal failure, CNS), lactic acidosis	Vasodilators, inotropic agents, ventilator support

support governed by measurements of pulmonary artery occlusion pressure (PAOP) and cardiac output is the foundation of resuscitation of the hypotensive septic patient. Some patients require alpha-adrenergic agonists such as norepinephrine or phenylephrine when SVR is decreased, others need beta-adrenergic inotropic support in the later stages of the sepsis syndrome.

The pulmonary effects of sepsis include increases in vascular permeability, shunting, and the gradient between the partial pressure of oxygen in the alveolus and blood. Increased inspired oxygen concentrations or positive end-expiratory pressure (PEEP) are often necessary. The minute ventilation of a spontaneously breathing patient can increase dramatically at the onset of sepsis, probably owing to an increase in alveolar dead space. Under anesthesia, these patients often require increased minute volumes. Septic patients exhibit increased gradients between end-tidal and Pa_{CO_2} as evidence of an increase in dead space. Patients in septic shock who require emergency operations usually have an abscess, gangrenous viscera, or gas gangrene. They come to the operating room on short notice and are desperately ill.

The approach to anesthesia in the patient with sepsis and shock is similar to that used in hemorrhagic and cardiogenic shock. Drugs and doses for induction and maintenance of anesthesia are chosen for their lack of hemodynamic effects. Early and continuing fluid therapy is important. The pulmonary arterial catheter is preferable to central venous pressure monitoring because septic shock affects preload, cardiac contractility, and afterload. An arterial and urinary catheter are used to monitor perfusion. Trends in left ventricular filling pressures guide fluid and inotropic therapy (Table 29–10).

Appropriate antibiotics are continued throughout operation on schedule. The level of neuromuscular blockade is monitored carefully because many of the antibiotics used in septic patients potentiate nondepolarizing muscle relaxants.

In some cases, regional anesthesia is appropriate. The amputation of a septic limb or drainage of a perirectal abscess are two examples of procedures that can be done with a regional anesthetic. Some anesthesiologists are concerned about seeding the epidural space or the cerebrospinal fluid (CSF) in a bacteremic patient while performing a spinal or an epidural injection and avoid these procedures in septic patients. Other practitioners feel the benefits of regional anesthesia outweigh the risks.

TABLE 29–10. Cardiovascular Support for Septic Shock

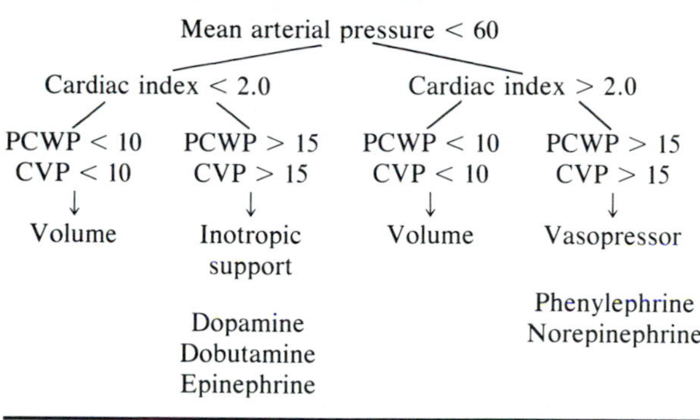

An interesting and not uncommon observation is that some patients improve dramatically with drainage of an abscess or amputation of a septic extremity. Typically, however, there is a period of hours to days before all evidence of organ dysfunction disappears.

SHOCK AND TRAUMA

Management of the patient who has suffered massive trauma is similar to management of hemorrhagic shock, but is complicated by a variety of confounding factors. Blood loss is accompanied by intracranial, intrathoracic, intra-abdominal, and long-bone injuries. Hypotension can be due to hypovolemia from blood loss, to cervical spine and cord injury, to pericardial tamponade or, in the 12 to 24 hours after injury, to undiagnosed fecal contamination of the peritoneal cavity with resultant sepsis. A systematic approach to the diagnosis and management of trauma patients is necessary to direct appropriate therapy (Table 29–11).

In the many areas that have organized trauma systems, emergency medical personnel transport injured patients by ground or air to a regional trauma center where the patient is evaluated and treated according to established protocols. Assessment of the patient's airway, breathing, circulation, and neurological status occurs immediately. All clothing is removed and the extent of

TABLE 29–11. Trauma and Shock

Type of Injury	Signs and Symptoms	Anesthetic Management
Injured with intoxication	Combative, uncooperative, alcohol on breath	Paralysis and intubation may be necessary for staff and patient safety
Exsanguination	Tachycardia, hypotension, vasoconstriction	Volume and hemoglobin replacement, hemostasis
Cervical spine	Mechanism of injury, cervical spine collar, neurological examination	In-line stabilization during intubation, collar on during surgery
Closed head injury	Mechanism of injury, obtundation, low Glasgow Coma Scale	Airway control, hyperventilation, ICP monitoring
Burn/inhalation	Facial burns, hoarseness, carbonaceous sputum, unconscious at scene	May need hyperbaric O_2, intubate early while stable

injuries is ascertained. Oxygen therapy, blood pressure, pulse, and electrocardiographic monitoring are begun. At least two large-bore intravenous catheters are inserted.

Early control of the patient's airway is of major value in the management of critically injured patients, and an area in which the anesthesiologist's judgement and skills are tested. Indications for tracheal intubation include airway obstruction, obtundation, combativeness, hemodynamic lability, or to allow hyperventilation in the event of increased intracranial pressure. Tracheal intubation in trauma patients is complicated by the coexistence of hypovolemia, injuries which distort the airway, suspected cervical spine injury, intracranial hypertension, or a full stomach (Fig. 29–1).

Hypotensive patients require volume repletion and modified doses of induction agents. Pericardial tamponade and tension pneumothorax must be considered.

Patients with suspected cervical spine injuries often require endotracheal intubation before radiologic examination is available. The trachea is intubated while the neck is stabilized, without extending the neck. Neck stabilization is distinguished from cervical traction (which was once

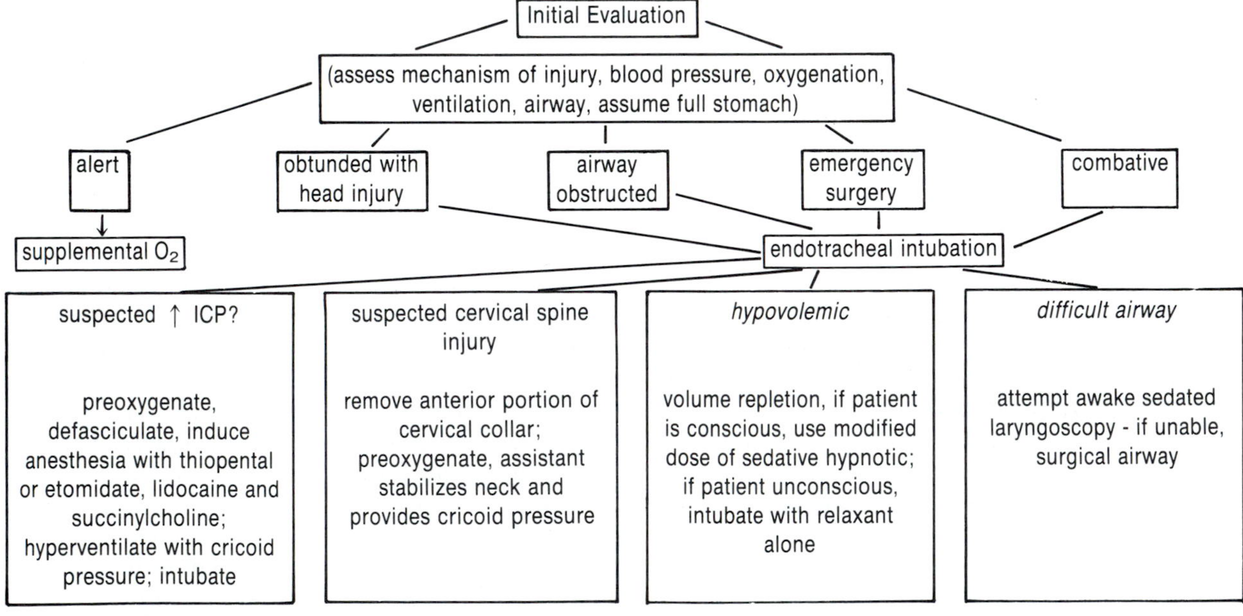

FIGURE 29–1. Airway management in the injured patient.

recommended), and implies prevention of rotational or anterior-posterior movement. It is appropriate to remove the cervical spine collar during intubation to allow simultaneous application of Sellick's maneuver (cricoid pressure) and cervical spine stabilization by an assistant.

Tracheal intubation in an injured patient suspected to have increased intracranial pressure (ICP) and assumed to have a full stomach involves a compromise among competing goals. Whereas patients with increased ICP usually undergo hyperventilation prior to intubation, patients with full stomachs are preoxygenated and then allowed to be apneic (to prevent any stimulus that might cause vomiting or regurgitation). Elective induction of anesthesia in patients with intracranial hypertension generally involves slow, titrated administration of drugs, whereas rapid sequence induction to prevent gastric aspiration requires the use of induction regimens that can precipitate significant changes in blood pressure or ICP. Succinylcholine is an ideal muscle relaxant for rapid sequence induction because of its speed of onset, although it can cause brief increases in intracranial pressure. The approach to the head-injured trauma patient used at many trauma centers includes preoxygenation, the administration of a defasciculating dose of a nondepolarizing muscle relaxant followed by judicious doses of thiopental and succinylcholine, hyperventilation while cricoid pressure is applied, and rapid intubation of the trachea (see Chapter 30).

The Advanced Trauma Life Support protocol recommends blind nasotracheal intubation for unconscious, spontaneously breathing patients, and patients in whom there is strong suspicion or proof of cervical spine injury, because it is less likely to require movement of the spine. Despite this recommendation, the vast majority of such patients and nearly all apneic patients can be safely intubated (orally) by experienced anesthesiologists. Nasal intubation risks injury to patients with basilar skull fractures, and it can provoke bleeding in the pharynx, resulting in airway compromise. In the hands of anesthesiologists experienced in managing trauma patients, oral intubation with cervical stabilization is safe, with few complications.

Paramedics are now trained to institute early, aggressive airway management at the scene of an accident. They are experienced at nasal or oral intubation. The esophageal obturator (EOA) or gastric tube airway (EGTA), and pharyngeotracheal lumen airways (PTL) are used less frequently. The anesthesiologist must verify proper position of a previously placed endotracheal tube as part of the initial airway management. Esophageal of pharyngeal airways are replaced by an endotracheal tube as soon as possible.

Hypotension often follows endotracheal intubation and positive pressure ventilation. It can be due to drugs, hypovolemia, pericardial tamponade, tension pneumothorax, or some combination. Positive pressure ventilation can convert a pneumothorax to a tension pneumothorax. The decrease in venous return with positive pressure ventilation in a hypovolemic patient can cause a decrease in cardiac output. Venous air embolism, a vasovagal response, or air trapping are other unusual causes of hypotension after intubation. Prompt diagnosis and treatment of each of these problems is critical.

Poor capillary refill, tachycardia, and hypotension are seen with most trauma patients and indicate a decrease in cardiac output. Successful resuscitation depends on differentiation between hypovolemia and impaired venous return. Blood loss can be obvious, as with major vascular lacerations and head wounds; or occult, in the case of hemothorax, abdominal bleeding, and pelvic fractures. Impaired venous return, but way of contrast, can cause hypotension and decreased output even when circulating blood volume is adequate. Pericardial tamponade or tension pneumothorax are two causes of impaired venous return that must be recognized promptly and treated appropriately.

The anesthesiologist must have a fundamental understanding of the implications of mechanisms of injury in the trauma patient. Blunt injuries (motor vehicle accident, falls from height), penetrating wounds (stabbings, shootings), burns (thermal, electrical, chemical), and mixed injuries produce different effects, requiring different care.

Blunt injuries result from the combination of several forces: direct impact, contrecoup, shearing, and rotary forces all contribute. Shearing injuries go beyond those sustained from direct contact. Blood vessels, nerves, and the musculoskeletal system are disrupted. Patients with blunt injuries are at risk for cervical spine injury, intracranial injuries, respiratory insufficiency (from lung contusion, thoracic injury), and aortic damage, each of which requires special management.

Penetrating injuries are more localized, although a high-velocity projectile also produces blunt injury. Stab wounds injure along the path of the blade. Bullets and shotgun pellets are less predictable; they do not necessarily follow straight lines through tissue. These patients can develop occult pneumothorax, hemopneumothorax, and pericardial tamponade. The anesthesiologist must suspect these problems in injured patients who develop otherwise unexplained hypotension or hypoxemia intraoperatively.

Burns represent a heterogeneous group of injuries, consisting of chemical, thermal, or mixed insults to the airway and skin. Toxic chemical gases such as carbon monoxide, carbon dioxide, nitrogen dioxide, hydrogen chloride, hydrogen cyanide, benzene, aldehydes, or ammonia are released from combustion. Carbon monoxide and cyanide interfere with cellular respiration. Thermal burns from heated gases or steam cause upper airway swelling and possible obstruction. Early endotracheal intubation is appropriate, as it is easier to intubate before edema affects the pharynx, vocal cords, and tracheal mucosa.

Immediate operative intervention for burn patients is seldom necessary in the absence of other injuries or a constricting eschar that interfere with respiration or circulation. Carbon monoxide inhalation is treated with oxygen therapy. Indications for hyperbaric therapy after carbon monoxide inhalation include loss of consciousness at the scene of injury, angina, or increased carboxyhemoglobin level (see Chapter 12).

The operating room is the second venue in which the anesthesiologist cares for trauma patients. Unlike other areas of anesthetic management, anesthesia for trauma requires preparedness for any degree of injury, type, and duration of the operation, and the ability to proceed despite limited information. An organized regional trauma system assures the immediate availability of surgical subspecialists at trauma centers, and the trauma anesthesiologist must be prepared to manage orthopedic, intra-abdominal, cardiac, and neurosurgical emergencies on an instant's notice.

Successful trauma anesthesia depends on adequate preparation. A specific operating room is designated for trauma cases and equipped for major procedures. Ideally, the room is large enough to accommodate more than one operating team, as well as fluoroscopy, perfusionists, and cardiopulmonary bypass equipment. The room temperature is maintained at 80° F because trauma patients are often hypothermic on arrival, and they become more so during the operation.

Anesthetic management is dictated by the nature of the patient's injuries and prior treatment. For example, the patient may have been sedated and paralyzed and the trachea intubated in the trauma area, in which case airway management in the operating room is simplified (although the position of the endotracheal tube must be verified). In many cases, the trachea has not been intubated, and the choice between regional and general anesthesia must be made. Regional anesthesia offers the advantage of retained protective airway reflexes in a patient with a full stomach; it improves perfusion to limbs with compromised blood flow, and it provides good postoperative analgesia. Disadvantages in trauma patients are that the airway remains unprotected should the patient lose consciousness or the condition worsen; the sympathectomy may compromise the circulation, and the anxious, possibly uncooperative patient remains awake.

Most critically ill patients receive general anesthesia and intubation. In rare cases, when massive intra-abdominal blood loss is present, intubation is deferred until the patient is draped, to minimize the delay between the induction of anesthesia and operative control of bleeding.

The choice of drugs to induce anesthesia in the trauma patient is similar to that for any hemodynamically unstable patient. Succinylcholine deserves special consideration, as it can provoke lethal hyperkalemia in patients after burns or crush injuries. Potassium release is presumed to result from abnormal muscle cells with an increased number of acetylcholine receptors (and therefore, sites for potassium exchange during succinylcholine-induced depolarization). Receptor proliferation does not occur in the first 48 hours following injury. It develops and persists for an indefinite period afterwards. Succinylcholine is therefore safe and appropriate in the immediate management of an injured patient, but must be avoided two days or more after major burns, massive crush injuries, or spinal cord injuries. The use of succinylcholine in patients with increased intracranial pressure has been discussed previously and in Chapter 30.

Invasive monitoring for operations after major trauma usually includes an arterial and central venous catheter, temperature measurement, and a urinary catheter.

Timing the placement of intravascular cannulae requires judgement. The use of an arterial catheter during induction can be quite helpful, and central venous routes are reliable paths by which to administer drugs in patients with circulatory impairment. However, delays in establishing vascular access must not prevent definitive surgical intervention. A radial arterial catheter can be placed after induction of anesthesia, for example, while draping or the operation proceeds.

Temperature monitoring is important. Coagulopathy, arrhythmias, and shivering result from hypothermia and are life threatening to the critically ill patient. Injured patients are draped so as to allow easy access to the trunk and extremities. Large incisions are the rule so that intraoperative heat loss conspires with fluid administration and preexistent hypothermia to further decrease body temperature. A warm operating room, humidifier or artificial nose and low flows in the anesthetic circuit prevent heat loss from the respiratory system. Intravenous fluids must be warmed. In cases of major blood loss, a rapid infusion device can be used, whereby large volumes of warmed blood products are given by a perfusionist (freeing the hands of the anesthesiologist). Standard blood warmers are an alternative.

The management of multiply-injured trauma patients requires assessment of the extent and severity of injuries and a schedule of treatment. The stabilization of a bleeding pelvic fracture takes precedence over the repair of a small intimal tear in the aorta, for example. Several surgical teams operate simultaneously in certain circumstances: an intracranial hematoma can be evacuated while a ruptured spleen is removed.

Operations for traumatic injuries are by their nature long and attended by hemodynamic and respiratory instability. The anesthesiologist must function as an intensivist, attending to critical organ systems while aware of the nature and implication of each of the patient's injuries.

Neurological injuries are seen frequently with blunt trauma and gunshot wounds. Preoperative neurological examination and radiographic studies are preferred; but when neurological evaluation is deferred owing to the severity of coexistent injuries, it is appropriate to empirically hyperventilate a patient with head injuries. In some circumstances, early intracranial pressure monitoring is instituted to improve management during long surgical procedures, and in anticipation of prolonged ICU care.

Renal hypoperfusion or direct injuries to the kidney and urinary tract are frequent causes of decreased urine output during anesthesia for trauma. Rhabdomyolysis with crush injuries can cause crystal deposition in the renal tubules. Some clinicians advocate the use of osmotic diuretics such as mannitol to increase urinary blood flow during the post-traumatic period. Alternatively, a loop diuretic can be used to differentiate renal from prerenal failure: the conversion of a low-output state to a high-output state is consistent with prerenal causes and a better prognosis.

Conclusion

Success in managing anesthesia for the critically ill patient depends on applying simultaneously two apparently contradictory philosophies. First, protocols, routines, and highly practiced skills must be employed to save time and ensure that nothing is overlooked. Second, analysis and imagination are required to resolve diagnostic dilemmas and successfully treat multiple disorders, especially when therapeutic goals conflict.

References

Advanced trauma life support course for physicians. American College of Surgeons, 1984.

Grande CM, ed. Trauma anesthesia and critical care, Critical Care Clinics. WB Saunders, 1990.

Parillo JE. Septic shock in humans: Clinical evaluation, pathogenesis, and therapeutic approach. *In* Shoemaker WC, Ayres S, Grenvik A, Holbrook PR, Thompson WL, ed. Textbook of critical care. Philadelphia: WB Saunders, 1989:1008.

Shoemaker WC. Physiologic monitoring of the critically ill patient. *In* Shoemaker WC, Ayres S, Grenvik A, Holbrook PR, Thompson WL, ed. Textbook of Critical Care. Philadelphia: WB Saunders, 1989:145.

CHAPTER THIRTY

NEUROANESTHESIA AND NEUROLOGIC DISEASES

This chapter begins with a brief review of relevant biochemistry and physiology, followed by a discussion of the anesthesia management of patients undergoing neurosurgical procedures and of patients who have incidental neurologic diseases but who are undergoing non-neurosurgical operations.

BRAIN BIOCHEMISTRY AND PHYSIOLOGY

Intracranial Pressures

Cerebral perfusion pressure (CPP) is the net blood pressure supplying the brain.

$$CPP = MABP - ICP$$

or

$$CPP = MABP - CVP$$

when

$$CVP > ICP$$

where MABP = mean arterial blood pressure
ICP = intracranial pressure
CVP = central venous pressure

Normal CPP is 80 to 90 mm Hg and normal intracranial pressure (ICP) is 0 to 10 mm Hg. Acute increases in ICP above 20 mm Hg warrant treatment.

The adult has about 150 ml of cerebral spinal fluid (CSF), made at a rate of about 0.35 ml per min (500 ml per day). The volume of intracranial contents can be rapidly increased by obstructing CSF outflow, reducing CSF reabsorption, increasing arterial CO_2 ($Paco_2$), administering anesthetic drugs, or obstructing venous drainage. The mostly fluid contents of the intracranial vault are incompressible, and cranial rigidity allows only minimal increases in brain volume. Increases in brain volume may increase ICP. As shown in Figure 30–1, an initial increase in brain volume does not change ICP; this is because of compensatory changes, which include decreases in intracranial venous blood volume, displacement of intracranial CSF, and some compression of brain tissue. Once the limit of compensation is reached, further small increases in volume sharply increase ICP. Increased ICP may reduce CPP, preventing adequate cerebral blood flow (CBF), or may produce brain herniation.

Brain Oxygen Demand

Relative to other organs, the brain has a large metabolic requirement, about 50 per cent of which

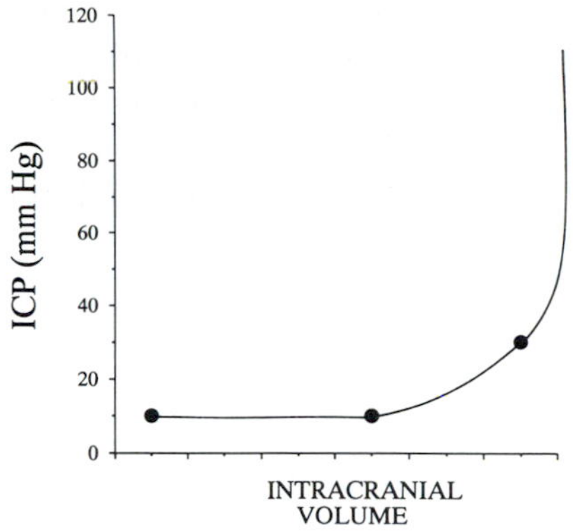

FIGURE 30–1. An idealized curve of the relationship between the volume of intracranial compartments and intracranial pressure (ICP). (Reproduced with permission from Miller JD, et al. Arch Neurol 1973; 28:266.)

is used to maintain the electrochemical gradients required for neurologic activity. The cerebral metabolic rate for oxygen ($CMRo_2$) averages 3 ml per 100 gm brain per min. The brain cannot meet its metabolic requirements though anaerobic glycolysis. As CBF decreases below a critical value, oxygen extraction from arterial blood increases; the conversion of glucose to lactate also increases; but $CMRo_2$ remains unchanged until oxygen delivery is severely compromised.

Cerebral Blood Flow

Whole brain CBF in unanesthetized, normothermic humans averages 54 ml per 100 gm brain per min. Cortical CBF less than about 20 ml per 100 gm per min in anesthetized patients is associated with decreased electroencephalogram (EEG) activity, and at CBF less than about 15 ml per 100 gm per min EEG activity ceases. Brain damage may occur if CBF decreases further (the threshold for neuronal depolarization due to energy depletion is about 10 ml per 100 gm per min). Normally the brain can tolerate a 50 per cent reduction in CBF before there is a significant risk of irreversible brain damage. This margin is decreased in patients with hypertension, carotid occlusion, or increased ICP.

Autoregulation of CBF

Through autoregulation, cerebral vascular resistance changes in response to changing blood pressure, so that CBF remains nearly constant despite large changes in CPP. In a normal person, CBF is autoregulated over a CPP of about 50 to 150 mm Hg (Fig. 30–2A). Below a CPP of 50 mm Hg CBF decreases as CPP decreases. As CPP exceeds 150 mm Hg, cerebral vessels dilate and CBF increases dramatically. There is significant individual variation with respect to the upper and lower limits of autoregulation (Fig. 30–2A).

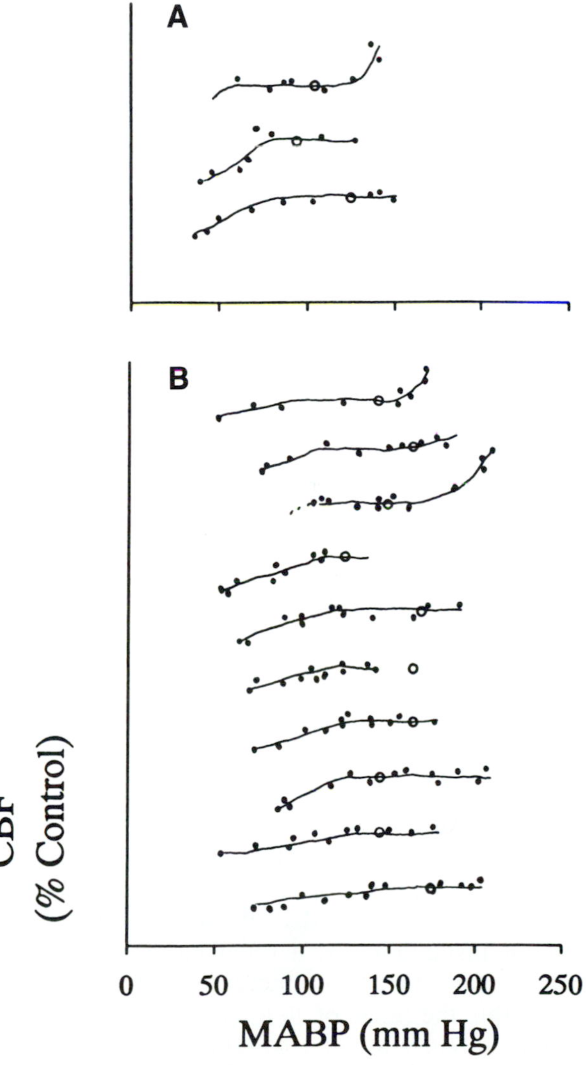

FIGURE 30–2. Autoregulation of cerebral blood flow (CBF) in response to changes in mean arterial blood pressure (MABP). Each curve shows relative CBF from an individual patient. The curves are offset from each other. The open circle represents a subject's typical MABP. In the hypertensive subjects (A) the autoregulation curve is shifted to the right so that the lower limit of autoregulation occurs at a greater MABP than in the normotensive subjects (B). (Reproduced with permission from Strandgaard S, et al: Br Med J 1973; 159:509.)

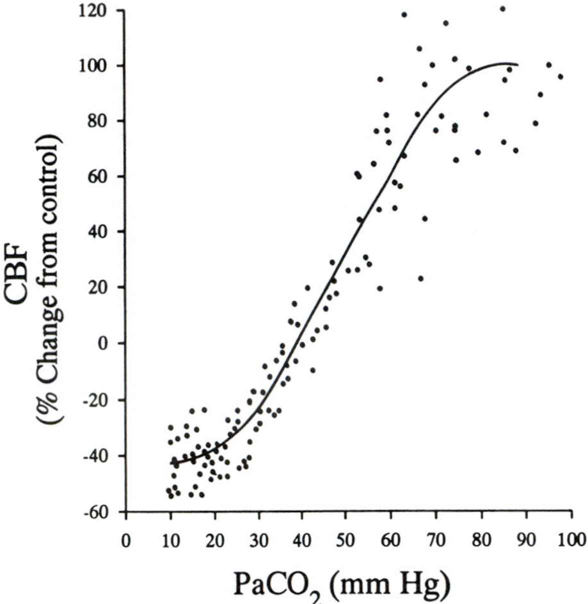

FIGURE 30–3. The relationship between $Paco_2$ and CBF. These data were obtained from dogs but human data are similar. Between a $Paco_2$ of 25 mm Hg and 75 mm Hg; the relationship is nearly linear. In the linear range there is roughly a 4 per cent change in CBF for each mm Hg change in $Paco_2$. (Reproduced with permission from Harper AM, Glass. J Neurol Neurosurg Psychiat 1965; 28:450.)

In hypertensive patients, the blood pressure limits for autoregulation are shifted to the right so that, compared to a normotensive person, autoregulation and CBF might fail at a greater mean arterial blood pressure (MABP) (Fig. 30–2B). With therapy, the hypertensive patient's autoregulation curve returns toward normal. In the elderly, autoregulation may be compromised because of occlusive vascular disease or loss of vessel distensibility. Autoregulation is lost after hypoxic or ischemic insults and in brain tissue near tumors. With impaired autoregulation, CBF depends more directly upon the MABP. Because autoregulation is not instantaneous, a rapid increase in MABP may result in transient increases in CBF.

Within the range of 20 to 60 mm Hg, changes in $Paco_2$ directly affect CBF (Fig. 30–3). Increases in $Paco_2$ tend to increase brain vascular volume, thereby increasing ICP. Decreases in $Paco_2$ have the opposite effect. In patients with brain swelling or increased ICP, hyperventilation is the most effective initial treatment to decrease ICP. With continued hyperventilation, vasoconstriction diminishes over 8 to 24 hours because of compensatory changes in serum bicarbonate. Rapid return to normocarbia after prolonged hyperventilation may increase cerebrovascular volume and ICP.

Changes in arterial oxygen tension between values of 50 and 300 mm Hg have little effect on CBF. As Pao_2 decreases below 50 mm Hg, CBF increases dramatically. Decreases in brain temperature decrease CBF and reduce $CMRo_2$ about 5 per cent for each 1°C.

Effects of Drugs Used During Anesthesia on CBF, ICP, and $CMRO_2$

Anesthetic drugs alter cerebrovascular volume. Intravenous anesthetic drugs, except ketamine, acutely produce cerebral vasoconstriction, reduce cerebrovascular volume, and decrease ICP (Table 30–1). Inhalational anesthetics produce acute cerebral vasodilation and may increase ICP. In pa-

TABLE 30–1. Effects of Drugs on Brain Blood Flow, Metabolism, and ICP

Drug	$CMRo_2$	CBF	ICP
Inhalational drugs			
N_2O	↑	↑	↑
Halothane	↓↓	↑↑↑	↑↑↑
Enflurane	↓↓	↑↑	↑↑
Isoflurane	↓↓↓	↑	↑
Desflurane	↓↓	?	↑↑
Intravenous induction drugs			
Barbiturates	↓↓↓	↓↓↓	↓↓↓
Etomidate	↓↓	↓↓	↓↓
Propofol	↓↓	↓↓	↓↓
Midazolam	↓	↓	↓
Ketamine	↑↑	↑↑	↑↑
Narcotics			
Morphine	±	±	↑
Fentanyl	±	±	0
Sufentanil	±	↑	↑
Alfentanil	?	↑	↑
Muscle Relaxants			
Tubocurarine	0	?	↑
Pancuronium	0	0	0
Atracurium	0	?	0
Vecuronium	0	0	0
Succinylcholine	↑	↑	↑↑

These data have been compiled from a variety of sources of primarily human but also animal data to serve as an initial guide. This table does not show changes in CPP, which is a function of both ICP and MABP; any drug that tends to decrease MABP may produce a decrease in CPP. $CMRo_2$, cerebral metabolic rate for oxygen; CBF, cerebral blood flow; ICP, intracranial pressure; CPP, cerebral perfusion pressure; MABP, mean arterial blood pressure.

tients with cerebral edema, intracranial masses, or obstructive hydrocephalus, drugs that increase brain volume may increase ICP enough to compromise cerebral perfusion or produce herniation. In contrast, drugs that reduce brain volume and ICP may improve cerebral perfusion, and the decreased brain volume may allow better surgical access.

Nitrous oxide (N_2O), 50 to 70 per cent, produces a 36 per cent increase in CBF and CMR_{O_2} in human volunteers and increases ICP by 100 to 200 per cent in patients with brain masses. However, when used with other anesthetic drugs, N_2O does not increase ICP. Increased ICP after dural closure in sitting patients occurs occasionally, presumable due to N_2O diffusing into entrapped air. Nitrous oxide is useful during neurosurgery because of its analgesic effects, rapid elimination, and lack of significant effects on blood pressure.

At less than 1 minimum alveolar concentration (MAC), isoflurane has minimal effects on ICP; an increase in ICP from isoflurane appears to be prevented by hyperventilation. Isoflurane and other halogenated drugs may also decrease MABP, producing a significant decrease in cerebral perfusion. In patients with brain tumors both sufentanil and alfentanil have been associated with increases in ICP that are usually insignificant.

Succinylcholine increases ICP under many conditions, but this may be prevented by blocking fasciculations. This intracranial hypertension may be produced by an afferent stimulus generated by mass activation of muscle spindle fibers during the initial depolarization, which produces a central arousal response accompanied by increases in CBF and cerebrovascular volume. Although succinylcholine may be avoided in patients at risk for intracranial hypertension, it may be used with defasciculating doses of nondepolarizing relaxant when rapid tracheal intubation is required. The nondepolarizing muscle relaxants pancuronium, vecuronium, and atracurium do not increase ICP. Histamine release with d-tubocurarine administration may cause cerebral vasodilatation and increased ICP.

Drugs used to control blood pressure may also alter ICP. In general, adrenergic agonists such as ephedrine, dopamine, and phenylephrine, or adrenergic antagonists such as propranolol, labetolol, or esmolol have no direct effect on ICP, nor does the ganglionic blocking drug trimethaphan. Direct-acting vasodilator drugs such as hydralazine, sodium nitroprusside, nitroglycerine, and adenosine increase cerebrovascular volume, as do calcium antagonists, which act on the cerebral vasculature (e.g., nimodipine).

Diuretics also alter ICP. Mannitol (0.25 to 1 gm per kg) increases plasma osmotic pressure relative to brain osmotic pressure. The movement of water from brain to blood reduces brain volume. Initially, rapid infusion of mannitol may increase vascular volume and ICP. Furosemide appears to be a less effective means of decreasing brain size, but it enhances the diuretic effect of mannitol and may inhibit mannitol-induced intracranial hypertension.

The effect on ICP is an important consideration in selecting a drug for use during neurosurgery; however, effects on blood pressure and post-operative alertness are also important. Anesthetics alter brain volume in varying degrees, and these effects may be countered by other drugs or hyperventilation. Thus, medications have proved useful during neurosurgery despite the fact that they can increase ICP. Cerebral compliance, hyperventilation, steroids, and diuretics may all modify the effects of an anesthetic. To choose anesthetic drugs only by their effects on ICP may eliminate some having unique benefits for a particular patient.

Electrophysiologic Monitoring

Electroencephalogram electrodes reflect localized cortical electrical activity and provide useful information about brain function and possible ischemia. With compromise of cerebral perfusion, the EEG will show a loss of high frequency activity (>14 Hz), possibly an increase in low frequency activity (2 to 4 Hz), and eventually loss of all activity. The EEG is sensitive to CPP, Pa_{CO_2}, anesthetic drugs, and electrocautery. The interpretation of the EEG is eased by computer processing, which emphasizes frequency changes and compresses the data. In anesthesia practice, the EEG is most commonly used to monitor brain activity during carotid endarterectomy or to monitor efficacy of barbiturate-induced metabolic suppression.

Evoked potentials (EP) are EEG signals triggered by electrical stimulation of a sensory nerve. Commonly used nerves are the median, ulnar, posterior tibial, or auditory; the resulting signals are detected by repeated stimulation and signal averaging and are sensitive to ischemia, anesthetics, and electrocautery. Evoked potentials indicate only the integrity of the sensory pathway and not adjacent motor pathways that might be independently compromised. During major spine operations EP monitoring reveals compromise in spinal cord function; during operations near the brainstem, monitoring the facial or auditory nerves is useful.

Brain Ischemic Damage, Protection, and Resuscitation

Complete loss of cerebral perfusion, such as during cardiac arrest, produces unconsciousness within six to seven seconds in normothermic subjects, loss of EEG activity within 15 to 25 seconds, and almost complete loss of brain high-energy metabolites such as adenosine triphosphate within two minutes. The disappearance of high-energy metabolites appears to set into motion a series of events that makes neuronal loss irreversible. The transition to irreversible damage occurs more slowly when regional CBF is compromised (focal ischemia, stroke), perhaps because of collateral flow.

Considerable research has produced neither a mechanism to explain the details of ischemic neuronal damage nor generally accepted approaches to increasing tolerance of an ischemic insult (protection) or to treatment after ischemia (resuscitation). In the operating room, decreasing the oxygen demand may be a useful strategy. Profound hypothermia (18°C) slows cerebral metabolism enough to allow periods of circulatory arrest during cardiac operations. Recent animal data suggest that moderate hypothermia (30 to 34°C) may also reduce neurologic damage during less severe compromises in oxygen delivery.

Thiopental at doses that abolish EEG activity or produce EEG patterns of burst suppression decreases neurobehavioral deficits after normothermic cardiopulmonary bypass. Although the use of intraoperative barbiturates during carotid endarterectomy or cerebral aneurysmectomy has been advocated, there are no prospective studies demonstrating clinical efficacy. Etomidate has also been suggested, but remains unproven. Isoflurane (about 1.5 per cent) decreases the level of regional CBF at which EEG changes occur. In addition, during carotid endarterectomy the incidence of EEG changes suggestive of ischemia appears to decrease with use of isoflurane compared to halothane.

A large number of animal studies suggest that hyperglycemia superimposed on an ischemic insult increases the neurologic damage. Because withholding glucose does not appear to produce hypoglycemia, this has become common practice during neurosurgical operations.

ANESTHESIA FOR PATIENTS WITH INTRACRANIAL MASSES

The Acutely Decompensating Patient

Patients with rapidly increasing ICP require emergency treatment to secure the airway, to provide oxygenation and ventilation, and to reduce ICP. Patients with subdural, epidural, or subarachnoid hemorrhage, severe head injury, or large tumors may present with acute loss of consciousness, seizures, and decorticate or decerebrate posturing.

The management of these patients for emergency neurosurgery begins by establishing oxygenation and hyperventilation by mask. If vascular volume appears adequate, and a rapid examination of the airway does not suggest difficulty, give 2 to 5 mg per kg thiopental and a large dose of vecuronium and intubate promptly. If there has been trauma, assume there is spinal cord injury and manage the intubation appropriately (see later section, Spinal Cord Injury). Treat transient increases in blood pressure with additional thiopental. Begin mannitol therapy before or after tracheal intubation; hyperventilation and thiopental have more immediate effects. If the need for continued neurologic evaluation rules out vecuronium, succinylcholine with small doses of a nondepolarizer to prevent fasciculations may be used instead. Invasive monitoring is helpful, but must not delay surgical decompression of a treatable lesion. Anesthesia may be maintained with additional thiopental or narcotic and, after decompression, with low doses of isoflurane.

Intracranial Masses

The etiology of an intracranial mass is not as important as its volume, speed of formation, and anatomic location. Thus, tumors or accumulations of blood may have similar effects, although rapidly expanding masses create greater neurologic impairment than do more slowly progressing lesions. The goals of anesthetic management include maintaining cerebral perfusion without increasing intracranial volume.

PREOPERATIVE EVALUATION

Drowsiness, obtundation, unconsciousness, nausea, vomiting, and papilledema all indicate increased ICP and a patient at significant risk for herniation or cerebral ischemia. The preoperative computed tomographic (CT) scan or magnetic resonance image (MRI) can help identify patients at special risk for intraoperative intracranial hypertension, as indicated by cerebral edema, obliterated, small, or massively dilated lateral ventricles, and a 5-mm or more midline shift. Narcotic or heavy sedative premedications are avoided because they may depress ventilation and increase ICP.

Monitoring for most intracranial neurosurgical procedures includes capnography, pulse oximetry, electrocardiogram, temperature, and urine output. An arterial catheter allows accurate assessment of blood pressure and sampling for $Pa{CO_2}$, serum electrolytes, and serum osmotic pressure. Central pressure monitoring for vascular volume replacement is often used if significant blood loss is expected.

Elevating the patient's head 10 to 15 degrees above the heart promotes venous drainage and avoids venous engorgement. Excessive rotation of the head or flexion of the neck may interfere with venous drainage, as may pressure on the anterior neck.

INDUCTION OF ANESTHESIA

Prior to induction of anesthesia, a brief period of voluntary hyperventilation may decrease brain volume. Induction of anesthesia with intravenous drugs that decrease cerebrovascular volume and ICP is followed immediately by hyperventilation, avoiding hypercapnia, hypoxia, coughing, or excessive peak inspiratory pressures, all to prevent increases in brain volume. Because abrupt increases in MABP may increase ICP, fentanyl (5 μg per kg in divided doses) may be given to obtund the response to tracheal intubation and other stimuli; this does not prevent rapid emergence after a three- to four-hour operation. Local anesthetics injected subcutaneously before the skin incision or placement of head fixation devices ameliorate hypertensive responses.

Vecuronium is an appropriate choice to ensure immobility. It not only has minimal cardiovascular effects, but its short duration of action minimizes residual neuromuscular blockade, even though these patients must often be kept paralyzed until the surgical dressing is in place.

Many of these patients have decreased intravascular volumes that may contribute to intraoperative hypotension. In adults, maintenance fluid replacement at rates of 1 to 1.5 ml per kg per hour with an isosmotic crystalloid or colloid solution causes minimal additional brain swelling. Maintaining hemoglobin concentrations between 8 and 10 gm per dl further decreases the risk of increased ICP or brain swelling. Glucose-containing solutions are avoided, as described earlier.

INTRAOPERATIVE MANAGEMENT

Nitrous oxide combined with amnestic doses of isoflurane (much less than MAC) and hyperventilation produce, at worst, minimal brain swelling. For massive brain swelling or severe intracranial hypertension, it may be wise to avoid the halogenated anesthetics and substitute thiopental by intermittent injection (50 to 100 mg) or as an infusion at 0.02 to 0.2 mg per kg per minute. The major risks of barbiturate anesthesia are hypotension and excessive postoperative sedation.

Because the concentration of inhalational anesthetic must be held to a minimum, hypertension occurring at the time of the incision is treated with narcotic or trimethaphan. During the operation hypertension responds to labetalol, usually in 5- to 10-mg increments. The mixed alpha- and beta-adrenergic antagonist action of this drug has no effect on ICP and may allow better control of MABP with less bradycardia than pure beta-adrenergic antagonists do.

BRAIN VOLUME

Surgical manipulation of the brain may produce swelling, treatable by hyperventilation ($Pa{CO_2}$ of 25 mm Hg) and osmotic or loop diuretics. Mannitol given at the time of skin incision will take effect in the 45 minutes the surgeon usually requires to reach the dura. Brain swelling can be treated by elevating the head, giving thiopental (100 to 300 mg), and discontinuing inhalational anesthetics.

EMERGENCE FROM ANESTHESIA

Large doses of sedatives or narcotics, or large concentrations of halogenated anesthetics may delay emergence from anesthesia and interfere with the prompt recognition of intracranial bleeding or other causes of increased ICP. During emergence, hypertension is best controlled with antihypertensive drugs rather than by adding anesthetic. Esmolol does not increase CBF or ICP and may work well in this situation.

Usually, the endotracheal tube is removed while the patient is still in the operating room. Exceptions include patients with preoperative obtundation or severe intraoperative brain swelling or ischemia. Changes in neurologic status that may indicate postoperative problems such as bleeding can best be detected in alert extubated patients. As the patient emerges from anesthesia, coughing may increase ICP or cause intracranial bleeding. Early signs of reaction to tracheal stimulation, such as swallowing or irregular ventilation, may be treated with small doses of additional narcotic or lidocaine, 20 to 40 mg IV.

Pituitary Tumors

Pituitary tumors tend not to increase ICP. Patients with acromegaly have increased jaw size, enlarged tongues, and overgrowth of laryngeal soft tissue, often requiring awake sedated intubation.

The most common surgical approach to pituitary tumors is a sublabial transsphenoidal route. A right-angle oral or wire spiral tracheal tube allows surgical access without compromise of airway control.

Posterior Fossa

Anesthesia for operations in or near the posterior fossa requires managing the occasional need to avoid muscle relaxants, the specific risks associated with the surgical position, increased ICP, brainstem compression, and brainstem stimulation. Operations include removal of cerebellar or brainstem tumors, removal of acoustic neurinomas, microvascular decompression for pain, and decompression of the brainstem. Preoperative considerations, induction, and maintenance of anesthetic are similar to those described for intracranial tumors.

POSITIONING

A variety of operative positions may be used, including supine with the head turned; lateral; 3/4 lateral (park bench); prone; or sitting (See Chapter 16).

INTRAOPERATIVE MONITORING

Monitoring is similar to that for intracranial tumors. The sitting position increases the risk of air embolism, requiring special monitoring. Resection of acoustic neurinoma and other procedures may require evoked potential monitoring, possibly limiting the use of greater concentrations of N_2O or halogenated anesthetics.

AIR EMBOLISM

When the surgical site is above the heart, there is a risk of air entry into the venous system. Air embolism occurs in about 40 per cent of posterior fossa operations performed in the sitting position, and less often in the prone position. Patients placed in the sitting position are monitored for air embolism by a precordial Doppler device and continuous capnography. End-tidal nitrogen detected by mass spectrometry appears to be a less sensitive monitor. Transesophageal echocardiography is the most sensitive detector of intracardiac air, but it is expensive. It can also detect air movement from the right to the left side of the heart. Hypotension, murmurs, and hypoxemia are late signs.

In order to remove air from the heart, many anesthesiologists place a right atrial catheter in these patients, using changes in the P wave of the EEG (monitored through the saline-filled catheter) as a guide. Optimal position of the catheter is just above the right atrium. Multi-orifice catheters are more efficient than single-orifice catheters for capturing intravascular air, including that trapped in the superior vena cava.

Maintaining adequate intravascular volume may decrease the incidence of air embolism. If air embolism occurs, the surgeon occludes open vessels or sinuses and covers the surgical field with saline. The anesthesiologist stops giving nitrous oxide, aspirates air via the right atrial catheter, and supports blood pressure with vasopressors and fluids. Persistent air entry or hypotension may require lowering the patient's head.

INTRAOPERATIVE MANAGEMENT

When muscle relaxants cannot be used, such as when the facial nerve is monitored, the dose of anesthetic is increased to prevent patient movement. This may produce hypotension, requiring vasopressors to maintain blood pressure and cerebral perfusion.

During posterior fossa operations, nitrous oxide may increase the size of air emboli. Because of its other favorable features, one may choose to use N_2O until an air embolus occurs, or until the dura is closed, in circumstances when air might be trapped beneath the dura.

CEREBROVASCULAR OPERATIONS

Carotid Endarterectomy

This operation is done to remove plaque that has produced a critical decrease in the diameter of the carotid artery or which may be a source of cerebral emboli. The carotid artery is exposed near its bifurcation, crossclamped above and below the lesion, and opened so that the plaque can be removed. The patient may have hypertension, coronary artery disease, or chronic obstructive pulmonary disease. Common complications include postoperative stroke and myocardial infarction.

Anesthetic choice may depend upon local preference. Under regional anesthesia the awake patient may provide information about mental function, and intraoperative hemodynamic instability may be lessened. Patient comfort and control of the airway are guaranteed with general anesthesia. Outcomes are similar. The majority of carotid endarterectomies are done using general anesthesia.

General anesthesia must be managed to allow smooth, rapid emergence with minimal postoperative sedation and close control of cardiovascular responses. For this reason, monitoring usually includes an arterial cannula. Infiltration of the carotid body with local anesthetic under direct vision can decrease intraoperative fluctuations in heart rate and blood pressure. The decrease in CBF that accompanies hyperventilation is avoided by maintaining Pa_{CO_2} between 35 to 40 mm Hg.

During the period of carotid artery crossclamping, systemic blood pressure is often maintained at the upper end of the patient's normal range to facilitate cerebral perfusion. Three approaches are used to maintain cerebral perfusion: relying on collateral circulation; routinely placing a plastic shunt to carry blood from the common carotid artery to the internal carotid artery; and selective shunting based on some measure of cerebral perfusion adequacy. Complications of shunting include embolization and increased operating time.

Cerebral perfusion in awake patients can be monitored by asking the patient to follow commands or answer questions, although untested pathways may suffer unrecognized compromise. Changes often occur within 30 seconds of crossclamping, if collateral circulation is inadequate. Other measures of cerebral perfusion have included jugular venous oxygen saturation, carotid artery stump pressure, oculoplethysmography, Doppler ultrasound, and intraoperative arteriography. Many of these techniques are intermittent and some are inaccurate. Cerebral blood flow measurements have been used, but the EEG is the most commonly used monitor.

Cerebral Aneurysms and Arteriovenous Malformations

Cerebral aneurysms occur most commonly at bifurcations of vessels, most frequently along the anterior and posterior communicating arteries, as well as the anterior and middle cerebral arteries. Patients who bleed from an aneurysm have a significant risk of bleeding again. They also suffer hypertension and cerebral vasospasm (thought to be related to extravascular hemoglobin decomposition), which reduces blood flow to the local tissue. Initial therapy consists of sedatives, anticonvulsants, and antihypertensive drugs. The calcium channel blocker nimodipine has been shown to reduce the incidence of neurologic complications from vasospasm. The antifibrinolytic drug aminocaproic acid can retard clot lysis and potentially reduce the risk of further bleeding, but it also increases cerebral ischemia.

The risk of bleeding is greatest during the first 72 hours, and operation within this period has become increasingly common. Most aneurysms are attached to the parent vessel by a narrow neck, across which the surgeon places a metal clip to isolate the aneurysm. Postoperative problems include cerebral vasospasm resulting in stroke, stroke from clip placement, continued hypertension, seizures, brain swelling, and bleeding because of clip dislodgement.

Arteriovenous malformations are masses of abnormal vessels that may present with bleeding, seizures, headache, or focal neurologic deficits. The operation involves isolation and ligation of the arterial supply and venous drainage followed by resection of the malformation. The risk of sudden intraoperative bleeding is considerably less than for aneurysms.

ANESTHETIC CONSIDERATIONS

The major anesthetic goals are as follows:

1. Induction of anesthesia and tracheal intubation without hypotension that might compromise cerebral perfusion or hypertension that might cause bleeding.
2. Brain relaxation to allow surgical exposure.
3. Occasional use of intraoperative hypotension to facilitate exposure and to control bleeding.
4. Maintenance of vascular volume to decrease the effects of vasospasm.
5. Emergence from anesthesia and extubation in the operating room, allowing early assessment of neurologic state.

In some patients, blood accumulation and edema from the initial bleeding may create a mass effect, and considerations similar to patients with brain tumors apply.

Many regimens have been used to avoid hypertension during induction and intubation; each has its advocates. The plan described for patients with intracranial mass lesions works well. Body temperature is allowed to decrease to about 33°C to decrease $CMRO_2$. In addition to the usual measures to prevent brain swelling, a lumbar drain may be used to allow removal of CSF during the operation.

To ease exposure of the aneurysm, the surgeon may temporarily clip the vessels feeding the aneurysm or request reduction in arterial blood pressure. Used together, these two maneuvers create extra risks of brain ischemia; arterial pressure must be maintained and clipping must be as brief as possible, typically less than four minutes. Pharmacologic measures might improve brain tolerance of inadequate oxygen delivery, but as yet none have been demonstrated to be effective in this situation.

Deliberate hypotension has been used in some institutions to reduce wall tension in the aneurysm and to decrease the rate of blood loss from ruptured aneurysms and from arteriovenous malformations or vascular tumors. As described in the section on brain physiology, normotensive patients tolerate decreased MABP to 50 to 60 mm Hg, whereas in hypertensive patients, an induced decrease in MABP of 35 to 45 per cent of the preoperative MABP is acceptable. Isoflurane and sodium nitroprusside, with beta-adrenergic blockers for reflex tachycardia, provide controllable hypotension.

After the aneurysm is clipped, MABP is increased above the patient's normal MABP to overcome vasospasm, by decreasing the depth of anesthesia and infusing fluids; occasionally a vasopressor is needed. Adequate volume replacement and the use of vasopressors, if needed, continues into the immediate postoperative period, but during emergence from anesthesia and extubation, excessive hypertension must be prevented.

ANESTHESIA FOR NEURORADIOLOGIC PROCEDURES

Patients may require anesthesia or sedation for radiologic diagnostic procedures. Planning must take into account the degree of neurologic compromise and diminished cerebral compliance. Sedation may be contraindicated if increased ICP is present. Tracheal intubation and controlled ventilation may be required.

Magnetic resonance imaging is unique because of the strong magnetic field. Ferrous objects can be drawn toward the magnet at high velocities, damaging equipment and people. Noninvasive blood pressure monitors, sidestream capnographs, and ECG oscilloscopes may be usable if placed sufficiently far from the magnet and immobilized. Because there is no ionizing radiation, the anesthesiologist can sit near the patient to provide sedation and reassurance, which are often sufficient. If needed, the induction of anesthesia and tracheal intubation take place outside the magnet area. Although MRI-compatible anesthesia machines have been described, they are unnecessary. Oxygen and intravenous drugs such as propofol, narcotics, and muscle relaxants provide adequate maintenance of anesthesia.

NEUROLOGIC DISEASE

Anesthetic management of patients for other than neurosurgical procedures often must include consideration of neurologic or muscular diseases which present as depressed levels of consciousness, weakness, or autonomic nervous system dysfunction.

Loss of Consciousness

Coma usually results from a diffuse insult to both cerebral hemispheres because, except for brainstem lesions involving the reticular activating system, isolated focal lesions do not impair consciousness. Preoperative sedation for comatose patients is usually unnecessary and may be harmful; hypoventilation may increase ICP. If intracranial compliance is decreased, induction and tracheal intubation are conducted as described for patients with intracranial masses. Because the comatose patient's ability to protect the airway may be impaired, careful evaluation is needed before extubation.

Seizures

The patient with seizures that recur without recovery (status epilepticus) is at risk for hypoxic injury and pulmonary edema from increases in systemic and pulmonary vascular resistance. Neuromuscular blocking drugs halt the motor activity and permit airway control but do not stop seizure activity, which is treated with barbiturates, phenytoin, or benzodiazepines. General anesthesia has been used to stop seizures that are refractory to other therapies.

For the patient with a known seizure disorder, important preoperative information includes the nature and frequency of the seizure activity, the etiology of the seizures, if known, and current medication. Blood levels of antiepileptic drugs can be obtained and compared to the patient's usual levels (most agents can be increased to therapeutic levels within 24 to 48 hours). Antiepileptics are continued on the day of operation; unexpected recurrence of seizures on the day of surgery is not a common problem. The pro- and anticonvulsant effects of anesthetic drugs are summarized in Table 30–2.

TABLE 30–2. Pro- and Anticonvulsant Effects of Anesthetic Drugs

Proconvulsants
- Methohexital (in complex partial seizures only)
- Etomidate
- Enflurane (in greater concentrations with hypocapnia)
- Meperidine and its metabolite, normeperidine
- Ketamine
- Local anesthetics*
- Laudanosine (metabolite of atracurium)

Questionable
- Fentanyl (myoclonic activity; minimal evidence for convulsive activity in humans)

Anticonvulsants
- Barbiturates
- Benzodiazepines
- Propofol
- Halothane
- Isoflurane
- Local anesthetics*

* Rapidly increasing blood levels of local anesthetics tend to suppress inhibitory neurons and promote seizures, but intravenous infusions of local anesthetics have been employed for their anticonvulsant effects.

Head Injury

The Glasgow Coma Score (GCS) is used to characterize neurologic impairment after head injury (Table 30–3). The GCS does not substitute for a

TABLE 30–3. Glasgow Coma Scale

Response	Characteristics	Score
Eye opening	Spontaneous	4
	To speech	3
	To pain	2
	Nil	1
Verbal response	Oriented	5
	Confused conversation	4
	Inappropriate words	3
	Incomprehensible sounds	2
	Nil	1
Best motor response	Obeys	6
	Localizes	5
	Withdraws (flexion)	4
	Abnormal flexion	3
	Extensor response	2
	Nil	1

Reproduced with permission from Teasdale, Jennett. Lancet 1974; 2:81.

minute-to-minute record of neurologic function, because it does not include signs of lower brainstem function such as respiratory rate, pattern and depth, and blood pressure. Coma corresponds to a GCS of 8 or less; these patients do not open their eyes, speak, or respond to commands.

The first step in the care of the patient with head injury is airway control, which is often complicated by facial or cervical spine injuries, bleeding into the mouth, a full stomach, or hypovolemia. Neck flexion or hypertension must be prevented throughout, unless there is an unequivocal radiologic diagnosis of cervical spine stability.

Blind nasotracheal intubation without muscle relaxants offers minimal neck movement, but also carries the risk of failure, blind passage into the cranial vault in the presence of a basilar skull fracture, epistaxis, and paranasal sinusitis with prolonged intubation. Orotracheal intubation after anesthesia and paralysis is often successful and carries other advantages as well. Movement, coughing, and hypertension in response to laryngoscopy and tracheal intubation can be prevented. Hyperventilation and rapid-sequence induction with thiopental or etomidate and vecuronium allows prompt intubation while minimizing the risk of aspiration or of increasing ICP. In the absence of brainstem injury, hypotension does not result from the head injury; decreased blood pressure prompts a search for bleeding or spinal cord injury.

Patients with head injury may present for craniotomy or other operations. Anesthetic management depends on ICP. If ICP is normal, simply avoiding measures that increase ICP is adequate. Management of brain swelling or intracranial hypertension is the same as that of intracranial masses.

The patient with diffuse bihemispheric cerebral impairment may be at risk for a lethal hyperkalemic response to succinylcholine. Brain injury can also produce ECG changes, such as QT prolongation and T wave and ST segment changes, despite the absence of myocardial ischemia.

Brain Death

Brain death is defined as the irreversible absence of cortical and brainstem function; cardiac death usually follows within 48 to 72 hours. Management of the brain-dead organ donor includes supporting the cardiopulmonary system after loss of central control, and protecting the organs to be donated from hypertension and tachycardia provoked by surgical stimuli (Table 30–4).

TABLE 30–4. Perioperative Management for the Brain-Dead Organ Donor

Problem	Recommended Treatment
Hypotension due to neurogenic shock and hypovolemia	Copious fluid therapy Vasopressors if needed
Bradycardia	Atropine
Hypoxemia due to atelectasis or neurogenic pulmonary edema	Oxygen PEEP (positive end-expiratory pressure)
Diabetes insipidus	Replace water PRN
Organ hypoperfusion	Maintain perfusion pressures, cardiac output; Treat reflex pressor responses with appropriate vasodilators

Weakness

It is useful to group disorders of motor function by the location of the lesion. Chronic upper motor neuron deficits (i.e., above the level of the anterior horn cell) present with spastic paresis with hyperreflexia and pathologic reflexes (upgoing toe). Interruption of neuromuscular transmission at the lower motor neuron or the peripheral nerve causes flaccid paralysis and hyporeflexia. Interference with transmission at the neuromuscular junction produces a fatigable weakness that may improve with anticholinesterase therapy. Finally, weakness may result from dystrophic changes within the muscle cell.

Spinal Cord Injury

Injured patients can have significant vertebral column instability without neurologic damage. Definitive cervical spine films are difficult to obtain; when results are equivocal, the patient's neck is splinted against movement. Neck flexion appears to increase the risk of further damage, whereas minimal neck extension may be tolerated. Hard and soft collars do not restrict the neck's range of motion adequately; a combination of a hard collar and bilateral sandbags joined with wide tape across the forehead most effectively controls neck motion. Excessive traction may cause vertebral dislocation, as can excessive cricoid pressure. Muscle relaxants, intravenous induction agents and adjuvant drugs are used as dictated by the clinical situation. For patients with unstable necks in traction who require elective operations, fiberoptic intubation with adequate sedation and topical anesthesia is preferred.

Methylprednisolone (30 mg per kg intravenously over 15 minutes followed by a 24-hour infusion at 5.4 mg per kg per hour) is started within eight hours of spinal cord injury. This improves neurologic recovery with no additional morbidity.

The early autonomic response to spinal cord injury is called spinal shock and is the result of depression of neurons below the level of injury. The acute clinical manifestations depend on the level of injury and include hypotension, bladder and bowel paralyses, and gastric dilation. Pulmonary edema may result from aggressive fluid loading. Hypotension is corrected by a combination of fluid and vasopressors, such as dopamine. In addition, many advocate the use of pulmonary artery catheters as a guide to fluid replacement.

After recovery from spinal shock, autonomic hyperreflexia may follow with injuries above T_5. This syndrome is also known as mass reflex; noxious stimuli trigger vasoconstriction, producing relative intravascular volume overload and extreme hypertension. Bladder irrigation, childbirth, defecation, or anal dilation and intra-abdominal procedures are potent stimulators. A few patients respond to cutaneous stimulation, and a small minority trigger spontaneously, requiring chronic treatment with ganglionic blocking drugs. Intraoperatively, autonomic hyperreflexia occurs with local anesthesia, sedation and light nitrous oxide-narcotic techniques, but not usually with sufficiently deep general anesthesia using halogenated anesthetics or spinal anesthesia of adequate extent. Episodes of hypertension can be treated by deeper anesthesia, direct-acting vasodilators, or ganglionic blocking drugs.

Denervation produces changes in the muscle membrane that alter the response to neuromuscular blocking drugs as described in Chapter 11. Severe hyperkalemia, ventricular arrhythmias, and cardiac arrest have been reported after succinylcholine as early as three days after spinal cord injury; the risk persists for six months to a year.

TABLE 30–5. Clinical Problems Caused by Spinal Cord Injury

Pathologic Process	Etiology
Impaired temperature regulation	Increased cutaneous blood flow due to sympathectomy
Atelectasis	Acutely due to pulmonary contusion; later, due to hypoventilation, decreased vital capacity, and inadequate cough
Pulmonary emboli	Dilated veins, immobility
Urinary tract infections	Bladder dysfunction
Nephrolithiasis, hypercalcemia	Immobility, calcium wasting
Decubital ulcers	Immobility, muscle atrophy

Succinylcholine has been used within the first 24 to 36 hours after injury without untoward response. Other management issues arising from spinal cord injury are listed in Table 30–5.

Myasthenia Gravis

Myasthenia gravis causes a functional decrease in acetylcholine receptors of the neuromuscular junction. Weakness affecting muscles of the airway, the chest wall, and the diaphragm, and the concomitant risks of postoperative respiratory failure are of first concern in anesthesia management. Tests of muscle strength, such as the vital capacity or the maximal inspiratory pressure, warn of impending ventilatory failure before dyspnea, hypercarbia, or hypoxia occur. Preoperative medical management to improve respiratory muscle function has been shown to reduce the need for postoperative mechanical ventilation.

There is no consensus on whether the anticholinesterase drugs used to treat myasthenia are best withheld or given just before operation; management has been successful with either approach. Withholding anticholinesterase drugs for a prolonged period risks respiratory failure. Excessive doses of anticholinesterase drugs can cause cholinergic crisis, which is marked by weakness and muscarinic symptoms such as salivation, bradycardia, and miosis.

Drugs which affect the neuromuscular junction, such as the type I-a antiarrythmic drugs (procainamide, quinidine) and aminoglycoside antibiotics, may worsen myasthenia. Intravenous lidocaine accentuates the neuromuscular blocking properties of other anesthetic drugs, but the use of lidocaine for regional or local anesthesia does not seem to exacerbate myasthenia.

Patients with myasthenia gravis respond variably to succinylcholine and tend to develop Phase II block. Myasthenic patients are sensitive to competitive neuromuscular blocking drugs and require doses only 20 to 50 per cent of those required by healthy patients. Elimination pharmacokinetics are normal; prolonged drug effect results from relative overdoses. Administration of exceedingly small increments of short-acting muscle relaxants, guided by monitoring of the response to a nerve stimulator, yields appropriate doses for each patient.

Myasthenic patients can also be managed with regional anesthesia or general anesthesia without relaxants. Regardless of the anesthetic employed, these patients require extra vigilance at the end of the procedure, because even if they meet conventional criteria of adequate strength and ventilatory function, fatigue often sets in rapidly and unexpectedly.

Myopathies

Patients afflicted with one of the progressive muscular dystrophies that present in childhood, most commonly Duchenne's, require operations for diagnostic biopsy as well as for orthopedic procedures such as Achilles tendon transfer and Harrington rod placement for scoliosis. Endomyocardial fibrosis with conduction abnormalities and other cardiac abnormalities are common. Restrictive respiratory disease results from weakness and kyphoscoliosis. Life-threatening gastric dilation under anesthesia has been described, suggesting use of a nasogastric tube.

Case reports and in vitro contracture testing indicate that many patients with myopathy, particularly of the Duchenne type, are susceptible to malignant hyperpyrexia, but the magnitude of this risk is unknown. An anesthetic plan for a myopathic patient might well include capnography, close temperature monitoring, and avoiding drugs known to trigger malignant hyperthermia. Prophylaxis with dantrolene is not indicated and may be harmful, as it exacerbates weakness.

Dysautonomia and Mixed Disorders

Movement disorders can involve deterioration of central dopaminergic or cholinergic pathways, which can cause diminished movement (bradykinesia), as with Parkinson's disease, or increased movements, as in Huntington's chorea. Cerebellar degeneration causing ataxia may involve other organ systems, as in cardiomyopathy in Friedreich's ataxia. Other degenerative conditions may impair protective airway reflexes.

Initially, Parkinson's disease responds to oral L-dopa combined with carbidopa to block the systemic effects of dopamine. Butyrophenones and phenothiazines exacerbate parkinsonism. Both droperidol and metoclopramide have been reported to cause severe rigidity that requires postoperative respiratory support. Parkinsonism can cause dyskinesias of airway musculature and functional airway obstruction.

Multiple sclerosis is a demyelinating disease characterized by exacerbations and remissions. Exacerbations occur spontaneously and with systemic stress, particularly fever. Because of these unpredictable exacerbations, and because of possible direct neurotoxic effects of local anesthetics, it may be prudent to avoid regional anesthesia in patients with demyelinating diseases.

Disorders of the autonomic system can be congenital or acquired and are often characterized as central or peripheral. Diseases associated with autonomic neuropathy are listed in Table 30–6. Autonomic neuropathy may produce orthostatic hypotension or syncope. Other clinical features include a relatively fixed heart rate, gastroesophageal reflux, disturbances in intestinal motility, and episodic hypertension. The cardiac output depends on preload and the systemic vascular resis-

TABLE 30–6. Diseases Associated with Autonomic Neuropathy

Congenital (Riley-Day syndrome)
Idiopathic (Shy-Drager syndrome or multisystem atrophy)
Peripheral neuropathies
- Guillain-Barré syndrome (acute idiopathic polyneuritis)
- Diabetes mellitus
- Alcohol abuse
- Vitamin B_{12} deficiency
- Heavy metal toxicity

tance is typically decreased. With a peripheral autonomic neuropathy, denervation hypersensitivity may cause an abnormal response to direct-acting sympathomimetic drugs.

Case reports of patients with significant autonomic neuropathy have identified possible approaches to anesthetic management based on know pathophysiology. Preoperative intravenous hydration and premedication with metoclopramide and cimetidine seem wise. Elastic stockings may be useful, especially for surgical positions that cause venous pooling. Gastroparesis may warrant rapid-sequence induction of general anesthesia. When dysautonomia is also associated with a peripheral neuropathy that produces significant motor denervation (such as Guillain-Barré syndrome), succinylcholine may cause hyperkalemia. Doses of direct-acting vasopressors must be reduced to avoid severe hypertension, and indirect-acting vasopressors may be unreliable in peripheral dysautonomias. General anesthesia with halogenated anesthetics, narcotics, or ketamine have all been reported to be safe. Regional anesthesia has been rejected by some because hypotension may be difficult to treat.

Overall Management of Patient with Neurologic Disease

Many neurologic diseases are rare, therefore experience is limited to case reports or small series of patients. Furthermore, many conditions, particularly degenerative disorders, are characterized by relapsing and remitting courses that make it difficult to draw inferences based on a small group of patients. Thus, detailed recommendations for the anesthesia management of these patients are likely to be based on personal preference as much as on scientific data. For example, regional anesthesia is often cited as contraindicated, but there is little direct evidence for such recommendation, which may reflect primarily medicolegal concerns. Successful anesthesia management of patients with neurological diseases depends on a thorough appreciation of the pathophysiology of the disease and a cautious approach more than it does on adherence to absolute caveats.

REFERENCES

Albin MS, ed. Acute spinal cord injury. *In* Critical care clinics. 1987; 3:441-697.

Azar I. The response of patients with neuromuscular disorders to muscle relaxants: A review. Anesthesiology 1984; 61:173-187.

Bruce DA. Management of severe head injury. *In* Cottrell JE, Turndorf H, eds. Anesthesia and neurosurgery. St. Louis: CV Mosby, 1986: 150-172.

Cucchiara RF, Michenfelder JD, eds. Clinical neuroanesthesia. New York: Churchill Livingstone, 1990.

Martz DG, Schreibman DL, Matjasko MJ. Neurological diseases. *In* Katz J, Benumof JL, Kadis LB, eds. Anesthesia and uncommon diseases. Philadelphia: WB Saunders, 1990: 560-589.

Schurr A, Rigor BM, eds. Cerebral ischemia and resuscitation. Boca Raton: CRC Press, 1990.

CHAPTER THIRTY-ONE

Management of Anesthesia for Specialty Procedures

Otorhinolaryngology, Extracorporeal Shock Wave Lithotripsy, Radiology, Electroconvulsive Therapy, Ophthalmology, Cancer Chemotherapy

Anesthesiologists face unique problems when operative procedures involve the airway. Further, anesthesiologists provide care for patients undergoing special procedures not only in traditional settings like operating rooms and obstetrical suites, but also in remote locations like lithotripsy facilities, radiology suites, and catheterization laboratories. This chapter describes the special concerns involved in managing anesthesia for these patients.

Otorhinolaryngology

Procedures in otorhinolaryngology (ORL) are unique because the anesthesiologist and the surgeon share the airway. Management of anesthesia in these patients centers on control of the airway. Preoperative airway assessment is as described in Chapter 13, with emphasis on a review of prior airway operations, airway management during these procedures, radiation treatment, and progression of the disease. If any uncertainty remains after these data have been evaluated, it is mandatory to pursue study of the anatomy of the patient's airway in consultation with the surgeon until all of the information is on hand to plan the induction of anesthesia and airway management. Indirect laryngoscopy, conventional x-rays, computed tomography scans, and nuclear magnetic imaging provide information on airway impingement by tumors, infection, or foreign bodies.

Cooperation between the surgeon and the anesthesiologist is essential. Prior to induction of anesthesia, both must agree on a plan for airway management with a clear determination of their respective roles. In the management of ORL patients with compromised airway anatomy, the available airway management schemes may be arranged in a hierarchy, from those which depend the most on normal anatomy to those that cope best with airways distorted or obstructed by disease.

Four rules apply in all cases. First, the patient with a compromised airway must not be given muscle relaxants unless control of the airway is assured. Second, almost all of these patients benefit for premedication to provide a dry mouth, which simplifies airway management by avoiding one stimulus to laryngospasm and by facilitating the effect of topic anesthetics. Third, pulse oximetry is essential to provide warning that airway obstruction is producing hypoxemia; efforts to intubate the trachea must stop from time to time to allow for ventilation and oxygenation. Fourth, supplemental oxygen given by insufflation can prevent hypoxemia during laryngoscopy (see also Chapter 13).

Conventional Intravenous Induction of Anesthesia. This is appropriate when airway anatomy is normal, with no bleeding, abscess, friable tumor, or area of tracheomalacia which might produce obstruction after anesthesia or paralysis.

Small-Dose Intravenous Induction. When the airway is likely to be adequate and the patient is free of cardiopulmonary disease and has a normal FRC, preoxygenation is followed by very small doses of thiopental (1 to 2 mg per kg), given so as to just cause the patient to lose consciousness. If the airway is obstructed, preoxygenation allows time for the patient to recover before becoming hypoxemic. If the airway can be maintained, anesthesia may be deepened with injectable anesthetics or gases. Also, a small dose of succinylcholine can be given and laryngoscopy performed; if the prospects for intubation are favorable, additional anesthetic and relaxant are given before passing the endotracheal tube. This strategy is appropriate only under limited circumstances: there must be no systemic illness and the anesthesiologist must be nearly certain of an intact airway. Gentle technique is required to manipulate the airway of such lightly anesthetized patients.

Gas Induction. Induction of anesthesia by breathing a mixture of oxygen and a potent anesthetic offers the prospect of an induction that automatically reverses itself when the airway becomes obstructed. Halothane is not unpleasant to smell and does not irritate the upper or lower airway in contrast to enflurane and isoflurane; despite the theoretical advantage offered by these two less soluble agents, in practice, the greater concentrations possible with halothane make it easier to perform smooth induction of anesthesia. Nitrous oxide is usually not used for gas induction of anesthesia in patients with compromised airways so that the maximum amount of oxygen may be used. This technique is applied to the same patients as are the two intravenous techniques described previously, but may be somewhat safer because inadvertent overdoses are less likely. The scheme works best in the hands of an experienced individual.

Awake Laryngoscopy. For patients with even more distortion of the airway, one may begin the sequence of an awake intubation, with opioids, sedatives, topical anesthetics and supplemental oxygen given so as to produce a responsive but calm and spontaneously breathing patient. If direct laryngoscopy demonstrates that intubation is possible, the laryngoscope may be withdrawn and the anesthetic completed before proceeding with intubation. If it does not seem possible to intubate with direct laryngoscopy, one may proceed with one of the techniques described below. This technique amounts to completing the preoperative evaluation by performing a sedated laryngoscopy.

Awake Fiberoptic Laryngoscopy. When poor mouth opening, a large tongue, or other distortions of normal anatomy make it evident that direct laryngoscopy will fail, one may begin with fiberoptic laryngoscopy through the nose or mouth, depending on anatomy, and proceed to intubation by passing the tube over the fiberscope (see Chapter 13).

Blind Nasal Intubation. This technique, also described in Chapter 13, is less popular since the advent of fiberoptic techniques. It is applicable to the same patients—those in whom conventional laryngoscopy is impossible. When secretions and bleeding make fiberoptic laryngoscopy difficult, blind nasal intubation may be preferred.

Operative Laryngoscopy of Bronchoscopy. Experienced surgeons can sometimes identify the glottic opening with an operating laryngoscope, or intubate the trachea with a rigid bronchoscope, when swelling or a mass in the airway make it otherwise impossible to see the larynx or to pass a tube blindly.

Transtracheal Needle Ventilation. This temporizing measure applies when unexpected airway obstruction cannot be resolved, and rarely is needed in the ORL setting if the patient has been well evaluated preoperatively and the surgeon is present to assist with a difficult airway. See Chapter 13 for details of this technique.

Tracheotomy Under Local Anesthesia. When upper airway distortion is severe, or when swelling, bleeding, or a friable tumor threaten complete obstruction if the airway is manipulated, planned tracheotomy under local anesthesia as the first part of the operative procedure is the safest course.

Although patient comfort is a concern in managing these patients, airway obstruction and death can result from the abrupt induction of anesthesia or paralysis, from excessive manipulation of swelling tissue and from persisting inappropriately with efforts to intubate.

Pharyngoscopy, Laryngoscopy, and Bronchoscopy

Pharyngoscopy, laryngoscopy, and bronchoscopy are diagnostic procedures that require direct visualization and, frequently, small-tissue biopsies. Anesthetic considerations include (1) thorough airway assessment for pathology; (2) suppression of secretions, cough, gag, and laryngeal reflexes; (3) protection of teeth and relaxation of jaw muscles; (4) rapid return of protective airway reflexes; and (5) airway management.

Premedication with an anticholinergic helps to minimize oral secretions. With proper patient selection and surgical skill some of the endoscopic and minor airway procedures like biopsies, vocal cord stripping, and Teflon injections can be accomplished under local anesthesia. This can be administered topically by means of sprays, nebulizers or soaked applicators, by regional block and by the transtracheal route. Lidocaine is the most commonly used local anesthetic; because of rapid absorption from the trachea, doses must be limited to prevent toxic reactions.

General anesthesia is used when a protected and controlled airway is essential, for the patient's comfort, in extended procedures, or because of the surgeon's preference. Volatile anesthetics provide adequate suppression of upper airway reflexes, allow increased concentrations oxygen, and in specific cases like foreign body removal when positive pressure ventilation may be harmful, allow for spontaneous ventilation. For endoscopy and laryngoscopy, a small endotracheal tube (5 mm ID) protects the trachea, facilitates ventilation, and allows for extended surgical time. Muscle relaxation for these procedures can be accomplished with succinylcholine infusion or intermediate-acting muscle relaxants such as atracurium or vecuronium.

When the endotracheal tube interferes with the operation, methods of airway management without an endotracheal tube are used. One method is to allow the patient to breath spontaneously a mixture of oxygen and a potent inhaled anesthetic, insufflated into the pharynx through a port on the laryngoscope or via a plastic tube lying in the pharynx. It can be difficult to control the depth of anesthesia with this technique because the patient entrains room air with each breath. Also, the surgeon and others in the operating room breath the anesthetic, too.

Another method is jet ventilation via a port on the laryngoscope, or via a metal cannula. It is essential that the vocal cords be fully relaxed and no airway obstruction exists to prevent proper inflow and egress of the gas. Oxygen, mixed with anesthetic if necessary, is delivered intermittently at 50 psi, with a rate of 6 breaths per minute. This method also contaminates the operating room atmosphere and entrains room air, but it does allow the use of muscle relaxants. Ventilation is adequate for good oxygenation, but carbon dioxide sometimes accumulates, especially in patients who are difficult to ventilate.

Another method is apneic oxygenation by insufflation of oxygen and anesthetic gas through a small catheter that is placed between the vocal cords just above the carina. This does not isolate the trachea nor does it allow for positive pressure ventilation or carbon dioxide elimination; apneic times are limited to ten minutes because of hypercarbia. See Chapter 13 for details of this technique.

Bronchoscopes most commonly used are the flexible fiberoptic and rigid ventilating types. The flexible fiberoptic scope is placed through a large (8.0 mm ID) endotracheal tube permitting reliable ventilation during the procedure. With rigid bronchoscopy, oxygen flows in through a side port of the bronchoscope; when the proximal end of the bronchoscope is occluded by a window or by the surgeon's thumb, ventilation through the sideport is possible. Jet ventilation can also be used. Because patient movement can result in a tracheal tear, complete paralysis with a muscle relaxant is appropriate.

Laser Surgery of Structures in the Airway

Lasers produce intense, monochromatic beams of light that can be focused to vaporize tissue. In addition to the usual measures described above, anesthetic management includes measures to protect the patient and operating room personnel from misdirected laser beams, and to lessen probability of fire during laser surgery. Laser beams through reflection or scatter can burn unprotected skin and mucous membrane. The patient's eyes are taped shut and covered with moist gauze, and operating room personnel wear protective goggles that absorb the radiation frequency of the laser in use.

Fire is the most serious danger during laser surgery. Endotracheal tubes made of flammable polyvinylchloride are avoided for this procedure. Special tracheal tubes made of rubber, silicone, or metal have been designed to afford protection by harmlessly absorbing the energy and providing a nonflammable airway. Wrapping an endotracheal tube in reflective aluminum tape reduces its vulnerability to the laser beam, but the cuff of the endotracheal tube may still be punctured. Inflating the cuff with saline enables it to absorb more energy, and the escaping fluid will alert the surgeon to cuff perforation and may extinguish a fire. The atmosphere the patient breathes can be made less combustible by eliminating nitrous oxide, substituting nitrogen or helium, and by decreasing the concentration of oxygen to the minimum level safe for the patient.

TONSILLECTOMY

In cooperative patients, tonsillectomy can be accomplished under local anesthesia. General anesthesia provides reliable control of the airway, suppression of laryngeal reflexes, and avoids reflex-induced hypertension, tachycardia, and arrhythmias. Extreme care is taken with the endotracheal tube as it is moved from side-to-side during the procedure. Rapid recovery with a return of the airway reflexes prior to extubation is desirable. Postoperatively, these patients are placed in the head-down lateral position to allow drainage of blood through the mouth.

The most common complication is postoperative bleeding, occurring most often within eight hours after operation, and sometimes requiring reoperation. Unsuspected hypovolemia owing to hidden blood loss, a full stomach, and airway obstruction are problems encountered during reoperation.

PHARYNGEAL ABSCESS

An abscess in the mouth or pharynx can cause severe pain, trismus, and respiratory obstruction. Sometimes, the abscess can be drained or decompressed by aspiration under local anesthesia. General anesthesia must address respiratory obstruction, difficult endotracheal intubation because of distorted anatomy and trismus, and the danger of rupture of the abscess with pus entering an unprotected airway. Any of the hierarchy of airway management plans described above may be applied, but gentle technique is required to avoid rupturing the abscess. If visualization is impossible, tracheostomy under local anesthesia may be the safest means of securing the airway.

TRACHEOSTOMY

Tracheostomy is best performed in the operating room. By intubating the trachea first, the airway may be protected from bleeding and the tracheostomy performed in a meticulous fashion. When the surgeon places the tracheal tube, the anesthesiologist withdraws the endotracheal tube so that the tip remains in the larynx, just above the tracheal incision; in case of difficulty in passing the tracheostomy tube, the anesthesiologist's tracheal tube can be advanced to secure the airway again.

Head and Neck Operations

Patients undergoing head and neck operations for carcinoma often have a history of cigarette smoking and chronic obstructive pulmonary disease. The airway may present a problem owing to distortion of normal structures by the tumor, by inflammation and edema, or fibrosis caused by radiation therapy. The hierarchy of airway management described previously applies in these cases. Tracheostomy under local anesthesia may be required if the tumor is extremely friable or exophytic, to avoid dislodging cancerous tissue into the tracheobronchial tree or provoking bleeding.

Intraoperative anesthetic considerations specific for head and neck operations include (1) manipulation around the carotid sinus causing vagal responses of hypotension and bradycardia (treatable with atropine or by infiltration of local anesthetic around the carotid sinus); (2) cardiac dysrhythmia and prolonged QT interval during right radical neck dissecton because of damage to the cervical sympathetic system; and (3) venous air embolism due to open neck veins. Laryngectomy and radical neck dissection are prolonged procedures (six to eight hours), involving substantial blood loss. Careful fluid management and prevention of hypothermia are required.

OTOLOGIC SURGERY

Most otologic procedures involve the middle ear and the mastoid air cells, and are performed for hearing loss resulting from scarring and fibrosis of the tympanic membrane, cholesteatoma of the ossicular chain, and occasional involvement of the labyrinth and the facial nerve.

The middle ear represents an air-filled noncompliant space; pressure is vented by the eustachian tube under normal conditions. As it does in other closed spaces, nitrous oxide can accumulate in the middle ear. Tympanic membrane rupture and dislodgement of tympanic grafts have occurred during nitrous oxide use. Until the surgeon begins to close the middle ear, there is no closed space and nitrous oxide use does not present a problem; discontinuing nitrous oxide 30 minutes before the tympanic membrane graft is placed ensures that there will be neither ingress or egress of nitrous oxide after the graft is placed.

The facial nerve is adjacent to structures of the ear, and it may be injured during ear operations. If muscle relaxants are used, some skeletal muscle response to direct nerve stimulation must be allowed to remain so that the surgeon can use mechanical or electrical stimulation to help identify and preserve the facial nerve.

A bloodless operating field is essential for microsurgery of the ear. To achieve this, many surgeons infiltrate the area with epinephrine solutions. This may produce hypertension and dysrhythmia, particularly with halothane, less so with isoflurane and enflurane. Other measures are controversial. Raising the head above the level of the heart aids in venous drainage and reduces cerebral venous pressure but increases the risk of venous air embolism. Induced hypotension reduces bleeding, but may introduce additional morbidity.

Volatile inhalation anesthetics are logical choices for ear operations as they produce adequate levels of anesthesia without the use of nitrous oxide, muscle relaxants, or narcotics. Nausea and dizziness are postoperative problems common to patients undergoing ear operations. Avoiding opioids and prophylactic administration of droperidol are helpful measures to decrease the incidence of nausea and vomiting.

NASAL SURGERY

During operations on the nose, the surgeon uses topical vasoconstrictors to minimize bleeding, most often cocaine, neosynephrine, or epinephrine. Cocaine is widely used as a local anesthetic in intranasal operations because it blocks reuptake of norepinephrine and serves as a vasoconstrictor; the safe dose is 3 mg per kg. Equally as effective, and not a controlled substance, is lidocaine 4 per cent with phenylephrine added as a vasoconstrictor.

Pharyngeal packs aid in absorption of blood intraoperatively and nasal packs are used for hemostasis postoperatively. It is important to verify that all pharyngeal packs have been removed and the pharynx cleaned by suction before the endotracheal tube is removed.

Extracorporeal Shock Wave Lithotripsy

During extracorporeal shock wave lithotripsy (ESWL), sound waves are focused on kidney and ureteral stones. The R wave of the electrocardiogram (ECG) triggers each shock wave. The stone location and the state of stone disintegration is confirmed by fluoroscopy. Newer versions of the lithotripter require no water bath and inflict less pain than do the older models, so that analgesia can be provided by short-acting narcotics like fentanyl and alfentanil.

In other models of the device the shock wave is transmitted through water and human tissue that have similar acoustic impedance, thus allowing its propagation without dissipation of energy. The shock wave produces cutaneous pain at the entry and exit points and visceral pain at the peritoneum and the renal capsule. A single shock wave can be tolerated, but 2000 shocks may be necessary to pulverize the stone, requiring some form of analgesia for the procedure.

Access to the patient who is secured to a frame in a water bath is difficult, and it can be impossible to hear heart breath sounds as the machine's noise is in the range of 90 to 100 db. Monitoring consists of ECG, automated blood pressure, pulse oximetry, and during general anesthesia, capnography.

Hemodynamic changes occur with immersion. Cardiac preload is increased as a result of compression of peripheral vessels by hydrostatic pressure, which shifts blood into the central vascular compartment. In healthy volunteers immersed to the clavicles, an increase of up to 700 ml in central blood volume, an increase in stroke volume (30 to 79 per cent), and cardiac output (30 to 62 per cent) with no change in heart rate are noted. Increases in central venous pressure and pulmonary artery pressure are directly related to the degree of immersion. Patients with cardiovascular compromise are immersed gradually and only partially for the treatment.

Hydrostatic pressure on the chest decreases functional residual capacity by 30 to 36 per cent and vital capacity by 20 per cent. Intrapulmonary pressure and the work of breathing increase, owing to the altered compliance.

Patients may require procedures such as retrograde catheterization to aid in visualization of the stone or manipulation of a stent. Continuous epidural anesthesia allows for safe transfer of these patients from the cystoscopy room to the ESWL room, and is the preferred anesthetic procedure for many of these patients. The epidural catheter site is protected with a simple waterproof dressing because bulkier dressings can absorb and attenuate the shock wave.

When regional anesthesia is contraindicated, a general anesthetic is administered. High-frequency jet ventilation or high-frequency (20 to 25 breaths per minute), small-volume (300 ml) positive pressure ventilation minimizes movement of the diaphragm and the stone.

Radiology

Anesthesia may be required to allow patients to tolerate the increasingly complex procedures performed by radiologists. The same operating conditions may be required as during open surgical procedures, but the setting is remote and unfamiliar. The usual supplies, drugs, anesthesia equipment, oxygen, suction, and support personnel must be provided. The anesthesia requirements focus on the special needs for each procedure. Position changes are integral to the many procedures: to allow movement of the contrast material, for example. Radiation hazards require that the anesthesiologist wear protective lead shields. Most procedures are not particularly painful, and many can be accomplished with local infiltration, sedation, and a minimum of opioids; some interventional procedures involve visceral stimulation as well.

Most procedures are done in dark rooms to allow fluoroscopy and imaging. The radiology procedure room is a confined area with bulky equipment that limits access to the patient. Frequently, there are no piped gases, wall suction, or isolated power supplies. The anesthesiologist must therefore plan carefully to ensure the availability of all the features of a safe anesthetizing location: oxygen, suction, means for positive pressure ventilation, airway equipment, anesthetics, pulse oximetry, blood pressure and ECG monitoring, capnography, resuscitative drugs, and assistance.

Radiographic dye provokes adverse reactions, occasionally fatal, in 2 to 3 per cent of patients. These may vary from pruritus, rashes, and vasomotor phenomena such as flushing and burning on injection, to anaphylactic reactions including dyspnea, wheezing, syncope, and cardiovascular collapse. Complement activation has been implicated, causing degranulation of mast cells and basophils, release of histamine, increased vascular permeability, release of chemotactic activators, cell membrane disruption, and thrombin activation. There may be evidence of an antigen-antibody explanation, but this is not substantiated in all severe responses to dye administration.

Preparation of a patient known to be allergic to dye includes a steroid preparation at least 18 hours prior to the study and antihistaminic premedication. Intradermal and skin testing are not predictive. Intravenous pretesting may be of little benefit in identifying a group at increased risk, because severe anaphylactoid reactions have occurred after 1 ml of dye. Table 31–1 lists the drugs and dosages for treatment of contrast media reactions.

Contrast medium (usually Hypaque, a hypertonic, iodinated solution), is a hyperosmolar solution that may result in transient hypervolemia, bladder distention, and vigorous diuresis. The osmolarity may cause shrinkage and clumping of erythrocytes, resembling agglutination, and necessitating proper hydration of patients with sickle cell disease. Intravenous contrast material competes with other drugs such as barbiturates, warfarin, and isoniazid for protein binding sites, thus causing temporary alterations in plasma concentrations of these drugs after intravenous dye administration. Nonionic dye preparations are available and are less likely to produce reactions in dye-sensitive patients. These new low osmolality contrast agents with nonionic-substituted amides offer better tolerance, lesser incidence of pain, nausea, vomiting or light-headedness, and fewer cardiovascular effects.

Anesthetic management for most radiology procedures is limited to monitoring and sedation, because discomfort is experienced only transiently during placement of a cannula, injection of the contrast material, or balloon dilation of a vessel or hollow viscus. Regional anesthesia may be indicated for visceral pain, such as occurs during nephrostomy, nephrolithotomy, cholecystostomy, or biliary duct drainage and cannulation. Often, epidural analgesia for the segments involved, peripheral nerve blocks, intercostal blocks, or celiac plexus block are ideal. Sensory analgesia without motor involvement is preferred so that position changes can be accomplished with the patient's help. General anesthesia may be needed for patients with movement disorders, or when communication and cooperation are a problem.

TABLE 31–1. Treatment of Contrast Media Reactions*

Adrenergic agonists	Epinephrine 3–5 μg/kg IV bolus Epinephrine 1–4 μg/min IV infusion
Methylxanthines	Aminophylline 5–6 mg/kg/20 min initial dose Aminophylline 0.5–0.9 mg/kg/hr maintenance
Anticholinergics	Atropine 0.5–2 mg IV
Antihistamines	Diphenhydramine 25–50 mg IV
Steroids	Methylprednisolone 100–1000 mg IV Dexamethasone 4–20 mg IV
Intravenous fluids	Normal saline (infuse to maintain normal blood pressure)

* Reproduced with permission from Goldberg M. Systemic reactions to intravascular contrast media. A guide for the anesthesiologist. Anesthesiology 1984;60:46–56.

ELECTROCONVULSIVE THERAPY

Electroconvulsive therapy (ECT) is used to treat depression in patients who have not responded to antidepressant drugs. Generalized electrically-induced seizures have a therapeutic effect, with biochemical changes at the regional, cellular, and subcellular levels as possible mechanisms of action. The treatment results in 30- to 60-second seizures, and is administered two or three times weekly for a total aggregate of 210 to 1000 seconds. No benefits are seen below this dose, and more side effects (memory loss, confusion) are noted beyond it.

The electrical stimulus, consisting of 500 to 800 ma of bidirectional square waves applied with scalp electrodes to the nondominant hemisphere, causes a grand mal seizure with increased cerebral blood flow and cerebral oxygen consumption. The autonomic nervous system is activated with a transient parasympathetic outflow followed by sympathetic effects such as hypertension and tachycardia.

The most common cardiac changes noted are sinus and ventricular tachycardia with a rate increase of 20 to 115 per cent, bradycardia (especially among patients taking beta blockers), premature atrial contractions, premature ventricular contractions, and ST segment depression. These are self limited and generally do not require treatment in most patients, but may be harmful to those with cardiovascular disease.

The incidence of medical complications is 0.4 per cent and the mortality rate is 0.3 per cent. Complications include myocardial ischemia, arrhythmias, laryngospasm, prolonged apnea, oral lacerations, and pulmonary aspiration. The most common causes of death are arrhythmia, infarction, and congestive heart failure occurring during the recovery period. Electroconvulsive therapy can be safe and effective with proper selection, pretreatment, and careful clinical management.

The anesthetic management starts with a thorough preoperative evaluation of the patient, with appropriate medical consultations as indicated. Drug interactions must be considered because patients often take drugs such as tricyclic antidepressants, monoamine oxidase inhibitors, benzodiazepines, and lithium.

The anesthetic requirements include: (1) rapid induction and rapid recovery; (2) amnesia for the procedure; (3) prevention of seizure sequelae such as long bone or vertebral fractures, injuries to tongue and lips, increased intraocular pressure, and increased intragastric pressure; and (4) attenuation of the hemodynamic effects of ECT. The combination of methohexital, succinylcholine, and ventilation with oxygen is the most widely used anesthetic.

Short-acting intravenous induction drugs given in hypnotic doses satisfy the requirements of rapid onset and minimal recovery time. Increasing the dose of the drug to control hypertension and tachycardia also increases seizure threshold and shortens seizure time. Retrograde amnesia results from effective seizures, even without an anesthetic. Attenuation of the parasympathetic response to ECT by atropine or glycopyrrolate also provides a dry mouth. The table of intravenous hypnotics for ECT (Table 31–2) uses methohexital as the standard for induction, but lists the dosages used and the observations made by various investigators for other drugs also.

The dose of succinylcholine (0.25 to 0.75 mg per kg) is adjusted to attentuate tonic-clonic motor responses that may result in fractures in susceptible patients, yet minimize the postictal apnea period. Routine intubation is not recommended because of increased drug requirements and cardiovascular responses provoked by intubation, but a protective device such as a "bite block" is used to prevent damage to teeth, lips, and tongue. Verification of seizures after complete neuromuscular blockade can best be ascertained by electroencephalographic (EEG) monitoring, or alternatively, by occlusion of arterial flow to a limb prior to administering succinylcholine, allowing seizure activity in the unparalyzed extremity. Intermediate-acting nondepolarizing muscle relaxants such as vecuronium and atracurium are not recommended because of their longer durations of action.

Table 31–2. Effects of Induction Drugs Used for ECT

Hypnotic	Dosage (mg/kg)	Observations
Methohexital	(0.7–1.2)	Minimal postictal side effects, hiccups, muscle twitches, some venous irritation
Thiopental	(2.0–3.0)	Longer sleep time, more ECG abnormalities, less K^+ elevation
Propofol	(1.5–1.6)	Less increase in heart rate and BP, decrease seizure time, pain on injection
Etomidate	(0.2–0.3)	Involuntary movements, increased muscle tone, pain on injection
Ketamine	(1.0–2.2)	Slow onset, increased duration of seizure, delayed recovery, nausea, ataxia; postoperative delirium and confusion
Diazepam	(0.3–0.5)	Slow onset, prolonged recovery, increases seizure threshold, shortens seizure time, more ECG abnormalities; venous irritation and phlebitis

Intense stimulation of the sympathetic nervous system and an increase in catecholamines result in tachycardia and hypertension, insignificant in most cases, but catastrophic in a few, causing cardiovascular and cerebral injury. Sinus tachycardia and most arrhythmias are short lived (ten minutes) and revert to normal as catecholamine levels decrease. Pharmacological intervention includes the use of beta blocking agents (esmolol, propanolol, or labetalol), ganglionic blocking agents (trimetaphan), or vasodilating agents (nitroprusside or nitroglycerine), sufficiently short acting to control increased blood pressure and heart rate but avoiding undesirable hypotension later. Intravenous lidocaine is effective in preventing arrhythmias, but suppresses or shortens beneficial seizure activity in a dose-related manner. Termination of a prolonged seizure (greater than 90 seconds duration) may be accomplished by administering additional intravenous short-acting barbiturates.

Ophthalmology

Anesthesia for ophthalmic operations is based on a knowledge of ocular anatomy and physiology, and with an understanding of factors influencing intraocular pressure, interaction between ophthalmic drugs and perioperative medications, and appreciation of the oculocardiac reflex. Patients represent extremes of age, with a preponderance of the elderly with coexisting medical conditions such as coronary artery disease, hypertension, diabetes, and chronic lung disease.

Normal intraocular pressure (IOP) is 10 to 22 mm Hg. Aqueous humor is formed in the ciliary body by active filtration on the anterior surface of the iris, and eliminated via the canal of Schlemm at the episcleral venous network with connecting channels to the superior vena cava. Thus, central venous pressure directly affects IOP, whereas arterial pressure has minimal influence because of autoregulation of the blood supply. Straining, coughing, vomiting, and the Valsalva maneuver can increase IOP as much as 40 mm Hg. Another physiologic determinant of IOP is intraocular (choroidal) blood volume. Hypocarbia decreases IOP by vasoconstriction of the choroidal blood vessels and reduces formation of aqueous humor through diminished carbonic anhydrase activity. External pressure on the eye or contraction of the orbicularis oculi muscle also causes increased IOP.

Most anesthetics decrease IOP by relaxing extraocular muscle tone, improving outflow of the aqueous humor, and decreasing venous and arterial blood pressure. A summary of the effects of anesthesia drugs on IOP is outlined in Table 31–3. Succinylcholine and ketamine increase IOP. Anatomically, ocular muscles have multiple motor nerve endings that respond to succinylcholine by a sustained tonic contracture instead of flaccid paralysis as in skeletal muscle, resulting in ocular hypertension. Nystagmus and blepharospasm limit the use of ketamine for ophthalmic operations.

Ophthalmic drugs may produce systemic effects that must be accounted for in planning anesthesia. Concentrated topical medications are absorbed systemically by way of the conjunctiva, or via the nasal mucosa following drainage through the nasolacrimal duct. Topical eye medications and systemic medications administered during eye operations that can cause systemic effects are listed in Table 31–4.

The oculocardiac reflex is a trigeminal-vagal reflex arc characterized by a 10 to 50 per cent reduction in heart rate precipitated by pressure on the globe or traction on the extraocular muscles, especially the medial rectus. Other manifestations include junctional rhythm, A-V block, premature ventricular contractions, ventricular fibrillation, or asystole. The reflex occurs most often during strabismus operations, during the injection of a retrobulbar block, or when pressure is exerted on the eyeball. Premedication with atropine or glycopyrrolate reduces the incidence but does not abolish it. The treatment is removal of the stimulus, and if bradycardia persists, intravenous atrophine (0.006 mg per kg).

General requirements of anesthesia for ophthalmic operations include an unmoving globe (akinesia), profound analgesia, minimal bleeding, and a smooth emergence. Specific clinical situations may dictate special anesthetic management.

Patients with glaucoma need special attention. Ophthalmic medications are continued to ensure miosis through the perioperative period. Anticholinergics used for premedication and for reversal of the effects of depolarizing muscle relaxants are safe, because too little drug reaches the eye to dilate the pupil. However, topical application of mydriatics such as atropine and scopolamine are contraindicated.

A sulfur hexafluoride (SF_6) bubble is injected into the vitreal cavity during retinal reattachment;

Table 31–3. Effects of Medications on Intraocular Pressure

Anesthesia Drugs	Intraocular Pressure Effect
Inhalation Agents	
Halothane	18–33% decrease
Enflurane	21–40% decrease
Isoflurane	Decrease, similar to halothane
Perioperative Drugs	
Thiopental 3 mg/kg IV	Decrease, baseline after 6 minutes
Innovar 1 ml/kg IV	12% decrease
Ketamine 5 mg/kg IM	37% increase, normal after 30 minutes
Etomidate 20 μg/kg/min IV	Decease 61%
Midazolam IV	Decrease similar to thiopental
Diazepam IV	Decrease
Muscle Relaxants	
Succinylcholine bolus or IV infusion	Increase 33%, normal after 7 minutes
Succinylcholine IM	Increase IOP for 15 minutes
Pancuronium IV	70–84% decrease
Atracurium IV	No effect
Vecuronium IV	Slight decrease

TABLE 31–4. **Anesthetic Implications of Ophthalmic Drugs**

Medication	Ophthalmic Use	Anesthetic Implication
Topical Drugs		
Acetylcholine	Miotic used after lens extraction	Bradycardia, hypotension, bronchospasm, salivation
Betaxolol	Beta adrenergic blocker oculospecific for glaucoma	Additive effects with beta blockers
Cocaine	Analgesia, vasoconstriction in dacryocystorhinostomy	Triggers dysrhythmia
Cyclopentolate	Mydriatic	CNS toxicity: dysarthria, convulsions, psychosis
Echothiophate	Long-acting anticholinesterase miotic for glaucoma	Prolongs succinylcholine and local anesthetic ester action
Epinephrine	Mydriatic used for open angle glaucoma	Tachycardia, nervousness, PVCs, caution with halothane
Phenylephrine	Pupillary dilatation, capillary decongestion	Hypertension, headache, tremulousness
Timolol	Beta adrenergic blocker (nonselective)	Bronchospasm, bradycardia, postoperative apnea in infants, exacerbation of myasthenia gravis
Systemic Drugs		
Glycerol po	Reduces IOP	Nausea, vomiting, risk of aspiration
Mannitol IV	Reduces IOP by decreasing aqueous humor formation	Cardiovascular and renal effects
Acetazolamide IV	Reduces IOP	Renal tubular effects, loss of HCO_3 and K ions

the bubble remains in place for ten days, holding the retina in place. Newer gases may persist as long as 28 days. Nitrous oxide is 117 times more soluble than SF_6 and rapidly enters the bubble, causing it to expand, increasing IOP. Nitrous oxide is discontinued 20 minutes before SF_6 injection, and not employed in the anesthetic gas mixtures for four weeks after retinal operations.

Anesthesia for emergency treatment of penetrating eye injuries involves conflicting goals between prevention of aspiration of gastric contents and prevention of increases in IOP that may cause further eye damage and loss of vision. Succinylcholine is used in rapid sequence induction of anesthesia to protect the airway, but it increases IOP and risks extrusion of ocular contents. A modified rapid sequence has been advocated that includes a dose of thiopental to ensure adequate depth, an intermediate acting nondepolarizer in large doses, cricoid pressure, and intubation when profound muscle relaxation has occurred. Measures to blunt the cardiovascular and IOP responses to laryngoscopy and intubation are similar to those used to manage increased intracranial pressure and may include lidocaine, a beta-adrenergic blocking drug, and a short-acting narcotic.

Strabismus operations are the most common pediatric ocular operations. In addition to oculocardiac reflex, these patients seem to have an increased incidence of malignant hyperthermia. Forced duction testing (FDT) is often done to differentiate between a paretic muscle and a restriction preventing ocular motion. Succinylcholine administration affects the results of FDT for a time longer than the duration of skeletal muscle relaxation. If FDT is planned, it is best to avoid the drug completely, or to perform the test before or at least 20 minutes after succinylcholine administration. Vomiting after strabismus operations is common (85 per cent). Droperidol (0.075 mg per kg) given at induction of anesthesia before manipulation of the eye has decreased the incidence to 10 per cent.

Cataract extraction is the most common ophthalmologic procedure done for the elderly, and anesthesia planning must address the presence of associated diseases. Analgesia and akinesia are provided by a local or general anesthesia. If general anesthesia is given, a smooth intraoperative course must occur with no coughing or straining to increase IOP. Extubation is accomplished under "deep" anesthesia and coughing attenuated by intravenous lidocaine administration. Prophylactic intravenous droperidol is helpful in minimizing the occurrence of postoperative nausea and vomiting.

Most cataract operations are performed with retrobulbar block, which provides local anesthesia and akinesia of the globe. Complications associated with the block include the oculocardiac reflex, hemorrhage, local anesthetic toxicity owing to intravascular injection, and inadvertent intraocular injection. An impressive record of safety is associated with local anesthesia, and available data do not demonstrate any difference in ocular morbidity between local and general anesthesia.

CANCER CHEMOTHERAPY

Multiple side effects, interactions, and complications are associated with chemotherapeutic agents. Anesthesiologists must be familiar with these side effects, because they can complicate the management of anesthesia in cancer patients who have received these drugs. Table 31–5 lists cancer medications with the most commonly associated systemic effects. The immediate side effects are nausea and vomiting, chills and fevers, tissue necrosis, phlebitis, rash, renal failure, and hypocalcemia. Complications occurring later (days to weeks) are bone marrow depression, paralytic ileus, hypercalcemia, disseminated intravascular coagulation, pulmonary infiltrate, and fluid retention. Side effects delayed for months are anemia, hepatocellular damage, pulmonary fibrosis, inappropriate secretion of antidiuretic hormone, peripheral neuropathy, and cardiac necrosis. Secondary malignancies, hepatic fibrosis, and encephalopathy can occur years later.

Administration of chemotherapeutic agents to specific tumor sites by means of regional perfusion (a modification of cardiopulmonary bypass) is done to minimize systemic side effects. Regional perfusion represents a single operative chemotherapeutic exposure. The best responses have occurred with melanomas and soft-tissue sarcomas of the limbs.

A variety of specific organ or system involvement occurs with cancer therapy. Myelosuppression caused by all the chemotherapeutic agents is usually resolved six weeks after the termination of therapy. A complete blood count, including platelet count, may provide the guide for component replacement therapy during the perioperative period. Coagulation defects not associated with thrombocytopenia can occur with mechlorethamine, mithramycin, and L-asparaginase. Immunosuppression occurs with the alkylating agents and a majority of the chemotherapeutic agents. Thus, meticulous aseptic technique must be observed to prevent infections.

The two types of cardiac effects noted with anthracycline antibiotic therapy (doxorubicin and daunorubicin) are the acute transient ECG abnormalities that occur during the course of therapy and a chronic cumulative dose-related (>500 mg per m^2) congestive heart failure. Loss of myocardial cells accounts for the cardiac effects. Cardiotoxicity is irreversible, and the fibrotic heart responds poorly to ionotropes and digitalis. Within three weeks of onset of symptoms, mortality is 59 per cent.

Pulmonary fibrosis and pneumonitis can be induced by alkylating agents, methotrexate, cytabrine, and bleomycin. Synergistic lung damage can occur when radiation therapy is combined with bleomycin. Case reports have suggested that the lung exposed to bleomycin is susceptible to oxygen toxicity and that the F_{IO_2} must be limited to 30 per cent in these patients, but some of these patients may have suffered fluid overload. It is prudent to limit both oxygen and fluids in these patients to the doses required.

Hepatotoxicity occurs with the use of the most antimetabolites, mithramycin, L-asparaginase, and the nitrosoureas. Relevant factors that can cause hepatic insult in cancer patients are multiple blood transfusions, immunosuppressive infection, and other drugs related to the chemotherapeutic protocol. The usual precautions for patients with compromised hepatocellular function are appropriate (see Chapter 23).

Nephrotoxic antineoplastic agents include cisplatin, streptozocin, vincristine, cyclophosphamide, and mithramycin. The nephrotoxic effects of these drugs are ameliorated by diuresis with saline and mannitol when urinary output is maintained at 100 ml per hour. Hyponatremia can occur with cyclophosphamide and vincristine. Hypomagnesemia, hypokalemia, hypocalcemia, and hypophosphatemia can often be encountered with cisplatin therapy. Potentially nephrotoxic anesthetics are withheld from these patients, and the anesthetic management includes perioperative monitoring of urinary output and central venous pressure to guide fluid and electrolyte replacement.

Neurotoxicity of chemotherapeutic agents must be considered when administering an anesthetic. Intrathecal methotrexate and cytosine have been reported to cause transient paraplegia and changes in sensorium. Peripheral neuropathy is caused by the plant alkaloids: vincristine, vinblastine, and vindesin; cisplatin, cytosine, and procarbazine.

TABLE 31–5. Side Effects of Chemotherapeutic Agents

Chemotherapeutic Agents	Side Effects
	General
Alkylating Agents (Interfere with normal mitosis by alkylating DNA)	Bone marrow suppression is dose-limiting factor, mild immunosuppression Hemolytic anemia and increased skin pigmentation Inhibit pseudocholinesterase resulting in prolonged succinylcholine action, Pneumonitis and pulmonary fibrosis
	Drug Specific
Melphalan (Alkeran, L-PAM)	Side effects as listed for alkylating agents
Thiotepa	Side effects as listed for alkylating agents
Mechlorethamine (nitrogen mustard)	CNS toxicity
Busulfan (Myleran)	Pulmonary toxicity, renal toxicity, minor GI effects like diarrhea and stomatitis
Chlorambucil (Leukeran)	Hepatic, CNS toxicity
Cyclophosphamide (Cytoxan)	Strong immunosuppression, hemorrhagic cystitis, inappropriate ADH secretion, stomatitis
	General
Antimetabolites (Inhibit enzymes thus producing aberrant, nonfunctioning molecule)	Strong immunosuppressant Liver dysfunction, reversible with cessation of therapy
	Drug Specific
Methotrexate (MTX)	Severe GI effects: stomatitis, diarrhea, hemorrhagic enteritis; occasional renal tubular necrosis, mild pulmonary toxicity
Mercaptopurine (6-MP)	Severe hepatotoxicity, occasional renal toxicity, mild diarrhea and stomatitis
Thioguanine (6-TG)	Severe hepatotoxicity, mild GI effects: diarrhea and stomatitis
Fluorouracil (5-FU)	Severe GI symptoms: diarrhea and stomatitis; rare CNS effect: cerebral ataxia
Cytarabine	Mild pulmonary toxicity, mild GI symptoms
	General
Plant Alkaloids (Bind to microtubule, arrest mitosis, affect protein synthesis)	Major side effect: leukopenia Moderate immunosuppression Peripheral and autonomic neuropathy
	Drug Specific
Vincristine (VCR)	Mild CNS toxicity, renal toxicity; inappropriate ADH secretion
Vinblastine (Velban)	Moderate diarrhea; mild stomatitis
	General
Anthracycline Antibiotics (Inhibit DNA and RNA formation by forming stable DNA complex)	Moderate stomatitis; leukopenia, thrombocytopenia and anemia
	Drug Specific
Doxorubicin (Adriamycin)	Moderate cardiotoxicity, mild hepatic toxicity, red urine
Daunorubicin (DNR)	Cardiotoxicity; mild immunosuppression and hepatic toxicity, red urine
Bleomycin (BLM)	Pulmonary toxicity, acts synergistically with radiation therapy in producing lung damage
Dactinomycin	Mild immunosuppression
Mithramycin	Moderate hepatic and renal toxicity; coagulation defects
	General
Nitrosoureas (Alkylation of nucleic acid and carboxylation)	Moderate leukopenia, thrombocytopenia, and anemia
	Drug Specific
Streptozocin	Severe hepatic and renal toxicity; selective destruction of pancreatic beta cells causing hyperglycemia
Carmustine	Mild pulmonary, hepatic, renal, GI effects
Enzymes and Random Synthetics	
L-Asparaginase	Moderate hepatic dysfunction, mild immunosuppression, coagulopathy
Cisplatin	Severe renal tubular damage; myelosuppression, peripheral neuropathy, seizures, loss of sense of taste
Procarbazine	Moderate myelosuppression, weak MAO inhibitor, lethargy, depression, synergism with sedatives

The earliest, most consistent sign is loss of achilles tendon reflex, and the most common complaint is paresthesia of the hands and feet. Cranial nerve involvement, autonomic neuropathy, and ototoxicity are other effects of chemotherapy. Preoperative documentation of neurological deficits provides a baseline for assessment of the patient postoperatively. Conduction anesthesia may be inadvisable in these patients with preexisting, possibly progressive, neurologic defects.

Gastrointestinal effects such as nausea, vomiting, and diarrhea may cause fluid and electrolyte abnormalities that require correction. Stomatitis is caused by the antimetabolites and some of the alkylating agents and plant alkaloids. Trauma and excessive manipulation of the upper airway must be avoided.

Anticholinesterase effects of the alkylating agents, most notably thiotepa, mechlorethamine, and cyclophosphamide may produce prolonged apnea after succinylcholine. Monoamine oxidase inhibition and synergistic action with barbiturates, antihistamines, and phenothiazines occur with procarbazine.

REFERENCES

Goldberg M. Systemic reactions to intravascular contrast media. A guide for the anesthesiologist. Anesthesiology 1984; 60:46–56.

Krementz ET. Regional perfusion, current sophistication, what next? Cancer 1986; 57:416–432.

Murphy DF. Anesthesia and intraocular pressure. Anesth Analg 1985; 64:520–530.

Selvin BL. Electroconvulsive therapy—1987. Anesthesiology 1987; 67:367–385.

Selvin BL. Cancer chemotherapy: Implications for the anesthesiologist. Anesth Analg 1981; 60:425–434.

Weber W, Madler C, Keil B, et al. Cardiovascular effects of ESWL. *In* Gravenstein JS, Peter K, eds. Boston: Extracorporeal shock wave lithotripsy for renal stone disease. Butterworth's; 1986:101–112.

CHAPTER THIRTY-TWO

Diagnosis and Therapy of Chronic Pain

Chronic pain exceeds in duration and magnitude the acute pain normally associated with tissue injury. Secondarily, chronic pain is associated with behavior adaptations that eventually become part of the chronic pain syndrome. Patients experiencing chronic pain become depressed, sleep deprived, and socially maladjusted; there may be secondary gain associated with the pain. Pain management involves the unravelling of the behavior from the physiology of the pain experience, finding an etiology for the pain, and planning a rational treatment program to interrupt the cycle of chronic pain and disability.

Physiology of Acute Pain and Nociception

Pain includes not only the sensation that results from tissue injury, but also the complex neurologic, hormonal, and psychological responses that ensue. A simple conceptual model consisting of a sensory receptor, an afferent neuron, and a chain of neurons to transmit the sensation to an area of the cerebral cortex corresponding to the site of pain fails to explain the sometimes unexpected responses to pain and to pain therapy, especially in the case of chronic pain. The following paragraphs provide an outline of current understanding of the physiology of acute pain perception.

Nociception, or the neurologic perception of and response to unpleasant, toxic, and threatening events, is dependent on small C- and A-delta fibers. The unmyelinated free endings of these fibers are called nociceptors; they respond to mechanical, chemical, and local stimuli. Tissue injury causes mechanical distortion, local disturbances in the chemical environment, the synthesis and release of algesic substances, and changes in the microvascular supply to the injured area that promote clotting. Resulting nociceptor activity increases impulses conducted along A-delta fibers, providing the first, or localizing pain perception. Cell bodies of these somatosensory nociceptive A-delta fibers are in the dorsal root ganglia and project onto dorsal horn neurons in laminae I, II, V, and X.

Secondary activation of C fibers results in the poorly localized visceral pain phenomenon. The neurons of the visceral nociceptive C fibers are also located in the dorsal root ganglia, and project onto substantia gelatinosa neurons (spinal cord dorsal horn laminae I and II) as well as onto wide-dynamic range neurons (spinal cord dorsal horn lamina V). Unmyelinated C fibers are closely associated with the myelinated autonomic (efferent)

B fibers. Like the autonomic innervation, branches of the dorsal root neurons of the C fibers first ascend and descend in Lissauer's tract before decussating to terminate on dorsal horn neurons, resulting in a dermatomal overlap of five segments.

The neural response to pain and injury is mediated in part at the spinal cord level. Segmental sympathetic efferent responses to injury are initiated by the grey and white rami communicantes in response to dorsal root ganglion activity.

Central nervous system stress responses begin as soon as A-delta activity localizes the noxious event. Production of central hypothalamic-pituitary stress hormones (ACTH, ADH, growth hormone) increases. The central hypothalamic-pituitary-limbic endorphin system is independently activated during times of tissue injury and extreme stress. Endorphin production within limbic structures enhances stress-induced analgesia. Increased cerebrospinal fluid (CSF) concentrations of endogenous opioids correlate with lesser requirements for exogenously administered opiates. Descending opioid (dynorphin and enkaphalin) and monoamine pathways are activated in the reticular activating system, brainstem, periaqueductal grey matter, and spinal cord to balance stress-induced peripheral norepinephrine release.

Under normal circumstances, the localized vasospasm near the injured tissue promotes blood clot formation in the area of trauma. Further changes in vasoactivity cause blood to be shunted away from the injured tissue, and enhance nociceptor activity by promoting the local accumulation of tissue toxins. Secondary muscle contraction constitutes a protective response; immobility reduces the extent of injury and promotes healing.

Nociception both promotes and is limited by peripheral and central humoral responses to stress and injury. The experience of pain is normally limited by the same segmental sympathetic and musculoskeletal reflexes that limit the extent of the injury, and simultaneously by the enhanced central production of endorphin.

PHYSIOLOGY OF CHRONIC PAIN

Chronic pain syndromes are the result of inappropriate or prolonged sympathetic, musculoskeletal, or central responses to tissue injury. Some theories of chronic pain mechanisms have postulated that untreated peripheral dysfunction results in chronic functional or structural changes in proximal neurons, thereby resulting in continuing pain. However, studies of animal models only support the appearance of neuraxial changes following injury to peripheral nerves, and not to other tissues.

Acute and chronic inflammation of muscles, tendons, joints, and nerves, tissue ischemia, and nerve compression of even short duration result in chronic somatosensory pain. When there is no associated injury to a peripheral nerve, the pain is due to exaggerated musculoskeletal reflexes independent of the sympathetic nervous system. When there is associated peripheral nerve damage, the symptoms may represent chronic deafferentation pain. Deafferentation implies interruption of impulses from the target tissue to the central nervous system, and is accompanied by burning pain, dysesthesias, and hyperalgesia. These are termed "sympathetically maintained pain." Sympathetically maintained pain is associated with reflex sympathetic dystrophy, causalgia, herpes zoster infection, the cranial neuralgias, amputation, nerve root compression of more than four weeks duration, and cancer.

There is clear evidence of structural and functional change in neurons following nerve injury. Changes in the central nervous system occurring in response to peripheral nerve damage represent "plasticity." In the periphery, nerve damage can result in formation of a neuroma. Neuromata have demonstrated intrinsic electrical activity and enhanced sensitivity to norepinephrine.

At the level of the spinal cord, there are permanent changes in the spontaneous activity and receptive fields of the wide-dynamic range (lamina V) neurons within days following section of a peripheral nerve. In cats, conduction velocity is slowed in the axons central to the injury immediately after cutting a mixed peripheral nerve (e.g., the sciatic). The corresponding dorsal root ganglion cells, and their terminals onto neurons in laminae I, II, and V of the dorsal horns, lose their normal peptide content.

Within minutes, the receptive fields of the affected dorsal horn cells reorganize to amplify messages from the injured target tissue. Days later, following C-fiber transport of abnormal substances and a decrease in tonic central inhibition, there is further reorganization of receptive fields so the deafferented dorsal horn cells may respond to inputs from adjacent undamaged peripheral nerves. There is enhanced sensitivity to pressure from target and adjacent tissues (allodynia). Normally nonnoxious stimulation of adjacent A-delta mechanoreceptors can elicit high frequency bursts of firing from deafferented lamina V neurons; these same neurons also exhibit spontaneous high-frequency bursts of discharge. Thus, injury to a nerve alters the behavior of other neurons to produce sensations that do not relate in an obvious way to the original injury.

Once peripheral nerve injury has resulted in neuraxial receptive field changes, peripheral interventions (such as nerve blocks) used alone do not usually result in prolonged relief of pain. Behavior modification is used to enhance the production of endorphins, as in an exercise program with emphasis on the stimulation of neighboring and contralateral A-delta mechanoreceptors, hypnosis, or relaxation training. Repeated nerve blocks, trigger point injections, physical therapy, transcutaneous or implanted electrical nerve stimulation, or acupuncture may all contribute to prolonged relief of deafferentation pain. Psychological issues must be addressed as well.

PSYCHOLOGY OF CHRONIC PAIN

Chronic pain is associated with maladaptive behavior, at least as compared to societal norms. Psychological aberrations accompanying persistent pain can be divided into primary psychiatric or nervous system illness (central pain), or secondary lifestyle adaptations that provoke abnormal behavior (chronic pain behavior).

Central Pain

Damage to central nervous tissue, (such as occurs in multiple sclerosis, thalamic stroke, paraplegia, quadriplegia, tabes dorsalis, AIDS, or Lyme disease) can result in spontaneous burning pain. Psychiatric disorders, such as schizophrenia and conversion hysteria (somatization disorder), are also associated with spontaneous burning pain, particularly when there is coincident depression. Psychogenic pain results from an overwhelming fear of bodily harm, in which anxiety and pain become indistinguishable.

Chronic Pain Behavior

Behavioral responses are judged in conjunction with the duration, intensity, and periodicity of the pain. The early phase of chronic pain begins with the first month after healing, and lasts up to six months after onset of the pain. There is associated evidence of sympathetic responses to tissue injury.

The intermediate phase occurs from six months to two years after onset of the pain, and is associated with variable sympathetic responses. Mood changes become evident, with an increase or decrease in appetite, decreased physical activity, more time spent in bed, and gradual social withdrawal. More time is spent in doctors' offices, physical therapy, the home, and the pharmacy; multiple drug prescriptions may compound symptoms.

Vegetative signs are part of the chronic pain syndrome after two years, in the "late phase." There is disturbance of sleep, appetite, mood, bowel habits, and sexual function. Psychomotor retardation and a decreased pain tolerance are evident. In addition to the central depletion of monoamines associated with chronic pain, maladaptive behavior is enhanced by secondary gain. Family members, physicians, and lawyers may reward pain-related behavior out of sympathy or to further their own goals. Pain becomes a habit and patients happily consent to procedures that reinforce the learned behavior.

PAIN MANAGEMENT

Chronic pain is a complicated, costly illness that demands multidisciplinary treatment. The complexity of the syndrome and its management increases with its duration. Adequate comparisons of therapies have been difficult because of the many medical specialists involved in the care of pain patients, and because of a lack of objective measures of chronic pain.

Diagnosis

Following work begun by J.J. Bonica, the International Association for the Study of Pain has completed a taxonomy of diagnoses to overcome the inherent interpretive problems imposed by communication differences among the various specialties involved. Pain diagnoses are coded according to region (I), system (II), temporal characteristics (III), intensity and time from onset (IV), and etiology (V). The interdisciplinary use of consistent diagnostic groups will provide a foundation for outcome comparisons of various treatments.

Pain Measurement

The methods used to assess pain objectively can be divided into three categories. Scales, such as the visual analogue scales and descriptive scales, provide useful data but are time consuming, and marked by frequent patient misunderstanding of the underlying concept. Studies of pain language give insight into ways in which words can reflect individual coping behavior during pain. Chronic pain patients are better at reliably reporting the relative pain intensity than they are at judging the relative unpleasantness of the experience. Ratios comparing subjective pain to experimentally induced pain have been used with such controllable forms of pain as tourniquet ischemia of variable duration or the intensity of electrical tooth pulp stimulation, but inevitably involve extrapolation.

Although these tests are useful for scientific studies, the outcome of treatment of individual patients is best measured in terms of return to an active, functional lifestyle. Restoration of normal circadian patterns of sleep, eating, and sexual behavior, the resumption of work duties, and an improved mental outlook are indications of successful chronic pain management.

Prescription Drugs

Patients with chronic pain often take a variety of sedative, hypnotic, narcotic, and antidepressant medications prescribed by several physicians. They may be unaware of potential drug interactions, and of the frequency with which some drugs exacerbate many of the symptoms associated with a particular chronic pain syndrome. Narcotics are ineffective for deafferentation pain. The perception of chronic musculoskeletal pain is attenuated by narcotics, but their administration seldom enhances an exercise-based rehabilitation program. Long-term narcotic administration is most useful for chronic cancer pain and may be combined with nonsteroidal anti-inflammatory drugs, tricyclic antidepressants, and nerve blocks.

Sedatives and hypnotics prevent normal sleep, exacerbating the sleep disturbance that accompanies chronic pain. Patients with pain and agitation often benefit from treatment with a small dose of a tricyclic antidepressant at bedtime. Larger doses of antidepressant medications may be administered under psychiatric supervision when depression is associated with chronic pain.

Anti-inflammatory Medication

Inflammation is part of many chronic musculoskeletal and cancer pain syndromes. Aspirin limits prostaglandin synthesis, effectively interrupting nociception due to an underlying inflammatory process. Ibuprofen-containing medications are available over the counter; doses of 600 to 800 mg every six hours can control many of the symptoms associated with arthritic and myofascial pain syndromes.

Exercise

Immobility and a progressively sedentary lifestyle commonly accompany chronic pain. The initial musculoskeletal reflexes associated with injury or visceral disease are exaggerated, and secondary muscular pain may eventually mask the initial problem. Daily exercises help restore a normal range of motion to dysfunctional muscle groups. Additional physiological, psychological, and social benefits are realized when patients participate in a daily aerobic exercise program outside the home.

Diagnostic Nerve Blocks

In the multidisciplinary management of chronic pain patients, anesthesiologists are primarily diagnosticians.

Diagnostic evaluation of chronic pain focuses on determining the neural pathways involved in the pain, using a sequence of sympathetic, somatosensory, and peripheral motor nerve blocks. Such blocks can distinguish placebo responders, demonstrate the role of sympathetically maintained pain, differentiate somatic from visceral pain, and establish that pain is centrally mediated.

Differential spinal anesthesia was used in the past to diagnose pain syndromes in the lower body. After a needle is placed in the CSF (see Chapter 18), a dose of saline is followed by increasing concentrations of a local anesthetic solution (saline, followed by 0.2 per cent, 0.5 percent and 1 per cent procaine) injected in sequence to produce a progressively more profound subarachnoid block. Because the tracts of Lissauer are separated from the CSF by one cell layer, local anesthetic injection into the intrathecal space results first in sympathetic preganglionic and corresponding C-fiber neural blockade. Somatosensory axons are more peripherally located at each spinal cord segment than are motor fibers, so increasing concentrations of local anesthetic result next in sensory, then motor blockade.

The results of differential spinal anesthetics were often inconsistent and confusing because objective correlates of discrete sympathetic or somatosensory blockade were never developed or applied to clinical pain syndromes. A more common practice is the provision of a diagnostic spinal anesthetic in which anesthesia is produced and pain return is correlated with regression of motor and somatosensory blockade. Patients who get no relief from a profound subarachnoid anesthetic with motor block require therapy centering on their psychological adaptation to pain.

Similar evaluations can be carried out using a series of paravertebral sympathetic ganglion blocks and peripheral somatosensory or motor nerve blocks. In the upper extremity, this involves combinations of brachial plexus block (somatic) and stellate ganglion block (sympathetic).

Diagnostic nerve blocks must be performed by a skilled operator without adjunctive sedative, narcotic, or hypnotic medications, any of which can interfere with assessment of pain relief or sympathectomy. Patient responses to nerve block procedures are indicative of coping behaviors and duration of the chronic pain syndrome.

Stellate Ganglion Block

The stellate ganglion is the fusion of the inferior cervical and first thoracic sympathetic ganglia and lies anterior to the prevertebral fascia and posteromedial to the vertebral artery and cupola of the lung, anterior to the transverse process of C7. The postganglionic sympathetic supply to the face, upper chest, thoracic viscera, and arm traverses the stellate ganglion.

A direct approach to the stellate at C7 risks pneumothorax; depositing the local anesthetic within the fascial space containing the cervical sympathetic ganglia at C6 produces as effective a block, without the risk of pneumothorax. There is a risk of injection into the vertebral artery. Because phrenic or recurrent laryngeal nerve block may result as well, only one side is blocked at a time.

The patient lies with the neck extended over a pillow, and looks up and behind at a spot on the wall. The mouth is open to allow relaxation of the sternocleidomastoid muscles. The operator's nondominant index and middle fingers retract the sternocleidomastoid muscle and vascular bundle laterally, with the carotid pulse beneath the index finger, at the level of the anterior tubercle of the transverse process of C6 (cricothyroid membrane). With a 23- to 25-gauge, 1- to 1.5-inch needle, on a 10-ml syringe, the tubercle is approached perpendicular to the plane of the table on which the patient lies until the tubercle is reached a few millimeters below the skin surface.

After aspiration to test for blood return, a test dose of no more than 1 ml of 0.25 per cent bupivacaine is injected. If there are no signs of intraarterial injection, the remaining 9 ml of solution are injected slowly. Sympathectomy renders the skin warm and dry and produces venodilation within 20 minutes.

Lumbar Sympathetic Block

Sympathetic outflow to the retroperitoneum, pelvis, perineum, and lower extremities can be blocked paravertebrally at L2 with a single injection. The patient is positioned with the side to be blocked uppermost; a pillow beneath the iliac crest opens the space between the transverse processes of L2 through L4. A skin wheal is made halfway between the tip of the eleventh rib and the tip of the spinous process of L2. This corresponds to the lateral border of the paravertebral muscles, and often lies just inferior to the tip of the twelfth rib.

For all but children and morbidly obese adults, a 5-inch 22-gauge spinal needle suffices. Starting from the point described, the needle is advanced perpendicular to all planes of the skin toward the umbilicus. As the edge of the paravertebral muscle is encountered there may be a slight contraction visible at the skin. As the quadratus lumborum is traversed there is a slight loss of resistance upon leaving the muscle. Patients then begin to expe-

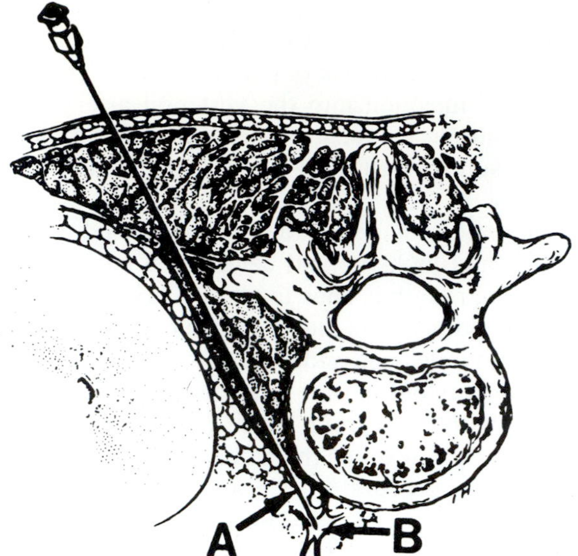

FIGURE 32–1. The relationship of the needle (A), the sympathetic chain (B), and the body of L2, during lumbar sympathetic block. (From Carron H, Korbon GA, Rowlingson JC with permission. Regional anesthesia, techniques and clinical applications. New York: Grune & Stratton, 1984:138)

rience paresthesias, first to the hip and later to the knee and below as the psoas is entered. At a depth of 4 to 5 inches, the needle exits the psoas fascia. There are no further paresthesias (Figure 32–1). A test dose (5 ml) of local anesthetic produces a sensation of pressure but no paresthesias.

If genitofemoral paresthesias are encountered, the needle is advanced 1 mm. If there is resistance to injection, the needle is advanced slowly until the prevertebral fascia is passed. If bone is encountered at 2.5 to 3 inches depth, the needle is repositioned cephalad or caudad to miss the transverse process. If the vertebral body is encountered at 3.5 to 4 inches, the needle is angled more laterally, while visualizing the relationship between the needle, the kidney and the vena cava, in order to avoid penetrating either of these structures.

Twenty to thirty ml of local anesthetic injected slowly produce sympathetic blockade. Risks include epidural, subdural, intrathecal, intrarenal, and intravascular injection. Patients are observed for at least half an hour following injection; the appearance of unilateral lower extremity sympathectomy is verified and documented. Other than incorrect needle position during injection, the most common reasons for producing sensory blockade are passage of the needle beneath the periosteal arcades that connect the vertebral bodies, tracking of local anesthetic along the needle during rapid injection, and injection into the psoas sheath because of incomplete penetration of the deep fascia.

Celiac Plexus Block

An extended periaortic ganglion, the celiac plexus sends postganglionic sympathetic fibers to the abdominal organs and also carries pain information from organs such as the pancreas. Blocks of the celiac plexus can be used to produce diagnostic sympathetic blockade and neurolytic blocks to relieve pain from upper abdominal cancer. Hypotension is an expected effect.

A number of approaches can be used to place the end of a needle inside the periaortic fascia at the level of T12, from which injected solution spreads to the anterior side of the aorta to block the celiac plexus. A single-needle, lateral technique is described.

The patient lies in the lateral position as described for lumbar sympathetic nerve blockade, with the left side upward. Following skin preparation and sterile draping, a skin wheal is made opposite the L2 spinous process, in the midaxillary line. A 22-gauge, 7-inch needle is advanced from beneath the tip of the eleventh rib following the midaxillary line at an angle to place the tip of the needle opposite the body of L1 or T12 (Fig. 32–2).

At a depth of 3 inches, the trochar of the needle is replaced with liquid (saline or local anesthetic) so that pulsations will be more easily felt. The needle is advanced another inch to an inch and a half, with the thumb of the operator on the liquid-filled hub. One mm beyond a noticeable loss of resistance, pulsations will be felt through the hub of the needle. Thirty ml of local anesthetic are injected in 5 ml increments.

A constant resistance to injection implies location of the needle tip within a fascial space. Increasing resistance to injection signals placement of the needle tip within the aortic muscularis; and the needle is pulled back 1 mm before proceeding with the injection. It is crucial to the success of the block that the solution be placed anterior and lateral to the aorta. For neurolytic blocks, confir-

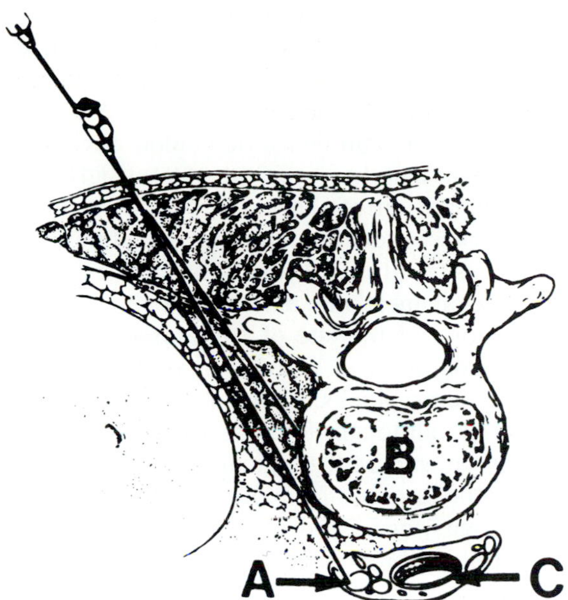

FIGURE 32–2. The placement of the needle adjacent to the celiac ganglia (A) and the aorta (C) at the level of the body of L1 during celiac plexus block. (From Carron H, Korbon GA, Rowlingson JC with permission. Regional anesthesia, techniques and clinical applications. New York: Grune & Stratton, 1984:138)

mation of needle position by radiographs, and a test dose of local anesthetic, are appropriate.

A therapeutic relationship develops during the performance of repeated nerve blocks. When this relationship continues beyond the time when nerve blocks are indicated, it is necessary to transfer the patient to someone better suited to teaching behavioral modification (such as a psychologist, psychiatrist or social worker, who may be part of a multidisciplinary pain clinic); otherwise the nerve blocks become incorporated into the chronic pain behavior.

Generalized Pain Syndromes

Because generalized pain syndromes often include the central neuraxial changes described previously, physical therapy and analgesics may be ineffective. Depending on the nature of the syndrome, a series of nerve blocks to interrupt sympathetic or somatic innervation may permit restoration of normal motion and end the cycle of disuse and pain. For some of the other syndromes described here, direct interruption of pain pathways may be required as therapy.

Sympathetically Maintained Pain

REFLEX SYMPATHETIC DYSTROPHY

Causalgia was the name given by S. Weir Mitchell in 1864 to the burning pain following peripheral nerve injury after gunshot wounds. Reflex sympathetic dystrophy is the term now used to describe any clinical syndrome consisting of burning pain, hyperesthesia, inappropriate and exaggerated sympathetic activity, allodynia, dystrophy, and eventual atrophy of an extremity following injury. It is presumed that neurovascular damage always underlies the perpetuation of the burning pain, hyperesthesia, and inappropriate sympathetic activity. Central nervous system changes are implied by the presence of allodynia.

The syndrome consists of three distinct stages. The acute stage lasts approximately three months following the onset of symptoms, which begin within weeks of injury. During the acute stage, normal vasoactive responses to healing do not persist, as if peripheral responsiveness to sympathetic efferent control has been exhausted. The extremity becomes red, hot, dry, edematous, and hyperesthetic. Skin, hair, and nail growth may be accelerated. Normal range of joint motion can be restored following one or more sympathetic ganglion blocks; resolution of symptoms is anticipated in at least 85 per cent of cases.

The syndrome may progress to the second or dystrophic stage in the first six months following the onset of symptoms. Allodynia is characteristic, indicating that changes have occurred in central neuronal receptive fields. Hyperactivity of the sympathetic nerves is evident: the extremity is cold, blue, sweaty, and stiff. Dystrophic features include early subcutaneous atrophy, shiny hairless skin, and slow-growing and brittle nails. Radiographically, periarticular demineralization is present. The patient protects the extremity assiduously; a classic presentation is the patient with an affected hand that is constantly cradled on a pillow. Secondary immobility of the shoulder or hip exacerbate symptoms.

Treatment emphasizes the restoration of function and relief of pain. Up to ten blocks of the sympathetic ganglia may facilitate a plan of therapy that includes the learned restoration of function. Continuous catheter techniques resulting in both sympathetic and somatosensory brachial plexus blockade for up to a week at a time have been advocated in desperate cases. Vasodilators may be administered either orally or using a Bier block (intravenous regional anesthesia) technique to restore capillary blood flow.

A few patients enter the third or atrophic stage of reflex sympathetic dystrophy within two years after the onset of symptoms. The affected extremity becomes a useless, painful appendage. Psychologically based treatments emphasizing improved coping and learning of health-oriented behavior are favored. There is no role for nerve blocks at this late stage.

Postherpetic and Cranial Neuralgias

Herpes zoster infection and cranial nerve compression result in deafferentation pain that is more successfully prevented than treated. More prevalent among the elderly, the initial peripheral nerve injury rapidly results in central neuraxial changes, after which treatment hinges on enhancement of central inhibition. The time from the onset of acute pain until central changes occur is estimated to be two to four weeks.

Following acute herpes zoster infection, the development of postherpetic neuralgia occurs in the majority of elderly patients. Once established, the pain may persist for years before spontaneously resolving. The virus travels from the skin along the axons of peripheral visceral and somatosensory nerves to the dorsal root ganglion, where neurons are destroyed. It is thought that the pain that follows results initially from the sympathetic efferent response to the destruction of dorsal root ganglion neurons.

Repeated local anesthetic sympathetic blockade (of the sympathetic ganglia or within the epidural space) during the acute phase of infection reduces the incidence of postherpetic neuralgia to zero. Without treatment, central neuraxial changes occur within two weeks of healing of the lesions. Once established, the pain does not respond to topical treatments, or to peripheral, sympathetic, and epidural nerve blocks. Patients suffering from persistent pain may respond to tricyclic antidepressants or to very–low–frequency stimulation of adjacent and contralateral skin mechanoreceptors to enhance central antinociception.

Of the cranial neuralgias, tic douloureux, or trigeminal neuralgia has been the most widely studied. Compression of the nerve peripheral to the nucleus causes deafferentation; sometime after four weeks, central neuronal changes are established. Local anesthetic nerve blocks are useful in the diagnosis of the site of compression, but are seldom prognostic of favorable responses to destructive nerve blocks. Carbamazepine treatment is effective, although doses as great as 1600 mg/day may be required. Surgical nerve decompression may be required for patients intolerant of anticonvulsants, or for those who do not respond to the central inhibitory effects of medical therapy.

Phantom Pain

The amputation of a painful limb often leads to phantom limb pain afterward; the mechanisms are similar to those involved in other peripheral nerve injuries discussed previously. Because the limb has been removed, physical therapy to stimulate adjacent mechanoreceptors is impossible, leaving tricyclic antidepressants or anticonvulsants as the best available therapy. Prevention of phantom pain is possible if blockade of the sympathetic and somatosensory nerves is carried out before amputation.

Such prophylactic treatment is unlikely for trauma victims, but treatment may begin promptly after amputation. Like the other situations in which peripheral nerve injury results in central pain, the time period during which peripheral neural blockade is helpful probably does not extend beyond two to four weeks following injury.

Cancer Pain

Cancer is associated with distortion of tissues, enhanced synthesis or release of algesic substances, and injury to peripheral nerves. These patients may also suffer postoperative (scar or myofascial) pain, peripheral neuropathy from chemotherapy or radiation, or opportunistic infections, such as herpes zoster.

Neoplastic pain is most often described as constant; features of both somatosensory and deafferentation pain are present. The somatosensory component of cancer pain is amenable to treatment with narcotic and anti-inflammatory medications. Local anesthetic peripheral nerve blocks can be used to treat secondary musculoskeletal symptoms. When there are associated tender trigger points in the musculature, they can be treated as described below. Accessible bony metastatic disease is amenable to treatment with local injections of mixtures of corticosteroids and local anesthetic. Radicular pain resulting from vertebral metastatic disease with epidural extension is responsive to the epidural injection of local anesthetic and a depot formulation of corticosteroid.

Visceral tumors are more often associated with deafferentation pain secondary to tumor invasion or the local synthesis of neurotoxins. The pain is initially sympathetically maintained, and if treated promptly (before central neuronal changes occur), it is amenable both to repeated local anesthetic blockade, or to neurolytic block of the associated sympathetic ganglia. Central changes probably occur within two to four weeks after onset of the pain.

Myofascial Pain

Injury can result in localized areas of hardened, tender muscle, called trigger points. It is speculated that these represent prolonged and inappropriate segmental muscle contraction, resulting in ischemia and edema. Referred pain results from pressing on these areas. Trigger points may occur where a peripheral motor nerve ending and the corresponding artery and vein pass between two fascial layers.

Chronic pain at trigger points is called the myofascial pain syndrome. Aggravating factors include poor posture. Therapies include restoration of normal muscle range of motion, daily exercise, and correction of posture. Stretching of the involved muscles to restore range of motion after a coolant spray to inactivate trigger points is the mainstay of physical therapy. Improvement also results from placing a needle in the trigger point, or injecting saline, local anesthetic, or a small amount of corticosteroid. Increased ability to exercise and to participate in muscle stretching physical therapy is the rationale of the injections. Patients are not offered repeated injections in the absence of significant effort on their part to restore normal muscle range of motion.

Localized Pain Syndromes

The anesthesiologist may be asked to help in the search for the etiology of localized pain. The data to be gathered from the patient include:

1. The history of the pain: when it began, associated injuries or illnesses, whether it is constant or intermittent.
2. The patient's choice of words to describe the pain.
3. The severity of the pain, as compared to other pain the patient has experienced and as it affects function, such as work, favorite activities, or sleep.
4. The location of the pain; the patient draws the location of the pain on a diagram of the body.
5. The diagnoses the patient has been given before.
6. Previous treatment and its effect.
7. The patients previous history of chronic pain.
8. Any litigation or workman's compensation that is involved.
9. History and physical finding of somatosensory deficits in affected parts, including close sensory neurological examination.
10. Range of motion of the affected parts.
11. Neurological examination for motor function.
12. Symptoms and physical signs of sympathetic overactivity: sensations of heat or cold, sweating, skin and hair changes, skin temperature, color, galvanic responses.

If pain might be attributed to a particular syndrome, a strategy involving various nerve blocks can be constructed to elucidate the pain pathways involved.

Herniated or Leaking Nucleus Pulposus

Intervertebral discs may bulge, herniate, or leak onto spinal nerve roots. Bulging discs that produce localized back pain and secondary paravertebral muscle spasm are treated with an exercise program designed to promote maximum axial mobility.

Facet nerve blocks with local anesthetic may be

used for pain relief to allow exercise therapy. Bed rest of more than ten days' duration owing to disc disease is associated with worsening of symptoms.

The epidural injection of depot steroids is sometimes used to reduce inflammation of nerve roots in patients with herniated discs. This therapy is controversial, because there are no controlled studies to support its efficacy and some studies that have failed to demonstrate positive effects. Ill effects include temporary exacerbation of the pain and the risk of possible neurotoxicity from depot steroid preparations inadvertently injected into the CSF. At best a palliative therapy, epidural steroid injections have been associated in recent studies with an earlier return to work and improved rehabilitation, indicating limited application to patients with radiculitis.

References

Bonica JJ, Loeser JD, Chapman CR, Fordyce WE, eds. The management of pain. Philadelphia: Lea and Febiger, 1990.

Carron H, Korbon GA, Rowlingson JC. Regional anesthesia, techniques and clinical applications. New York: Grune & Stratton, 1984.

CHAPTER THIRTY-THREE

Hazards of Anesthesia

Is it safe?

William Goldman

The Overall Risk of Undergoing Anesthesia

The question Babe Levy could not answer for Christian Szell is one patients often ask. How safe is anesthesia? For several reasons, this question cannot be answered with precision. "Anesthesia" encompasses multiple drugs, techniques, and anesthetists, and the outcome depends on the patient as well; it is likely that valid estimates of risk can only be made for narrowly defined patient cohorts. Also, the risks are those of anesthesia and operation combined. Patients never undergo anesthesia without also undergoing an operation or diagnostic procedure; control groups of patients who undergo anesthesia without operation or who undergo operation without anesthesia are equally inconceivable. Instead, series of cases are analyzed in retrospect. Risk is usually defined as the risk of dying, and the contribution of anesthesia to the outcome is determined through retrospective analysis by a panel of experts.

The major limitation of such studies lies in the retrospective analyses, which are limited by the unrecognized prejudices and state of knowledge of the expert analysts. In such studies, unknown pathological processes go unrecognized (e.g., malignant hyperthermia in any studies conducted before 1960), and conclusions about causation are likely to be erroneous, at least when viewed in retrospect. This occurred in the early 1950s when Beecher and Todd found an increased death rate in patients receiving curare and concluded that the drug had an inherent toxic effect, missing the fact that inadequate postoperative ventilation was causative. Through medical progress, deaths once attributed entirely to patient diseases come to be seen as due in part to excusable suboptimal management, and eventually, to inexcusable error. Our understanding of the hazards of anesthesia derives from studies such as these, from case reports, and from analyses of untoward events.

The overall death rate within the first 30 days after operation ranges from 1 to 2 per cent. Of these deaths, the majority are attributed to the patients' diseases; a smaller fraction are said to be due to surgical mismanagement; very few are attributed solely to anesthesia. In recent studies, the rates of death owing to anesthesia range from 0.01 per cent (1:10,000) to 0.0005 per cent (1:185,000). Long series of anesthetics without deaths have been reported from outpatient surgery centers. Given that 20 to 25 million operations are performed in the United States each year, there may be as many as 2000 or fewer than 100 (presumably preventable) anesthesia-related deaths each year. These are many fewer deaths than are attributable to cardiovascular disease, cancer, or automobile accidents, but are more than the number dying in airplane accidents each year.

These studies, and the studies of "critical incidents" begun by Cooper, also have described the epidemiologic profile of death or harm from anesthesia. Even when other confounding factors are taken into account, the overall risk of dying after operation varies by as much as a factor of ten from hospital to hospital. Various studies of mortality after repair of fractured hip report postoperative mortalities ranging from 6 to 25 per cent. Equipment malfunction is not a common cause of death or critical incidents attributed to anesthesia, but human error is. Hypoxic gas mixtures, airway management problems, errors in drug administration, and failures of vigilance are most often reported as causative.

The overall death rate is greater for patients undergoing more invasive operations. The death rate from anesthesia appears not to be increased in the elderly, but is greater in the ill, perhaps because they cannot recover as well from episodes of hypotension or hypoxemia. No convincing large-scale studies have shown a specific safety advantage for general or regional anesthesia; the retrospective studies that have been done were unlikely to detect small differences in safety of various techniques, especially given that anesthetics are chosen to be as safe as possible for each patient. Perhaps because of recent reports of large series of cases with anesthesia-related death rates markedly less than the formerly accepted value of 1:10,000, some have claimed that the death rate from anesthesia is decreasing. This has been attributed to improved training and equipment such as inspired oxygen analyzers and pulse oximeters, but convincing proof of an improvement in the death rate or of its cause is lacking.

When patients ask about the safety of a proposed anesthetic, the anesthesiologist can offer not only detailed information about the plans for anesthesia management, but also general reassurance based on the information presented above and on comparisons to travel by automobile and airplane. Although the assertion cannot be tested, patient safety is enhanced by the rational application of scientific principles, not only to the development of new drugs, equipment, and procedures, but to the day-to-day care of patients. In this sense, the whole of this text is about the hazards of anesthesia and the steps needed to reduce these hazards to a minimum. The remainder of this chapter discusses some specific hazards not discussed elsewhere in this volume.

MALIGNANT HYPERTHERMIA

Pathophysiology

Malignant hyperthermia is a rare inherited myopathy characterized by ineffective uptake of calcium by sarcoplasmic reticulum or inappropriate release from intracellular storage sites in muscle. The syndrome is almost always inapparent in humans until certain anesthetics or succinylcholine ("triggering agents") are administered. Under the influence of the anesthetic, intracellular calcium metabolism is further deranged; the massive muscle depolarization characteristic of succinylcholine probably overwhelms available mechanisms for uptake of intracellular calcium. Onset may be prompt or delayed after exposure to the responsible agent; the diagnosis is sometimes first made in the recovery room.

Because of increased calcium concentrations, there develops a hypermetabolic state in the muscle, with or without marked increases in tone. This increased metabolism is manifested at first by increased CO_2 production, tachycardia, and increased cardiac output, mimicking light anesthesia. As the hypermetabolic state continues, body temperature increases, at times rapidly and to dangerous values (40 to 43°C). Anaerobic metabolism, metabolic acidosis, cellular hypoxia, muscle cell breakdown, hyperkalemia, myoglobinemia, cardiac failure, and renal failure follow. Early series reported mortalities as great as 70 per cent; with better therapy and improved detection of the syndrome early in its course, mortality now may be less than 10 per cent.

Preoperative Evaluation; Diagnostic Testing

The incidence of susceptibility to malignant hyperthermia may vary, depending on the makeup of the gene pool and perhaps the degree of inbreeding in the population studied. In one study, the incidence of fulminant malignant hyperthermia was 1 in 62,000 anesthetics involving agents known to trigger the syndrome. Preoperative findings in the patient or the patient's family suggesting an increased likelihood of susceptibility include a history of a previous episode, a history of unexplained fever in the operating room or recovery room, a history of an aborted anesthetic, Duchenne's muscular dystrophy, or other muscular dystrophies.

The gene for malignant hyperthermia has not been identified yet. In humans, the disease seems to be inherited as an autosomal dominant trait with variable penetrance. This, along with the fact that even susceptible patients may undergo several anesthetics uneventfully, makes the patient's history useful for suggesting susceptibility, but not for ruling out the possibility of malignant hyperthermia.

Preoperative diagnosis of patients suspected of being susceptible, or of patients who have suffered an event resembling malignant hyperthermia, depends at present on observing in vitro greater-than-usual contractile responses to halothane, caffeine, or a combination of the two in a fresh, viable muscle specimen taken from the patient. Testing is performed at a limited number of centers,[1] and results are inconsistent. There is debate as to whether these inconsistent results signify variable severity of the syndrome or inconsistent testing; standards for testing have been established that may improve the reliability of this testing. There are no specific noninvasive tests for malignant hyperthermia.

A telephone call to the North American Malignant Hyperthermia Registry[2] may provide information if the patient or a relative has been documented as having malignant hyperthermia previously.

Neuroleptic malignant syndrome occurs following long-term exposure to phenothiazines or haloperidol and includes fever, muscle rigidity, acidosis, and rhabdomyolysis. Although there is no obvious inherited basis for this syndrome, muscle from these patients exhibits enhanced susceptibility in the halothane-caffeine contracture test used to diagnose malignant hyperthermia, suggesting that it is prudent to avoid the use of succinylcholine when they require anesthesia for electroconvulsive therapy or other procedures.

Clinical Presentation; Early Detection

Malignant hyperthermia often presents in an insidious fashion; the hyperdynamic circulation that occurs in response to the increased metabolic rate resembles light anesthesia. The earliest reliable sign of malignant hyperthermia is inappropriate CO_2 production, manifested by increased end-tidal CO_2 during controlled ventilation, increased minute ventilation in a patient breathing spontaneously under anesthesia, or warmth and rapid exhaustion of the CO_2 absorbent. These are never normal findings and deserve close investigation. Fever is a later and inconsistent sign of hypermetabolism. Routine monitoring of temperature is of little use for brief anesthetics, but a necessary part of routine care for operations lasting more than a few minutes.

Another presentation sometimes associated with malignant hyperthermia is masseter spasm: after succinylcholine, the jaw is clenched and the mouth cannot be opened. If the patient has received succinylcholine in adequate doses and was capable of opening the mouth preoperatively, this finding is suggestive of malignant hyperthermia. If the anesthetic is continued, and the patient is indeed to develop malignant hyperthermia, the jaw may relax after the succinylcholine effect dissipates and the signs of the hypermetabolic state may be delayed for 10 to 30 minutes. In one series, 50 per cent of patients who had developed masseter spasm had positive caffeine-halothane contracture tests. On the other hand, as many as 1 per cent of all children receiving halothane and succinylcholine developed marked increases in masseter tone, a finding that casts doubt on the specificity of this sign. Some authorities recommend treating all patients with masseter spasm as though they had malignant hyperthermia; others recommend proceeding with the anesthetic, using nontriggering anesthetics and monitoring temperature and CO_2 production.

An anesthetized patient who shows signs of unexplained hyperdynamic circulation, increased CO_2 production, increasing temperature (or one that is not decreasing as fast as usual for the temperature of the operating room and the size of the

[1] Malignant Hyperthermia Association of the United States (MHAUS), PO BOX 3231, Darien, Conn. 06820, (phone 209-634-4917, ask for "Index Zero"). MHAUS is an organization of patients and families involved with MH. By calling the phone number, one can obtain immediate referral to physician experts.

[2] The North American Malignant Hyperthermia Registry, Department of Anesthesiology, Pennsylvania State University Medical Center, Hershey, Pa (phone 717-531-6936). The registry responds to inquiries about patients.

patient), with or without increased muscle tone and with or without masseter spasm, must be treated as though developing malignant hyperthermia to avert tissue damage and death resulting from the fully developed syndrome.

Treatment

Treatment of an episode of malignant hyperthermia consists of halting the anesthetic and the operation as soon as possible, eliminating the triggering agents immediately, administering dantrolene (which blocks calcium release), enhancing the monitoring (arterial and urinary bladder catheters, core temperature probe at the minimum), treating the biochemical abnormalities described above, and cooling the patient (Table 33–1). Bicarbonate and hyperventilation are needed to treat acidosis and hyperkalemia. Because of expected myoglobinuria, mannitol for diuresis is indicated. Cooling measures include administration of iced intravenous fluids, surface cooling with ice, gastric lavage with iced solutions, and heat exchange with a pump oxygenator. It has been recommended that the anesthesia machine be changed because of residual volatile anesthetic in the breathing circuit. This recommendation is not well founded, as the increased fresh gas flows (6 to 10 L per minute) quickly wash out residual anesthetic, and time taken obtaining an uncontaminated anesthesia machine is better spent on specific therapy. Appropriate supplies for treating malignant hyperthermia, including ice and iced solutions, dantrolene, and a flow sheet describing the appropriate therapy must be maintained for ready use near all anesthetizing locations.

TABLE 33–1. Treatment of an Acute Episode of MH

1. Discontinue all anesthetics; if the operation cannot be concluded immediately, narcotics and nondepolarizing muscle relaxants are safest.
2. Intubate the trachea and establish controlled hyperventilation to prevent hypercarbia and treat acidosis; insert esophageal temperature probe at the same time.
3. Administer dantrolene 2 mg/kg intravenously every 5 minutes to a total dose of 10 mg/kg.
4. Give intravenous sodium bicarbonate 2 to 4 mEq/kg; more may be required, depending on results of arterial blood gas analysis.
5. Apply ice to groin, axilla, neck, and apply iced irrigating solutions to stomach, bladder and open body cavities as needed to maintain temperature below 40° C.
6. Insert arterial cannula, and draw blood for gas analysis, electrolyte determinations, glucose, BUN, creatinine coagulation studies, acute CPK values, and urine and blood myoglobin and hemoglobin; treat abnormalities as required.
7. Telephone the malignant hyperthermia hotline (209-634-4917, ask for "Index Zero") for consultation as required.
8. Continue biochemical treatment as required, intravenous dantrolene and monitoring in recovery room or intensive care unit at least overnight.

After the initial episode abates, intravenous dantrolene is continued at 12-hour intervals for at least a day, and the patient is observed in a recovery room or intensive care unit, because recurrence is possible. After the acute episode, an informative visit with patient and family, and referral to the Malignant Hyperthermia Registry and a center where biopsies are offered, are appropriate.

Anesthesia for Malignant Hyperthermia-Susceptible Patients

Patients known to be susceptible to malignant hyperthermia can be anesthetized safely. Prophylactic dantrolene, 2.5 mg per kg intravenously shortly before beginning anesthesia (oral dantrolene is sometimes ineffective), is effective in blocking the onset of malignant hyperthermia. Anesthesia may be provided with nerve blocks, spinal or epidural anesthesia, or general anesthesia. The drugs recommended in Table 13–2 have established records of safety in human patients and in malignant hyperthermia-susceptible swine. Flushing the anesthesia machine, ventilator, and breathing circuit with oxygen at moderate flows (10 L per minute) for an hour, and removing or flushing until dry the vaporizers containing volatile anesthetics ensures that the inspired gas will not contain a triggering agent. Close monitoring of end-tidal CO_2 and temperature are required.

In some instances, a patient may have preoperative findings that suggest the possibility of susceptibility, but do not warrant a biopsy. For example, a patient with bulky muscles and a family history of unknown difficulties with anesthesia in the distant past who requires a minor operation might not wish to obtain a biopsy. In these cases, anesthesia with an agent that does not trigger malignant hyperthermia is prudent, but prophylactic dantrolene is not warranted; monitoring of temperature and CO_2 production are required.

TABLE 33–2. Malignant Hyperthermia and Drugs Used in Anesthesia

Safe
- Barbiturates
- Etomidate
- Droperidol
- Opioids
- Nondepolarizing muscle relaxants (possible exception: curare)
- Anticholinesterases
- Local anesthetics, esters and amides
- Nitrous oxide
- Antihistamines
- Propranolol
- Catecholamines and sympathomimetics

Known triggering agents, unsafe
- All inhalational anesthetics except nitrous oxide
- Depolarizing muscle relaxants: succinylcholine, decamethonium

Controversial, or insufficient experience
- Curare
- Phenothiazines (increase intracellular calcium)
- Ketamine (likely a safe drug, but the hypertension and tachycardia of ketamine anesthesia would confuse the management of a patient susceptible to MH)

TOXICITY OF ANESTHETICS

Until relatively recently, it was thought that inhaled anesthetics were biologically inert; it is now clear that they all are metabolized to a variable extent and that they and their metabolites sometimes can react with tissues to produce deleterious effects. Toxic effects are reproducible, dose-related, and predictable; allergic reactions and those that depend on genetic predisposition (e.g., malignant hyperthermia) are discussed elsewhere. The toxic effects of intravenous agents (e.g., etomidate and adrenal function) and the acute toxic effects of inhaled agents on the liver and kidney have been described previously. Other toxic effects have been proposed, usually related to long-term exposure or to exposure during vulnerable periods of fetal development.

Carcinogenic Effects

Several surveys have raised the possibility that anesthesiologists, anesthetists, and dentists chronically exposed to small concentrations of anesthetics in the work place may suffer an increased incidence of cancer. Many of these surveys are open to criticism for their design, and show either no statistically significant increase in the incidence of cancer in exposed workers, or small increases (50 per cent increase in incidence, of borderline statistical significance). Nitrous oxide differs from the other inhaled anesthetics. First, it inhibits methionine synthetase, impairing synthesis of deoxyribonucleic acid (DNA) and producing bone marrow depression during prolonged exposure. Second, in a survey of dentists and chairside assistants, there was a marginally significant increase in the rate of cancer in those exposed to nitrous oxide.

The inhaled anesthetics are structurally similar to chemicals known to be carcinogens. In the initial animal testing of isoflurane, an increased incidence of liver tumors was observed in mice; this finding delayed the approval of isoflurane for human use by several years. However, it became apparent that the animals had been exposed to known carcinogens, and the studies were repeated. These studies, and others in which rats and mice have been exposed to the greatest concentrations of anesthetics they will tolerate over nearly their entire life spans, have failed to show any carcinogenic effects from inhaled anesthetic agents.

At present, it is clear that patients are at no increased risk of cancer from therapeutic exposures to inhaled anesthetics. Although the risks of long-term exposure to trace concentrations of anesthetic for those in the operating room seem minimal, there is no reason to abandon inexpensive measures that reduce the contamination by anesthetics of the operating room atmosphere.

Teratogenesis and Anesthesia for Pregnant Patients

Some older anesthetics (divinyl ether and fluroxene) alter DNA in vitro, but of the agents now in use, only nitrous oxide and halothane sometimes have been found to have weak effects in animal studies. No chromosomal aberrations have been found in patients or operating room workers exposed to anesthetics. These findings suggest that anesthetics are unlikely to alter genetic material.

Rats and mice exposed to anesthetics during the period of pregnancy that corresponds to the first trimester in humans produce an increased number of malformed fetuses. Similar effects for isoflurane, enflurane, and halothane occur only for prolonged exposures and very large doses. These findings of weak teratogenic potential suggest that human exposure to inhaled anesthetics during early pregnancy might result in fetal malformations.

Retrospective surveys among those who work in the operating room suggest small increases in the rate of spontaneous abortion (20 to 30 per cent), but not in the rate of congenital defects. However, these studies depend on recall and do not differentiate between the effects of trace anesthetics and the effects of other elements in the operating room environment, including stress, activity, work hours, and radiation exposure.

Of the many surveys of the outcome of pregnancy in women exposed to operation and anesthesia, the most thorough involved a review of 2500 women in Manitoba Canada who underwent general anesthesia for operations during pregnancy. As compared to a matched cohort of pregnant women who did not undergo operation, the group of women studied suffered an increase in the rate of spontaneous abortion when operations and general anesthesia occurred during the first two trimesters, but there was no increase in the occurrence of congenital malformations among their babies. As with others, this study could not differentiate the effects of anesthesia from other effects of operation.

Thus, there appears to be little risk of harmful effects on the fetus from exposure to typical amounts of inhaled anesthetics in patients or in those who care for them. Nevertheless, because of remaining uncertainty in the results of these studies, certain precautions are indicated in providing anesthesia for pregnant women. Because the risk of harm in animal models is greatest early in pregnancy, it is appropriate during preanesthetic evaluation to ask women of childbearing age whether they are likely to be pregnant. Elective operations can be postponed until after the pregnancy. More urgent operations can be performed safely. Especially later in pregnancy, management includes measures to ensure adequate uterine blood flow (see Chapter 26). Regional anesthesia may offer the advantage of minimal physiologic effects, but general anesthesia appears to be safe as well.

Table 33–3. Precautions to Reduce Environmental Exposure to Anesthetics in the Operating Room

1. Avoid leaks around face masks.
2. Use waste gas scavenger to collect gas from pop-off valve of breathing circuit and anesthesia ventilators.
3. Ensure regular inspection and maintenance to detect and repair leaks in gas machines, piped gas supplies, connections and fittings.
4. Regularly assay anesthetic gas concentrations in operating rooms.
5. Shut off vaporizer and nitrous oxide when breathing circuit is not attached to patient.
6. Provide adequate operating room ventilation.

Preventing Occupational Exposure to Anesthetics

There are still no data to establish a safe concentration of anesthetic vapors to which those who work in the operating room may be exposed for long periods. In surveys, some operating rooms have been found to have peak concentrations of nitrous oxide of 5000 parts per million (ppm) and of halothane, 50 ppm. By employing simple precautions (Table 33–3), these can be reduced to the concentrations that the government has recommended (but not required by regulation): 0.5 ppm for volatile agents, and 25 ppm for nitrous oxide.

Infections

Infection of Patients

In the hospital, patients may acquire infections from other patients or from those caring for them. This hazard is reduced in anesthesia practice by the routine use of aseptic precautions, gloves, and other elements of sterile technique, as well as disposable needles and other equipment for vascular access. A sometimes neglected precaution is to discard syringes and contaminated multi-dose vials at the end of each anesthetic. The prevention of the spread of infections via airway equipment is not so straightforward. Sterile, disposable endotracheal tubes and single-use oral and nasal airways are now standard. Whether breathing circuits used in anesthesia are sources of infection for patients is difficult to establish, but it is also now standard practice to use disposable breathing tubes, to interpose a filter between patient and breathing circuit, or to wash the breathing circuit in germicidal solutions between uses. Laryngoscope blades require cleaning in germicidal solution between uses, as well.

Varicella is a particular hazard to immunosuppressed patients, such as those with transplanted organs or human immunodeficiency virus (HIV) infection. It is important to protect patients from hospital personnel who might spread varicella virus.

Infection of Anesthesia Personnel

Although one can acquire almost any infection from a patient in the course of anesthesia practice, the two that are of greatest concern at present are hepatitis B and HIV. Although transmission of HIV from patient to anesthetist has not yet appeared as a major vector for this virus, the well-documented risk of hepatitis B infection makes it appropriate to take precautions against both viral diseases (Table 33–4). The routine testing of patients for HIV remains controversial; because tests based on antibody formation may not identify patients in the latent phase of the infection, it is appropriate to employ these precautions in managing all patients, with or without HIV testing.

Electrical Accidents

Because of the large number of electrical devices attached during anesthesia and operation, patients are vulnerable to electrical burns and shocks. A complete review of the physics of electrical currents lies beyond the scope of this chapter, but the precautions required for safety are uncomplicated.

Table 33–4. Precautions to Prevent the Spread of Blood-Borne Viral Illness Such as HIV or Hepatitis B in Anesthesia Practice

1. Hepatitis B immunization
2. Eliminate the use of needles as far as practical: stopcocks in intravenous sets instead of injection ports
3. Safe handling and disposal of needles, scalpels, and other sharp objects
4. Routine use of gloves for all procedures such as intubation, placing intravenous catheters, handling patient's secretions; avoid injury by patients' teeth
5. Frequent hand washing
6. Proper disposal of contaminated waste
7. Already standard methods of cleaning and sterilizing instruments and surfaces suffice
8. Goggles, eyeglasses, or other protection for eyes during awake intubation or during surgical procedures that scatter bone, blood, or tissue fragments

Table 33–5. Significant Electrical Currents in Humans

Current	Biological Effect in Humans
0.010 ma	Maximum leakage current allowed for devices in contact with the heart; designed to prevent microshock
0.020 ma	Probably lower limit of current that will produce fibrillation if applied directly to heart
0.1 to 10.0 ma	Typical implanted pacemaker current
0.3 ma, 60 Hz	Threshold for sensation
1 ma, 60 Hz	Threshold for pain
2 ma	Maximum whole-body current permitted by isolated power before line isolation monitor sounds alarm
10–100 ma, 60 Hz	"Let go" current: subject is unable to relax grasp and let go of current source
100 ma	Usual whole-body resistance of 100 Ω, when connected to household current supply of 110 V, permits current of about 100 ma
100–2500 ma, 60 Hz	Whole-body current required to produce ventricular fibrillation
100 ma/cm^2	Current density (current per unit area) at which burns occur

Microshock and Macroshock

The mechanisms of death from increasing electrical current are due progressively to arrhythmias, respiratory paralysis, or massive tissue injury from heating (rare except in industrial accidents or legal electrocution). The biological effects of various currents are given in Table 33–5. Electrical effects on the heart depend on current density; whereas very small currents of a few microamperes delivered directly to the heart can produce electrical responses, much larger whole-body currents greater than 100 ma are needed before the current passing through the heart is great enough to do harm to that organ.

Macroshock in the operating room is prevented by attaching the chassis of equipment to ground, by routine maintenance of equipment, and, in some hospitals, by isolated power supplies. These devices consist of a transformer interposed between the power line from the local electrical company and the distribution system for the operating room. In contrast to ordinary power distribution systems, neither of the arms of the circuit in an isolated supply is connected to ground. Thus, even if a patient or a worker touches a piece of equipment that has become "live" through a fault in the insulation, a circuit is not completed if the power system is isolated. A monitoring device called a line isolation monitor constantly monitors the system for failure of insulation between either arm of the circuit and ground; insulation faults that could allow currents of 2 ma or more trigger the alarm. When the alarm sounds, there is only the potential for an electrical hazard and the current is not shut off, but it is appropriate to investigate immediately the cause of the fault and disconnect the responsible equipment. The alarm threshold of 2 ma is low enough to guarantee against the hazard of macroshock, but does not guarantee against possible microshock.

Microshock occurs when currents as small as a few microamperes pass through low-resistance pathways such as external pacer wires or saline filled catheters directly to the heart. Because these pathways offer so little resistance to current flow, very small potential differences may produce lethal currents. Devices that might cause microshock are now designed with internal isolated power supplies, high-impedance patient connections, and optically isolated signal paths to reduce the chance of this complication, which now seems to be rare. When external pacemaker wires are exposed or saline-filled catheters are used to obtain intracardiac electrocardiogram (ECG) signals, special care must be employed.

Electrosurgery

Radiofrequency electrosurgery units cut or coagulate tissue with electrical current. Because the tip of the operating electrode is small, local current densities are great; the return electrode attached to the patient's skin with adhesive and a conductive gel is large, keeping current density below the threshold for damage to tissue. The current is supplied at 0.3 to 2 MHz, to reduce the chance of ventricular fibrillation. Unwanted burns can occur at the site of an improperly applied return pad, if the path for the return of current to the electrosurgical unit offers greater than usual impedance. In the same situation, high-frequency electrocautery currents may pass through capacitive coupling to ECG wires or other devices that offer a return path to ground, causing burns at these sites. Careful attention when attaching the electrocautery ground pad and placing it as close to the operative site as possible help prevent burns.

Pacemakers

Patients with implanted pacemakers often require operations. Usually, no difficulties are encountered. However, current from the electrocautery may induce a signal in the pacemaker leads that a demand-type pacemaker may interpret as cardiac electrical activity, causing it to stop pacing; this induced current may also produce microshock, but this seems rare. Risks are minimized by using a bipolar electrocautery, in which current flows only between two small electrodes in the cautery wand. The anesthesiologist must be prepared to convert the pacemaker to fixed-rate operation if necessary.

ADDICTION

Addiction to opioids and other drugs does not seem to be a significant hazard for patients in the operating room, but there is increasing awareness of the problem of addiction among those who administer anesthesia. Listing addiction as a "hazard of anesthesia" implies that choosing anesthesia as a career increases one's liability to addiction. This proposition has not yet been proved; data about the true prevalence of drug abuse among the population at large, among physicians, and among anesthesiologist are so difficult to gather that it is impossible to state with certainty that anesthesiologists are more likely to be addicted than are other physicians, or the general populace. There is also some indication that those who choose anesthesia as a career are more likely to have personalities that predispose them to becoming addicts: the addict may make anesthesia a career instead of the career making the addict. Indeed, several surveys of causes of death among anesthesiologists have found a disproportionate incidence of suicide.

Nevertheless, the data that are available are worrisome. Anesthesiologists are disproportionately likely to be found in drug rehabilitation programs, as compared to other physicians, and they seem to use a wider variety of drugs and to be more likely to take drugs intravenously. The anesthesiologist's job may increase the risk of substance abuse, both because of the tension and anxieties of providing or supervising anesthesia, and because of the unique availability of drugs. Death owing to inadvertent or intentional overdose is frequently reported in surveys of drug abuse among anesthesiologists.

Departments of anesthesia and individual anesthesiologists can take steps to reduce the prevalence of the problem and the severity of its consequences. First, individuals can seek counseling when emotional problems seem overwhelming or when there is a temptation to experiment with drugs. Although this simple advice is notoriously futile (because of the strong effects of denial), it is worth giving, and worth heeding. Second, departments can establish programs to detect and treat addicted individuals (an example of such a policy has been published by the ASA; another example appears in Lecky et al., 1986). The limits of these programs are established by the rights of the individual against unreasonable surveillance, and at the other extreme by the department's obligation to ensue that those who provide care for patients do so with their mental faculties unimpaired.

REFERENCES

Buring JE, Hennekens CH, Mayrent SL, et al. Health experiences of operating room personnel. Anesthesiology 1985; 62:325–330.

Cooper JB, Newbower RS, Kitz RJ. An analysis of major errors and equipment failures in anesthesia management: considerations for prevention and detection. Anesthesiology 1984; 60:34–42.

Duncan PG, Pope WDB, Cohen MM, et al. Fetal risk of anesthesia and surgery during pregnancy. Anesthesiology 1986; 64:790–794.

Goldman W. Marathon man. New York: Delacorte Press, 1974.

Lecky JH, Aukburg SJ, Conahan TJ, et al. A departmental policy addressing chemical substance abuse. Anesthesiology 1986; 65:414–417.

Orkin FK, Cooperman LH. Complications in anesthesiology. Philadelphia: JB Lippincott, 1983.

CHAPTER THIRTY-FOUR

The Law and Anesthesia Practice

Today, many who practice anesthesia can expect to be involved in legal action alleging malpractice, either as defendant or expert witness. Even if one does not come to be part of a suit, the cost of malpractice insurance and the threat of legal action now influence the ways in which physicians practice, relations with patients, fee structures, and equipment purchases. This chapter reviews briefly some relevant legal principles (in the United States), the means of minimizing legal risk, and what to do in the event of an accident or untoward medical outcome.

Suits for Medical Negligence

Torts

Malpractice concepts are part of tort law. A tort is an action or inaction that society has declared to be unlawful through a series of decisions in court; these are wrongful acts even though no formal contract or statue is violated. For example, the courts have consistently required a professional to act "reasonably" and with the care required to similar members of the profession. Some courts have also held that failure to adopt a new procedure that would clearly increase safety at little or no risk is negligent, even if the new procedure is not yet widely used.

Variations Among States

Conditions of law under which malpractice suits may be pursued successfully vary among the states. Where the legislature has spoken by passing a statute, the courts are obligated to follow the clear language of that statute. For example, so called "statutes of limitations" are virtually always laws passed by the state's legislature to define the permissible time after an alleged injury occurs during which a person retains their right to sue. This period varies considerably from state to state. Courts can effectively alter statutes by the process of interpreting that statute. Based purely on this process of judicial interpretation, in many states the period of time before the plaintiff first has reason to suspect that an injury has occurred does not count against the time during which a plaintiff still retains the right to file suit.

Because the plaintiff has the "burden of proof," plaintiffs often have considerable more choice about where a lawsuit is adjudicated than do defendants. This can be very important to outcome, since the forum selected can be important with regard to which state's law will govern the outcome, what types of pretrial discovery will be permitted, what rules of evidence will govern trial procedure, how soon the case is likely to come to trial, and whether the jury is likely to favor economic "haves" (usually the defendant physicians in a medical malpractice suite) or the economic "have-nots." If the suit is of sufficient financial magnitude and all plaintiffs come from a different state than do all the defendants, either the plaintiff or the defendant may be able to have the suit adjudicated in federal rather than state court.

Trials and Appeals

In theory, judges decide what the law is, and the jury decides what the true facts are. For example, the judge in some states will instruct the jury that, as part of informed consent, a doctor will be required by the law to provide only that information that a "reasonable doctor" will provide. In other states the judge will instruct the jury that a doctor must provide those facts that a "reasonable patient" would require to make an intelligent decision. This can turn out to be a quite different standard. If there is a dispute as to what facts a doctor did or did not provide, or about whether the facts provided were sufficient for a reasonable patient to make an informed decision, this dispute is resolved by the jury.

For the most part, only decisions about what the *law* is, rather than what the *facts* were, can be appealed. Except on the rarest occasions, courts of appeal do not second guess the jury as to what the facts actually were, since the appellate judges are not able to listen to the witnesses and to weigh their credibility. While juries are generally given great deference about what was or was not "reasonable," this deference is not absolute, and both the trial and appellate judges occasionally overrule juries when their decisions are completely inconsistent with undisputed evidence. Nevertheless, it is by far the exception for either side to lose a civil case in court and then win it on appeal.

Nature of Malpractice

Malpractice, or to use the preferred term, medical negligence, consists of failure to employ methods, agents, or skills ordinarily considered appropriate, and having that failure result in harm. Unfortunately, any practitioner sooner or later does something negligent. Usually, these errors are discovered and corrected before they cause serious harm. Physicians who are sued when such a careless act does produce harm need not be completely unforgiving with themselves; none of us is without fault.

Just because a hoped-for result does not follow or complications occur after an anesthetic does not imply liability, unless the complication arises from improper care or the physician is foolish enough to have promised a specific result. Physicians must also recognize that they may be sued without merit. When that happens they must not take to heart the inflammatory language of the usual legal complaint. These are only accusations, and are overstated for effect.

On the other hand, many malpractice actions are justified, particularly when results are both catastrophic and unanticipated. In a recent study of 104 cases drawn at random from an insurance company's files, 26 cases involved cardiac arrest during anesthesia or immediately after anesthesia; the anesthetic care afforded was unacceptable in all 26, and this group accounted for 99 per cent of the total cost of the settlements and judgments rendered in the 104 cases.

Judgments concerning medical negligence hinge on the requirement of reasonable behavior by a physician, but what is reasonable depends on circumstances and the state of the art at the time. Thus, experts disagree on what is reasonable, and the result of a trial often depends largely on the jury's choice of which experts to believe.

Understandably, many physicians are uncomfortable when nonphysician jurors decide what constitutes reasonable professional behavior. However, physicians can take comfort from the fact that well over two thirds of the medical cases brought to plaintiff lawyers for possible suit are rejected by the lawyers, after consultation with doctors, for obvious lack of merit. Further, well over two thirds of the medical negligence cases that are tried result in a verdict in the favor of the defendant physician.

Settling Out of Court

Once begun, a medical negligence suit may be interrupted at any point: the plaintiff may learn through counsel's advice that there is no legitimate basis for a suit; the defendant may be forewarned that there is unquestionable liability and settlement is advisable; after hearing depositions, either party may make settlement; the plaintiff may not find experts to testify that there was malpractice; finally, a settlement can be arranged with the aid of the judge during the trial, prior to the jury's verdict. Plaintiffs may be motivated to settle by the guarantee of a financial return as opposed to the uncertainty of a trial. Defendants may be motivated to settle not only to avoid the uncertainty of a trial, but because the expense of defending successfully against a suit (defendant's expenses are not incorporated in the award through contingency arrangements, as are the plaintiff's expenses) can be as costly as an adverse verdict. Only a small proportion of malpractice suits proceed to trial and a court verdict.

Conflicts of Interest Between Physician and Insurer

One recent change in federal law is likely to make physicians less likely than before to follow recommendations for settlement in cases where negligence remains clearly in dispute. Since January 1991, a federal statute has required every adverse judgment or settlement to be reported to a national registry. Every hospital is required to query that registry at the time of any new staff appointment or reappointment. Fear of an adverse entry in the registry might prompt a physician to defend against a suit despite the insurance company's recommendation that it might be less expensive to settle the case without trial. Some insurance policies specify that a suit may not be settled by the insurance company without the defendant physician's consent. A conflict between the physician and the insurance company may also arise when an insurer refuses to offer an amount equal to the limits of the policy to settle a meritorious case, thereby exposing the physician to personal liability in excess of insurance protection.

Even though it is the insurance company that is paying the defense attorney's bill, that attorney is required to represent the physician's best interests, and to inform the physician of any possible conflict of interest between the insurance company and the defendant physician. In case of a significant conflict, the defense attorney is wise to suggest that the physician obtain independent representation. Failure to make such a suggestion when appropriate can expose both the defense attorney and the insurance company to legal liability. Physicians can raise these issues themselves, as well; if consultation with the defense attorney is not adequately reassuring, it is wise to seek independent counsel. Lawyers, just as do doctors, have the professional obligation to give their clients enough information to participate in informed decision making.

Proof of Malpractice: Expert Opinion, *Res Ipsa Loquitur*

Proof of malpractice can be established in several ways. Most commonly, the plaintiff and defendant produce expert testimony to establish the standard of care for the specialty involved. Once, physicians were notably reluctant to testify against colleagues; today, more are willing to do so, especially when standards of patient care have not been met. Thus, the accusation of a "conspiracy of silence" is of less merit now than it was. Sometimes, expert witnesses recruited by the plaintiff provide evidence in favor of the defendant and vice versa, but this is rare in court, except in fiction.

Because physicians were once reluctant to participate, the law developed the doctrine of *res ipsa loquitur*, which in certain cases, for practical purposes, eliminates the need for expert testimony. Literally, the *res ipsa* doctrine says, "the act speaks for itself." This has usually been applied in situations wherein harm could not possibly have occurred except through negligence. However, except when foreign objects are left in the body after a surgical or diagnostic procedure, expert testimony is still needed to establish the proposition that a given result would not have occurred except through negligence.

Patient Rapport and the Chances of Being Sued

The chance of a suit increases greatly when physicians fail to establish rapport with their patients. Anesthesiologists are at special risk, as opportunities for contact with patients outside the operating room are few and visits too often are completed hastily. If one anesthesiologist performs the preoperative evaluation and then another anesthetizes the patient without first having established rapport, the liability for misunderstanding is increased further. When a preoperative examination has been omitted and postoperative visits are not made, the patient may not remember the anesthesiologist at all, until the bill arrives. Obviously, under these circumstances a bond of understanding between patient and physician has not been established and the stage is set for resentment if anything goes even a bit wrong.

RESPONSIBILITIES OF MEDICAL STUDENTS, RESIDENTS, AND NURSE ANESTHETISTS

Students and Residents

Medical students and resident physicians are not immune to court action and must be protected by malpractice insurance. Rarely are they named as sole defendants; more likely, they are named as one of several, including the supervising anesthesiologist, perhaps the surgeon, and the hospital. Medical students pursuing courses for credit and registered with a university or college are usually protected against suit through the institution, sometimes by the hospital and occasionally by both, provided that they act under the supervision of a faculty member on the staff at the hospital.

However, students who are under preceptorships, who are taking elective courses not approved by the medical school, or who are training in hospitals or working with physicians unaffiliated with a medical school, should inquire as to their protection rather than assume that they are protected and therefore bear no risk. House staff, likewise, are protected through the hospital or medical center in which they are training, but they can inquire as to insurance protection and, if need be, secure it for themselves. Residents who engage in extramural part-time work must recognize that they are not protected outside the parent institution unless they have made prior arrangements with an insurance carrier.

Nurse Anesthetists

A nurse anesthetist can be held liable for negligence in the administration of anesthesia, and it would appear that the incidence of malpractice cases against nurses is increasing. This person is assumed to be responsible for the technical administration of the anesthetic, for the observation and recording of vital signs, and for the welfare of the patient. Most certified registered nurse anesthetists (CRNAs) avail themselves of malpractice protection.

When a suit involves the actions of a nurse anesthetist, the likelihood is that legal responsibility for those actions will be shared at least in part by others. If a surgeon or anesthesiologist supervises a nurse in the administration of an anesthetic, under the "borrowed servant" doctrine the nurse is an assistant of the physician and the latter must assume responsibility. If an anesthesiologist or surgeon employs the nurse or advises the hospital as to the qualifications or conditions of employment, the anesthesiologist is responsible, even though not directly concerned in supervision at the time of an alleged act of negligence. Under the doctrine of "joint and several" responsibility, where multiple defendants share any responsibility for negligence, a plaintiff is free to collect the entire judgment, if he wishes, from the defendant with the greatest resources ("deepest pockets," rarely the nurse or resident) even if that defendant bears relatively minor responsibility. The defendant who pays is then free to try to seek reimbursement from others for their proportional share, but that is of little practical importance if a more responsible defendant has few assets.

Hospital's Liability and Quality Assurance

The last two decades have seen an important expansion of two theories of law, *respondeat superior* and "corporate liability," within the doctrine of hospital liability. The impetus for change came from the case of *Darling v Charleston Community Hospital* (1966), in which hospital liability was extended to include failure, through control of staff membership and clinical privileges, to monitor the care provided by attending physicians. To hold a hospital liable on corporate liability theory, a plaintiff must show that the hospital knew, or should have known, that the physician (and presumably the resident or nurse), whose negligence caused the plaintiff's injury, was providing substandard care.

The implications of this doctrine include the need for hospitals, through their responsible physicians, to routinely survey the clinical privileges and clinical competence of professional staff. In a recent malpractice action against a southwestern for-profit hospital and a CRNA, the hospital made a large pretrial settlement on behalf of the brain-damaged plaintiff, acknowledging that its Board of Trustees neither established guidelines for quality control in hiring and overseeing CRNAs nor delineated the supervising responsibilities of surgeons and anesthesiologists for those CRNAs employed by the hospital.

Minimizing Legal Risk

Preparation for Anesthesia and Informed Consent

Pertinent points of the history must always be summarized on the patient's chart along with results of the physical examination and interview, including a statement of any unusual risk involved, the type of anesthesia planned, and the reasons for the choice if the choice has possible disadvantages. If such a procedure were always followed, many a lawsuit would be avoided.

The problem of "informed consent" must be considered at the time of the interview with the patient, and a notation made on the chart. Patients not only must sign a statement authorizing operation and anesthesia but also must thoroughly understand what is to be done. The patient is given the opportunity to ask questions or to make a choice if any is to be made. This does not mean that the anesthesiologist presents the patient with a "shopping list" of agents and techniques; few patients have the competence to make such a selection. Informed patient choices are more likely to involve regional versus general anesthesia, intravenous induction versus inhalation induction, premedication versus no premedication, and so on.

What constitutes adequate informed consent? The various states have different interpretations, some insisting that every possible complication be described to the patient, others recommending to speak only of likely complications and tempering what is said. In general, a physician may not withhold facts or even minimize risks to induce the patient's consent. At the same time, the physician must place the welfare of the patient first; this requirement may conflict with the need to inform the patient. One alternative is to explain to the patient every risk no matter how remote, risking alarming the patient and thereby doing harm. The other alternative is to recognize that each patient presents a separate problem, that the patient's mental and emotional condition may be crucial, and that in discussing the element of risk a certain amount of discretion must be employed. The physician may choose in unusual instances to share certain information only with the patient's family, but this must clearly be the exception rather than the rule.

The anesthesiologist must go into detail about possible complications if an unusual drug or technique is to be used or if the patient is susceptible to a particular complication, such as the dislodging of loose or diseased teeth during laryngoscopy. The note on the record includes a statement that the anesthesiologist has described the proposed anesthetic and that the patient understands. When new drugs or techniques are to be used, or when patients are in critical condition or are to undergo prolonged, complicated operations, it is best to have them sign for both understanding and consent.

Shared Responsibility with Surgeon

Once a patient has been delivered into the hands of the anesthesiologist, the anesthesiologist assumes responsibility for the patient, except when this is shared by the surgeon. Depending on the specific situation, positioning of the patient for operation may be the responsibility of the surgeon, the anesthesiologist, or both. In this and other matters of shared responsibility, differences of opinion are best resolved promptly, but without writing in the chart accusatory notes likely to harm all potential defendants, including the writer.

The surgeon is not usually responsible for the conduct of anesthesia because the anesthesiologist is in effect an independent contractor. However, both physicians have a duty to protect the patient, to the extent they can, against obvious negligence on the part of the other.

Legal Aspects of Monitoring

In the event that new techniques, equipment, or agents are employed, anesthesiologists should be able to substantiate their familiarity with these methods and an understanding of any complications that may arise from their use.

What monitoring devices are required during general anesthetic procedures? There is no unanimity on this question; this text's recommendations appear in Chapter 6, and the American Society of Anesthesiologists has approved standards for basic intraoperative monitoring. In the opinion of many experts, pulse oximetry and capnography are now so cost effective at preventing catastrophe that routine failure to employ them might be considered presumptive negligence.

Anesthesiologists are not ordinarily responsible for maintenance of nonanesthetic equipment in operating rooms although they must be certain that a routine, preventive inspection program is in place. They are responsible for seeing that anesthesia equipment is regularly inspected and serviced.

Anesthesiologists are wise to point out to the hospital administration improper control of humidity and ventilation, inadequate disposal of waste gases, and obvious electrocution hazards associated with electrocautery, electrocardiography, and other devices. If anesthesiologists find that such equipment is defective and continue to use it, they are quite likely to be held liable for resulting accidents.

Records

The best protection an anesthesiologist can devise against suit is an accurate and complete anesthesia record with written observations at regular intervals as the operation and anesthesia progress. A record must never be altered after the fact. If items of information are subsequently recorded, these must be clearly indicated as additions. In at least some states it is a presumption of law that anything that would customarily be recorded but was not recorded, was not done.

Blood Component Infusion

The kinds and quantities of parenteral fluids given during operation are best determined by consensus between surgeon and anesthesiologist. The physician who starts a transfusion is responsible for identifying each unit of blood or component given and determining that it has been properly matched. The anesthesiologist must be aware of the hazards of blood transfusion and must be certain that the indications for transfusion are valid.

Postoperative Care

Responsibilities of the anesthesiologist do not cease when the patient is transported from the operating room; observation continues until care is assigned to another competent person. If dissatisfied with the patient's condition, the anesthesiologist is responsible for remaining in attendance. In most institutions the recovery room is supervised by an anesthesiologist. A detailed record of the patient's progress in the recovery room is essential and the release of a patient from the recovery room must be signed by a physician.

During postoperative visits, discussion of the anesthetic experience can be encouraged; if the patient is dissatisfied, this is usually apparent. It is the disgruntled patient not given the opportunity to express dissatisfaction who may ultimately sue. An appropriate note is written on the patient's record after each visit.

Testimony at Deposition or Trial

If called upon to testify at a deposition, a physician is well advised to set aside the time for one or more preparation sessions with the attorney, the first at least a week in advance of the deposition. Of the greatest importance is to tell the truth, but avoid speculation. What may seem like a helpful answer in context may be devastating if it is shown to be untrue or it is employed by the plaintiff's attorney in some unanticipated way. Cases with otherwise relatively minor damages have been converted into economic catastrophes for physicians when juries became convinced that those physicians had given false testimony or made a self-serving change in a record.

If called to testify at trial or at a video deposition, the physician's greatest enemy is likely to be any appearance of arrogance. A patient one makes unnecessarily angry is far more likely to sue; similarly, a jury can be antagonized by a defendant's manner. Doctors need good bedside manners to help stay out of court and to win when they cannot.

There are hard choices faced by an anesthesiologist called upon to provide expert testimony in a medical negligence case. Experts have an obligation to other members of their specialty to distinguish between a failure to follow their own particular preference and a failure to follow defensible practice. They must also distinguish between a breach in the standard of care that has no ill consequences and one that caused the harm of which a plaintiff complains. Frivolous malpractice cases are rarely initiated in the absence of frivolous or poorly thought out expert reports. However, when care is indeed improper, physicians with the time and expertise to do so have a moral obligation to testify on behalf of an injured plaintiff. Moreover, a physician who is willing to testify for plaintiffs when indicated is far more effective and believable when he appears as a defense witness in another case than is a physician who never testifies except for the defense.

IN THE EVENT OF AN ERROR OR A COMPLICATION

Medicine cannot be practiced without accident or complication. Most patients are understanding and are satisfied by frank discussion of problems. However, if the physician belittles or ignores a complication or fails to impart sympathetic understanding, the stage is set for malpractice action.

In the event of an accident or complication definitely or possible related to anesthesia, the anesthesiologist must document the facts on the patient's chart in chronological order during or immediately following administration of anesthesia. The notes include the treatment employed and the consultative opinions obtained. Subsequent notes are made on the chart periodically during the remainder of the patient's course.

The anesthesiologist must immediately provide the hospital and the insurer with a complete account of an accident, but must be aware that the contents of such reports may be discoverable by the plaintiff. Should a suit be threatened or legal inquiry made, the physician must also notify the insurer and, where appropriate, seek legal assistance. Many large hospitals now retain full-time attorneys, whose advice may be sought. Failure to carry out these obligations within a reasonable period has resulted in loss of protection from insurers.

The anesthesiologist's best protection against medicolegal action lies in the thorough and up-to-date practice of anesthesia, coupled with sympathetic interest in the patient and maintenance of detailed records on the course of anesthesia. One must keep in mind that sickness does not deprive the patient of legal rights and that physicians cannot impose what they think is advisable simply because they know what is in the patient's best interest. Patients and their families must be given the information on which to base decision.

REFERENCES

Peters JD, Fineberg KS, Kroll DA, et al. Anesthesiology and the law. Ann Arbor: Health Administration Press, 1983.

Weisbard AJ. Defensive law: A new perspective on informed consent. Arch Intern Med 1986; 146:860.

SECTION 7

POST-ANESTHETIC CARE

CHAPTER THIRTY-FIVE

Recovery from Anesthesia: The Postoperative Visit

The anesthesiologist's responsibility for the care of the surgical patient does not end at the conclusion of the operation, but extends to the transport of the patient to the recovery room, management of recovery room problems, continued care of complications resulting from anesthesia, and a final assessment, called the postoperative visit. In the first few hours after operation, the patient suffers pain, the effects of blood loss, and hypothermia, while responses are impaired by the remaining effects of anesthesia. This phase of the anesthetic depends on what has gone before; the management of emergence and recovery must be incorporated in the overall anesthesia plan.

Awakening From Anesthesia

As patients emerge from general anesthesia, they pass in reverse order through the stages of anesthesia: from a surgical plane in which even sympathetic responses to pain are minimal; through a stage of excitement in which responses to stimuli may be exaggerated and harmful; then a stage of awake sedation when they may follow orders and respond to questions, but may not remember events; to a stage when they appear to return to their preoperative mental state. Even at this point, residual impairment in cognitive functions persists for days, due in part to residual concentrations of anesthetic drugs. The moment at which the patient is declared awake depends on the stimuli applied and the level of response desired. Patients who attempt to cough because the endotracheal tube is in place, yet who do not respond to commands, are awake only in the sense that they have recovered at least one reflex characteristic of awake patients. Patients passing through the stage of hyperreflexia during emergence are at risk of vomiting, laryngospasm, hypertension, tachycardia, and violent movement and require the anesthesiologist's full attention.

In most cases, the patient can be declared to have awakened from general anesthesia when immediate supervision by a person skilled in anesthesia is not required (sedated or paralyzed patients requiring mechanical ventilation are exceptions). This usually implies that the endotracheal tube has been removed, the patient breathes spontaneously, maintains a patent airway without assistance, and responds to simple commands and questions.

Just as the minimum alveolar concentration (MAC) is defined as the alveolar concentration of anesthetic at which 50 per cent of patients do not respond with movement to skin incision, MAC awake is the end-tidal concentration of anesthetic agent at which 50 per cent of patients respond appropriately to a verbal command (open eyes on request). MAC awake is determined for inhaled anesthetics by maintaining a given alveolar anesthetic concentration for about 15 minutes to achieve equilibrium prior to determining the patient's response.

MAC awake applies to conditions of pure inhalation anesthesia without supplementation with adjuvant drugs such as narcotics, barbiturates or benzodiazepines. When adjuvant drugs are used, MAC awake is found to be about 50 per cent of MAC for most pure inhalation anesthetics. In patients emerging from typical general anesthesia, it is more usual not to see them open eyes to command until end-tidal concentrations of halothane, enflurane, or isoflurane have decreased to 10 to 20 per cent of MAC. This discrepancy is accounted for by associated drugs and by differences between the conditions under which MAC awake is determined and those prevailing in the clinical setting, where the concentration of the agent is decreasing rapidly and end-tidal concentrations may not reflect brain concentration accurately. Hypothermia and the residual effects of intravenous drugs also decrease the patient's responsiveness.

When to Awaken the Patient

The timing of emergence from anesthesia depends on circumstances. At one extreme, a patient who has just undergone a minor procedure in the day surgery unit is awakened as rapidly and promptly as possible. At the other extreme, no measures at all may be taken to end anesthesia after a complex cardiac procedure, because in the intensive care unit the patient may still benefit from analgesia, amnesia, and muscle relaxation. The need to control intracranial pressure, intraocular pressure, coughing, or hypertensive responses modifies plans for the end of anesthesia: a slower, more controlled awakening may be preferable in these cases, even at the expense of delayed emergence. Patients with difficult airways or full stomachs, on the other hand, may benefit from the most rapid, complete awakening possible, to prevent airway obstruction or aspiration of gastric contents.

In most cases, it is desirable to have the patient awaken as soon as possible after the operation ends, usually in the operating room. This practice is not universally followed, but it makes transport from operating room to recovery room safer, because it avoids the excitement stage or the need for extubation of the trachea during transport. Routinely admitting patients to the recovery room asleep with endotracheal tubes in place means that one of the most critical phases of the anesthetic—emergence and removal of the endotracheal tube—is likely to be managed in the anesthesiologist's absence.

Determining the Timing of Awakening

Preparing for prompt awakening requires taking into account a number of factors. First, all those factors that make patients more sensitive to the effects of anesthetics also make them susceptible to relative anesthetic overdose and delayed emergence. These include alterations in the sensitivity to anesthetic drugs and alterations in pharmacokinetics (organ dysfunction, hypoproteinemia, age). These influences need not delay emergence, if small doses of anesthetics are used and titrated according to need.

Second, hypothermia, along with its other ill effects, delays emergence.

Third, premedicants, as well as drugs not ordinarily thought of as sedatives, cross the blood-brain barrier and exert central sedative effects. Antihypertensives, beta blockers, and atropine are examples, especially in the elderly. Some studies have shown that small doses of benzodiazepines used as premedicants need not delay emergence, but these results may not apply to sicker, older patients.

Fourth, the level of stimulation affects awakening. Even with an endotracheal tube in place, a patient may lie quietly with their eyes closed, yet respond if asked a question.

Pain-free Emergence from Anesthesia

It is appropriate to administer narcotics at the end of a general anesthetic, so that the patient may awaken as comfortably as possible, but this may delay emergence also. The risk of slow awakening with its attendant effects on the operating room schedule, delay in removing the tracheal tube, and possible increased nursing requirements in the recovery room, must all be balanced against the benefits to the patient of awakening with a minimum of pain. As a general rule, if the respiratory rate is greater that 15 per minute, and the minute ventilation is appropriate for the patient, then intravenous morphine can be given before emergence, beginning with 0.05 to 0.1 mg per kg, giving more or less according to the patient's needs and tolerance.

Neurological Findings During Emergence

Abnormal findings on the neurological examination are common among normal patients emerging from anesthesia. These signs must be distinguished from inadequate reversal of neuromuscular blockade and from neurologic conditions requiring intervention. Transient hyperreflexia, sustained ankle clonus, and upgoing plantar responses are all seen following the use of inhalation agents. Although these abnormal responses to neurologic examination can persist for 40 minutes or even longer after anesthesia, they disappear rapidly as the patient awakens, which distinguishes them from the signs of some neurologic insult suffered during anesthesia.

TRANSPORTING THE PATIENT

The patient's journey from the operating room to the recovery room or the intensive care unit can be a hazardous one. The need to begin the next operation demands that the patient leave the operating room as soon as possible after the operation is completed and that the anesthesiologist return from the recovery room promptly. Because the patient's condition is quite unstable after awakening, the anesthesiologist's full attention must remain with the patient during these minutes. As always, the precautions required depend on circumstances.

The healthy young patient from the day surgery unit, who was described previously as awakening in the operating room, may need no monitoring beyond a sustained conversation during the trip to the recovery room. The sick patient still anesthetized after cardiac surgery may require all monitoring and therapy to be continued during the transfer to the ICU, including invasive cardiovascular monitoring data displayed on portable equipment and continuing infusions of cardiovascular drugs by battery-operated pumps.

For the usual patient who has undergone general anesthesia or regional anesthesia with sedation, a safe transfer to the recovery room begins with a determination that the patient's condition permits moving him from the operating table to the bed or litter. This requires that blood pressure, oxygenation, and the airway all be satisfactory and unlikely to deteriorate in the next few minutes. The move from the operating table to the litter must be well organized, with enough assistants to prevent accidents.

Once the patient is on the bed or litter, a second evaluation (recorded on the anesthesia record) includes the following, depending on circumstances:

1. Strength: head lift test.
2. Airway patency, tidal volume: by examination.
3. Oxygenation: a pulse oximeter reading.
4. The level of a spinal or epidural anesthetic.
5. Blood pressure.
6. Intravenous catheter in place and functioning.
7. Availability of emergency drugs or supplies likely to be needed during transport (ephedrine for a patient with a high level of subarachnoid anesthesia for example).

Hypoxemia is common in the immediate postoperative period. The use of battery-operated pulse oximeters has shown that patients who do not receive oxygen during transport to the recovery room may become hypoxemic far more often than was once suspected. Oxygen administration during this period is an appropriate precaution.

During transport to the recovery room, an assistant pulls the litter while the anesthesiologist stands by the patient's head, monitoring the patient as needed by giving simple commands, holding a conversation, watching the chest, feeling for exhaled gas at the mouth and nose, supporting the chin, or feeling a pulse.

RECOVERY ROOM CARE

The recognition that the patient is in a vulnerable state immediately after operation led to the development of specialized postoperative nursing units, where patients could be observed after operation instead of being returned to the ward. Previous editions of this text relate that a recovery room opened at the Mayo Clinic in March 1942, and one opened at the Hospital of the University of Pennsylvania is 1946. At present, standards for recovery room care are set in the United States by organizations such as the Joint Commission on Accreditation of Hospital Organizations, the American Society of Anesthesiologists, and the American Society of Post-Anesthesia Nurses.

On arrival at the recovery room, the anesthesiologist simultaneously performs two duties: to reevaluate the patient and to transfer care of the patient to the recovery room nurse (and anesthesiologist, if one is assigned). The anesthesiologist and the admitting recovery room nurse perform the reevaluation together. The evaluation is the same as that performed at the end of the operation, with the addition of measuring body temperature. The results and the time of admission to the unit are recorded at the end of the anesthesia record and the beginning of the recovery room record. The transfer of care requires that the anesthesiologist provide the recovery room personnel with a concise history of the patient, the anesthetic, and the perioperative management (Table 35–1).

To assist in the rapid assessment of the patient, various scoring methods have been developed. The PARS score takes into account activity, respiration, circulation, awareness, and color. An arbitrary number (0.1, or 2) is assigned to each of these characteristics (see Table 35–2). The PARS score is analogous to the Apgar; patients with lesser PARS scores need more intense nursing care that do those with greater scores.

The anesthesiologist leaves the recovery room only when satisfied that the patient can be cared for by the personnel there. Many recovery rooms have an anesthesiologist in attendance, but the anesthesiologist who cared for the patient intraoperatively is notified as well when problems arise postoperatively.

TABLE 35–1. Reporting to Recovery Room Personnel

1. Patient's name, brief medical history
   - Drugs
   - Allergies
2. The operation
   - Site
   - Bleeding
   - Anticipated problems in recovery room
3. The anesthetic
   - Anesthetic agents, sedatives, narcotic
   - State of alertness
   - Muscle relaxants, recovery
   - Expected vital signs
4. Summary of fluid balance
   - Blood and fluids given
   - Urine output
   - Blood loss
5. Expected problems and plans
   - Oxygen required
   - Fluid therapy
   - Pain, plan for management

TABLE 35–2. The PARS Score

	Score	Criterion
Activity	2	Moves 4 extremities
	1	Moves 2 extremities
	0	Unable to move extremities
Respiration	2	Breathes deeply, coughs
	1	Dyspnea, limited breathing
	0	Apnea
Circulation	2	BP within 20% of preop, no ECG change
	1	BP changed 20–50%, minor ECG changes
	0	BP changed 50%, major ECG changes
Awareness	2	Fully awake
	1	Aroused by voice
	0	Unresponsive
Color	2	Pink
	1	Pale, dusky
	0	Cyanotic
Total score	0–10	

COMMON RECOVERY ROOM PROBLEMS

Failure to Awaken

On occasion, a patient may fail to emerge from anesthesia when expected. The differential diagnosis is similar to that for coma. When patients fail to awaken from anesthesia as expected, these diagnoses are considered, in this order:

1. Hypercarbia, hypoxemia, hypotension, hypoglycemia, electrolyte disorders, other metabolic problems.
2. Preexisting coma (was the patient awake before anesthesia?).

3. Residual effects of injectable drugs, including premedications: Atropine and scopolamine have profound effects.
4. Other drugs, including illicit ones.
5. Residual anesthetic agents.
6. Hypothermia.
7. Brain damage.
8. Biological variation.

A systematic approach begins by ensuring adequate cardiac output, oxygenation, and ventilation, and then considers such metabolic derangements as hypoglycemia before moving to less urgent concerns such as hypothermia. Appropriate antagonists of narcotics, anticholinergic agents, and benzodiazepines can be used, but doses must be small to avoid unwanted withdrawal effects. Even if an antagonist is successful, continued observation is needed because sedation may recur.

Hyperthermia and Hypothermia

Increased body temperature postoperatively can represent fever or hyperpyrexia. With fever, there is an increased body temperature with an alteration of the hypothalamic set point. It is usually associated with an infection, toxin, allergen, or immune state. It is still unclear whether fever itself is a desirable response to such an event; nevertheless, it is usually treated. Hyperthermia is similar to fever in that it is a state in which the heat production is not matched by the ability to dissipate it. It differs from fever in that the hypothalamic set point is not changed.

Both states are unusual in the postanesthetic patient. When increased temperature occurs, the question of malignant hyperpyrexia must be considered, because therapy must begin immediately for this lethal (but rare) disorder. An otherwise unexplained marked increase in CO_2 production is the hallmark of malignant hyperpyrexia. Malignant hyperpyrexia can occasionally present postoperatively, but usually it manifests itself first in the anesthetizing location.

Hypothermia is a more frequent concern in the recovery room. Heat loss occurs in the operating room because anesthesia obtunds thermoregulatory mechanisms and operating rooms are usually too cold for patients to maintain their body temperatures while breathing dry gases or while body cavities are open. It is now accepted that the operating rooms must be kept warm (26°C or greater) for infants and for seriously ill patients, such as the victims of major trauma or those undergoing liver transplantation. Nevertheless, many patients still arrive in the recovery room cold.

In addition to discomfort and slowed emergence from anesthesia, hypothermia causes harm because of the patient's efforts to conserve and produce heat. Shivering and nonshivering thermogenesis increase oxygen consumption severalfold. This results in increased cardiac output and (in the elderly) hypoxemia resulting from increased oxygen extraction when cardiac output fails to keep pace with total body oxygen consumption. At the same time, the vasoconstriction that occurs as part of the reflex response to hypothermia enhances the vasoconstriction caused by sympathetic responses to pain. Supplemental oxygen is required, infrared warming lights and warm blankets are used, and small doses of meperidine (12.5 to 25 mg IV) are uniquely effective in halting shivering. However, the most appropriate approach is prevention of hypothermia. prevention begins in the operating room, with careful attention to preventing heat loss and use of warming techniques.

Agitation

Although many patients pass through a brief period of excitement as they awaken from anesthesia, some remain agitated for a prolonged period. The following are possible causes of agitation in patients in the recovery room:

1. Hypoxemia or airway obstruction.
2. Pain.
3. Full bladder.
4. Incomplete reversal of neuromuscular blockers.
5. Withdrawal from alcohol or other drugs.
6. Central anticholinergic syndrome (especially scopolamine).
7. Residual anesthetics or sedatives.
8. Senile dementia.
9. A return to preoperative agitation.

The diagnosis should be established first, because agitation often signals dangerous underlying disorders. After these problems have been treated, opioids, benzodiazepines, or a combination of them will usually calm the patient. Anticholinesterases (physostigmine 1 to 2 mg IV) are sometimes required as specific treatment for the central anticholinergic syndrome.

Postoperative Pain Management

In the taxonomy of pain, early postoperative pain occupies a place of its own, with its own characteristics and its own treatment. The responses to the pain immediately after operation are often not recognized, and a patient in severe pain may show little distress to the casual observer. Cultural and learned behaviors all play a part in the outward demonstration of the inner feeling called pain and in the observer's interpretation of the patient's complaints. Postoperative pain can come from a variety of sources, including incision pain (usually not severe), localized muscle spasm, unrecognized full bladder, or swelling under a tight dressing or cast. Unrelated and perhaps new conditions can also appear, such as angina or peptic ulcer pain. Iatrogenic conditions such as corneal abrasion, tongue or lip edema from instrumentation of the airway, or the effects of fluid extravasation, can also give more discomfort to the patient than the surgical condition itself. Anxiety also can cause a patient to appear to be experiencing pain.

Before beginning empiric treatment of postoperative pain, these diagnoses are considered. If the pain is the result of the operation, an opioid may be used to treat it. Small intravenous doses, such as 2.5 to 5 mg of morphine, can be given to produce the desired effect, or patient-controlled analgesia may be started (see Chapter 36). Pain from the surgical incision can be prevented by continued regional anesthesia or the prophylactic use of spinal or epidural opioids (see Chapter 36).

Nausea and Vomiting

Nausea and vomiting are common problems after anesthesia and operation. The patients most at risk for nausea and vomiting are (1) those with histories of vomiting after anesthesia; (2) those with gastric distension caused by gas forced down the esophagus during efforts at positive pressure ventilation with a mask; (3) those who have received narcotics; (4) those who have undergone ophthalmic, otologic, laryngoscopic, or gastrointestinal procedures; and (5) younger women.

Treatment of nausea and vomiting begins early, by avoiding distention of the stomach during mask ventilation or by emptying the stomach with a gastric tube after intubation. Someone who gives a history of significant previous nausea is a candidate for prophylactic treatment with a drug such as metoclopramide, prochlorperazine, or droperidol, drugs that are also useful for treating vomiting (see Chapter 4).

Bleeding and Hypovolemia

Hypotension, oliguria, and decreasing cardiac filling pressures may result from continued bleeding or third-space losses. Appropriate fluid therapy is the same as during anesthesia (see Chapter 15); serial determination of hematocrit or hemoglobin values during fluid replacement will differentiate blood loss from third-space losses. If volume loss is significant, a search is begun to find the cause.

Hypertension

Hypertension is a common reaction in patients in the recovery room, most often occurring in patients with preexisting hypertension (see Chapter 21). The differential diagnosis is similar to that for postoperative pain and agitation. Although the reaction is usually short lived (hours), treatment may be required to avoid myocardial ischemia, bleeding, disruption of vascular anastomoses, or stroke. After other causes of pain and hypertension have been ruled out, treatment with analgesics, vasodilators, and beta blockers (if tachycardia is present) is appropriate (see Chapter 21).

Hypervolemia

Although continued bleeding and third-space losses predispose patients to hypovolemia, hypervolemia can occur in the recovery room following vigorous infusion of fluid during operation. Pain and hypothermia often result in peripheral vasoconstriction. Following spinal or epidural anesthesia, the capacitance vessels contract as the sympathetic block recedes. Thus, a volume of fluid that was appropriate earlier may now be too great, resulting in pulmonary edema.

Treatment requires diuretics and mechanical ventilation if respiratory failure occurs. Prevention begins intraoperatively, with careful attention to fluid management. The judicious use of pressors in the treatment of hypotension as a partial alternative to the infusion of fluids may prevent postoperative fluid overload.

DISCHARGE FROM RECOVERY ROOM

The patient who has awakened from anesthesia, has acceptable vital signs, is alert, aware, responsive, and free from significant nausea and pain is ready to be discharged from the recovery room. Patients who do not meet these criteria may still leave the recovery room, but may require postoperative care in an ICU, a step-down unit or in a location that allows intermediate care such as ECG monitoring. At no time can a patient be discharged simply because an arbitrary time has elapsed.

THE POSTANESTHETIC VISIT

After anesthesia, a postoperative visit is performed and the results recorded in the chart, just as with the preoperative visit. This serves several purposes. First, it alerts the anesthesiologist to complications of anesthesia that can be treated and whose course can be followed. Examples include headache after subarachnoid block, injury to the lips or teeth, vomiting, or backache. Second, evaluating the outcome of the anesthetic and comparing it to the preoperative assessment helps the individual practitioner improve standards of care. Third, answering patients' questions can serve to correct misconceptions and misunderstandings that might otherwise lead to litigation. Indeed, if there has been a complication of anesthesia, or the question of such a complication has been raised, then close contact with the patient must be maintained until the problem is resolved.

Postoperative visits are difficult to arrange for day surgery patients. Sometimes, the postoperative visit is accomplished by a phone call from a nurse or trained secretary. Provided that the results of the conversation are communicated with the anesthesiologist, this compromise may be acceptable. If the anesthesiologist is not made aware of actual problems or complaints, the practice must be revised.

REFERENCES

Edwards TW, Breed RJ. Acute post-operative pain in the post-anesthesia care unit. Anesthesiol Clin North Am 1990; 8:235–265.

Rosenberg H, Clofine R, Bialik O. Neurologic changes during awakening from anesthesia. Anesthesiology 1981; 54:125–130.

Stoelting RK, Longnecker DE, Eger EI. Minimum alveolar concentrations on awakening from methoxyflurane, halothane, ether and fluroxene in man: MAC awake. Anesthesiology 1970; 33:5–9.

CHAPTER THIRTY-SIX

MANAGEMENT OF POSTOPERATIVE PAIN

Patients suffer pain after almost any operation. Until recently, the anesthesiologist's responsibility for pain relief ended in the recovery room, and the recuperating patient received intermittently oral or parenteral narcotics, which often give only partial relief. Recently, techniques such as patient-controlled intravenous narcotic infusions, spinal and epidural narcotics, and prolonged regional anesthetics have offered effective relief of postoperative pain, as well as of the risk of new complications and requirements for closer supervision of patients.

Although convincing evidence that it improves patient outcome is lacking, there are well-recognized benefits of effective postoperative pain management. Intercostal nerve block and epidural or interpleural analgesia significantly increase lung volumes and the ability to cough after major abdominal or thoracic operations. The detrimental effects of tachycardia and hypertension resulting from unrelieved pain may also be reduced by effective analgesia. Effective management of postoperative pain clearly relieves human suffering and may ameliorate some complications; provision for postoperative analgesia can be part of any plan for anesthesia management.

PAIN PATHWAYS

The central nervous system includes interconnected neural circuits that provide information about noxious stimuli. At several points in this system the flow of information may be interrupted to produce analgesia.

Information signalling painful stimuli from somatic and visceral structures is transmitted primarily by two nerve types. A-delta fibers are thinly myelinated neurons that respond primarily to intense mechanical stimulations. C fibers are unmyelinated neurons that respond to mechanical, thermal, and chemical irritation. A-delta and C fibers transmit information about noxious input through the dorsal spinal roots and into the dorsal horn of the spinal cord. At the level of the spinal roots, afferent pain impulses are amenable to interruption by local anesthetics administered via the epidural or spinal route.

From the dorsal horn, sensory information is transmitted through the dorsal columns and the spinothalamic tract, whose cells of origin arise from the laminae of the dorsal horn, including the substantia gelatinosa, which is richly populated with opioid receptors. Through a complex network involving brain to spinal cord descending systems and dorsal horn interneuron pools, information about painful stimuli arriving at the spinal cord is amplified or attenuated. The attenuation mechanisms, including opioid and adrenergic inhibition of noxious input, provide the basis for selective blockade of pain at the spinal level.

A specific neurotransmitter for nociception released in response to painful stimuli by primary afferent neurons terminating in the dorsal horn has not been identified unequivocally. It has been

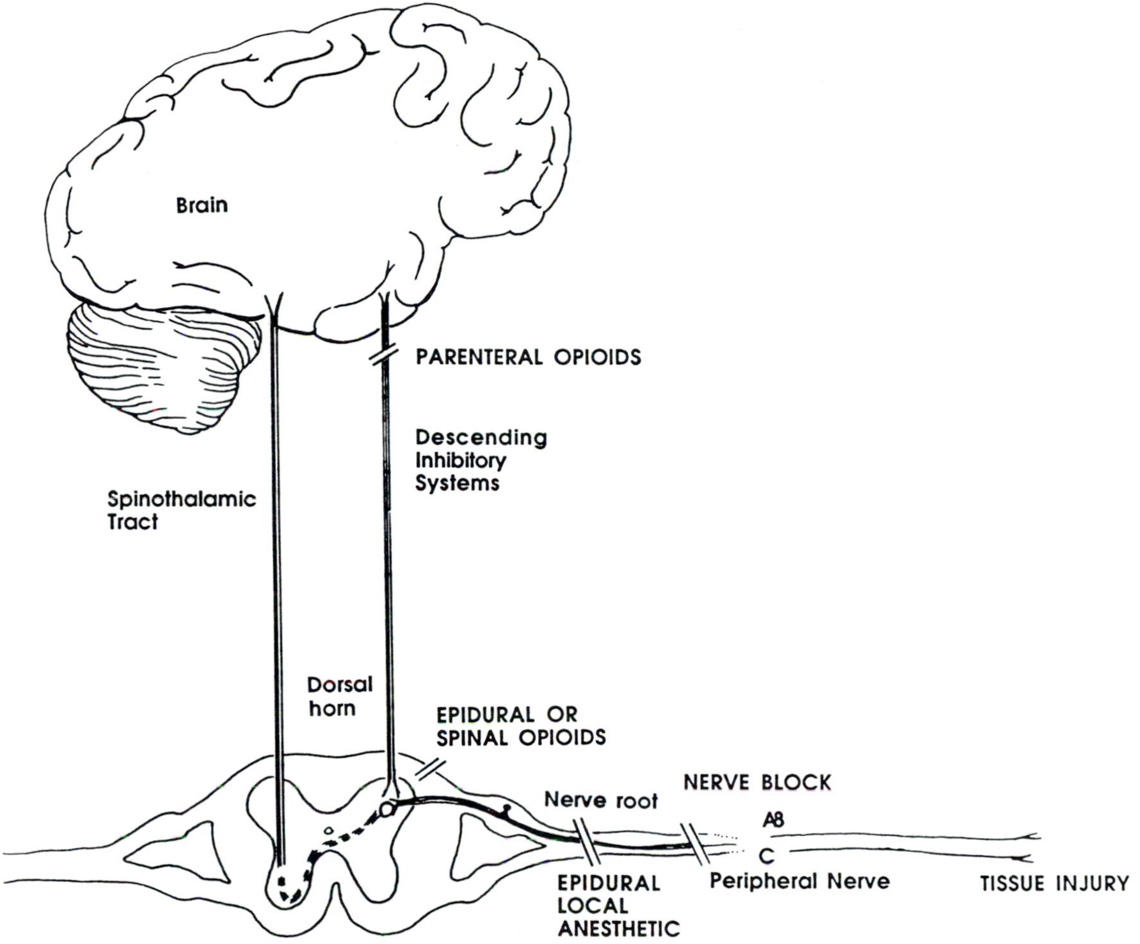

FIGURE 36–1 Sites of potential interruption of acute pain pathways. Descending inhibitory systems are simplified but are probably activated by central effects of parenteral opioids. Epidural local anesthetic-opioid mixtures act at dorsal horn and nerve root level. Adrenergic agonists (e.g., clonidine) also act at dorsal horn level. Nerve block includes various blocks described in text, as well as interpleural technique.

shown that substance P, a small peptide neurotransmitter, is released in response to noxious stimuli. This release is blocked by application of opioids to the dorsal horn, which may explain the action of opioids at the spinal level. Multiple opioid receptor subtypes are involved in this selective spinal analgesia, as different opioids produce qualitatively different effects when applied to the dorsal horn. Figure 36–1 summarizes these neural pathways and the sites where analgesia may be produced.

PATIENT-CONTROLLED ANALGESIA

The intramuscular (IM) administration of narcotics for acute pain is standard practice, because intravenous access is not needed and the tissue depot releases drug over three to six hours. Serious drawbacks limit the effectiveness of IM injections. Large depot doses of opioid (e.g., meperidine 75 mg or morphine 10 mg) often result initially in excessive blood levels of drug and corresponding side effects such as nausea, pruritus, or unwanted sedation. A few hours after IM injection, blood levels decrease to subtherapeutic values, and analgesia is adequate. This cycle of side effects and pain results from the variable and erratic absorption of the drug from the muscular depot (Figure 36–2). The cycle is accentuated by the time required to respond to the needs of the patient in pain.

To circumvent these difficulties, self-adminis-

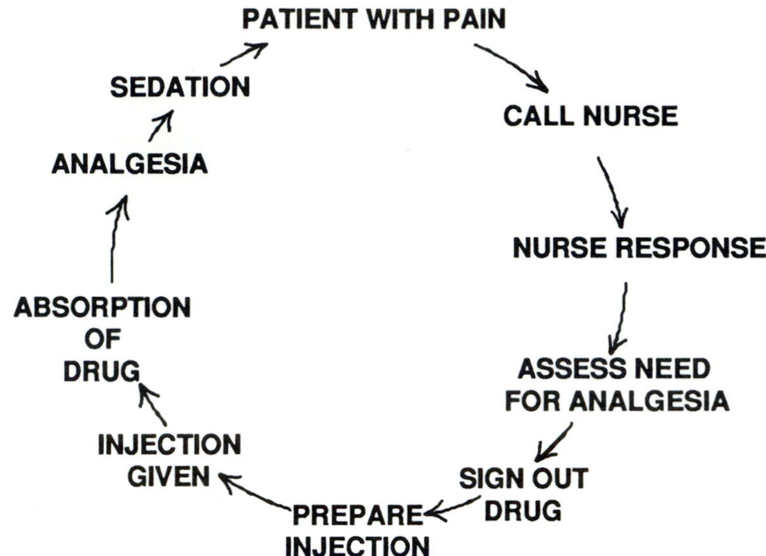

FIGURE 36–2 The cycle of conventional intramuscular (IM) opioid analgesia. (Modified with permission from Graves DA, Foster TS, et al. Patient-controlled analgesia. Ann Intern Med 1983; 99:360–366.)

tration by patients of intravenous opioids was developed in the 1970s. These patient-controlled analgesia (PCA) devices overcome the drawbacks of intermittent IM injection techniques by administering opioids intravenously at the request of the patient, with limits set by the physician.

PCA Devices and Indications for Use

Although the technology is new and designs differ according to manufacturer, a complete PCA device incorporates the design features shown below.

Features of a PCA Device

1. **A programmable microprocessor that is set by the physician to determine drug doses, minimum intervals between doses ("lockout interval"), background constant infusion rate, if any, and limits on maximum total dose.**
2. **An easily accessible control button by which the patient registers with the PCA device a request for drug.**
3. **A drug cartridge or syringe connected by tubing to the patient's intravenous site.**
4. **A drive mechanism controlled by the microprocessor.**
5. **A compact design that permits the patient to move about.**
6. **Simultaneous delivery of intermittent demand doses and a continuous infusion (background infusion) of small amounts of opioid.**

Nearly all patients are candidates for PCA, including the old and the young, provided they understand the need to request drug themselves, and are physically able to do so. Patients with histories of narcotic dependency may require large doses and may be managed more easily with epidural or spinal analgesic techniques, in combination with baseline opioid therapy.

Management of PCA

Patient-controlled anesthesia is best begun in the recovery room as soon as the patient is alert enough to use the demand button, while the patient is still comfortable, either from perioperative opioids or a regional anesthetic technique. Patients in severe pain usually do not obtain effective an-

TABLE 36–1. **Guidelines for PCA Opioid Doses**

Drug	Demand Dose	Lockout Interval (Minutes)
Morphine	1–3 mg	5–15
Meperidine	10–30 mg	5–15
Methadone	0.5–3 mg	10–20
Fentanyl	15–75 μg	3–10
Hydromorphone	0.1–0.5 mg	5–15

algesia from demand doses alone and require an intravenous loading dose of opioid prior to starting PCA. Morphine, meperidine, and hydromorphone are the most common opioids used for PCA; Table 36–1 lists typical demand doses and lockout intervals for several different drugs.

Adjustments in PCA Therapy

Because opioid requirements vary among individuals, doses and lockout intervals must be adjusted when the patient complains of pain or side effects. If analgesia is inadequate, demand dose size may be increased or the lockout interval decreased, to allow more drug in a given time. A background continuous infusion, for example 0.5 mg morphine per hour, may also improve analgesia, especially for pain associated with movement such as walking, coughing, or physical therapy, but such continuous infusions may increase the incidence of opioid-related side effects. Ideally, one change in one PCA parameter is made at a time; the appropriate change must be tailored to the specific patient problem. Complete pain relief is unlikely in most patients; an appropriate goal is a tolerable amount of pain with no side effects.

Side effects also require adjustments in dose schedule, as excess opioid delivery is nearly always the cause of untoward effects associated with PCA. Sedation, nausea, pruritus, urinary retention, or respiratory depression are the usual presenting problems. If side effects occur soon after each demand dose, then the dose is too great. If side effects are present continuously, then the background infusion rate likely is excessive. Severe side effects may require therapy beyond simply adjusting the doses. For nausea, an antiemetic may be prescribed. Also effective are small incremental intravenous doses of naloxone (0.05 to 0.1 mg) or partial agonist-antagonists such as butorphanol (0.25 to 0.5 mg) and nalbuphine (1 to 3 mg).

TYPICAL ORDERS FOR PATIENTS RECEIVING PCA THERAPY

Opioid used, concentration	**Morphine, 1 mg per ml**
Demand dose	**1.5 mg**
Lockout interval	**Seven minutes**
Four-hour dose limit	**30 mg**

Monitor respiratory rate every two hours.

Call pain treatment physician for:

- **Nausea**
- **Pruritus**
- **Respiratory rate less than 10 breaths per minute**
- **Somnolence**
- **Inadequate pain relief**

Naloxone available at bedside at all times.

No other narcotics to be given unless ordered by pain treatment physician.

Patients on PCA therapy can experience side effects through overdose, because lockout intervals are often shorter than the time to maximum opioid effect following intravenous administration. For severe sedation or respiratory depression, PCA is discontinued temporarily and an intravenous infusion of naloxone begun. Although this phenomenon is the exception rather than the rule, it reinforces the need to tailor PCA therapy to the needs of the individual patient.

Patient-controlled anesthesia is discontinued when pain is amenable to oral analgesic therapy, usually one to three days after operation. After abdominal operations, PCA may continue until a liquid diet is tolerated.

EPIDURAL ANALGESIA TECHNIQUES

Single doses or prolonged administration of local anesthetics or opioids to the epidural space provides excellent postoperative analgesia. The required techniques for epidural anesthesia appear in Chapter 18.

TABLE 36–2. **Commonly Used Epidural Opioids**

Drug	Relative Lipid Solubility	Bolus Dose	Onset (Minutes)	Duration (Hours)	Infusion Rate (mg/hr)
Morphine	1	2–5 mg	30–45	12–24	0.1–0.8
Meperidine	30	50–75 mg	5–10	5–8	10–30
Fentanyl	700	50–100 μg	5–10	5–8	0.030–0.100
Hydromorphone	1	1 mg	15	10–15	
Methadone	80	5 mg	10–15	5–10	

Epidural Opioids

Opioids applied to the dorsal horn of the spinal cord produce analgesia without loss of sensation or motor function. Because sympathetic nerve fibers are not affected, hypotension does not result. This selective analgesia constitutes the advantage of epidural or subarachnoid administration of opioids for pain management. Although the epidural injection of local anesthetics produces more profound analgesia, hypotension, motor blockade, and sensory loss also follow. When early mobility is essential, or even a mild degree of hypotension is unacceptable, opioids alone are given without local anesthetics. Epidural opioids may be unsuitable for patients in whom the risk of respiratory compromise is greatest, such as those with chronic obstructive pulmonary disease (COPD) or sleep apnea.

Although knowledge of epidural opioid pharmacokinetics and pharmacodynamics is incomplete, enough data exist to guide clinical applications. Table 36–2 lists the properties of opioid drugs commonly used in the epidural space.

The pharmacokinetics of epidural opioids are best predicted by their lipid solubilities. Lipid-soluble drugs enter neural tissues more readily than do lipid-insoluble drugs. The lipid-soluble opioids, fentanyl, sufentanil, and meperidine, reach their sites of action rapidly and take effect quickly (5 to 30 minutes). Morphine, being relatively lipid insoluble, has a much longer time to onset, usually 30 to 60 minutes.

The duration of action of an epidural opioid is determined by movement of drug away from spinal cord receptors, and its continued presence in the cerebrospinal fluid (CSF). Movement away from the spinal cord results from dissociation of drug from opioid receptors and removal by local spinal cord blood flow.

Lipid-soluble agents may pass into spinal cord blood vessels more easily than do lipid-insoluble drugs, so that fentanyl, sufentanil, and meperidine have short or intermediate durations of action, while drugs such as morphine have a much longer duration of action. Lipid solubility accounts for another important clinical feature of epidural opioids; their cephalad migration in the CSF. Less lipid-soluble opioids accumulate in CSF, migrating with CSF up the spinal fluid column. Thus, drugs like morphine tend to produce analgesia over multiple dermatomes, regardless of the site of epidural injection. Morphine given in the lumbar epidural space relieves thoracic pain, for example.

TYPICAL ORDERS FOR PATIENTS RECEIVING EPIDURAL NARCOTICS

Patient received (*dose*) mg epidural (*opioid*) at (*time*).

Measure respiratory rate, sedation level every hour for first 24 hours.

Call pain treatment physician for:

- **Nausea**
- **Pruritus**
- **Respiratory rate less than 10 breaths per minute**
- **Somnolence**
- **Inadequate pain relief**

Naloxone available at bedside at all times.

Infuse (*opioid*) into epidural catheter at (*mg or μg*) per hour via pump.

No other narcotics to be given unless ordered by pain treatment physician.

When lipid-soluble opioids are given via the lumbar epidural approach, the doses required to relieve thoracic pain are so great that systemic blood levels are appreciable and may account for much of the drug's effect. The cephalad migration of lipid-insoluble drugs increases brain CSF opioid levels, thereby promoting nausea, pruritus, sedation, and respiratory depression.

Bolus Versus Continuous Infusion

Epidural opioids may be given by bolus or continuous infusion. A single bolus is given either with the dose of epidural local anesthetic or at the end of the operation, the opioid chosen according to the duration of postoperative analgesia desired. Morphine reliably gives 10 to 24 hours of analgesia; fentanyl and meperidine last four to six hours. Subsequent doses given through an indwelling epidural catheter extend the period of analgesia, as does infusing opioids continuously. Table 36–2 lists the opioids commonly employed for epidural infusion.

Continuous administration of lipid-soluble opioids minimizes side effects expected with the more water-soluble drugs by limiting spread of the drug to distant dermatomes and avoiding cephalad spread in the CSF. This requires placing an epidural catheter as close as possible to the relevant nerve roots.

If the epidural catheter is distant from the critical nerve roots, or if the surgical incision is extensive, lipid-insoluble opioids are preferred as they produce effective and reliable pain relief at moderate doses. The large doses of lipid-soluble drugs required to produce analgesia in the same circumstance lead to excessive blood levels and more side effects.

Complications of Epidural Opioids

Respiratory depression, nausea, sedation, and pruritus result from significant concentrations of opioid reaching the brainstem, usually by cephalad migration in CSF but also from excessive blood levels of drug secondary to large epidural doses of opioid. They appear to be mediated by mu opioid receptor agonist activity, as mu-antagonist drugs reverse these effects.

Respiratory depression may be fatal. The likelihood of ventilatory compromise is probably greatest for the lipid-insoluble drugs, because of their propensity for cephalad spread to brainstem respiratory centers. A progressive decrease in respiratory rate to the range of four to ten breaths per minute is the common clinical presentation. However, significant respiratory depression (increased arterial CO_2 tension and decreased tidal volume) may occur despite a normal respiratory rate. Other evidence of excessive brain CSF opioid such as somnolence or pruritus usually accompanies ventilatory depression.

Unless the epidural dose of opioid is excessive, or accidental intrathecal injection has occurred, respiratory depression develops slowly and can be detected well before an emergency ensues. Respiratory depression after a single dose usually has an early and a late phase. The early phase occurs within an hour of injection and represents vascular uptake and delivery of opioid to the brain via the circulation. Later respiratory depression begins several hours after the epidural dose, and occurs almost exclusively with the lipid-insoluble opioids. It results from the cephalad movement of drug in CSF, and persists as long as brain CSF concentrations are substantial. Respiratory depression during continuous epidural opioid infusions may occur regardless of the drug used; with water-soluble drugs it is due to opioid in the CSF; with lipid-soluble drugs, to opioid in the circulation.

Moderate degrees of respiratory depression are dangerous for some patients, but safe for many. Clearly, markedly decreased respiratory rates (less than six per minute), apnea, and severe obtundation require immediate treatment in all patients. Healthy patients with moderate respiratory depression (i.e., six to ten breaths per minute, arterial CO_2 tension 45 to 55 mm Hg) require only increased observation and supplemental oxygen. All patients who receive opioids require monitoring for respiratory depression, ranging in intensity from frequent determinations of respiratory rate to apnea detectors or intensive care; the choice depends on the general condition of the patient and the presence of risk factors such as obesity, sleep apnea syndrome, lung disease, or advanced age. After conventional doses of epidural opioids, and absent special risk factors, simple monitoring of breathing rate alone in a non–intensive care setting is safe for most patients.

Epidural opioid-induced respiratory depression is treated with narcotic mu-receptor antagonists, of which naloxone is the prototype. Small intravenous doses (0.05 to 0.1 mg) are given until the desired respiratory rate or level of alertness is achieved. In most cases, respiratory depression can be expected to recur, requiring that an intravenous infusion of small amounts of naloxone (0.05 to 0.1 mg per hour) be started. This is adjusted according to the patient's respiratory rate, and discontinued as the expected duration of action of the epidural opioid is exceeded. Small doses of opioid antagonists reverse most side effects without reducing pain relief, perhaps because of the relatively lesser opioid concentrations in the brainstem (respiratory depression) than in the spinal cord (analgesia).

Nausea also results from excessive brain CSF opioid, presumably stimulating the vomiting centers and chemoemetic trigger zone. Though antiemetics may be useful for treatment, small doses of intravenous naloxone readily eliminate nausea without affecting analgesia.

Pruritus occurs when opioid spreads over the spinal cord, perhaps owing to extensive alteration of sensory input. It is not due to histamine release, and responds poorly to antihistamines. Naloxone, nalbuphine, and butorphanol all relieve pruritus.

Urinary retention owing to opioid receptor-mediated inhibition of normal micturition mechanisms may require use of a bladder catheter after epidural opioids. Urinary retention is readily reversed by naloxone.

Intrathecal Opioids

Opioids injected directly into the CSF produce analgesia, also. The implications of lipid solubility for duration of action are identical to those for epidural opioids, but the doses required are smaller because opioids injected directly into the CSF are not lost to vascular and tissue absorption, as happens with epidural opioids. Intrathecal morphine in doses of 0.25 to 0.5 mg produces excellent pain relief of long duration. Doses of 1 mg or more produce long periods of analgesia but result in many side effects, especially respiratory depression. Because subarachnoid catheters are not popular, this route is not used for continuous treatment of postoperative pain.

The opioid-related side effects of respiratory depression, pruritus, nausea, and urinary retention also occur with intrathecal administration. Their etiologies and treatment are the same as those described for epidural opioids.

Epidural Anesthetics

Epidural anesthesia with lesser concentrations of local anesthetics provides good relief of postoperative pain. Bupivacaine 0.25 per cent to 0.5 per cent is chosen for its long duration of action and relatively selective sensory blockade. Continuous infusion rates of bupivacaine are usually between 5 ml per hour and 15 ml per hour in adults. Tachyphylaxis, the progressive reduction in effect seen when local anesthetics are given for prolonged periods, may make treatment difficult when local anesthetic is used alone.

Because of tachyphylaxis, the frequency of doses or the infusion rate increases during therapy. Hypotension, numbness, weakness, and urinary retention may all occur during epidural local anesthetic therapy; this may eliminate this technique if the risk of hypotension is unacceptable or if the patient must walk. As with epidural opioids, the catheter site is best placed as close as possible to the nerve roots innervating the surgical wound. This helps limit the extent of epidural blockade and attendant risks of hypotension. Less severe hypotension, and sensory and motor block may follow use of combinations of dilute local anesthetic and opioid mixtures described below.

Combined Local Anesthetic and Opioid Epidural Infusions

Mixtures of subanalgesic doses of local anesthetics and opioids produce profound analgesia with minimal side effects. The two drugs act at different sites in the pain pathway (nerve roots and dorsal horn), raising the possibility of greater than additive effects. Synergy has been demonstrated in animals, but conclusive evidence in humans is lacking.

The usual mixtures consist of bupivacaine 0.1 per cent to 0.25 per cent, and any of the several commonly used epidural opioids. Morphine, 0.05 to 0.1 mg per ml, meperidine 1.0 to 2.5 mg per ml, and fentanyl 5 to 10 μg per ml have all been used effectively in this regimen. Typical infusion rates are from 4 to 12 ml per hour, depending on the location of the epidural catheter (lesser rates for thoracic catheters) and the size of the surgical wound (greater rates for large incisions). Just as with opioid infusions, hourly doses of morphine in excess of 1 mg, fentanyl in excess of 0.1 mg, and meperidine in excess of 30 mg, may result in excessive blood levels or CSF levels of drug, producing sedation or respiratory depression.

Although lesser doses of local anesthetic and opioid might result in fewer side effects, complications related to each drug do occur. Opioid-induced side effects are treated as described earlier. Local anesthetics produce sympathetic blockade and hypotension, treated with intravenous fluids or vasoactive drugs. Motor and sensory block are unlikely unless bupivacaine concentrations of 0.25 per cent or greater are used; nevertheless, these patients are not expected to walk or stand unassisted.

Epidural local anesthetic and opioid infusions are not used if mild hypotension is unacceptable or early mobility is essential for postoperative care. It may be difficult to achieve analgesia with these solutions when the epidural infusion site is distant from the nerve roots serving the surgical incision. In these instances, less lipid-soluble opioids without local anesthetic may be useful (Table 36–3).

PERIPHERAL NERVE BLOCKS FOR ACUTE PAIN

Peripheral nerve blocks provide profound postoperative pain relief. These can be performed in the operating room, or postoperatively, as specific treatment for acute pain; they are particularly useful when epidural or spinal techniques are contraindicated or difficult to perform. Because these techniques are often used for patients who have undergone orthopedic procedures, special precautions are required. The profound analgesia and motor block may make it impossible for the surgeon to evaluate a limb after operation or for the

TABLE 36–3. Techniques of Postoperative Pain Relief

Therapy	Indications	Contraindications	Advantages/Benefits	Disadvantages/Risks
Patient-controlled analgesia (PCA)	Postoperative pain that is: Severe; Prolonged; Not amenable to oral analgesics	Narcotic allergy Patient cannot activate PCA History of drug abuse or drug-seeking behavior	Drugs given on time Dose titrated to need Patient satisfaction Little physician or nurse labor required	Opioid-related side effects Incomplete analgesia Overdose due to errors
Epidural and subarachnoid opioids	Pain relief after any major operation below shoulder girdle Early patient mobility required	Narcotic allergy Risks of respiratory depression, especially in COPD, sleep apnea, obesity	Good analgesia Motor, sensory, sympathetic functions intact Continuous block	Nausea Pruritus Urinary retention Respiratory depression
Local anesthetic with or without opioids in epidural space	Pain relief after any major operation below shoulder girdle when early patient mobility not required	Narcotic allergy Patient mobility required Risk of hypotension unacceptable	Most profound analgesia Less severe opioid-related side effects Continuous block	Hypotension Nausea Pruritus Urinary retention Respiratory depression
Peripheral nerve block	Procedures on the extremities, or in areas served by thoracic dermatomes	When early neurovascular evaluation of limb is required Circumferential cast	Most profound analgesia Possibly improved blood flow to ischemic areas such as skin flaps	Motor & sensory deficits in distribution of block Continuous analgesia difficult to provide
Interpleural analgesia	Unilateral incisions through areas served by thoracic dermatomes	Pleural effusion or fibrosis Pleural inflammation	Technical simplicity Profound analgesia Avoids hypotension Continuous techniques possible	Pneumothorax Local anesthetic toxicity Frequent repeat injections

Note: Contraindications to regional anesthesia are also contraindications to all of these techniques except PCA.

patient to report pain; both increase the risk of compartment syndromes and nerve damage from tight casts. Nerve blocks of an extremity for postoperative pain relief are inappropriate when the limb is to be placed in a cast or when there is risk of neurovascular compromise. Directions for specific nerve blocks are found in Chapter 19.

Brachial Plexus Blockade

The simplest method of providing postoperative analgesia for operations on the upper extremity is to perform a brachial plexus block with an epinephrine-containing local anesthetic. When 0.5 per cent or 0.75 per cent bupivacaine with epinephrine is used for brachial plexus blockade, analgesia usually persists for 10 to 15 hours after the operation. Of course, the site of the operation determines the preferred approach to the brachial plexus.

If extended analgesia is needed, a brachial plexus catheter permits giving additional doses or a continuous infusion. This technique is not popular, perhaps because it is difficult to fix brachial plexus catheters in place. Continuous infusions of 0.25 per cent bupivacaine at 6 to 12 ml per hour or intermittent injections maintain analgesia. In the axillary approach to the brachial plexus, it is best to place the catheter nearest the nerve or cord innervating the surgical site. Thus, for analgesia after reimplantation of the fifth finger, the catheter is placed near the medial cord and ulnar nerve.

Femoral Nerve Block

Blockade of the femoral nerve provides significant analgesia after operations on the knee or distal femur. A reliable method for easily locating the femoral nerve is with a peripheral nerve stimulator, as discussed in Chapter 19. Peripheral nerve stimulation is especially useful during or just after an operation, when the patient may be unable to report a paresthesia. This block provides useful but incomplete pain relief after knee operations, because the obturator, lateral femoral cutaneous, and sciatic nerves also innervate the knee area.

Intercostal Nerve Block

Intercostal nerve blocks can provide excellent pain relief for areas served by the thoracic dermatomes; when 3 to 5 ml of 0.5 per cent bupivacaine with epinephrine are used, analgesia persists for 6 to 12 hours. Continuous subpleural intercostal block has been described, but is technically difficult. Because of the rich vasculature, local anesthetic toxicity is a risk, particularly when several nerves must be blocked repeatedly. Finally, pneumothorax is a risk, especially if multiple injections are performed. This complication is rare when block are performed by trained persons.

Interpleural Analgesia

A recent innovation is the interpleural injection of local anesthetics, which produces the equivalent of unilateral multiple intercostal blocks, thus giving analgesia after cholecystectomy, splenectomy, nephrectomy, or breast operations. Simple techniques allow placement of an interpleural catheter, through which intermittent injections or a continuous infusion of local anesthetic can be given.

TECHNIQUE OF INTERPLEURAL BLOCK

An epidural needle filled with saline is advanced over the cephalad margin of the fifth, sixth, or seventh rib until it pierces the parietal pleura and the saline is drawn into the pleural cavity. This is analogous to the "hanging drop" method of epidural placement; do not substitute the loss of resistance technique, which may lead to puncture of the visceral pleura and pneumothorax. An epidural catheter is threaded 5 to 6 cm into the thoracic cavity, the needle is removed over the catheter, and the injection site covered with an adhesive sterile dressing.

Bupivacaine, 20 to 30 ml of 0.25 per cent or 0.5 per cent, is injected through the catheter and the patient placed supine or tilted slightly to the nonoperative side, so that local anesthetic solutions are in contact with pleura where it is nearest the intercostal nerves. Analgesia reaches its maximum within 30 minutes. The block is maintained with injections repeated every four to six hours or an infusion of 0.25 per cent bupivacaine at 10 to 12 ml per hour.

Even when efforts are made to ensure that local anesthetic is not lost through chest tube drainage, the analgesia obtained with this technique is often unsatisfactory after thoracotomy. Perhaps pleural reaction or dilution of drug by pleural fluid contribute to this problem.

Although pneumothorax is unusual, it must be

considered if the patient develops dyspnea. Aspiration of air through the interpleural catheter is diagnostic. In severe cases, a chest tube may be necessary.

CONTRAINDICATIONS TO INTERPLEURAL BLOCK

Contraindication	Expected problem
Thoracotomy	Failed block
Pleural fibrosis	Inadequate spread of drug
Pleural inflammation	Rapid uptake; toxicity
Pleural effusion	Dilution of local anesthetic; ineffective block
Blebs	Pneumothorax
Bleeding disorder	Hemothorax
Bilateral block required	Excessive drug needed; toxicity

Interpleural analgesia may be preferred over epidural anesthesia when thoracic epidural puncture is difficult or when hypotension is to be avoided. Although interpleural blocks can produce unilateral thoracic sympathetic or splanchnic nerve block, this has not been associated with hypotension.

FUTURE ADVANCES IN POSTOPERATIVE PAIN THERAPY

Current research on the physiology and pharmacology of pain is likely to have more impact on the treatment of postoperative pain than on anesthesia for surgical procedures. Potent receptor-specific opioids may produce powerful analgesia when given into the epidural space, without depressing respiration. Alpha-2 adrenergic agonist drugs such as clonidine produce epidural analgesia and reduce minimum alveolar concentration (MAC) by affecting nonopioid receptors. The new amide local anesthetic ropivacaine may block sensory fibers without producing motor block in lesser concentrations, although it has yet to undergo clinical trials as a postoperative analgesic agent. Transcutaneous electrical nerve stimulation (TENS) is usually not effective when given alone for acute pain, but has been shown to reduce narcotic requirements when used postoperatively.

THE POSTOPERATIVE PAIN TREATMENT SERVICE

The treatment of postoperative pain with these newer techniques is appealing to both patients and anesthesiologists, but comprehensive acute pain services are not widely established. Favoring this approach are the clear opportunities to relieve human suffering, the less certain physiologic benefits such as improved pulmonary function and reduced cardiovascular stress, and the potentially favorable (yet speculative) effects on perioperative mortality. Against it are a number of factors. Third-party payers are reluctant to pay for novel therapies, especially when routine methods of pain treatment are already reimbursed as part of postoperative care. The lack of clear improvements in outcome makes it more difficult to establish funding. Lastly, the added risks of novel complications make these procedures less appealing to some.

Nevertheless, when the environment and funding permit, an organized postoperative pain treatment service can offer considerable benefits to patients. Anesthesiologists skilled in the techniques of epidural and peripheral nerve blockade, and knowledgeable in the area of pharmacokinetics of narcotic drugs, are logical choices to be physicians in charge of postoperative pain therapy, but the concurrent treatment of numerous patients is demanding and labor intensive. Participation by surgeons, other consultants, pharmacists, and nurses is necessary for success, but the gratitude expressed by satisfied patients is just reward for the effort.

REFERENCES

Bridenbaugh LD. The upper extremity: Somatic blockade, neural blockade in clinical anesthesia and management of pain. 2nd ed. Philadelphia: JB Lippincott, 1987:387–416.

Bridenbaugh PO. The lower extremity: Somatic blockade neural blockade in clinical anesthesia and management of pain. 2nd ed. Philadelphia: JB Lippincott, 1987:417–441.

Cousins MJ, Mather LE: Intrathecal and epidural administration of opioids. Anesthesiology 1984; 61:276–310.

Mather LE, Owen H. *In* Ferrante FM, Ostheimer GW, Covino BG, ed. The pharmacology of patient-administered opioids, Patient-Controlled Analgesia. Boston: Blackwell Scientific Publications, 1990:27–50.

Reiestad F, Stromskag KE. Intrapleural catheter in the management of postoperative pain—a preliminary report. Reg Anesth 1986; 11:89.

Sjöström S, Hartvig P, Persson MP, Tamsen A. Pharmocokinetics of epidural morphine and meperidine in humans. Anesthesiology 1987; 67:877–888.

CHAPTER THIRTY-SEVEN

Critical Care of the Surgical Patient

Critical care medicine has evolved during the past 25 years to provide care for patients in whom potentially reversible life-threatening changes in clinical condition may occur very quickly. The major indication for admission to the intensive care unit is potentially reversible cardiorespiratory instability, present or impending, that could cause death if not treated promptly. Regardless of the underlying illness, all critically ill patients are susceptible to a number of common problems, including sepsis, renal failure, gastrointestinal bleeding, cardiovascular failure, and respiratory failure.

Intensive care of the surgical patient requires attention to all organ systems, and a broad understanding of medical and surgical illness that cannot be described in detail in an introductory text. Respiratory function is the major determinant of survival: patients in respiratory failure requiring more than 24 hours of mechanical ventilation at inspired oxygen concentrations exceeding 50 per cent have a greater than 50 per cent chance of in-hospital death. Thus, this chapter emphasizes clinical management of respiratory failure in the surgical patient.

The role of the anesthesiologist in caring for critically ill surgical patients varies widely, from consultant to primary physician. Because airway management, close monitoring, and maintenance of cardiorespiratory stability are central issues in these illnesses, anesthesiologists were among the pioneers in developing critical care medicine. These continue to be the areas of anesthesiologists' greatest interest and expertise.

Transportation of the Critically Ill Surgical Patient

The critical care of the surgical patient begins in the operating room. During transport to the intensive care unit (ICU), the patient requires the same monitoring and support as in the operating room.

Portable mechanical ventilators have advantages when transportation time is prolonged or when end-expiratory pressure is required, but such equipment may malfunction. Self-inflating bags function even when the oxygen supply fails, but clinical assessment of oxygen delivery and ventilation are less certain than with a flaccid rebreathing bag because the sensation of the bag filling and emptying is obscured. In addition, there is the possibility of valve malfunction in all self-inflating bags (see also Chapter 20). During transportation, respiratory monitoring may be limited to patient observation, but battery operated pulse oximeters are preferred for many of these patients.

The hemodynamic monitoring used during transportation depends on the patient's condition. Because movement often provokes hypotension or hypertension, those who need indwelling arterial pressure monitoring during operation require similar monitoring during transportation to and from the ICU. Likewise, the vasoactive drugs available to support the circulation during anesthesia are brought with the patient during transportation to the ICU.

The anesthesiologist notifies the intensive care unit before moving the patient, so that preparations can be made. On arrival in the intensive care unit, hemodynamic and respiratory monitoring are restored immediately; greater minute ventilation and F_{IO_2} than are thought necessary are provided until proper monitoring provides data that justify lesser values. Endotracheal tube position is reconfirmed immediately by auscultation and chest x-ray.

MANAGEMENT OF RESPIRATORY FAILURE

Table 37–1 lists the changes in pulmonary function that lead to respiratory failure in critically ill patients after operation. It is usually impossible to distinguish specific causes in a given patient, as all of these defects may coexist. Pathophysiologic processes worsen pulmonary gas exchange in these patients; the most common are listed in Table 37–2.

Aspiration Pneumonia

In critically ill patients, general debility, neuromuscular dysfunction, and the blunting of airway reflexes from oversedation and from the presence of oropharyngeal tubes and airways create circumstances favorable for aspiration of oropharyngeal contents. Despite recent widespread adoption of precautions for prevention of aspiration of gastric contents, (see Chapters 4, 13, 25, and 26) this problem still causes significant morbidity and mortality in critically ill patients. Endotracheal tubes limit but do not eliminate the risks of aspiration of gastric or oropharyngeal contents. Further, the 24-hour period immediately following removal of endotracheal tubes is a period of great risk owing to residual laryngeal dysfunction caused by the tracheal tube.

Treatment of aspiration pneumonia includes meticulous removal of secretions, postural drainage, antibiotic treatment based on culture sensitivities, maintenance of fluid and nutritional balance, and therapy for ventilatory failure as needed. Acid aspiration may result in severe lung injury with massive extravasation of fluid into lung parenchyma and the need for intravascular fluid replenishment. Neither steroids nor prophylactic antibiotics have been shown to be efficacious in the treatment of aspiration pneumonia.

TABLE 37–1. Changes in Pulmonary Function in Postoperative Critically Ill Patients

Compromised lung volumes
- Functional residual capacity
- Residual volume
- Vital capacity
- Total lung capacity

Diminished flow rates
Decreased compliance
V/Q mismatching
- Intrapulmonary shunting
- Dead space

Increased work of breathing
Increased demand for oxygen

TABLE 37–2. Disease Processes Worsening Gas Exchange in Critically Ill Patients

Aspiration pneumonia
Atelectasis
Airway obstruction
Sepsis
Bacterial pneumonia
Obstructive pulmonary disease
Pulmonary embolism
Pulmonary edema
Neuromuscular dysfunction

Atelectasis

Atelectasis, the collapse of lung parenchyma that can be seen on chest x-ray, occurs commonly after major operations (50 per cent of patients after abdominal procedures). In critically ill patients, it may impair oxygenation through intrapulmonary shunting. Atelectasis in debilitated patients commonly leads to pneumonia and respiratory failure. The distinction between pneumonia and atelectasis is never clear. Fever in excess of 38°C with purulent sputum, intracellular bacteria on sputum gram stain, radiographic evidence of infiltrates, and positive sputum cultures strongly suggest a bacterial pneumonia.

A syndrome of progressive loss of lung volume and hypoxemia without x-ray evidence of atelectasis has been referred to as microatelectasis. In spontaneously breathing patients, a program of getting the patient out of bed and deep breathing exercises (with appropriate analgesics or regional anesthesia to reduce splinting) has been shown to limit the development of atelectasis. In mechanically ventilated patients, periodic sighing and clearing of the trachea by suction, coupled with ventilation with tidal volumes larger than 10 ml per kg of body weight, usually limits or reverses both types of atelectasis. Prophylactic positive end-expiratory pressure or bronchoscopy have not been shown to be superior to the above regimen. When significant atelectasis fails to respond to conservative therapy, bronchoscopy may be effective in removing large mucus plugs or particulate material from major bronchi.

Acute Airway Obstruction

Airway obstruction in patients who have not undergone intubation of the trachea is well described elsewhere (see Chapter 13). Obstruction in an endotracheal tube may present insidiously, often mimicking decreased lung compliance or bronchospasm. It is usually caused by inspissation of secretions owing to inadequate humidification of inspired gases or inadequate removal of secretions by suction. However, it may also occur for other mechanical reasons including overinflation of the tracheal cuff, biting on the tube, kinking in the posterior pharynx, or tracheobronchial disruption. Partial obstructions may produce increased airway pressures during inspiration (peak pressure) with normal static lung compliance (plateau pressure relative to tidal volume), calling attention to this possibility. Partial endotracheal tube obstruction sometimes can be differentiated from bronchospasm by the absence of wheezing, but expiratory wheezing may be present with partial obstruction, also. Failure to pass easily a suction catheter or fiberoptic bronchoscope through the endotracheal tube is a strong indication for replacement or repositioning of the tube, followed by x-ray confirmation of proper position.

Table 37–3. Common Causes of Sepsis in Critically Ill Surgical Patients

From Known Infection:
Pneumonia
Urinary tract infection
Postoperative infection (abscess, empyema)
Wound infection
Primary:
Intravascular cannulae
Implanted foreign material
Drainage tubes

Sepsis

The diagnosis of sepsis depends on signs of systemic infection such as fever, tachycardia, hemodynamic instability, leucocytosis, and altered mental status, regardless of culture proof of blood stream seeding. Table 37–3 lists common sources for septic contamination in critically ill patients. Sepsis is the major cause of death among patients developing the adult respiratory distress syndrome (ARDS), described in a later section of this chapter.

Survival depends on rapid recognition and treatment of the infection with antibiotics, prompt surgical drainage where possible, and fluid resuscitation to maintain renal function. Other supportive measures, including maintenance of hemodynamic function with inotropes and vasodilators, mechanical ventilation, and supplemental oxygenation allow time for definitive therapy to be effective (see Chapter 29).

Bacterial Pneumonia

Bacterial pneumonia is the most common fatal hospital-acquired infection; more than 50 per cent of critically ill patients with bacterial pneumonia do not survive to leave the hospital. In patients with the adult respiratory distress syndrome and bacterial pneumonia, mortality approaches 90 per cent. Common causes of bacterial pneumonia in the critically ill surgical patient include aspiration, atelectasis, hematogenous spread from extrapulmonary sources, and retention of secretions owing to lack of an effective cough mechanism. Patients in whom tracheostomy or prolonged tracheal intubation is necessary are at increased risk for development of bacterial pneumonia owing to aspiration of secretions and loss of upper airway defense mechanisms. Clearing these secretions from the trachea with suction, postural drainage, and early treatment with antibiotics (often gram-negative organisms) offer the best chance of success. In the presence of lobar pneumonia, positive end-expiratory pressure may worsen gas exchange (see later section on PEEP, CPAP).

Among ICU patients, sputum cultures usually reveal gram-negative organisms, even without clinical evidence of pneumonia. Treatment of this infestation leads to rapid appearance of antibiotic-resistant organisms, limiting therapeutic options should pneumonia occur later. It is important to not give antibiotics for positive cultures unless other evidence of infection is present, including fever, new pulmonary infiltrates, leucocytosis, and increased purulence of sputum. Early detection of bacterial pneumonia in a critically ill patient is required for successful treatment; any change in the patient's clinical condition, sputum quality or quantity, or chest physical findings, is an indication for sputum culture and chest x-ray.

Chronic Obstructive Lung Disease

Chronic obstructive lung disease consists of a spectrum of illnesses, the major types of which include chronic bronchitis, asthma, and emphysema. Though the severity of respiratory obstruction may be measured by pulmonary function testing, unless obstruction is severe, these tests do not correlate well with postoperative morbidity. Functional testing and exercise tolerance are more likely to give meaningful prognostic information regarding postoperative pulmonary complications (see Chapter 22).

The pathogenesis of these complications has its origin in the patient's reduced ventilatory ability, which may become severe enough postoperatively to produce CO_2 retention, requiring mechanical ventilation. In addition, inadequate cough associated with viscid pulmonary secretions results in progressive airway plugging and gas exchange abnormalities. Once the patient with chronic obstructive pulmonary disease (COPD) presents with respiratory failure following operation, the critical care physician is faced with a therapeutic dilemma. Often the respiratory muscles of the patient with severe obstructive disease were fully employed to support even minimal activities; subsequent mechanical ventilation results in disuse atrophy and alterations in respiratory control mechanisms. The return to spontaneous ventilation may require a prolonged period of reconditioning of both muscles and control systems. Thus, complete mechanical support of ventilation may make the patient ventilator dependent, whereas limited support may overburden an already compromised cardiovascular or pulmonary system.

The first choice is to avoid ventilatory support, carefully titrating pain control by treating with parenteral or epidural analgesics, controlling fluid excess with diuretics, relieving reversible airway obstruction with nebulized bronchodilators, limiting inspired oxygen concentration to the minimum so as to preserve hypoxic pulmonary drive, and ensuring adequate reversal of residual muscle relaxants. If these measures fail, then mechanical ventilation is limited to as short a time as is possible. Frequent brief intervals of maximal respiratory work, without allowing the development of fatigue, will often promote later weaning from mechanical ventilation. This may be accomplished by allowing the patient to breathe spontaneously without ventilatory assistance for short intervals. Newer modes of partial ventilatory support that provide graded exercise, such as intermittent mandatory ventilation or pressure support ventilation, may maintain respiratory muscle strength if excessive fatigue is not allowed to develop. Weaning is discussed more fully later.

In patients with acute ventilatory decompensation imposed on COPD there are several special considerations. First, many such patients compensate for their illness by increasing sympathetic tone to maintain cardiac output and by retaining bicarbonate to maintain a normal blood pH in spite of hypercarbia. Restoring normal CO_2 elimination by mechanical ventilation abruptly corrects respiratory acidosis without immediately affecting plasma bicarbonate concentrations, resulting in severe metabolic alkalosis. This may provoke dangerous hypokalemia and loss of sympathetic tone, leading to cardiovascular collapse. Deliberate initial underventilation and slow correction of the ventilatory disturbance over hours, with careful attention to maintenance of normal blood hydrogen ion concentrations, creates the least metabolic and hemodynamic disturbance.

Second, many of these patients have diminished ventilatory responses to carbon dioxide; ventilation may depend on blood oxygen tension ("hypoxic drive"). In these few patients, excessive oxygen, especially in combination with sedatives and narcotics, can decrease ventilatory drive, leading even to carbon dioxide narcosis and ventilatory arrest. Inadequate blood oxygenation in patients with chronic obstructive disease is usually due to ventilation/perfusion inequality in the lung. Unless significant shunting owing to some other process is present, adequate blood oxygenation can be attained with modest concentrations (usually less than 50 per cent) of inspired oxygen. In spontaneously breathing patients, the oxygen content of the inspired gas may be controlled by delivery through a venturi mask at a concentration dilute enough to preserve hypoxic ventilatory drive.

Pulmonary Embolism

Critically ill surgical patients are at risk for pulmonary embolism because they are bedridden and because circulatory insufficiency leads to peripheral venous stasis. Common signs and symptoms include the sudden onset of dyspnea, wheezing, diaphoresis, tachycardia, and a feeling of impending doom. These nonspecific findings are often seen with acute cardiogenic pulmonary edema; objective tests, including pulmonary angiography or radioisotopic ventilation/perfusion lung scans, may be necessary to confirm the diagnosis. Small pulmonary emboli may produce dramatic changes in hemodynamics, with hypotension, tachycardia, and hypoxemia that do not readily respond to oxygen therapy; this diagnosis must be considered whenever these findings occur. The classic electrocardiographic (ECG) and radiographic findings (right ventricular strain and abrupt termination of pulmonary vasculature or wedge-shaped infiltrates) may be absent. Pulmonary function testing reveals increased dead-space ventilation, but this finding also occurs in acute cardiogenic pulmonary edema.

Once pulmonary embolism has occurred, there is a significant likelihood of recurrent embolism and death. Absent contraindications, prophylactic therapy with small doses of heparin, and stockings or mechanical devices to improve venous emptying from the lower extremities are considered for all critically ill surgical patients. These measures failing, larger doses of heparin are required. If full heparinization fails to prevent recurrence or cannot be used, an intravenous filter or ligation of the inferior vena cava may prevent migration of large emboli to the lungs.

After large pulmonary emboli, mechanical ventilation combined with fluid therapy and inotropic support may allow time for more definitive therapies to be effective. In such circumstances, thrombolytic therapy must be considered despite risks of serious hemorrhage. All else failing, early operative pulmonary embolectomy may offer salvage rates of up to 50 per cent.

Pulmonary Edema

The diagnosis of pulmonary edema is based on history, physical examination, blood gas analysis and chest x-ray. Preexisting cardiac or renal dysfunction heightens suspicion as does a history of prolonged illness or extensive intraoperative fluid resuscitation. If fluid and sodium are given in excess of patient requirements, virtually all critically ill patients will retain fluid, unless given diuretics. On physical examination, aside from the usual findings related to respiratory distress and decreased lung compliance, moist bibasilar rales and wheezing are present. Although blood carbon dioxide tensions may remain normal or decreased until severe respiratory failure supervenes, the gradient between alveolar and arterial oxygen tensions always increases, and does not readily respond to oxygen therapy.

The major physiologic causes of pulmonary edema include hydrostatic edema owing to heart failure and fluid overload, and permeability edema, in which the pulmonary vascular bed is damaged by toxic or inflammatory processes. The latter type is often called the adult respiratory distress syndrome (ARDS) or more recently, acute lung injury.

It may be difficult to distinguish between hydrostatic and permeability edema of the lung; both types are often present in critically ill patients. In hydrostatic edema, chest x-rays show characteristic central venous congestion with alveolar and interstitial infiltrates. In edema owing to lung permeability changes, central vascular congestion is absent. Though permeability pulmonary edema (ARDS) has many causes, the majority of cases are associated with intra-abdominal sepsis or other major bacterial infections. Pulmonary edema associated with sepsis may occur without a clearly defined focus of infection, particularly when the patient is elderly, or debilitated and malnourished.

The response to treatment may help differentiate forms of pulmonary edema. Permeability edema usually clears slowly as the inciting cause resolves. Hence, rapid clinical improvement (within several hours) with treatment strongly supports a diagnosis of hydrostatic pulmonary edema. When the diagnosis is in doubt, measurement of cardiac output and pulmonary artery pressure may aid in both management and diagnosis. Normal left ventricular filling pressures are seen in permeability edema, but increased pressures characterize relative fluid overload and heart failure.

Despite the differences in course and causes of the two types of edema, management is similar and aims at maintaining gas exchange and cardiac output while decreasing pulmonary capillary hydrostatic pressure. Supportive treatment with assisted ventilation, supplemental oxygen, and positive end-expiratory pressure are the major temporizing maneuvers while awaiting response to more definitive therapy. Excessive sodium and water administration worsens pulmonary function in all forms of pulmonary edema; close control of fluid balance is required in the patient with pulmonary edema, regardless of cause. In hydrostatic edema, narcotics, diuretics, sodium and fluid restriction, vasodilators, and inotropic support usually result in rapid improvement. In permeability edema, the course to recovery commonly lasts several weeks, with a mortality approaching 75 per cent. Prognosis worsens as the course extends beyond several weeks.

CHOICE OF MONITORING

Respiratory Monitoring

Anticipated need for respiratory monitoring after operation depends on the predicted risk of pulmonary failure, according to factors outlined in Table 37–4. Although scoring systems have been established to predict the risk of respiratory difficulties, these have not been subjected to rigorous prospective evaluation. At one extreme, the alert patient without signs of respiratory distress may require no more than hourly assessment of vital signs. Patients with marginal ventilatory function or neuromuscular disease who are breathing spontaneously may suffer sudden respiratory collapse; such patients require constant observation or electronic apnea monitoring. At the other extreme, the desperately ill patient may require continuous monitoring of arterial oxygenation and carbon dioxide output, together with frequent monitoring of cardiovascular values including cardiac output and pulmonary artery pressures.

TABLE 37–4. Respiratory Failure—Predisposing Factors

Diminished ventilatory reserve
Advanced age
Malnutrition
Neuromuscular disorders
Impaired cardiovascular function
Pulmonary disease
Operation
Limiting ventilatory reserve:
Intra-abdominal operations
Thoracic operations
Affecting control of ventilation:
Intracranial operations
Residual anesthetic effects
Relative overdose of analgesics
Pain limiting vital capacity and functional residual capacity
Relative fluid overload
Increased metabolic demands, due to pain, fever, response to hypothermia

Physical Examination

Dyspnea, tachypnea, restlessness, and increased sympathetic tone may signal respiratory collapse, but it is not uncommon for these signs to be muted or missing owing to effects of anesthetics, sedatives, narcotics, and neuromuscular disease. Physical examination of the chest may detect some of the more common correctable physical abnormalities leading to respiratory failure such as pneumothorax, pleural effusion, bronchospasm, major atelectasis, or incorrect placement of endotracheal tubes. Auscultation of the chest will be required at regular intervals or at the time of any change in the patient's vital signs. This examination also indicates the need for bronchodilators or clearing of secretions from large airways by suction.

Blood Gas Measurement

Definitive diagnosis of respiratory failure is based upon abnormalities in arterial blood gas measurements, which are indicated whenever respiratory failure is suspected (see Chapters 2 and 22).

No reliable method now exists for continuous monitoring of arterial oxygen tensions in adults. For patients who require routine surveillance, and for those whose peripheral oxygen saturations are less than 100 per cent, pulse oximetry is of use. It is of particular value in patients in whom hypoxic drive supplies the major impetus to maintenance of ventilation. In these patients, careful titration of inspired oxygen concentrations is necessary to maintain saturation levels in the range of 88 per cent to 90 per cent, where hypoxic ventilatory drive is active. For critically ill patients in whom subtle changes in A–aDo_2 must be detected, especially when the arterial Po_2 exceeds 90 mm Hg, pulse oximetry is inadequate.

In the critically ill patients, capnography does not substitute for the measurement of arterial carbon dioxide tensions. Airway obstruction, alterations in dead space, and changes in cardiac output all affect the apparent end-tidal CO_2. As acute airway obstruction develops, isolated values of "end-tidal" carbon dioxide tension measured by capnography may decrease as ventilation and mixing of dead space and alveolar gas worsen. Hence, the end-tidal CO_2 value may suggest improvement as gas exchange deteriorates. In contrast to end-tidal CO_2 only, the continuous monitoring of expired carbon dioxide may provide subtle additional information about respiratory function that is not evident by other simple means. For example, the failure to achieve a plateau on the expirogram suggests bronchoconstriction or other forms of obstruction.

Balloon-tipped flow-directed pulmonary artery catheters can monitor both respiratory and cardiovascular functions. As use of flow-directed pulmonary artery catheters has increased, so has the use of mixed venous saturation and gas tension measurements. The expression derived from the Fick equation shown below demonstrates that mixed venous oxygen content is dependent on factors affecting total body oxygen delivery and consumption (see Chapter 29).

Much of the therapeutic effort to maintain cardiorespiratory stability in critically ill patients is derived from manipulation of the variables governing oxygen transport expressed in the Fick equation. Each variable is changed so as to keep to a minimum adverse effects while producing

FICK EQUATION

O_2 consumption

= cardiac output × A-V O_2 content difference

$$Qo_2 = CO \times K \times (Sao_2 - S\bar{v}o_2)$$

where K = 1.38 ml O_2/gm Hb × Hb gm/dl

Mixed venous O_2 Saturation

$$S\bar{v}o_2 = Sao_2 - Qo_2/(CO \times K)$$

Mixed venous oxygen saturation increases when arterial oxygen saturation, the hemoglobin concentration, or cardiac output increase, or when total oxygen consumption decreases. Management of patients with inadequate total oxygen delivery begins with this relationship, but insight into the patient's overall physiology is essential. For example, mixed venous oxygen saturation can be improved in a febrile patient, or in one moving about violently by decreasing oxygen consumption through appropriate measures to reduce fever or halt movement, but decreases in oxygen consumption resulting from cyanide toxicity also increase mixed venous oxygen saturation. Normal mixed venous blood, sampled in the pulmonary artery, has an oxygen saturation of 75 percent.

The values for the oxygen-carry capacity of fully saturated hemoglobin has been measured in adults as 1.31 ml/gm Hb; the theoretical value is 1.39; the value used here is an intermediate one.

therapeutic benefit. Factors affecting this balance, including metabolic rate, cardiac output and its determinants, arterial oxygen carrying capacity, and arterial oxygen saturation, all are reflected in changes in the mixed venous oxygen tension or saturation. This measurement can be made by sampling blood from the distal port of the pulmonary artery catheter or from direct measurement with a fiberoptic catheter. Mixed venous oxygen saturation is of particular value in determining the best positive end-expiratory pressure (PEEP) and in regulating cardiac output with volume replacement, inotropic agents, and vasodilators.

Ventilator Monitors

During mechanical ventilation in the ICU, monitoring of the ventilator and breathing circuit is even more necessary than in the operating room, where an anesthesiologist is in constant attendance. All recent ventilators provide these monitoring capabilities, including inspired oxygen content, minute ventilation, and airway pressures. These monitors also detect airway obstruction or disconnection from the ventilator, and are used whenever the patient is connected to the ventilator.

There are more sophisticated measurements of value in assessing severity of pulmonary disease and effects of treatment. These include static compliance, inspiratory: expiratory time ratio, and presence of breath stacking (auto-PEEP) to assess whether adequate time has been permitted during a ventilatory cycle for complete exhalation of each inspired breath. Many are included as part of the monitoring package provided with newer ventilators. Measurement of static compliance and peak inflation pressure are helpful in differentiating airway obstruction from changes in lung stiffness.

Monitoring Cardiovascular Function

The monitoring of cardiovascular function is described in Chapter 6. Heart and lung function are closely linked; to monitor cardiovascular function is to monitor respiratory function too. Although the uses of invasive cardiovascular monitors in the ICU are similar to those in the operating room, there are several special considerations.

In patients with severe ARDS, regulation within narrow limits of fluid balance, inotropes, and PEEP may be required to obtain satisfactory urine output, cardiac output, and oxygenation. Repeated measurement of pulmonary arterial pressures and cardiac output may be required to accomplish these goals. Long-term invasive arterial and venous monitoring presents special hazards including thrombosis, infection, bleeding, and misinterpretation of data. Thorough knowledge of waveforms and common artifacts, combined with sterile precautions, regular dressing changes, and replacement of indwelling cannulae (every four days) are required.

To reduce risks, development of noninvasive methods continues, including impedance cardiography, and transcutaneous and transesophageal Doppler echocardiography. These have yet to find widespread use in the intensive care unit because they still lack the precision and accuracy needed for long-term monitoring in this environment.

THE NEED FOR INTUBATION

In critically ill surgical patients, intubation of the trachea serves the same functions as in patients under anesthesia: it preserves airway patency, prevents aspiration, allows removal of pulmonary secretions, and provides a route for mechanical ventilation. Prolonged tracheal intubation is associated with significant morbidity; difficulties are listed in Table 37–5.

To avoid complications, the endotracheal tube is removed as soon as it is safe to do so. In general, intensive care patients who are awake with intact upper airway reflexes and who have no need for continued mechanical ventilatory support are candidates for tracheal extubation. If upper airway obstruction was related to an infection, resolution of the infection (decreased temperature, normalization of white blood cell count, decreased pharyngeal inflammation and neck swelling) usually indicates that extubation is safe. If the upper airway obstruction is due to edema and hemorrhage

TABLE 37–5. **Difficulties Related to Tracheal Intubation and Mechanical Ventilation**

Related to Intubation*
- Damage to teeth
- Pharyngeal or laryngotracheal damage
- Nasal necrosis, sinusitis, or otitis media
- Tube obstruction (secretions, kinking)
- Right mainstem bronchus intubation
- Cuff leak or rupture
- Tracheal hemorrhage
- Infection (pneumonia, tracheostomy infection)
- Retained secretions
- Tube dislodgement

Related to Mechanical Ventilator†
- Accidental disconnection of power source, gas supply, or patient from ventilator
- Tension pneumothorax, pneumomediastinum, pneumopericardium
- Inspissated secretions (inadequate humidification)
- Circuit leaks
- Air trapping or auto-PEEP
- Fluid retention
- Overventilation or underventilation
- Ventilator and patient's efforts not synchronous
- Hemodynamic instability due to hypovolemia
- Atelectasis

* Data on incidence from 158/354 patients.
† Data on incidence from 103/354 patients.
(Adapted with permission from Zwillich CW. Complications of assisted ventilation: A prospective study of 354 consecutive episodes. Am J Med 1974; 57: 161–165.)

related to operation, this usually resolves within 24 to 48 hours, permitting extubation. The precautions for extubation are described in Chapter 13, and include preparations for immediate reintubation if needed.

Because of the complications associated with the use of endotracheal tubes, there is controversy regarding the preferred route and duration of endotracheal intubation. Endotracheal tubes with cuffs of large volumes and minimal compliance have reduced the incidence of tracheal stenosis owing to cuff overinflation, allowing tubes to remain in place for three weeks or more. However, prolonged intubation by the oral route causes laryngeal damage and interferes with oral feeding, mouth care, and patient comfort. Trachcostomy allows oral feeding, easier mouth care and tracheal toilet, while reducing damage to the larynx. Adverse effects of tracheostomy include tracheomalacia and stenosis at the stoma site, and stomal infection with seeding of the lungs.

Nasal intubation is of value in managing the airway after certain operations and in some trauma patients (see Chapters 13, 29, and 31). In patients requiring intensive care, nasotracheal tubes are best left in place for only a few days because of the prevalence of purulent sinusitis with their continued use. Computerized tomographic scanning or sinus films may be the only clue that sinusitis is the source of sepsis in patients with nasal endotracheal tubes.

TABLE 37–6. Values Used to Assess Need for Mechanical Ventilation

Measurement	Normal	Mechanical Ventilation Indicated
Ventilatory reserve:		
Tidal volume (ml/kg)	5–80	<5
Respiratory rate (breaths/min)	12–20	>35
Vital capacity (ml/kg)	65–75	<10–15
Arterial P_{CO_2} (mm Hg)	35–45	>55
FEV_1 (ml/kg)	50–60	<10
Negative inspiration pressure (cm H_2O)	75–100	<25
Maximum voluntary ventilation (L/min)	150	$<2 \times V_E$
V_D/V_T ratio	0.25–0.40	>0.6
Resting V_E (L/min)	6	>15
Blood oxygenation:		
Intrapulmonary right-to-left shunt (%)	<5	>20
$P(A\text{-}a)O_2$ (mm Hg)	25–65	>450
Arterial P_{O_2}/alveolar P_{O_2}	0.75	<0.15
Clinical signs:		
Fatigue:		
Tachycardia		
Diaphoresis		
Accessory respiratory muscle activity		
Hemodynamic instability (hypertension, hypotension)		
Hypoxia:		
Cyanosis		
Restlessness, confusion		
Hypercapnia:		
Peripheral vasodilatation		
Headache, somnolence		

THE NEED FOR MECHANICAL VENTILATION

Mechanical ventilators are used to enhance alveolar ventilation, decrease work of breathing, and improve carbon dioxide elimination and oxygenation. The major indication for their use is acute or impending respiratory failure, usually manifested by changes in blood gas tensions and ventilatory fatigue. Table 37–6 lists criteria signaling the need for ventilatory assistance.

Single measurements of pulmonary function are of less predictive value than trends involving multiple indices; abnormalities occur together. While one minor abnormality may be well tolerated, two or more signs of impending failure (none of which is as severe as suggested in Table 37–6) may still indicate the need for mechanical ventilation.

Whereas arterial blood gas values provide the major criteria for the diagnosis of respiratory failure, often mechanical ventilation is begun before significant abnormalities appear. In patients with neuromuscular disease or acute asthma, the margin between adequate gas exchange and total respiratory collapse is very small. The signs of fatigue listed in Table 37–6, or clinical signs of excessive sympathetic activity, provide timely warning of respiratory failure in such patients, and indicate the need for intervention even if blood gas values are still acceptable. Conversely, in some patients with significant hypoxemia or hypocarbia, every effort is made to avoid assisted ventilation because of predictable difficulties in weaning later. Patients with progressive respiratory failure despite optimal treatment are less likely to derive long-term benefits from mechanical ventilation than are patients in whom mechanical ventilation provides short-term support during which an acute derangement can be treated. Thus, the patient with longstanding COPD who finally develops ventilatory failure with no acute precipitating cause (pneumonia, abdominal operations) is unlikely to be weaned from mechanical ventilation, whereas a young patient with the sudden onset of asthma can expect to recover.

Mechanical ventilators subject the patient to life-threatening risks. Table 37–5 outlines the more common problems, including not only those owing to mechanical failure, but to adverse effects of mechanical ventilation itself. Complications occur in almost 30 per cent of patients undergoing mechanical ventilation. New features added to mechanical ventilators also bring new possibilities for malfunction, requiring added vigilance in monitoring both patient and ventilator. Emergency equipment to maintain artificial ventilation, including self-inflating bags, must be available at the bedside in case of mechanical breakdown.

Other sequelae of mechanical positive pressure ventilation include reduced venous return to the heart, mismatching of pulmonary blood flow with ventilation, fluid retention, electrolyte and blood acid-base disturbances, and pulmonary barotrauma.

During inspiration, positive pressure ventilation increases intrathoracic pressure, limiting venous return to the right side of the heart and diminishing cardiac output. The magnitude of this effect depends on the fraction of the total respiratory cycle occupied by inspiration and the pressure applied. It is worsened by hypovolemia or when there is airway obstruction causing air trapping within the lung. In contrast, if the lungs are stiff and noncompliant, then only part of the airway pressure is transmitted to the intrathoracic space and the effect will be lessened. Shortening inspiratory time diminishes the impairment of venous return. In adult patients with normal lungs, positive pressure inspiration occupying less than half of the total cycle causes minimal depression of cardiac output because of compensatory increases in right heart output occurring during exhalation.

Mechanical ventilation increases physiologic and anatomical dead space owing to redistribution of blood flow away from well-ventilated areas of lung and airway distension by positive airway pressures. Airway obstruction or restrictive disease further alters distribution of gas flow to areas of lesser resistance or greater compliance. This augments collapse of alveoli distal to partially obstructed airways, causing atelectasis. This may be relieved by using large tidal volumes (>10 ml per kg) or periodic large breaths (sighs) to distribute gas back into those areas at risk for collapse.

Patients with preexisting metabolic alkalosis owing to diuretics, gastrointestinal drainage, or renal compensation for chronic respiratory acidosis may suffer acute increases in blood pH (alkalosis) as mechanical ventilation is begun and minute ventilation is increased. The ensuing derangements in oxyhemoglobin dissociation, electrolyte disturbances, and imbalance between brain oxygen delivery and consumption may occasionally precipitate convulsions, cardiac arrhythmias, and death. When such acid-base abnormalities exist prior to institution of mechanical ventilation, it is helpful to decrease arterial P_{CO_2} slowly to allow time for correction of the primary metabolic disturbance.

After several days of positive pressure ventilation, progressive fluid retention is likely, particularly when excessive quantities of sodium and free water are administered. This often occurs with intravenous hyperalimentation, because water must be given to dilute amino acids and glucose infusions. It is sometimes associated with clinical signs of pulmonary edema in the absence of increased venous pressures. Positive end-expiratory pressure worsens this phenomenon. It appears to be due to a number of mechanical and humoral mechanisms, including renal retention of sodium and water, partial intrathoracic venous obstruction, and interference with pulmonary lymphatic clearance. Control of sodium and fluid intake, use of diuretics, and careful monitoring of patient weight are necessary to avoid this complication.

In patients with stiff lungs or small airways obstruction, increased airway pressures may be required to deliver adequate tidal volumes. Increased airway pressures, particularly peak inflation pressure, increase the risk of pressure damage to the lung (pulmonary barotrauma). The major types of barotrauma include tension pneumothorax, mediastinal and pericardial air accumulation, and subcutaneous emphysema. Of these, tension pneumothorax is the most serious, occurring in about 5 per cent of all mechanically ventilated patients, and rapidly producing cardiovascular collapse. The clinical signs of tension pneumothorax are caused by accumulation of gas within the pleural space: increased airway pressures, hypoxemia, hypercapnia, diminished breath sounds, hyperresonance over the affected side, pulsus paradoxus, and decreased cardiac output. Although clinical signs may be equivocal, impending cardiovascular collapse may not permit time to obtain a chest x-ray. Immediate percutaneous placement of an interpleural catheter or tube is justified whenever a patient in distress is suspected of having a tension pneumothorax.

MODES OF MECHANICAL VENTILATION

For prolonged use in the critically ill surgical patient, a mechanical ventilator must maintain good exchange of warmed, humidified oxygen-enriched gas despite airways obstruction or greatly decreased compliance. It must be capable of positive end-expiratory pressures up to 30 cm H_2O, peak inflation pressures up to 100 cm H_2O, and peak inspiratory flows up to 100 L per minute. It must detect and sound alarms for disconnection from the patient, loss of power source or loss of gas supply. It must monitor continuously inspired gas temperature, oxygen concentration, airway pressure, exhaled gas volumes, rate, tidal volume, and minute ventilation. Ventilators of different types deliver different patterns of ventilation, all of which may be appropriate for use in the intensive care unit.

Ventilator Types

Today, the overwhelming majority of ventilators used for the prolonged ventilation of critically ill surgical patients produce positive airway pressures (positive pressure ventilation). Positive pressure ventilators are divided into three types, depending on the method used to stop inspiratory gas flow.

Pressure cycled machines end inspiration when a preset airway pressure is reached. *Time cycled* ventilators deliver a constant flow of gas during inspiration for a preset (variable) time interval. Most ventilators capable of delivering square wave flow patterns fit into this category. *Volume cycled* ventilators deliver a preset volume of gas per breath regardless of the flow wave form, which may be altered independently. Many newer ventilators provide all three methods of operation and all of the multiple modes of ventilatory support outlined below. Although each possesses advantages, with few exceptions all ventilators now manufactured for continuous use can be adapted to the majority of ICU patients.

Ventilatory Modes

Modern ventilators provide a wide variety of methods of augmenting minute ventilation in a graded fashion, most of which are reported to improve ease of use and patient comfort. However, there are no properly controlled studies showing differences in patient outcome. Table 37–7 outlines major features of these modes of ventilation.

CONTROLLED MECHANICAL VENTILATION

In controlled mechanical ventilation (CMV), the ventilator delivers a fixed tidal volume at a fixed respiratory rate regardless of the patient's efforts. This provides respiratory support when spontaneous ventilation is completely suppressed, as by muscle relaxants or other forms of paralysis of the respiratory musculature. It also provides a default mode during assisted ventilation as discussed below. The disadvantage of CMV is that it allows no control by the patient, who may not synchronize respiratory efforts with the machine. Also, the ventilator settings must be adjusted as metabolic demands and pulmonary function change to prevent marked blood gas abnormalities.

ASSISTED MECHANICAL VENTILATION

In assisted mechanical ventilation (AMV) mode, the machine determines the tidal volume, but the patient sets the ventilatory rate. Each inspiratory effort creates a negative pressure in the airway, triggering a breath from the ventilator. Synchronization of patient effort with the ventilator is facilitated, usually without need for additional sedation or paralysis. If the patient's respiratory rate is inadequate, the ventilator reverts to timed control as a default mode. Assisted mechanical ventilation allows the patient with intact respiratory control mechanisms to regulate ventilation to satisfy metabolic demands. Initiation of negative in-

TABLE 37–7. **Modes of Ventilation**

Factor	Continuous Mandatory Ventilation (CMV)	Assisted Mechanical Ventilation (AMV)	Intermittent Mandatory Ventilation (IMV)	Pressure Support Ventilation (PSV)	High Frequency Jet Ventilation (HFJV)
Default on apnea	CMV	CMV	IMV rate	CMV	Controlled
Patient's spontaneous breath	Uncoordinated with machine	Assisted	Spontaneous + assisted	Assisted	Spontaneous
Size of patient's breath	Fixed	Fixed	IMV fixed; variable size spontaneous breath	Variable	Fixed
Response to need for increased ventilation	None	Increased rate	Increased rate and tidal volume, if patient strong enough	Increased rate and tidal volume, if patient strong enough	None
Response to narcotics, neuromuscular blocker	None	Rate decreases to default	Minute ventilation decreases to IMV default	Minute ventilation decreases to CMV default	None
Respiratory muscle deconditioning	Maximal deconditioning	Not as marked as CMV	Minimal deconditioning, depending on IMV level	Minimal deconditioning, depending on CMV level	None
Respiratory muscle fatigue	None	Minimal	Fatigue likely	Fatigue likely	Minimal
Weaning	Abrupt	Abrupt	Graduated	Graduated	Graduated

spiratory pressure provides some (inadequate) exercise for the muscles of respiration. This mode of ventilation has been used for more than 30 years and is present on nearly all ventilators manufactured for use in intensive care settings.

To wean patients from AMV requires periodic cessation of ventilatory support while allowing the patient to breath spontaneously. During weaning, intervals of ventilatory support are gradually shortened, while intervals of spontaneous ventilation are progressively lengthened, based on the patient's ability to maintain adequate gas exchange without fatigue. The major disadvantage of AMV is that some patients' native respiratory rates are rapid, leading to respiratory alkalosis. A second disadvantage is the increased complexity of weaning efforts, requiring careful monitoring to avoid unexpected ventilatory collapse during periods of spontaneous breathing.

INTERMITTENT MANDATORY VENTILATION

Intermittent mandatory ventilation (IMV) provides breaths of fixed tidal volume at a (low) rate set by the operator. Between these breaths, the ventilator provides gas for the patient's spontaneous ventilation. In AMV, each of the patient's breaths is mechanically assisted and the machine provides a fixed rate of breathing only if the patient becomes apneic. In IMV, the patient's breaths are unassisted, but the fixed breaths are automatic and occur regularly even if the patient continues to breathe. In newer ventilators, the fixed breaths are synchronized with the inspiratory effort of the patient (SIMV) to avoid conflict between a spontaneous breath and one delivered by the ventilator. Numerous theoretical advantages are cited for IMV, including less ventilator-induced depression of cardiac output, improved acid-base balance, facilitation of weaning, and reduced incidence of pulmonary barotrauma. Theoretical disadvantages include respiratory muscle fatigue and hypoventilation (at the IMV default rate) should the patient receive muscle relaxants or ventilatory depressants. None of the studies of these advantages or disadvantages have been well enough controlled to provide definitive conclusions.

In older ventilators, the demand valves supplying inspiratory gas to the patient between IMV breaths were insensitive, slow to respond, and unable to match patient inspiratory flow requirements. The excessive work of breathing caused the rapid onset of fatigue during IMV. Newer inspiratory demand valves minimize these problems. Though IMV appears to have stood the test of time and provides an acceptable alternative to the older AMV mode, its superiority remains unproven.

PRESSURE SUPPORT VENTILATION

In pressure support ventilation (PSV) the ventilator delivers a flow of gas to the patient's airway until a set pressure is reached. This pressure is maintained until inspiratory flow decreases to a predetermined level, at which point flow ceases and the expiratory phase begins. The patient initiates each breath when the ventilator senses negative airway pressure. Thus, the patient sets both the tidal volume and the rate. Pressure support ventilation supplements the patient's effort, allowing breaths at varying rates and volumes. Further, like IMV, PSV can be discontinued gradually as patient gas exchange and respiratory muscle strength improve. Also like IMV, it allows the patient to exercise respiratory musculature. Theoretical disadvantages include respiratory muscle fatigue and ventilatory failure if drugs are administered without changing the amount of assistance, and lack of studies proving its efficacy.

HIGH-FREQUENCY JET VENTILATION

High-frequency jet ventilation (HFJV) provides high-pressure jet flow of gas at fast respiratory rates, between 60 to 150 breaths pr minute, and small tidal volumes not much greater than the anatomical dead space of the lung. The small tidal volumes minimize peak airway pressure and the consequent adverse hemodynamic effects of pulmonary barotrauma. Though it is effective in some patients with bronchopleural fistulae, there is no consensus as to its use in other disorders. Disadvantages include difficulty in monitoring the ventilation it produces, the lack of alarms, and poor warming and humidification of inspired gases. High-frequency oscillation, a mode of ventilation related to HFJV, is used only experimentally.

PEEP, CPAP

Limiting expiratory gas flow from the patient has long been considered as a method for minimizing airway collapse, improving ventilation/perfusion distribution, and reducing intrapulmonary shunting. Unfortunately, reduction in venous return to the heart limits the use of this technique. Positive end-expiratory pressure (PEEP) has been the most successful variant, improving oxygenation with minimal hemodynamic disturbance. An adjustable valve controlling pressure in the exhaled limb of the breathing circuit is included on all of the ventilators now manufactured for intensive care use. The valve applies constant airway pressure through the full exhalation cycle. When used in conjunction with a mode of ventilation that never allows airway pressure to decrease to ambient levels, PEEP is designated as continuous positive airway pressure (CPAP).

Positive end-expiratory pressure is beneficial when arterial hypoxemia exists despite use of increased inspired oxygen concentrations. PEEP minimizes risks of oxygen toxicity by allowing the patient to attain a given level of arterial P_{O_2} with a lesser F_{IO_2}. Some evidence suggests that it may reduce bleeding following thoracotomy. It has adverse effects, including depression of cardiac output, increased incidence of pulmonary barotrauma, fluid retention, and difficulties in interpreting pulmonary vascular pressure data obtained from indwelling pulmonary artery catheters. Of these, the most significant has proved to be depression of cardiac output: as PEEP improves arterial oxygen tension it may depress cardiac output, diminishing the quantity of oxygen transported to the body. It is useful to evaluate the effects of PEEP by calculating oxygen transport (the product of cardiac output and arterial oxygen content), or by measuring the oxygen saturation of mixed venous blood.

Because its adverse effects are directly related to the pressure applied, PEEP is limited to the level required to permit adequate tissue oxygen delivery while avoiding pulmonary oxygen toxicity. PEEP is best used to treat diffuse, homogeneous lung disease such as pulmonary edema. The salutary effect on arterial oxygenation is much less certain when disease in the lung is localized, as in atelectasis or lobar pneumonia. Although there is no well-documented explanation, the lack of efficacy in localized lung disease may be due to redistribution of pulmonary blood flow away from well-ventilated lung and into the impaired region during PEEP.

WEANING THE PATIENT FROM MECHANICAL VENTILATION

Weaning young patients without lung disease from mechanical ventilation is usually simple. Normal arterial blood gas values, a vital capacity in excess of 15 ml per kg, and negative inspiratory pressures of greater than 20 cm H_2O usually predict that it will be safe to discontinue mechanical ventilation. This is the case in the majority of mechanically ventilated patients in the surgical intensive care unit. Presence of debility and chronic or acute illness may prolong the need for ventilatory support and make weaning from mechanical ventilation more difficult.

The longer mechanical ventilation is continued, the more difficult it is to stop. For this reason, progressive weaning from the ventilator must begin as soon as possible. Quantitative criteria for weaning are sparse and largely empirical. The clinical state of the patient, along with periodic measurement of arterial blood gas tensions and tests of ventilatory adequacy usually provide enough information to assess effects of weaning efforts. Numerical indices of ventilatory adequacy are shown in Table 37–6. Because fatigue may limit weaning in elderly and debilitated patients who have been maintained on mechanical ventilation for even short periods of time, measurements of ventilatory performance are made during weaning trials. Failure owing to respiratory muscle fatigue during weaning often leads to further deterioration, requiring prolonged rest. Although there is no single clinical sign or number diagnostic of fatigue, increased sympathetic tone and respiratory rates greater than 30 breaths per minute suggest impending failure.

The most common cause of continued ventilator dependence is persistence of the pathophysiologic process requiring need for mechanical ventilation. Before patients can be weaned from ventilators, all organ systems must function as well as circumstances permit. Neurologic depression or coma may blunt airway reflexes, resulting in aspiration of pharyngeal contents. Weakened airway and respiratory muscles may be inadequate to maintain an unobstructed airway or adequate alveolar ventilation. Cardiovascular responses to discontinuing mechanical ventilation include increased venous return to the heart and the increased cardiac work needed to support the increased work of breathing. In borderline congestive heart failure these changes may precipitate pulmonary edema. It is important to adjust fluid balance, blood oxygen carrying capacity, and cardiac performance with inotropic support and vasodilators prior to weaning. Increased sympathetic tone associated with increased work and inadequate gas exchange, as well as electrolyte abnormalities may provoke life-threatening arrhythmias in some patients.

Patients with coexisting renal and respiratory failure are often troublesome to wean because stable fluid balance is hard to maintain. Weaning of the patient in acute or chronic renal failure is delayed until satisfactory fluid balance can be maintained for several days. Although poor nutritional status and cachexia are associated with a difficult weaning, no studies have demonstrated that acute nutritional support improves the likelihood of rapid weaning. Nevertheless, maintenance of respiratory muscle function, ventilatory drive mechanisms, and lung defense mechanisms against infection depend upon maintenance of nutrition, particularly in critically ill patients with increased nitrogen catabolism and loss of lean body mass. Perversely, nutritional support can also impede weaning, owing to increased CO_2 production from glucose and amino acid loading and fluid retention.

The three factors ultimately determining the success of weaning are pulmonary oxygen exchange, ventilation, and fatigue. A timed trial of unassisted ventilation is often helpful because it is impossible to predict with certainty whether fatigue and deterioration in pulmonary gas exchange will occur following discontinuation of ventilation. Though efficacy of arterial oxygenation can be expressed numerically in numerous ways (i.e., shunt or alveolar-arterial oxygen difference), the functional problem is to provide adequate oxygenation. Unless unassisted ventilation sustains an arterial Po_2 greater than 60 mm Hg with an inspired oxygen concentration of 60 per cent or less, successful weaning is unlikely for several reasons. First, it is quite difficult to maintain inspired oxygen concentrations above 60 per cent without intubation. Second, unintentional discontinuation of the oxygen supply in patients requiring more than 60 per cent oxygen can quickly lead to life-threatening hypoxia. Third, such patients may still suffer from the original disease that precipitated respiratory failure.

Assessment before weaning must also predict

the likelihood of hypoventilation induced by fatigue. Avoiding fatigue may be accomplished in several ways. The first is to gradually decrease assistance until it is no longer required, using IMV and PSV. Either the frequency of mandatory breaths or the amount of inspiratory pressure support can be reduced gradually while vital signs and arterial blood gas tensions are monitored. When signs of fatigue, including increased respiratory rate and hemodynamic signs of sympathetic nervous system activity, become pronounced, ventilatory assistance is increased until signs of fatigue diminish or are eliminated.

Another approach derives from the observation that patients with normal lung function can indefinitely sustain one half of their maximal voluntary ventilation. Based on this, the following method has proven to be helpful in assessing both adequacy of ventilation and predicting likelihood of fatigue. The patient is allowed to spontaneously breath humidified oxygen-enriched gas for a period of one hour. During that time, clinical signs of hypoxia, hypercarbia, or any marked increase in restlessness, sympathetic activity, or respiratory rate above 30 breaths per minute are considered signs of worsening respiratory failure or fatigue, indicating need for measurement of arterial blood gas tensions and possible return to assisted ventilation. If all goes well for an hour, arterial blood gas tensions, minute ventilation, and maximal breathing capacity are measured. If the patient cannot cooperate, maximum voluntary ventilation can be estimated by measuring vital capacity and multiplying it by 35. If the minute ventilation required to maintain an acceptable P_{CO_2} during the trial is less than one half the maximum voluntary ventilation, fatigue is unlikely to develop. If the patient cannot maintain adequate ventilation for the full hour, a shorter time period of unassisted ventilation during which unacceptable fatigue does not occur is interspersed with periods of rest, allowing adequate periods of time for sleep at night. As weaning progresses, the period of unassisted ventilation is progressively prolonged until there is no deterioration or fatigue.

Unfortunately, there are increasing numbers of patients who cannot be weaned after prolonged ventilatory support in critical care units. For these patients, the options for continued care are limited and extremely expensive. For some there is the possibility of productive activity despite the need for chronic ventilatory support. For others, options are much more limited. The financial and ethical dilemmas raised in the care of these patients remain unresolved.

Such concerns are not limited to those who have required prolonged ventilatory or circulatory support. Critical care is expensive, and it is clear that society cannot afford to provide unlimited intensive care to all who might possibly benefit. Yet it is through such intensive care that high-risk patients can recover from major operations and severe illnesses. Selection of appropriate candidates for admission to critical care facilities is a medical, legal, and ethical problem that is not yet resolved.

REFERENCES

Goldenheim PD, Kazemi H. Cardiopulmonary monitoring of critically ill patients. N Engl J Med 1984; 311:717–720, 776–780.

Morganroth ML, Grum CM. Weaning from mechanical ventilation. J Intensive Care Med 1988; 3:109–119.

Norwood SH, Civetta JN. Ventilatory support in patients with ARDS. Surg Clin N Am 1985; 65:895–916.

Perel A. Newer ventilation modes—hazards and pitfalls. Crit Care Med 1987; 15:707–709.

Ruark JE, Raffin TA, The Stanford University Medical Center Committee on Ethics. Initiating and withdrawing life support: Principles and practice in adult medicine. N Engl J Med 1988; 318:25–30.

Stauffer Jl, Olsen DE, Petty TL. Complications and consequences of endotracheal intubation and tracheostomy. A prospective study of 150 critically ill adult patients. Am J Med 1981;70:65–76.

Weisman IM, Rinaldo JE, Rogers RM. Positive end-expiratory pressure in adult respiratory failure. N Engl J Med 1982; 307:1381–1384.

CHAPTER THIRTY-EIGHT

The Further Study of Anesthesiology

This book is intended for all students of anesthesia, but the reader most directly addressed is the resident beginning the first year of clinical anesthesia training (CA-1). This final chapter contains suggestions for the study of anesthesia beyond the reading of an introductory text. Rather than cover all aspects of learning in anesthesia, it offers advice directly to the physician-student.

Residency Versus School

Physicians enrolled in residencies sometimes fail to make the progress in learning that they or their instructors might wish, despite the fact that such residents have long histories of success in school. Sometimes this is because the resident (or the teacher) does not understand the nature of postgraduate medical education and does not benefit fully from the available opportunities for learning. Residents and their instructors may wrongly model resident education after their prior education—school. Learning in school differs from learning in a residency because of several factors: the learners, the subject matter, the methods of learning, the teachers, and the environment.

Residents in training are adults whose educational needs differ from those of the less mature students found in schools. They are older, with less resilient and retentive minds; learning comes more slowly. Their financial and family responsibilities are greater than those of most students. Motivation comes from within; adults are not likely to learn simply because they are told to do so. Physicians come to residencies with widely varied backgrounds and plans, and it is from these that motivation best comes, not from outside pressures. An anesthesia resident planning a career as a laboratory investigator has learning goals different than does one with previous training in psychology who plans a clinical career in pain management. Further, residents often learn best if allowed to employ their own styles of learning as much as possible, rather than being forced into a lock-step program.

Before residency, learning in college and medical school is perceived largely as cognitive: a body of information is to be learned. In addition to simply acquiring information, residents must also learn complex behaviors, the intellectual foundations of their knowledge, and an array of skills (for some, this is the first opportunity to learn mechanical skills). To acquire this noncognitive material, residents must adapt to methods of learning little used in school. Classroom teaching becomes less important, and on-the-job training and independent study are more important. Teaching is less structured, and more responsibility falls on the student to ensure that such informal instruction is productive.

As compared to those in schools, instructors in residencies are not primarily teachers. Although well meaning, they have no formal training as teachers and receive their salaries in return for performing clinical care or research, not for instructing residents. Although the resident's instructor is likely to be an expert and to have a great deal of information to impart, the resident may have to contribute as much to the tutorial relationship as does the instructor.

The environment within which the resident learns differs markedly from that of school. A resident is an employee who receives a salary for providing the services of a physician; the job is so demanding, and the responsibility of taking care of patients is so important, that residents may forget their roles as students. In addition, everyone around residents (nurses, consultants, supervisors, peers) is likely to evaluate them as workers and not as learners. Fatigue, a constant factor in residents' lives, not only robs them of the time and energy for formal study, but may prevent them from learning from clinical experience.

All of these characteristics distinguish residents from students and residency from school. Residency more closely resembles continuing medical education for the practicing physician than it does college or medical school. Successful residents recognize the difference and adapt to the challenges.

Learning During Residency

Learning during residency requires that one not simply accept the instruction offered by the residency, but formulate plans for study that take advantage of situations that motivate learning, and follow an overall plan that takes into account individual goals and learning styles. Some of these opportunities and plans are described below.

Reading

Reading is by far the most important method of cognitive learning during residency. Readers may choose an appropriate level of instruction that takes into account their backgrounds and goals. A passage may be reread until understood. Articles in journals and texts are written and edited with more care than all except the best lectures. Reading during and after residency must become a regular habit; there is too much material to cope with by cramming.

An appropriate reading program begins after completing an introductory text, with reading one of the large comprehensive texts cover-to-cover well before the end of the CA-1 year. At present, no one textbook is clearly superior to the others, because all are multiauthored texts; direct comparison of chapters dealing with the same subject shows that each book has its own strengths. Even though not all of this material is retained at first, familiarity with the specialty provides a framework for other reading. The drawback to this suggestion is that motivation for daily reading is weak. Other reading, begun simultaneously, benefits from more immediate motivation.

First, a resident benefits from the habit of reading in some depth for at least one case each day. A new anesthetic drug or procedure, an intercurrent disease, an incidental medication, a new surgical procedure or an instructor's suggestion can all prompt additional study. Material learned in this way is retained well. Second, residents assigned to subspecialty rotations (such as obstetrical anesthesia) are well advised to take advantage of the motivation to read and remember material from specialty texts.

Third, residents can begin reading journals regularly at the start of the residency. In the United States, residents can begin with two major journals, *Anesthesiology* and *Anesthesia and Analgesia*, both of which are provided as part of inexpensive resident memberships in the sponsoring organizations. Other journals and the periodicals that provide review articles can be valuable additions to a reading program, but they may require more time and money than residents have to spend on them. To make the reading of journals more efficient, residents can form the habit of reading selectively, focusing on major scientific articles accompanied by editorial comment, medical intelligence articles, and the letters, which often expose the reader to a wide range of opinions expressed in a lively format. Rather than reading superficially, the resident must study each article,

TABLE 38–1. Questions About a Scientific Article in a Medical Journal

1. What type of article is it?
   - A report of a single case
   - A report of a series of cases
   - A retrospective study based on a series of cases
   - A controlled clinical trial
   - An in vivo laboratory study
   - An in vitro laboratory study
2. What hypothesis did the study test? Do the findings validate or reject the hypothesis? Summarize the findings in a single sentence.
3. Why was the study undertaken? Does it provide new information that reinforces or contradicts what the reader already knows? How does this article compare to others on related subjects?
4. Under what clinical circumstances are the findings of this study important? How and when will the reader put this information to use? Here, the reader must avoid the temptation to view animal studies as irrelevant, while also resisting the urge to apply laboratory information uncritically, without first evaluating the validity of the animal model.

At first, it will be difficult for the beginning resident to put articles in perspective; the discussion section of the paper, an accompanying editorial and reference to textbooks will help. Answering these questions will allow the resident to assimilate efficiently the information in an article. In a few cases, it may seem to the reader that the study did not provide a valid answer to an important question. This may be the fault of the article and not the reader.

making notes and filing them for later use (Table 38–1).

The Resident's Library

At first, the expense of buying medical texts makes accumulating a useful library seem impossible. However, a small personal collection of books and journals can be accumulated at relatively modest cost (Table 38–2). Books to be included in this library are those required for close study or for frequent reference. Less commonly used items may be found in departmental or hospital libraries.

Learning From Cases

Because the majority of the resident's time is spent in managing patients' anesthetics, this clinical experience must be made as educational as possible. To do so, each case begins with a thorough, problem-oriented note and a socratic discussion with the instructor. During this discussion, the instructor questions the resident in a manner resembling the oral examination used for Board certification, but also provides guidance designed to instruct the resident. Residents can improve this experience not only by participating willingly, but by drawing out reticent instructors with suggestions for alternative plans for managing anesthesia. Reading for the case also enhances learning, as does even a brief discussion with the supervising faculty after the anesthetic is concluded. Occasionally, something about the case suggests further study; from this beginning, a resident may prepare a case report, review article, or a scientific study.

Lectures, Conferences

Compared to reading and individual study, lectures are inefficient means of conveying information to learners; there is not time enough to impart by lecture all of the information residents are required to learn. Lectures are of greatest value when they convey a lecturer's unique insights, when their content is designed around local needs, or when the lecture serves to direct resident study. Resident attendance at lectures is sometimes poor, perhaps reflecting not only the residents' busy schedules, but also their perceptions that lectures are not as useful as reading or interactive conferences.

TABLE 38–2. A Minimum Personal Library in Anesthesia

1. An introductory text
2. The most recent edition of at least one comprehensive anesthesia text; two are better
3. The current edition of a comprehensive pharmacology text
4. One of the texts describing the anesthesia management of patients with uncommon diseases
5. Specialty texts (obstetrical anesthesia, etc.) according to the recommendations at the end of the various chapters in this book, or faculty preference at the time of the resident's assignment to the specialty service
6. Journals
   - Subscriptions
     - *Anesthesiology*
     - *Anesthesia and Analgesia*
     - *New England Journal of Medicine*
   - Read in library, or subscribe, as time and money permit
     - *British Journal of Anaesthesia*
     - *Canadian Journal of Anesthesia*
7. Comprehensive surgery and medicine texts

Interactive forms of group teaching, such as seminars and clinical case conferences, are more valuable than lectures because they make residents participants instead of spectators. These conferences, however, only reach their full potential when they are based on firm scientific information rather than simple recollections of prior experience. Residents can improve their learning by participating actively in these conferences. Journal clubs and opportunities to teach medical students provide residents with the same benefits of active participation.

Residents Helping Teachers

Residents must contribute to the tutorial relationship with their teachers. Usually, this simply requires that they participate in socratic teaching and be willing to use new anesthetic drugs and methods suggested by their instructors. Less often, a resident may take the lead, drawing out a reticent instructor who may have much to offer when stimulated by a curious learner.

Scheduling Elective Time During Residency

The structure of anesthesia residencies is determined by the American Board of Anesthesiology (ABA) and the Residency Review Committee (RRC), which certifies residencies. Postgraduate training in anesthesia begins with the clinical base year (CBY), similar to the internship year, and goes on to three years of clinical anesthesia training (CA-1, CA-2, CA-3). Although programs have some latitude in scheduling, the CA-1 year is meant to be spent in learning the basics of anesthesia care, the CA-2 year in learning advanced subspecialities such as cardiac anesthesia, obstetrical anesthesia, and the like, and the CA-3 year in advanced studies according to an elective schedule worked out through consultation between the resident and the program director.

There are three general categories of study in the CA-3 year: the Subspecialty Clinical Track (SCT) requires spending the majority of the year in the study of one or two anesthesia clinical subspecialties; the Advanced Clinical Track (ACT) involves spending the year in more diversified but still advanced clinical assignments; the Clinical Scientist Track (CST) involves spending six months in clinical work and six months in scientific studies. As of September 1992, an alternate CST will allow mixing equal portions of clinical and research work over 36 months of residency following completion of the CA-1 year. In no case will a resident spend less than 30 months of time in the study of clinical anesthesia following the CBY. To reap the advantages of these options, residents must consult early with faculty to design the optimum schedule of rotations and to choose the track that is most appropriate for their career interests.

The ABA/ASA In-Training Examination

The annual In-Training Examination sponsored by the American Board of Anesthesiology and the American Society of Anesthesiologists is open to all residents-in-training in anesthesiology. The written component of the ABA certifying examination is based on a subset of the questions from the In-Training Examination; the candidate's performance on this subset constitutes the score for the written examination. Data returned to the resident or to the program director in the In-Training Examination include the subject matter of questions the resident answered incorrectly, individual scores, and data that allow comparison between an individuals performance or a department's performance and national performance. This examination provides individual residents and their program directors with objective, comparative assessments of cognitive learning. The content outline of this examination has been carefully designed to represent the breadth of the specialty; it serves as an outline against which to compare personal and departmental education efforts.

Information Retrieval

Lecture handouts, notes, articles taken from journals, and other scraps of information soon accumulate to defeat casual storage and defy easy retrieval; storing and retrieving this sort of information is necessary for organized study and reference. Workable systems for individuals must be simple to administer and require as little clerical work as possible, so that the physician's time can be spent in study and not in managing a filing system. Tempting though they are in prospect, complex systems involving elaborate cross referencing or computerized database management do not meet this test and usually prove impractical.

A workable scheme consists of a collection of file folders labeled according to subject. The subject outline can be taken from the index of a text or the ABA/ASA content outline, but a better scheme is the indexing system used in common by *Anesthesiology* and *Anesthesia and Analgesia*. At the beginning of training, the number of folders is few and subjects are broad (for example: "ANESTHESIA, regional") As the user's interests become better defined and entries accumulate, individual folders contain too many items to search easily (40 items seems to be an upper limit). When that happens, additional folders are added to accommodate subheadings (for example: "ANESTHESIA, regional, brachial plexus"). This simple system requires little maintenance and answers the most common requirement for individuals, the need to review a given subject rather than to search according to authors' names, key words, or other criteria. Cross references depend on the user's familiarity with the subject matter.

For searches of the literature, residents can begin with a review of relevant articles in textbooks or recent reviews in journals. Also, automated searches of the National Library of Medicine are now made easy and inexpensive by computer programs such as Grateful Med. At present, the citations generated by this search usually are found in a local library; as more journals become available in electronic form, the articles themselves can be called to one's computer screen. These automated databases are already an important part of learning; they will soon be a routine part of practice.

New Drugs

Frequently, anesthesiologists are asked to use new drugs claimed by their makers to offer significant advantages over other similar drugs. Indeed, for residents, every drug is a new drug the first time it is used. Although information from the manufacturer represents a good-faith effort to provide complete information, more scholarly assessments can be found in the scientific journals. Even after studying all of the available information on a drug or technique, actually putting it to use remains a challenge. Using new drugs or new techniques invites the charge of "experimenting" on patients, especially because tried and true methods of anesthesia are often satisfactory. However, they are not perfect, and to shun the new is to reject progress.

To put a new drug into use safely, follow several rules. First, learn as much as possible about it beforehand, taking special care to compare it to more familiar drugs of the same family. Second, begin with patients and operations for which a certain awkwardness in using the drug will not compromise a successful outcome. Usually, these are healthy patients undergoing less severe procedures. Third, if possible, begin with lesser doses of the drug and study the effects carefully before progressing to greater doses. For example, a new muscle relaxant might be used first for a peripheral procedure expected to last several hours, so that unexpected prolongation of effect will not delay the end of the anesthetic.

Learning Technical Skills

In addition to learning facts and thought processes, residents learn technical skills. For some of them, this may be the first time they have been required to formally learn something that cannot be tested in a written examination. For most, obvious analogies with sports, mechanical trades, hobbies, or laboratory skills suggest how one goes about learning to do something instead of to know something. The hoary adage "watch one, do one, teach one" contains elements of truth, but does not describe the best way to go about teaching or learning a skill.

Consider as an example learning to intubate the trachea using a curved laryngoscope. To learn this efficiently, it is best first for the instructor or the text to break the task down into as many small discrete steps as possible. For example, one step might be positioning the head, the next might be opening the mouth, and the next inserting the laryngoscope. Sometimes, this sequence of steps can become a checklist (e.g., the checklist for preparing an anesthesia machine given in Chapter 5). This analysis of the task not only makes it easier to understand and demonstrate, but it also makes it easier for the learner and the instructor to assess performance at each stage. Also, even though few learners succeed at the entire task (intubating) at the first attempt, all will succeed at some portion of the task; this allows credible praise, providing the positive reinforcement that is more effective than negative reinforcement as a means of changing behavior. Another task of the instructor is to guarantee that the task will be completed safely and without undue delay; this allows the student to focus on learning. Even during residency, this sort of careful teaching may not be available; it is almost always unavailable to practitioners. This need not deter individuals from organizing their own learning along these lines by preparing notes and checklists as needed.

Learning after Residency

Residents who adopt the methods of learning described here, as opposed to limiting themselves to activities prescribed by the residency program, will have little difficulty with continuing medical education. An individual reading program, learning from cases, and attending departmental meetings at which clinical care is discussed (a JCAHO requirement) will provide abundant continuing education. Just as in residency, at national meetings practitioners will find it most valuable to attend lectures, conferences, or seminars that provide more than simple recitations of facts. Indeed, at the ASA's annual meeting, panel discussions and interactive learning opportunities are consistently oversubscribed, probably because those who attend recognize the value of these sessions.

Most reading programs for practitioners involve the same journals read in residency—subspecialty journals or those designed for continuing education. An often overlooked source of reading material for continuing education is the comprehensive textbook. It may not cover areas of special interest as thoroughly as subspecialists might like, but periodic rereading of such a book is a good way to keep up a broad familiarity with anesthesiology in general.

During residency, evaluation of the resident's performance comes from the faculty and from the In-Training Examination; it is a natural part of the resident's learning. Later, such evaluation is harder to obtain, but is just as important. Quality assurance programs are often perceived as threats or as bureaucratic nuisances, but they provide a possible avenue for such continued assessment. Even more important is one's own careful retrospective assessment of cases. Adverse outcomes and complications must never be accepted as inevitable; rather, they must provoke efforts to improve future care.

APPENDIX

ABA/ASA In-Training Examination Content Outline. Joint Council on In-Training Examinations. American Board of Anesthesiology–American Society of Anesthesiologists, 515 Busse Highway, Park Ridge, IL 60068.

The American Board of Anesthesiology booklet of information, January 1991. Office of the Board, 100 Constitution Plaza, Hartford, CN 06103-1721.

Anesthesia and Analgesia. Residents may join the International Anesthesia Research Society, Suite 140, 2 Summit Park Drive, Cleveland, Ohio 44131, at reduced rates.

Anesthesiology. Residents may join The American Society of Anesthesiologists, 515 Busse Highway, Park Ridge, IL 60068, at reduced rates.

GRATEFUL MED. U.S. Department of Health and Human Services. National Institutes of Health. National Library of Medicine, Bethesda, MD.

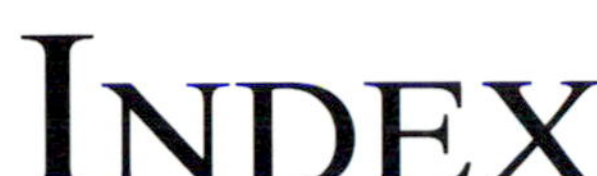

Index

Page numbers in *italics* refer to illustrations; numbers followed by t refer to tables.